BIOMARKERS FOR TRAUMATIC BRAIN INJURY

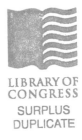

BIOMARKERS FOR TRAUMATIC BRAIN INJURY

Edited by

ALAN H.B. WU
Department of Laboratory Medicine, School of Medicine, University of California San Francisco, San Francisco, CA, United States

W. FRANK PEACOCK
Baylor College of Medicine, Houston, TX, United States

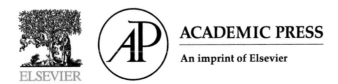

ACADEMIC PRESS
An imprint of Elsevier

ELSEVIER

Academic Press is an imprint of Elsevier
125 London Wall, London EC2Y 5AS, United Kingdom
525 B Street, Suite 1650, San Diego, CA 92101, United States
50 Hampshire Street, 5th Floor, Cambridge, MA 02139, United States
The Boulevard, Langford Lane, Kidlington, Oxford OX5 1GB, United Kingdom

Notices
Knowledge and best practice in this field are constantly changing. As new research and experience broaden our understanding, changes in research methods, professional practices, or medical treatment may become necessary.

Practitioners and researchers must always rely on their own experience and knowledge in evaluating and using any information, methods, compounds, or experiments described herein. In using such information or methods they should be mindful of their own safety and the safety of others, including parties for whom they have a professional responsibility.

To the fullest extent of the law, neither the Publisher nor the authors, contributors, or editors, assume any liability for any injury and/or damage to persons or property as a matter of products liability, negligence or otherwise, or from any use or operation of any methods, products, instructions, or ideas contained in the material herein.

British Library Cataloguing-in-Publication Data
A catalogue record for this book is available from the British Library

Library of Congress Cataloging-in-Publication Data
A catalog record for this book is available from the Library of Congress

ISBN: 978-0-12-816346-7

For Information on all Academic Press publications
visit our website at https://www.elsevier.com/books-and-journals

Publisher: Nikki Levy
Acquisitions Editor: Melanie Tucker
Editorial Project Manager: Kristi Anderson
Production Project Manager: Kiruthika Govindaraju
Cover Designer: Matthew Limbert

Typeset by MPS Limited, Chennai, India

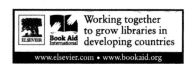

Contents

12. Traumatic brain injury biomarkers glial fibrillary acidic protein/ubiquitin C-terminal hydrolase L1

GARY JAMES MITCHELL

13. Neurofilaments light chain/ Neurofilaments heavy chain

SHOJI YOKOBORI, RYUTA NAKAE AND HIROYUKI YOKOTA

14. Tau protein, biomarker for traumatic brain injury

PABLO TOVAR

Section V

NOVEL TBI BIOMARKERS

15. Neurogranin

JULIAN POHLAN, BERND A. LEIDEL AND TOBIAS LINDNER

16. Myelin basic protein in traumatic brain injury   221

STANLEY L. WU

Section VI

ANALYTICAL TESTING CONSIDERATION

17. Antibody selection, evaluation, and validation for analysis of traumatic brain injury biomarkers

ROBERT J. WEBBER, RICHARD M. SWEET AND DOUGLAS S. WEBBER

24. Digital neurocognitive testing

KARINA M. SOTO-RUIZ, MD

25. Electroencephalographic as a biomarker of concussion

JERALD H. SIMMONS AND HARRY KERASIDIS

26. Neuropsychological testing

JEFFREY BRENNAN, KEVIN K. WANG, RICHARD RUBENSTEIN, CLAUDIA S. ROBERTSON AND HARVEY LEVIN

27. Outpatient risk stratification for traumatic brain injury

ZUBAID RAFIQUE AND RODMOND SINGLETON

28. Peptidomics and traumatic brain injury: biomarker utilities for a theragnostic approach

HAMAD YADIKAR, GEORGE A. SARKIS, MILIN KURUP, FIRAS KOBEISSY AND KEVIN K. WANG

List of Contributors

Fatimah Ahmad Department of Biochemistry and Molecular Genetics, Faculty of Medicine, American University of Beirut, Beirut, Lebanon

Imoigele P. Aisiku Emergency Medicine and Pulmonary Critical Care, Brigham and Women's Hospital, Boston, MA, United States

Peter Allfather Emergency Medicine and Pulmonary Critical Care, Brigham and Women's Hospital, Boston, MA, United States

Henriette Beyer Trauma Surgery Klinikum rechts der Isar, Munich, Germany

S. Bezek Emergency Medicine Baylor College of Medicine, Houston, TX, United States

Peter Biberthaler Department of Trauma Surgery, Klinikum rechts der Isar, School of Medicine, Technical University of Munich, Munich, Germany

Viktoria Bogner-Flatz Department of Trauma Surgery, Klinikum rechts der Isar, School of Medicine, Technical University of Munich, Munich, Germany; Department of General, Trauma and Reconstructive Surgery, Emergency Medicine, Ludwig Maximilians University, Munich, Germany

Jeffrey Brennan University of Texas School of Public Health, Houston, TX, United States

Victoria J. Dardov The Advanced Clinical Biosystems Research Institute, The Smidt Heart Institute, Cedars Sinai Medical Center, Los Angeles, CA, United States

Mahasweta Das Department of Molecular Medicine, College of Medicine, University of South Florida, Tampa, FL, United States; James A. Haley VA Hospital, Tampa, FL, United States

Elvisha Dhamala Weill Cornell Medicine, New York, NY, United States

Clara E. Dismuke-Greer Health Economics Resource Center (HERC), Ci2i, VA Palo Alto Health Care System, Palo Alto, CA, United States

Ryan Duggan Weill Cornell Medicine, New York, NY, United States

Donna J. Edmonds ImmunArray, Richmond, VA, United Kingdom

Daniel Fatovich Royal Perth Hospital, Perth, WA, Australia

Justyna Fert-Bober The Advanced Clinical Biosystems Research Institute, The Smidt Heart Institute, Cedars Sinai Medical Center, Los Angeles, CA, United States

Melinda Fitzgerald Curtin University, Bentley, WA, Australia

L. Foerschner Department of Trauma Surgery, Klinikum rechts der Isar, School of Medicine, Technical University of Munich, Munich, Germany

Aleksandra Gozt Curtin University, Bentley, WA, Australia

Putuma P. Gqamana Pathology and Laboratory Medicine University of Rochester Medical Center, Rochester, NY, United States

Samar Abdel Hady Department of Biochemistry and Molecular Genetics, Faculty of Medicine, American University of Beirut, Beirut, Lebanon; Faculty of Medicine, Alexandria University, Alexandria, Egypt

Hiba Hasan   Department of Biochemistry and Molecular Genetics, Faculty of Medicine, American University of Beirut, Beirut, Lebanon

Houssein Hajj Hassan   Department of Biological and Chemical Sciences, Lebanese International University, Beirut, Lebanon

Ayah Istanbouli   Departments of Emergency Medicine, Psychiatry, Neuroscience and Chemistry, University of Florida, Gainesville, FL, United States

Damir Janigro   FloTBI Inc., Cleveland, OH, United States; Case Western Reserve University, Cleveland, OH, United States

K.-G. Kanz   Department of Trauma Surgery, Klinikum rechts der Isar, School of Medicine, Technical University of Munich, Munich, Germany

Harry Kerasidis   Chesapeake Neurology Associates, Center for Neuroscience at Calvert Health, Prince Frederick, MD, United States

Firas H. Kobeissy   Department of Biochemistry and Molecular Genetics, Faculty of Medicine, American University of Beirut, Beirut, Lebanon; Departments of Emergency Medicine, Psychiatry, Neuroscience and Chemistry, University of Florida, Gainesville, FL, United States; Brain Rehabilitation Research Center, Malcom Randall Veterans Affairs Medical Center (VAMC), Gainesville, FL, United States

Barry Kosofsky   Weill Cornell Medicine, New York, NY, United States

Milin Kurup   Departments of Emergency Medicine, Psychiatry, Neuroscience and Chemistry, University of Florida, Gainesville, FL, United States

Bernd A. Leidel   Department of Emergency Medicine, Campus Benjamin Franklin, Charité—Universitätsmedizin Berlin, Berlin, Germany

Harvey Levin   Neurosurgery Department, Baylor College of Medicine, Houston, TX, United States; Michael E. DeBakey Veterans Affairs Medical Center, Houston, TX, United States

Kent Lewandrowski   Department of Pathology, General Hospital, Boston, MA, United States

Tobias Lindner   Department of Acute & Emergency Medicine, Campus Virchow-Klinikum, Charité—Universitätsmedizin Berlin, Berlin, Germany

Maximo J. Marin   Department of Pathology, Keck School of Medicine, University of Southern California, Los Angeles, CA, United States

I. Martinez-Espina   Emergency Medicine Baylor College of Medicine, Houston, TX, United States

Audrey McKinlay   University of Canterbury, Christchurch, New Zealand

Gary James Mitchell   Emergency Trauma Centre, Royal Brisbane and Womens Hospital, Brisbane, QL, Australia

Shyam S. Mohapatra   James A. Haley VA Hospital, Tampa, FL, United States; Department of Internal Medicine, College of Medicine, University of South Florida, Tampa, FL, United States

Subhra Mohapatra   Department of Molecular Medicine, College of Medicine, University of South Florida, Tampa, FL, United States; James A. Haley VA Hospital, Tampa, FL, United States

Robert M. Murcko   The Ohio State University, Columbus, OH, United States

Ryuta Nakae   Department of Emergency and Critical Care Medicine, Nippon Medical School, Tokyo, Japan

Takahito Nakagawa   Konica Minolta, Tokyo, Japan

Leila Nasrallah   Department of Biochemistry and Molecular Genetics, Faculty of Medicine, American University of Beirut, Beirut, Lebanon

David O. Okonkwo Department of Neurosurgery, University of Pittsburgh Medical Center, Pittsburgh, PA, United States

Rakhi Pandey The Advanced Clinical Biosystems Research Institute, The Smidt Heart Institute, Cedars Sinai Medical Center, Los Angeles, CA, United States

W. Frank Peacock Emergency Medicine Baylor College of Medicine, Houston, TX, United States

Julian Pohlan Department of Radiology, Campus Mitte, Charité—Universitätsmedizin Berlin, Berlin, Germany

Ava M. Puccio Department of Neurosurgery, University of Pittsburgh, Pittsburgh, PA, United States

Zubaid Rafique Emergency Medicine, Baylor College of Medicine, Houston, TX, United States

Lakshman Ramamurthy DxDevice Strategies LLC (formerly CDRH, USFDA), Rockville, MD, United States

Claudia S. Robertson Neurosurgery Department, Baylor College of Medicine, Houston, TX, United States

Richard Rubenstein Downstate Medical School, Brooklyn, NY, United States

Daisuke Saito Konica Minolta Healthcare Americas, Wayne, NJ, United States

George A. Sarkis Departments of Emergency Medicine, Psychiatry, Neuroscience and Chemistry, University of Florida, Gainesville, FL, United States; Department of Chemistry, Faculty of Science, Alexandria University, Alexandria, Egypt; Department of Biological Engineering, Massachusetts Institute of Technology, Cambridge, United States

Abdullah Shaito Department of Biological and Chemical Sciences, Lebanese International University, Beirut, Lebanon

Nour Shaito Department of Biochemistry and Molecular Genetics, Faculty of Medicine, American University of Beirut, Beirut, Lebanon; Department of Biological and Chemical Sciences, Lebanese International University, Beirut, Lebanon

Jerald H. Simmons Comprehensive Sleep Medicine Associates, Houston, TX, United States; Sleep Education Consortium, Houston, TX, United States

Rodmond Singleton Emergency Medicine, Baylor College of Medicine, Houston, TX, United States

Deborah Snell University of Otago, Christchurch, New Zealand

Karina M. Soto-Ruiz, MD Comprehensive Research Associates, Houston, TX, United States

Šárka O. Southern Saliva Diagnostics Gaia Medical Institute, La Jolla, CA, United States

Richard M. Sweet School of Medicine, University of California San Francisco and Renal Department, Zuckerberg San Francisco General Hospital, San Francisco, CA, United States

Martin Paul Than Emergency Department, Christchurch Hospital, Christchurch, New Zealand

James W.G. Thompson Evoke Neuroscience, Inc., New York, NY, United States

Pablo Tovar Emergency Medicine, Baylor College of Medicine, Houston, TX, United States

Jennifer E. Van Eyk The Advanced Clinical Biosystems Research Institute, The Smidt Heart Institute, Cedars Sinai Medical Center, Los Angeles, CA, United States

Timothy E. Van Meter ImmunArray, Richmond, VA, United Kingdom

Xander M.R. van Wijk Department of Pathology, Pritzker School of Medicine, The University of Chicago, Chicago, IL, United States

Kevin K.W. Wang   Departments of Emergency Medicine, Psychiatry, Neuroscience and Chemistry, University of Florida, Gainesville, FL, United States; Brain Rehabilitation Research Center, Malcom Randall Veterans Affairs Medical Center (VAMC), Gainesville, FL, United States

Jolewis Washington   FloTBI Inc., Cleveland, OH, United States

Douglas S. Webber   Research & Diagnostic Antibodies, Las Vegas, NV, United States

Robert J. Webber   Research & Diagnostic Antibodies, Las Vegas, NV, United States

Stanley L. Wu   Baylor College of Medicine, Houston, TX, United States

Hamad Yadikar   Department of Biological Sciences, Faculty of Science, Kuwait University, Safat, Kuwait; Departments of Emergency Medicine, Psychiatry, Neuroscience and Chemistry, University of Florida, Gainesville, FL, United States; Department of Chemistry, University of Florida, Gainesville, FL, United States

Zhihui Yang   Departments of Emergency Medicine, Psychiatry, Neuroscience and Chemistry, University of Florida, Gainesville, FL, United States; Brain Rehabilitation Research Center, Malcom Randall Veterans Affairs Medical Center (VAMC), Gainesville, FL, United States

Shoji Yokobori   Department of Emergency and Critical Care Medicine, Nippon Medical School, Tokyo, Japan

Hiroyuki Yokota   Department of Emergency and Critical Care Medicine, Nippon Medical School, Tokyo, Japan

John K. Yue   Department of Neurosurgery, University of California San Francisco, San Francisco, CA, United States

Y. Victoria Zhang   Pathology and Laboratory Medicine University of Rochester Medical Center, Rochester, NY, United States

Kazem Zibara   Biology Department, Faculty of Sciences, Lebanese University, Beirut, Lebanon

Foreword: The hit that would change football forever

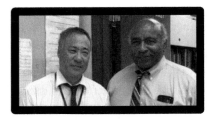

Traumatic brain injury event

On January 15, 1967, the Kansas City Chiefs lost to the Green Bay Packers in the first Super Bowl ever played. Three years later, the Super Bowl trophy would be named after the coach of that Packers team, Vince Lombardi. After that first game, it was clear to the Chief's leadership that their team's defense was not strong enough to win the top prize. So that spring, in the annual draft of the top college players each year, the Chiefs selected a linebacker in the second round from Morgan State University. His name was Willie Edward Lanier.

Lanier stood 6 foot, 1 inch and weighed 245 pounds. During training camp, Lanier showed his coaches that they made the right choice in selecting him. Willie was a quick learner of the game. His knowledge of his position made him a natural leader. He was inserted as the first African American linebacker to start an NFL game. They won three of the first four games in the fall of 1967, including two shutouts.

In the fifth game, something happened to Lanier that would alter how he played the position forever. A half century later, that same man would influence the rules of the game to make it safer today for all players. It was a running play. It was an away game against San Diego. The Chargers' quarterback handed off to his running back. An offensive lineman tried to block Lanier defending the play. The linebacker leaped over the lineman to greet the ball carrier behind the line of scrimmage. He had his arms outstretched to tackle the halfback who was running in a crouched position. The ball carrier's knee collided with Lanier's helmet causing injury to his forehead. Lanier came off the field and was momentarily dazed but he did not fall, he felt no pain, and he returned to finish the game. The Chiefs lost the Chargers that day by a score of 41−35.

Willie Lanier felt no ill effects from that hit. The next game was at home against the Houston Oilers. He was on the field in the defensive huddle when Lanier suddenly collapsed onto the field. Recently, some five decades later, Willie asked his former teammate, Emmitt Thomas, a cornerback for the Chiefs, if he remembered the incident while they were in the huddle together. Thomas said, "I thought you were dead." Willie was taken from the field and sent to the hospital. He would miss the next two games because of the symptoms he was suffering from. During the ambulance ride, Dr. Albert Miller, the Chief's team doctor noted that Willie's pulse had stopped three times. Emmitt was right, Willie was on the edge of death. Neither of these facts were told to Willie during his playing days.

Despite these medical problems, Willie was cleared to play in the next several games and returned to the starting lineup. Then in a rematch against the Chargers, Willie suffered double vision during the game. He saw two quarterbacks and attempted to tackle the second image and not the real player. It was then Willie and Dr. Miller decided to seek expert medical opinion and they traveled to the Mayo Clinic in Rochester, Minnesota. The neurologists diagnosed him as suffering from a subdural hematoma. The bleed was from that hit he suffered back in week 5. The brain injury near his optic nerve caused his vision problems. Willie was held out for the last four games of the 1967 season, and the Chiefs team did not make the playoffs.

Willie contemplated retirement after this rookie season. He determined that if he could adjust his playing style so that it would give him a 90% guarantee of safety, he would continue. At that time, and perhaps even more true today, a guarantee of 90% safety is absurd. Football is a violent sport where collisions and serious injury are unavoidable. Yet, Willie found ways to protect himself and his opponents, and played at an all pro-level for the next 10 years without missing a single game. Willie Lanier was an eight-time All Pro, was elected to the NFL Hall of Fame, had his jersey number 63 retired by the Kansas City Chiefs, and was named in the NFL's 75th Anniversary All-Time Team. I had the pleasure of interviewing Willie Lanier in my office and received permission from him to report on our meeting.

Detection of traumatic brain injury

According to statistics compiled by the Centers for Disease Control and Prevention, there are 1.5 million people who suffer from traumatic brain injury (TBI) each year, accounting for 50,000 deaths, 230,000 hospitalizations, and 80,000–90,000 patients exhibiting long-term disability. The most common cause of TBI is motor vehicle crashes, falls, and violence. Teens, young adults, and elderly subjects have the highest incidence, with more male cases than females.

There were no laboratory tests to diagnose concussion or traumatic brain injury in the 1960s and 1970s when Willie Lanier played professional football. It would be another 4 years before the first prototype head CT scanner would be installed at Atkinson Morely Hospital in London. While the electroencephalogram (EEG) was first studied in the latter part of the 19th century, the technique of sensory evoked potentials (EEG recordings following stimulation), would not be in routine medical use into the 1970s. Even today, there are no on-the-field laboratory diagnostics that can be conducted to determine if a player of any sport has suffered a head injury that puts them at risk for permanent disability. It is impractical to have imaging equipment and real-time testing available within the player's locker room. Even if the National Football League (NFL) could afford it, defects may not be detectable immediately after the injury. It would be ideal if a point-of-care testing lab blood testing device for brain injury biomarkers can be developed and used on the field of play. This could involve the use of a finger stick blood collection to detect multiple biomarkers. The devices may need to be more analytically sensitive than the current platforms that are used for other biomarkers.

An important issue for TBI survivors is stratification of risk for future adverse events and some objective measure for return to duty (or play). In this regard, all major league sports such as the NFL, National Basketball Association, Major League Baseball, National Hockey League, etc., have "concussion protocols." Of course, none of these were in place when Lanier played. The NFL's protocol calls for (1) rest and recovery, (2) light aerobic exercise, (3) continued exercise and strength training, (4) football-specific activities, and (5) full football activity. These assessments are made in the absence of objective clinical laboratory data that determine the likelihood of ongoing or recurring damage. Future risk stratification assessments may be based on the measurement of autoantibodies. Brain injury will release proteins from the central nervous system to the blood through damage to the blood−brain barrier. These biomarkers are normally not present in the blood in sufficiently high concentrations. If there is sufficient release of these proteins into the circulation, the individual's immune system might recognize it as foreign antigen and evoke an immune response. This could provide the basis of a test for long-term complications.

The primary objective of this textbook is to provide the state-of-the art knowledge of TBI biomarkers from discovery to possible clinical implementation. In February 2018, the US Food and Drug Administration used their Breakthrough Devices Program to clear the first blood test for mild traumatic brain injury. The test, Brain Trauma Indicator produced by Banyan Biomarkers Inc. (San Diego CA) measures ubiquitin C-terminal hydrolase-L1 (UCH-L) and glial fibrillary acidic protein (GFAP) to rule out the need for a head computed tomography (CT) scan in adults that present with a suspected head injury. Obviating the need for CT scan may eliminate unnecessary radiation exposure to patients and reduce the costs of obtaining CT scans. The approval of these biomarkers is the beginning of the TBI biomarker field. There have been dozens of proteins, peptides, and autoantibodies that have been studied regarding the medical management of TBI. As shown by Brain Trauma Indicator, a multimarker approach will be necessary to obtain the necessary sensitivity and specificity for current and future claims. This textbook provides the scientific and medical basis for many of the most widely studied of these tests, how they might be measured, and how they can be used in conjunction with other TBI tools.

Changes to playing style to avoid traumatic brain injury

Enrollments in high school football have declined by an average of 7% in the past 10 years according to the National Federation of State High School Associations. This is due to increasing concerns over concussions and TBI and other football-related injuries. Both of Lanier's sons played organized football. He currently does not have any grandsons, only granddaughters. When asked about whether he would encourage or discourage these children from participating, his response was, "It depends on the coaches' and school's commitment to safety over winning." He believes that football and other contact sports can be played to a higher safety standard with changes to rules and equipment.

So what actions did Willie Lanier take after his rookie season to protect himself from further injury to his brain? During his rookie season, the team equipment manager, Bobby Yarborough created a special padded helmet for Willie to wear. The padding was placed on the outside of the helmet to provide some additional protection to Lanier's head. While he wore this helmet for the remainder of this career, Lanier does NOT credit use of this helmet that protected him from further head injury. Instead, he took two other approaches.

The first was to take his head out of the game. He no longer used his skull as a tackling weapon. Given a prior diagnosis of subarachnoid hemorrhage, Lanier recognized that a second brain bleed could be fatal. Lanier was determined to stay healthy and remain on the field. His reasoning was that a player who is often injured is of little to no value to his team. His strategy as a defenseman was body on body contact, such as using his shoulders, instead of head on body or worse, using his head to collide with the opponent's head. The focal point was the opposing player's jersey number.

The result of his altered playing strategy adopted during his rookie season was safety and longevity. Lanier did not suffer any more significant head injuries. He played in almost every game for the remaining 10 of his 11-year career. This was more than triple the average NFL career of just 3.3 years. Today, some 40 years after the end of his career, Lanier has suffered no effects of his concussion. He reports no double vision, headaches, or seizures. His mental focus is sharp, with no changes in personality and he has no depression symptoms and is not a victim of posttraumatic stress syndrome.

The second approach toward avoiding injury was to play the game with compassion for his competitors. He never sought to physically harm or disable his opponents. This is contrary to some player's mentality of disabling their opponent to gain a competitive advantage. Lanier recognized that while knocking out a key player, such as the quarterback may have immediate advantages for that particular contest, in the long term, this strategy undermines the integrity of the game itself. Moreover, such brutal tactics make the offending team vulnerable for a retaliatory attack. Some fans of the sport seek the acts of violence that are produced by the sport. Lanier succeeded at the highest level without satisfying this primordial instinct.

In recent years, the NFL has adopted rule changes that followed Willie Lanier's playing style a half century earlier. "Roughing" penalties are now regularly assessed when the head and helmet are used in making a tackle. These rule changes are not a coincidence, Lanier was named in 2011 by the Commission to the NFL Player Safety Advisory Committee, cochaired by the former player Ronnie Lott and the former coach John Madden. The Committee were charged to improve player safety by reviewing playing rules and making recommendations on changes in protective equipment. This group were instrumental in pushing for rule changes regarding the use of the head for tackling.

Former players including Frank Gifford, Kenny Stabler, Dave Duerson, Junior Seau, and Mike Webster, all died from chronic traumatic encephalopathy or CTE, a progressive degeneration of the brain that is directly related to excessive blows to the head. These individuals suffered from cognitive decline, memory loss, and behavioral changes, including aggression and depression. With clinical implementation of TBI biomarkers and the development of effective therapies, it is hoped that TBI can be better diagnosed and treated to reduce the incidence of CTE.

December, 2019

Alan H.B. Wu[1] and Willie E. Lanier[2]

[1]San Francisco, CA, United States [2]Richmond, VA, United States

Introduction

Introduction—scope of the problem

David O. Okonkwo[1] and John K. Yue[2]

[1]Department of Neurosurgery, University of Pittsburgh Medical Center, Pittsburgh, PA,
United States [2]Department of Neurosurgery, University of California San Francisco,
San Francisco, CA, United States

1.1 Scope of the problem

Traumatic brain injury (TBI), caused by external force to the head, remains a leading source of morbidity and mortality worldwide. In the United States, 4.8 million persons seek medical care for TBI annually, with 2.8 million emergency department (ED) visits, 280,000 hospitalizations, and 56,000 deaths [1]—this translates to 6 deaths, 31 hospitalizations, 194 ED visits, and 457 concussions *per hour*. TBI is the leading cause of death in persons under age 45, and recent evidence shows that the incidence in the elderly is approaching epidemic proportions [2].

TBI clinical care, as well as TBI clinical trials, has been hampered by lack of objective measures of TBI pathophysiology. To date, more than 30 Phase III therapy trials have failed in translating to an FDA-approved treatment for TBI [3]. These failures have largely been driven by the fool's chase of one drug treating all TBIs. In fact, investigators have likely failed the drugs more than the drugs have failed the patients.

A fundamental reason for the lack of targeted treatment lies in the heterogeneity of TBI. While injuries may present similarly when assessed by the Glasgow Coma Scale (GCS) as mild (GCS 13–15), moderate (GCS 9–12), and severe TBI (GCS 3–8), neuroimaging features including lesion type, location, and volume are equally necessary in defining clinical severity and guiding management considerations. Severe TBI in a comatose patient may be due to extraaxial hemorrhage, intraparenchymal mass lesion, or diffuse brain swelling—different pathophysiologies requiring different forms of treatment. Similarly, on the mild end of the spectrum, the GCS shows ceiling effects, and subclassification of precise "mild" TBI clinical phenotypes (vestibular, cognitive, migraine, etc. disorders) for targeted treatment has been elusive.

Biomarkers for Traumatic Brain Injury
DOI: https://doi.org/10.1016/B978-0-12-816346-7.00001-4

The field of TBI has benefited immensely from the most widely used, and in many respects the only, biomarker available today: the CT scan. The head CT has saved countless lives across the world following trauma, and steered countless more toward effective medical management. Now, the field of TBI needs additional biomarkers in order to advance clinical practice. This next generation of biomarkers must reflect the complex pathophysiology of TBI, including excitotoxic damage, oxidative stress, and neuroinflammation, among others [4]. New biomarkers will derive from neuroimaging, biofluids, and electrophysiology. This textbook will discuss these and other developments as the field of biomarkers for TBI enters a golden era.

1.2 Candidate biomarkers

Biomarkers can advance TBI clinical care by improving diagnosis, triage, and treatment. Detecting the pathology of TBI using blood, cerebrospinal fluid (CSF), and other biofluidic biomarkers of sufficient sensitivity constitutes a paradigm shift for the field of neurotrauma. Over the past two decades, a range of candidate biomarkers have been studied extensively. The commercialization efforts to date have focused primarily on biomarkers that predict intracranial injuries visible on CT and prognostication of 3- to 6-month outcome. Biomarkers are also being studied in reference to specific injured cell types. These include markers of glial (GFAP: glial fibrillary acidic protein; S100B: calcium binding protein B; MBP: myelin basic protein), axonal and neuronal (UCH-L1: ubiquitin carboxyl-terminal hydrolase-L1; NSE: neuron-specific enolase; Tau protein and phosphorylated-Tau [p-Tau]; AIIS-BDP: alpha-II-spectrin breakdown products), and immunological (cytokines, autoantibodies) injury [5]. These and other biomarkers will be discussed in depth in the subsequent chapters of this text.

Biomarkers are already in routine clinical use for myocardial ischemia, kidney disease, infection, and cancer and have revolutionized clinical care and research in these diseases. As shown in Table 1.1, biomarkers are applied across several contexts of use, including

TABLE 1.1   Example FDA biomarker context of use definitions.

FDA context of use	Definition
Diagnostic biomarker	Categorizes a person by the presence or absence of a specific physiological or pathophysiological state or disease
Prognostic biomarker	Categorizes patients by degree of risk for disease occurrence or progression of a specific aspect of a disease
Predictive biomarker	Categorizes patients by their likelihood of response to a particular treatment relative to no treatment
Pharmacodynamic biomarker	Indicates a response to therapy and the change in biomarker level is indicative of the magnitude of response to therapy
Efficacy—response biomarker	Predicts a specific disease-related clinical outcome and can serve as a surrogate for a clinical efficacy endpoint

diagnostic, prognostic, predictive, pharmacodynamic, and efficacy—response biomarkers. Through its qualification process, the FDA provides a pathway for biomarkers to serve as endpoints in clinical trials. Biomarkers specific to their respective context of use can also enable early diagnosis in the field (prior to arrival to a medical facility), serial measurements to detect temporal evolution of injury, as well as prognostic and predictive capabilities to determine risk for disease progression and likelihood of response to treatment, respectively.

1.3 Blood biomarkers for traumatic brain injury

Since 2015, S100B has been included in an algorithm in the Scandinavian guidelines to triage patients with mTBI to CT after TBI [6]. In a landmark decision on February 14, 2018, the US Food and Drug Administration cleared marketing of the Banyan Brain Trauma Indicator (BTI) as the first diagnostic blood test to evaluate mild TBI (mTBI) in North America   (https://www.accessdata.fda.gov/cdrh_docs/reviews/DEN170045.pdf).   The FDA decision was based on the 2018 ALERT-TBI pivotal trial, where in 1959 mild-to-moderate TBI patients the combined panel of serum GFAP and UCH-L1 had a negative predictive value (NPV) of 0.996 for detecting intracranial injury on CT [7]. These data are summative of the research to date regarding the discriminability of GFAP and UCH-L1 for CT abnormalities, with areas under the receiver—operating characteristic (ROC) curve (AUCs) of 0.8—0.9 and 0.7—0.9, respectively [8,9]. The Banyan BTI test is a proprietary core lab assay which provides results in 4—6 hours, constituting a barrier for use in acute injury that must be overcome—ideally with point-of-care testing with rapid return of results.

Regarding prognostic biomarkers, Tau is a cytoskeletal protein that contributes to the stabilization of axon microtubules. After TBI, Tau may become hyperphosphorylated by kinases or undergo proteolysis by calpains and caspases to produce p-Tau, which is a precursor to long-term tauopathy. p-Tau has been found to be elevated not only in acute but also chronic TBI, with AUCs of 1.0 in distinguishing mTBI and chronic TBI from healthy controls in a 2017 report from the TRACK-TBI Pilot study [10]. Furthermore, p-Tau was able to weakly distinguish those with good versus less-than-good outcomes (e.g., able to return to work) on the Glasgow Outcome Scale Extended (GOSE) at 6 months (AUC 0.663). Other markers such as BDNF predicted complete versus incomplete recovery in mTBI (AUC 0.65) [11], and MAP-2 and cleaved-Tau in CSF predicted clinical outcome after severe TBI [12]. In severe TBI, monitoring biomarkers include S100B, which is associated with intracranial pressure (ICP) and cerebral perfusion pressure (CPP) [13], as well as GFAP and UCH-L1, which have the ability to distinguish mass lesions from diffuse injuries [14,15]. Several markers have been investigated to assess treatment efficacy, such as NSE and S100B for progesterone [16], and NSE for memantine [17].

Fig. 1.1 shows ranges of time for which biomarkers can become elevated in response to injury. The part of the time continuum that the treatment is affecting will dictate the efficacy—response biomarker to be used. For example, GFAP and UCH-L1 may be appropriate efficacy—response biomarkers on the order of hours, and demyelination markers such as MBP may be more appropriate on the order of weeks.

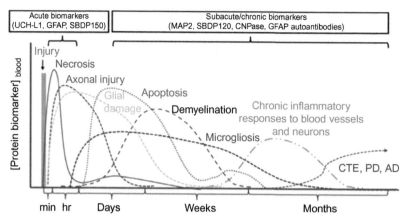

FIGURE 1.1   **Temporal trends of blood-based biomarkers after TBI.** *AD*, Alzheimer's disease; *CNPase*, 2′,3′-cyclic nucleotide 3′-phosphodiesterase; *CTE*, chronic traumatic encephalopathy; *GFAP*, glial fibrillary acidic protein; *MAP2*, microtubule associated protein 2; *MBP*, myelin basic protein; *PD*, Parkinson's disease; *SBDP15*, spectrin breakdown product 150; *SPDP120*, spectrin breakdown product 120; *UCH-L1*, Ubiquitin C-terminal hydrolase L1.

These data and others show the imminent promise of candidate biomarkers undergoing validation in large prospective studies for diagnostic, prognostic, and predictive contexts of use, which will be discussed in detail in the forthcoming chapters. The implications of these biomarkers extend beyond civilian trauma and hospital care. The capability to obtain an objective, diagnostic point-of-care result from a blood-based biomarker on the battlefield, or on the sport sidelines, have high potential to guide resource utilization to remove a soldier from combat and a player from play. Further, the temporal trend of monitoring biomarkers may judiciously triage at-risk patient to follow-up scans, referral to inpatient and outpatient TBI services, and follow-up with primary care.

1.4 Nonblood biomarkers

Other biofluids in addition to blood hold promise and will be explored in this text. For example, several salivary micro-RNAs from the inflammatory cascade are upregulated after concussion and correlate with sideline concussion testing [18]. Neurocognitive and functional testing will be explored in this text in the context of sideline concussion assessment and return-to-play decisions. Objective evaluations of brain function after concussion, such as electroencephalogram (EEG), may be important to compensate for the subjective nature of symptoms' assessment. The concussed brain produces decreased alpha, beta, gamma, and theta band amplitudes, increased delta band amplitude, and focal network dysfunction that can be evaluated with EEG in both acute and subacute periods after injury [19,20]. Risk stratification and management will be discussed in the context of biomarker qualification, implementation, and discriminability across the course of TBI recovery.

1.5 Conclusions

TBI is a global health epidemic and presents a public health crisis, given the paucity of available diagnostic tests and effective treatments. There is a critical need for TBI biomarkers to guide diagnosis, treatment, and triage to follow-up. The FDA clearance of the first diagnostic biomarkers for TBI (GFAP and UCH-L1) on February 14, 2018, represents a seminal moment in the advancement of TBI practice, which has long relied on the neurologic exam and CT scan. This FDA clearance and subsequent findings from large-scale prospective studies herald the beginning of a "Golden Age" in TBI research, in which clearing additional candidate biomarkers for clinical use will be a priority. The contents of this book are structured to highlight the promise of multimodal, blood and nonblood biomarkers for integration into TBI clinical care and research, across the spectrum of injury and continuum of care.

Disclaimers and Acknowledgments

None.

References

[1] Korley FK, Kelen GD, Jones CM, Diaz-Arrastia R. Emergency department evaluation of traumatic brain injury in the United States, 2009—2010. J Head Trauma Rehabil 2016;31(6):379—87.
[2] Taylor CA, Bell JM, Breiding MJ, Xu L. Traumatic brain injury-related emergency department visits, hospitalizations, and deaths—United States, 2007 and 2013. MMWR Surveill Summ 2017;66(9):1—16.
[3] Maas AIR, Roozenbeek B, Manley GT. Clinical trials in traumatic brain injury: past experience and current developments. Neurotherapeutics 2010;7(1):115—26.
[4] Galgano M, Toshkezi G, Qiu X, Russell T, Chin L, Zhao L-R. Traumatic brain injury: current treatment strategies and future endeavors. Cell Transpl 2017;26(7):1118—30.
[5] Wang KK, Yang Z, Zhu T, Shi Y, Rubenstein R, Tyndall JA, et al. An update on diagnostic and prognostic biomarkers for traumatic brain injury. Expert Rev Mol Diagn 2018;18(2):165—80.
[6] Undén L, Calcagnile O, Undén J, Reinstrup P, Bazarian J. Validation of the Scandinavian guidelines for initial management of minimal, mild and moderate traumatic brain injury in adults. BMC Med 2015;13:292.
[7] Bazarian JJ, Biberthaler P, Welch RD, Lewis LM, Barzo P, Bogner-Flatz V, et al. Serum GFAP and UCH-L1 for prediction of absence of intracranial injuries on head CT (ALERT-TBI): a multicentre observational study. Lancet Neurol 2018;17(9):782—9.
[8] Papa L, Brophy GM, Welch RD, Lewis LM, Braga CF, Tan CN, et al. Time course and diagnostic accuracy of glial and neuronal blood biomarkers GFAP and UCH-L1 in a large cohort of trauma patients with and without mild traumatic brain injury. JAMA Neurol 2016;73(5):551—60.
[9] Diaz-Arrastia R, Wang KKW, Papa L, Sorani MD, Yue JK, Puccio AM, et al. Acute biomarkers of traumatic brain injury: relationship between plasma levels of ubiquitin C-terminal hydrolase-L1 and glial fibrillary acidic protein. J Neurotrauma 2014;31(1):19—25.
[10] Rubenstein R, Chang B, Yue JK, Chiu A, Winkler EA, Puccio AM, et al. Comparing plasma phospho tau, total tau, and phospho tau-total tau ratio as acute and chronic traumatic brain injury biomarkers. JAMA Neurol 2017;74(9):1063—72.
[11] Korley FK, Diaz-Arrastia R, Wu AHB, Yue JK, Manley GT, Sair HI, et al. Circulating brain-derived neurotrophic factor has diagnostic and prognostic value in traumatic brain injury. J Neurotrauma 2016;33(2):215—25.

[12] Welch RD, Ayaz SI, Lewis LM, Unden J, Chen JY, Mika VH, et al. Ability of serum glial fibrillary acidic protein, ubiquitin C-terminal hydrolase-L1, and S100B to differentiate normal and abnormal head computed tomography findings in patients with suspected mild or moderate traumatic brain injury. J Neurotrauma 2016;33(2):203—14.

[13] Olivecrona Z, Bobinski L, Koskinen L-OD. Association of ICP, CPP, CT findings and S-100B and NSE in severe traumatic head injury. Prognostic value of the biomarkers. Brain Inj 2015;29(4):446—54.

[14] Posti JP, Takala RSK, Runtti H, Newcombe VF, Outtrim J, Katila AJ, et al. The levels of glial fibrillary acidic protein and ubiquitin C-terminal hydrolase-L1 during the first week after a traumatic brain injury: correlations with clinical and imaging findings. Neurosurgery 2016;79(3):456—64.

[15] Okonkwo DO, Yue JK, Puccio AM, Panczykowski DM, Inoue T, McMahon PJ, et al. GFAP-BDP as an acute diagnostic marker in traumatic brain injury: results from the prospective transforming research and clinical knowledge in traumatic brain injury study. J Neurotrauma 2013;30(17):1490—7.

[16] Shahrokhi N, Soltani Z, Khaksari M, Karamouzian S, Mofid B, Asadikaram G. The serum changes of neuron-specific enolase and intercellular adhesion molecule-1 in patients with diffuse axonal injury following progesterone administration: a randomized clinical trial. Arch Trauma Res 2016;5(3):e37005.

[17] Mokhtari M, Nayeb-Aghaei H, Kouchek M, Miri MM, Goharani R, Amoozandeh A, et al. Effect of memantine on serum levels of neuron-specific enolase and on the Glasgow Coma Scale in patients with moderate traumatic brain injury. J Clin Pharmacol 2018;58(1):42—7.

[18] Di Pietro V, Porto E, Ragusa M, Barbagallo C, Davies D, Forcione M, et al. Salivary microRNAs: diagnostic markers of mild traumatic brain injury in contact-sport. Front Mol Neurosci 2018;11:290.

[19] Jacquin A, Kanakia S, Oberly D, Prichep LS. A multimodal biomarker for concussion identification, prognosis and management. Comput Biol Med 2018;102:95—103.

[20] Munia TTK, Haider A, Schneider C, Romanick M, Fazel-Rezai R. A novel EEG based spectral analysis of persistent brain function alteration in athletes with concussion history. Sci Rep 2017;7(1):17221.

The need for traumatic brain injury markers

Martin Paul Than[1], Daniel Fatovich[2], Melinda Fitzgerald[3], Aleksandra Gozt[3], Audrey McKinlay[4] and Deborah Snell[5]

[1]Emergency Department, Christchurch Hospital, Christchurch, New Zealand [2]Royal Perth Hospital, Perth, WA, Australia [3]Curtin University, Bentley, WA, Australia [4]University of Canterbury, Christchurch, New Zealand [5]University of Otago, Christchurch, New Zealand

2.1 Introduction

Traumatic brain injury (TBI), and the subgroup of patients with mild traumatic brain injury (mTBI) represent an important public health system and societal burden. It is estimated that 42 million people worldwide experience an mTBI annually [1]. Males are 1.6 times more likely than females to present to the emergency department (ED) with a TBI [2].

In the United States, which has a population of ~327 million people, approximately 2.8 million people per year are affected by TBI, with 2.5 million of these injuries related to ED visits [3]. Similar burden is experienced in other developed countries; for example, in New Zealand (population ~5 million), a recent population-based incidence study reported a total incidence of TBI of 790 cases per 100,000 person-years [4]. A New Zealand government report states that there are approximately 14,000 people who are treated for TBI each year [5]. In Australia, which has a population of ~25 million, there were over 14,000 hospitalizations for TBI in 2004/2005 [6]. However, mTBI (or concussion) accounts for 70%–85% of TBI [7] and most of these patients do not attend hospital. Indeed, only 10%–25% of people seek medical attention for TBI, so these injuries are substantially underreported. The incidence rates in New Zealand of 790 cases per 100,000 person-years (which is greater than the incidence of cancer) [8] equates to 190,000 to 200,000 cases per year in Australia.

As TBI disproportionally affects young people, chronic disability following TBI is particularly costly both in terms of productive years lost and burden on the healthcare system. A recent Centers for Disease Control and Prevention (CDC) report estimated the

9

economic cost of TBI in the United States (including direct and indirect medical costs) to be approximately US$76.5 billion. Severe TBI accounted for approximately 90% of the total TBI medical costs. New Zealand government statistics estimate the annual cost of mTBI to be NZ$83.5 million. The lifetime cost of each TBI in Australia is estimated at AU$2.5 million for moderate and AU$4.8 million for severe injuries. New cases of moderate and severe TBI add more than AU$2 billion in lifetime costs to the Australian healthcare system annually, and the total annual cost of TBI in Australia is AU$8.6 billion [9]. The costs from mTBI are minimally documented and not included in these estimates.

2.2 Context

This chapter will focus upon the need for better tests in the assessment of TBI in three areas:

- The acute assessment of patients in the ED.
- The identification of who will have ongoing morbidity following their TBI.
- The prediction of the extent of such morbidity.

2.3 Probabilities, decision-making, and test thresholds

It is now almost 40 years since Stephen Pauker and Jerome Kassirer (a future editor-in-chief of the New England Journal of Medicine) wrote their article entitled "the threshold approach to clinical decision-making" [10]. The logic explained then remains relevant today. For a specific diagnosis of interest, clinicians are constantly determining and reevaluating the likely probability of that diagnosis. This process starts with the first information the clinician has available from the history (and also even from precontact information such as primary care, ambulance, or nursing records), and is then refined as new information, such as examination findings, laboratory results, and imaging, becomes available. Pauker and Kassirer described that at some point during medical assessment, the disease probability will either (1) pass a lower threshold at which more testing does more harm than good because the disease is very unlikely, or (2) pass above the threshold at which the probability of the disease is already high enough to begin treatment with confidence (Fig. 2.1). These thresholds will vary according to the clinical scenario. The test/treatment threshold concept is applicable to the assessment of patients with TBI.

2.4 Acute assessment of patients with traumatic brain injury in the emergency department

Patients presenting to the ED with TBI can do so via ambulance, primary care physician, or through self-presentation. Ambulance presentations are usually more serious. There is therefore a range of severity from very minor injury through to the comatose patient. In an isolated TBI, the primary ED decision-making focuses upon the identification of those

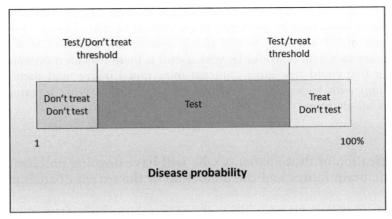

FIGURE 2.1 **Test/treat thresholds.** Medical assessment determines the probability of the disease of interest with each new piece of information making small or large adjustments to this probability. Below the test/no treatment threshold the optimal strategy is for no further testing because the harms outweigh the benefits. Above the test/treatment threshold the probability that the disease is present is enough to begin evidence-based treatment for that disease despite any potential side effects that might occur.

patients with significant intracranial injury, for example, epidural or subdural hematoma. The focus is identifying those patients who require neurosurgical intervention.

In the context of decision thresholds, a very high (near certain) degree of probability of major intracranial injury is required before the patient has neurosurgery. Fortunately, CT scanning is very specific for injury identification (very accurate for rule-in).

The decision of when to request CT scanning is heavily influenced by the fact that missed intracranial injury can be catastrophic. As a result, clinicians are motivated to request a CT scan in order to avoid the risk of missing intracranial injury. This has led to a progressive increase in usage of CT scanning in this context. The use of CT in the ED increased sixfold from 1995 to 2007 and the use of CT has increased at a higher rate in the ED than in other settings [11]. As many as 63% of patients with mTBI in the ED undergo CT scanning [12]. While up to 15% of ED patients with mTBI have an acute finding on CT, <1% require neurosurgical intervention [13,14]. This has also led to the development of clinical decision aids to identify which patients require imaging with the aim of rationalizing usage.

CT scan usage in the ED for TBI varies according to nation, health system, age, and setting [15–17]. Where CT scans are easily available with no resource or funding impediment then there is little downside (other than radiation dosage in children) to scanning large numbers of patients. In systems or settings where access to CT is problematic, then the decision to test must be weighed against other priorities.

In taxation-based health systems (such as New Zealand's National Healthcare System), requests for CT scans for TBI need to be balanced against CT scanning resource availability (particularly out of hours) and large numbers of requests for other clinical problems both from the ED and other hospital areas. The rational use of CT scanning for TBI in the ED has been strongly advocated by the Choosing Wisely movement. Choosing Wisely is a multinational initiative of the American Board of Internal Medicine (ABIM) Foundation which is strongly supported at a government level. It seeks to advance dialogue on avoiding unnecessary duplication of tests and procedures, and to empower patients to choose care that is supported by evidence, in the context of shared decision-making.

Since the use of CT scanning is still rising despite low numbers of a CT-identified intracranial injury in mTBI, it would be very useful if there was an inexpensive and accurate biomarker that could rule out significant intracranial injury (and therefore the need for CT scanning) with high accuracy. This need is already driving research, and this is described in other chapters.

2.5 Identification of those patients who will have ongoing problems following traumatic brain injury and the prediction of the extent of such problems

The assessment of patients with TBI in the ED has historically focused on the identification (and then onward treatment, especially neurosurgery) of serious intracranial injuries such as cerebral hemorrhage. Once such serious injury is ruled out, then if the patient is reasonably well, ambulant, coherent, and able to look after themselves, they are suitable for discharge with variable degrees of patient information guidance regarding possible ongoing injury symptoms [13].

It is now clear that mTBI is common and has significant impact on patients and society. As a result, research interest has reached fever pitch as more and more implications are discovered in multiple contexts such as the armed forces, contact sport, and workforce employment. The understanding of the pathology and science relating to ongoing symptoms from mTBI is now improving but remains substantially incomplete. This is compounded by the fact that management solutions for ongoing symptoms are poorly developed.

Most people recover fully after a mTBI, but 20% or more can have a delayed recovery due to persisting symptoms, more recently referred to as persisting post-concussion symptoms (PCS). Persisting PCS are known to occur following even the mildest forms of TBI, and there is currently no way of knowing which individuals will go on to develop persistent difficulties.

A range of physiological, structural, and neuropsychological outcomes have been assessed for their capacity to predict outcome following mTBI, most being limited to investigating a single type of measure. The results reported have been mixed [18–21]. Given that PCS is complex and multifactorial, affecting several important aspects of functioning, it is unlikely that any single measure will be able to predict the likelihood of an individual experiencing ongoing symptoms. Current predictors of outcomes following mTBI use algorithms that may be useful for groups of patients but are not helpful at the level of the individual [22–24]. It is thus becoming apparent that a suite of markers is likely to be required to effectively predict poor recovery at the level of the individual. Against this background there is a need for additional tests that can provide guidance in relation to the specific issues below.

1. *Prediction of the severity of injury and the likelihood of ongoing symptoms and disability*
   Some may argue that such a test is of little value if there is not a clear intervention that can then be applied to improve outcomes, but this is not completely true. Clarification of a diagnosis conveys information about injury severity and expected symptoms and can be beneficial for treatment providers, funders, and the patient. From a patient's

perspective, this can be reassuring. Early troubling and unexpected symptoms after mTBI have been associated with increased anxiety and risk for slow recovery [25–27]. Earlier prediction of injury severity and likely associated symptoms can guide return to work planning and expectations. If it were possible to give patients this information, it might be reasonable to provide it. In fact, accurate forewarning of specific problems might prompt an individual to change their career or life path or simply just rearrange their life (if possible), for example, from working full time to part time.

Such information could be valuable to the patient's employer and insurer, although the access to and use of this information would have to be handled with great care given the complexity of clinical issues especially over time, and with stringent safeguards. However, negative consequences of atypical outcomes, especially after mTBI, include unfair labels such as feigned symptoms or malingering; tests capable of determining ongoing injury-related impairment would be useful in this context. Further to this, it is important to recognize that most people recover in a timely fashion following mTBI and undue anxiety about continuing symptoms can contribute to poor outcomes. If a sufficiently accurate and specific predictive test could be developed it may allow unnecessary fears to be allayed.

2. *Identification of those patients who may benefit from specific interventions*

As previously mentioned, this is a rapidly developing field in which there is much to learn. mTBI covers a broad range of symptoms and likely differing underlying pathophysiology. As such, it is likely that for interventions to be beneficial they will need to be targeted to specific subgroups of symptoms [28]. Tests that can categorize patients into these subgroups can be utilized to focus specific interventions and related resources on the patients for whom they would be most beneficial.

3. *Identification of those patients who would benefit from delayed, structured, or tapered return to usual activities*

Historically, advice regarding return to work or sport has been variable. Many sports now have organized guidance processes for returning to partial or full participation, including the Zurich graduated return to play program [29,30]. The optimal guidance on returning to work is less clear and will obviously depend on the nature of the work and the extent of symptoms. It would be very useful to have an objective test or tests which provide measurable guidance measures for return to activity.

4. *Identification of patients at risk for development of subsequent mental health issues*

There is increasing evidence that there is an association between mTBI and development of subsequent mental health problems, including depression and suicide. In fact, there is a growing literature highlighting the impacts of a range of potentially modifiable psychological factors on injury outcomes [31]. It would be important to identify such patients early and potentially initiate early referrals for psychological support and/or specialist mental health monitoring.

5. *Identification of patients who might progress to neurological diseases in association with mTBI*

The best well-known case of a person with persistent mTBI and who then developed further neurological pathology is Muhammad Ali's progressive development of Parkinson's disease. Multiple mTBI, which can occur during sport, have generally been shown to lead to worse outcomes, increasing the risk of profound long-term consequences, including encephalopathy, mental health issues, and Alzheimer's disease [32,33].

2.6 Issues for children

Early childhood is one of the most common periods for mTBI to occur [3]. Predicting outcomes following mTBI in children is important for informing and reassuring their families and for directing rehabilitation services and return to school and play. Currently, evaluations of mTBI are based on imaging, and parent and child report. This is problematic as many children are injured while they are still preverbal. Biomarkers would also assist in determining whether there was a need for imaging procedures and also possibly in differentiating between children with intentional versus nonintentional injury.

Existing research reports correlations between biomarkers and injury severity measures, global outcomes, and neuroimaging abnormalities. However, methodologies of existing studies vary, making it difficult to combine different studies [34].

For many of the biomarkers currently being investigated in adults, there is little or no data for pediatric populations. This may be due to the difficulties in evaluating biomarkers in a pediatric population; biomarkers are expressed at different levels across the life span [35] and show different patterns in children. For example, S-100B and myelin basic protein have elevated normative concentrations in children [36]. Moreover, neuron-specific enolase (NSE) shows different patterns for children and S-100B is not sensitive for use with children [37].

Goldman and colleagues [35] pointed out that difficulties evaluating biomarkers for use in a pediatric population typically result in biomarkers that are developed in adult populations and then adapted for use in pediatric populations instead of child-specific markers [33]. Goldman and colleagues suggest the following as optimal characteristics of an ideal biomarker for children:

- Noninvasive
- Pediatric-specific
- Results correspond with age-dependent physiologic changes
- Cost-effective
- Well-established pediatric-specific norms

2.7 Issues for women

Some research has suggested that being female has been identified as a risk factor for both the occurrence of a concussion and prolonged recovery from the injury [38]. This increased risk may in part be due to actions of hormones on the brain's inflammatory response. Research has shown that menstrual cycle phase and progesterone concentration at the time of mTBI may affect symptoms [39] and length of time symptoms are present [40].

While hormonal changes may partly explain the higher report of concussive symptoms for females compared to males, more recently the architecture of the female brain has also been implicated. Female axons have been found to be thinner with fewer microtubules than male brains which creates less stability in the brain and more damage to axons when injury occurs. It has been suggested that the extended recovery time for females following concussion may be reflective of longer time taken to repair the axons [41]. It is likely that both hormonal changes and brain architecture play a role in outcomes following concussion for females [42,43]. The identification of accurate sex-specific biomarkers would provide individualized information about the impact of injury and its impact on recovery, thereby reducing patient stress and uncertainty. Biomarkers would also enable efficient allocation of rehabilitation services to those with prolonged recovery. Currently there is growing information regarding the impact of sex on biomarkers [44].

2.8 Issues for future research to consider

A range of issues hamper progress toward identification of a biomarker or combination of tests capable of detecting brain injury and identifying those with risk for development of persisting symptoms and disability after TBI. These include representativeness of cases captured by research, complexity of mTBI prognosis, and knowledge uptake considerations.

Firstly, many prognostic studies recruit from first healthcare presentation following a TBI, usually at the ED. However, the ED is not the first healthcare contact for many patients, especially for those sustaining mTBI [45]. Diverse recruitment methods and eligibility criteria across the research contribute to samples with diverse injury severity, likely favoring more severe injuries. Many studies and reviews of studies have shown that injury severity and mechanism are not consistently associated with mTBI outcomes. Thus the synthesis of findings, and confidence in resulting prognostic models and their applicability to a diverse mTBI population, remain areas of difficulty.

Secondly, evaluating risk for slow recovery after mTBI is complicated by interacting pre-, peri-, and postinjury factors resulting in individual variability; a biopsychosocial model is probably required [46]. Additional prognostic factors such as preinjury neuropsychological functioning, prior history of mental health symptoms, and previous TBI have all been associated with mTBI outcomes and need to be incorporated into prognostic algorithms.

Finally, many patients do not present to an ED promptly enough (or at all) for some tests to be effective, for example, early enough to have detectable levels of serum biomarkers. This risks problematic missing data and difficulties encouraging clinician uptake. Given the complexity of TBI recovery especially over time, prognostic algorithms or signatures may be better targets than an elusive test (e.g., combinations of clinical data, imaging data, serum biomarkers, and other physiological and/or neurocognitive assessment results) [47].

2.8.1 Summary—the importance of being able to predict post-concussion symptoms

Having the ability to determine which individuals may be at risk of developing PCS has implications for both clinical and research practice. PCS has been associated with disability and high utilization of healthcare services [48–52]. As such, it is useful for clinicians to be able to identify those patients that may be at risk of developing the disorder in order to optimize patient outcomes, that is, reduce number of missed days at work/school, and to reduce the overall burden on the healthcare system that is attributed to PCS [53]. Furthermore, the ability to predict which patients will have prolonged symptoms would help clinicians and patients by allowing proper anticipatory guidance, determining the need for academic or occupational accommodations, allowing athletic team members and coaches to plan for the prolonged absence of a player, and allowing patients and their coworkers to prepare for prolonged absences from work [54].

The formulation of clinician-friendly tools that can be easily translated into patient care, can empower healthcare providers to identify those patients that are in need of ongoing monitoring and/or whom could benefit from being prescribed specific pharmaceutical agents for recovery or triage to various other forms of early therapeutic intervention [55]. Furthermore, such tools can also be used to bridge the gap between clinical and research settings. For example, clinicians could use them to direct patients towards clinical trials of new therapies that may prevent or ameliorate the effects of PCS. This is particularly important given that research has found TBI to be linked to several chronic neurodegenerative diseases such as Alzheimer's disease and chronic traumatic encephalopathy [56–60]. Thus being able to predict who is at risk of developing PCS can also help researchers identify potential cohorts of people that can be involved in future studies of therapies that aim to prevent or ameliorate the cognitive impairments that characterize these associated diseases. Moreover, being able to identify which individuals are at risk of developing PCS can help increase the statistical power of randomized controlled trials though risk stratification and covariate adjustment [61,62].

2.8.2 Promising areas of predictive biomarker research

The ApoE genotype is the major apolipoprotein within the CNS synthesized by astrocytes and microglia [63]. It is involved in many intra- and extracellular processes in the CNS and has been proposed to affect cellular maintenance and repair [64]. The gene has three common alleles (e2, e3, and e4), coding for three protein isoforms (designated E2, E3, and E4). The APOE-e4 genotype is known to influence cognitive performance and decline. This is possibly because the least active E4-isoform confers a survival disadvantage to injured neurons [65,66]. A meta-analysis by Zhou et al. [67] reported an association between the presence of the APOE-e4 allele and the risk of poor outcome at 6 months after injury. A study by Müller and colleagues [64] found APOE-e4 to be the sole unique predictor of reduced improvement in neuropsychological performance at 6 months postinjury ($b = 0.08$ (95% CI = 0.03–0.14) $P = .006$) [64,67]. These findings suggested that APOE-e4-negative patients improved twice as much as the APOE-e4-positive patients. It is therefore possible that genetic factors such as ApoE genotype may play a moderating role in recovery following TBI.

Whilst there is a strong theoretical and empirical basis that supports the notion of using neuropsychological measures to evaluate the influence of mTBI on cognition, little is known about the ability of neuropsychological test outcomes alone to *predict* nonrecovery. A recent meta-analysis by Allanson et al. [18] found immediate verbal memory ($r = 0.43$; $P < .001$), delayed verbal memory ($r = 0.43$; $P < .001$), visuospatial construction

$(r = 0.29; P = .001)$, set-shifting $(r = -0.31; P < .001)$, and generativity $(r = 0.44; P < .001)$ to be correlated with a functional measure of disability experienced following moderate to severe TBI. These findings imply that it may be possible to predict the likelihood of an individual developing chronic symptoms after TBI by considering an individual's performance on neuropsychological tests of these particular cognitive domains when measures are obtained shortly after injury. However, it is increasingly understood that other measures of psychomotor test performance such as those involving visuomotor or oculomotor functions may be superior predictors of PCS and further comparative assessments are needed for validation [68].

Investigation into the extent to which magnetic resonance imaging and, in particular, diffusion tensor imaging scalars can predict PCS is also limited. In Mayer et al. [69] found that a model consisting of only diffusion tensor measures had superior classification accuracy (80% for mTBI patients; 70% for healthy controls), relative to that which featured neuropsychological measures (71.4% for mTBI patients; 60% for healthy controls). Fractional anisotropy measures the degree to which diffusion of water is unidirectional and serves as a proxy measure of white matter integrity. Fractional anisotropy values in the right hemisphere $(F_{2,18} = 6.84; P < .01)$ predicted variance in attentional deficits [69], while the severity of white matter lesions present at the acute stage of mTBI injury were related to cognitive impairment in the chronic disease stage [70]. Within a PCS-like context, Messé et al. [71] have reported similar findings using a two-step approach. Mean diffusivity quantifies average molecular motion in all directions, and can change with cellular responses to injury such as edema. Average values from six white matter tracts were able to distinguish between patients classified as poor or good outcome with 69% sensitivity and 77% specificity, respectively, if a patient had a 50% chance of developing PCS, which is not clinically useful.

Several blood-based biomarkers indicative of mechanical injury to cells, glutamate excitotoxicity and calcium ionic imbalance, have been evaluated thus far within the context of severe TBI, with those found to be elevated including calcium binding S100 protein β (S100β) [72,73], myelin basic protein (MBP) [74], glial fibrillary acidic protein (GFAP) [75], NSE [76], ubiquitin carboxy-terminal hydrolase 1 (UCHL 1) [77], Tau isoforms [78], and calpain-derived αII-spectrin N-terminal fragment (SNTF) [79]. Whilst several of these biomarkers have also been investigated in respect to mTBI, a consensus is yet to be reached regarding their utility in predicting PCS, particularly given concerns noted earlier about the proportions of mTBI patients who do not present to health services early enough to access such biomarker testing opportunities.

References

[1] Gardener R, Yaffe K. Males are 1.6 times more likely than females to present to the emergency department with a TBI. Mol Cell Neurosci 2015;66:75–80.

[2] Jager TE, Weiss HB, Coben JH, Pepe PE. Traumatic brain injuries evaluated in US emergency departments, 1992–1994. Acad Emerg Med 2000;7:134–40.

[3] Taylor CA, Bell JM, Breiding MJ, Xu L. Traumatic brain injury–related emergency department visits, hospitalizations, and deaths—United States, 2007 and 2013. MMWR Surveill Summ 2017;66(SS-9):1–16.

[4] Feigin VL, Theadom A, Barker-Collo S, Starkey NJ, McPherson K, Kahan M, et al. Incidence of traumatic brain injury in New Zealand: a population-based study. Lancet Neurol 2013;12(1):53–64.

[5] Traumatic brain injury strategy and action plan 2017–2021 published in September 2017 by ACC.

[6] Helps Y, Harrison J HG. Hospital separations due to traumatic brain injury, Australia 2004–05, in injury research and statistics series number 45. Adelaide: AIHW.; 2008.

[7] Government NSW. Children and infants—acute management of head injury. D.O. Health, editor, 2011.

[8] Australian Government CA. All cancers in Australia [cited 2018 29/10/2018], Available from: <https://canceraustralia.gov.au/affected-cancer/what-cancer/cancer-australia-statistics>.

[9] Access economics: a report to the Victorian Neurotrauma Initiative; 2009.

[10] Pauker SG, Kassirer JP. The threshold approach to clinical decision making. N Engl J Med 1980;302:1109–17. Available from: https://doi.org/10.1056/NEJM198005153022003.

[11] Larson DB, Johnson LW, Schnell BM, et al. National trends in CT use in the emergency department: 1995–2007. Radiology 2011;258:164–73.

[12] Mannix R, O'Brien MJ, Meehan WP. The epidemiology of outpatient visits for minor head injury. Neurosurgery 2013;73:129–34.

[13] Seabury SA, Gaudette É, Goldman DP, Markowitz AJ, Brooks J, McCrea MA, Okonkwo DO, et al. Assessment of follow-up care after emergency department presentation for mild traumatic brain injury and concussion: results from the TRACK-TBI study. JAMA Netw Open 2018;1(1):e180210. Available from: https://doi.org/10.1001/jamanetworkopen.2018.0210.

[14] Faul M, Xu L, Wald MM, et al. Traumatic brain injury in the United States: emergency department visits, hospitalizations and deaths 2002–2006 [Internet]. Centers for Disease Control and Prevention, National Center for Injury Prevention and Control; 2010 [cited 2013 Feb 6] <http://www.cdc.gov/traumaticbraininjury/>.

[15] Jones et al. <https://escholarship.org/uc/item/1630q5bn>.

[16] Jagoda AS, Bazarian JJ, Bruns Jr JJ, et al. Clinical policy: neuroimaging and decision making in adult mild traumatic brain injury in the acute setting. Ann Emerg Med 2008;52(6):714–48.

[17] Koning ME, Scheenen ME, van der Horn HJ, Hageman G, Roks G, Yilmaz T, Spikman JM, et al. Outpatient follow-up after mild traumatic brain injury: Results of the UPFRONT-study. Brain Inj 2017;31(8):1102–8. Available from: https://doi.org/10.1080/02699052.2017.1296193.

[18] Allanson F, Pestell C, Gignac GE, Yeo YX, Weinborn M. Neuropsychological predictors of outcome following traumatic brain injury in adults: a meta-analysis. Neuropsychol Rev 2017;27:187–201. Available from: https://doi.org/10.1007/s11065-017-9353-5.

[19] Bazarian JJ, et al. Epidemiology and predictors of post-concussive syndrome after minor head injury in an emergency population. Brain Inj 1999;13:173–89.

[20] Sheedy J, Geffen G, Donnelly J, Faux S. Emergency department assessment of mild traumatic brain injury and prediction of post-concussion symptoms at one month post injury. J Clin Exp Neuropsychol 2006;28:755–72. Available from: https://doi.org/10.1080/13803390591000864.

[21] Topolovec-Vranic J, et al. The value of serum biomarkers in prediction models of outcome after mild traumatic brain injury. J Trauma 2011;71:S478–86. Available from: https://doi.org/10.1097/TA.0b013e318232fa70.

[22] Health NMO. Adult trauma clinical practice guidelines: initial management of closed head injury in adults; 2011.

[23] Cnossen MC, van der Naalt J, Spikman JM, Nieboer D, Yue JK, Winkler EA, et al. Prediction of persistent post-concussion symptoms after mild traumatic brain injury. J Neurotrauma 2018;35(22):2691–8. Available from: https://doi.org/10.1089/neu.2017.5486.

[24] Faux S, Sheedy J, Delaney R, Riopelle R. Emergency department prediction of post-concussive syndrome following mild traumatic brain injuryan international cross-validation study. Brain Inj 2011;25(1):14–22.

[25] Snell D, Hay-Smith E, Surgenor L, Siegert R. Examination of outcome after mild traumatic brain injury: the contribution of injury beliefs and Leventhal's Common Sense Model. Neuropsychol Rehab Int J 2013;23(3):333–62.

[26] Snell D, Martin R, Surgenor L, Siegert R, Hay-Smith E. What's wrong with me? seeking a coherent understanding of recovery after mild traumatic brain injury. Disabil Rehabil 2017;39(9):1968–75.

[27] Broshek D, De Marco A, Freeman J. A review of post-concussion syndrome and psychological factors associated with concussion. Brain Inj 2015;29(2):228–37.

[28] Ellis MJ, Leddy JJ, Willer B, et al. Physiological, vestibulo-ocular and cervicogenic post-concussion disorders: An evidence-based classification system with directions for treatment. Brain Inj 2015;29(2):238.

Marshall S, Bayley M, McCullagh S, Velikonja D, Berrigan L, Ouchterlon D, et al. Updated clinical practice guidelines for concussion/mild traumatic brain injury and persistent symptoms. Brain Inj 2015;29(6):688.

[29] McCrory P, Meeuwisse WH, Aubry M, Cantu B, Dvořák J, Echemendia RJ, et al. Consensus statement on concussion in sport: the 4th International Conference on Concussion in Sport held in Zurich, November 2012. Br J Sports Med 2013;47(5):250−8.

[30] Leddy J, Baker JG, Haider MN, Hinds A, Willer B. A physiological approach to prolonged recovery from sport-related concussion. J Athl Train. 2017;52(3):299−308.

[31] Snell DL, Martin RM, Macleod AD, Surgenor LJ, Siegert RJ, Hay-Smith EJC, et al. Untangling chronic pain and post-concussion symptoms: the significance of depression. Brain Inj 2018;Feb 1:1−10. Available from: https://doi.org/10.1080/02699052.2018.1432894 [Epub ahead of print]. PMID: 29388838.

[32] Plassman BL, et al. Documented head injury in early adulthood and risk of Alzheimer's disease and other dementias. Neurology 2000;55:1158−66.

[33] Mez J, et al. Clinicopathological evaluation of chronic traumatic encephalopathy in players of American football. JAMA 2017;318:360−70. Available from: https://doi.org/10.1001/jama.2017.8334.

[34] Papa L, Ramia MM, Kelly JM, Burks SS, Pawlowicz A, Berger RP. Systematic review of clinical research on biomarkers for pediatric traumatic brain injury. J Neurotrauma 2013;30(5):324−38.

[35] Goldman J, Becker ML, Jones B, Clements M, Leeder JS. Development of biomarkers to optimize pediatric patient management: what makes children different? Biomark Med 2011;5(6):781−94.

[36] Glushakova AO, et al. Biomarkers for acute diagnosis and management of stroke in neurointensive care units. Brain Circul 2016;2:129−32.

[37] Kövesdi E, Lückl J, Bukovics P, Farkas O, Pál J, Czeiter E, et al. Update on protein biomarkers in traumatic brain injury with emphasis on clinical use in adults and pediatrics. Acta Neurochir 2010;152(1):1−7. Available from: https://doi.org/10.1007/s00701-009-0463-6.

[38] Iverson GL, Gardner AJ, Terry DP, Ponsford JL, Sills AK, Broshek DK, et al. Predictors of clinical recovery from concussion: a systematic review. Br J Sports Med 2017;51(12):941−8. Available from: https://doi.org/10.1136/bjsports-2017-097729.

[39] Kathryn BA, Hoeger MD, MPH KM, Wasserman BA Erin, Bazarian MD, MPH. JJ. Menstrual phase as predictor of outcome after mild traumatic brain injury in womenWunderle. J Head Trauma Rehab 2014;29(5):E1−8. Available from: https://doi.org/10.1097/HTR.0000000000000006.

[40] Davis-Hayes C, Gossett JD, Levine WN, Shams T, Harada J, Mitnick J, et al. Sex-specific outcomes and predictors of concussion recovery. J Am Acad Orthop Surg 2017;25(12):818−28. Available from: https://doi.org/10.5435/JAAOS-D-17-00276.

[41] Jean-Pierre D, Andrew J, Anderson Stewart A, Hossein A, Shenoy Vivek B, Smith Douglas H. Newfound sex differences in axonal structure underlie differential outcomes from in vitro traumatic axonal injury. Exp Neurol 2018;300:121−34.

[42] King N. Literature review mild head injury: neuropathology, sequelae, measurement and recovery. Br J Clin Psychol 1997;36(2):161−84. Available from: https://doi.org/10.1111/j.2044-8260.1997.tb01405.x.

[43] King NS. Post-concussion syndrome: clarity amid the controversy? Br J Psychiatry 2003;183(04):276−8. Available from: https://doi.org/10.1192/bjp.183.4.27.

[44] Strathmann FG, Schulte S, Goerl K, Petron DJ. Blood-based biomarkers for traumatic brain injury: evaluation of research approaches, available methods and potential utility from the clinician and clinical laboratory perspectives. Clin Biochem 2014;47(10−11):876−88.

[45] Silverberg ND, Gardner AJ, Brubacher JR, Panenka WJ, Li JJ, Iverson GL. Systematic review of multivariable prognostic models for mild traumatic brain injury. J Neurotrauma 2015;32(8):517−26. Available from: https://doi.org/10.1089/neu.2014.3600. Epub 2015 Jan 13.

[46] Iverson GL, Silverberg ND, Lange RT, Zasler ND. Conceptualizing outcome from mild traumatic brain injury. In: Zasler ND, Katz DI, Zafonre RD, editors. Brain injury medicine: principles and practice. 2nd ed New York: Demos Medical Publishing; 2012.

[47] Jeter CB, et al. Biomarkers for the diagnosis and prognosis of mild traumatic brain injury/concussion. J Neurotrauma 2013;30:657−70.

[48] Kirsch NL, de Leon MB, Maio RF, Millis SR, Tan-Schriner CU, Frederiksen S. Characteristics of a mild head injury subgroup with extreme, persisting distress on the rivermead postconcussion symptoms questionnaire. Arch Phys Med Rehab 2010;91(1):35−42. Available from: https://doi.org/10.1016/J.APMR.2009.09.019.

[49] Kristman VL, Borg J, Godbolt AK, Salmi LR, Cancelliere C, Carroll LJ, et al. Methodological issues and research recommendations for prognosis after mild traumatic brain injury: results of the International Collaboration on Mild Traumatic Brain Injury Prognosis. Arch Phys Med Rehab 2014;95(3):S265−77.

[50] Lundin A, de Boussard C, Edman G, Borg J. Symptoms and disability until 3 months after mild TBI. Brain Inj 2006;20(8):799–806. Available from: https://doi.org/10.1080/02699050600744327.

[51] Wojcik SM. Predicting mild traumatic brain injury patients at risk of persistent symptoms in the emergency department. Brain Inj 2014;28(4):422–30.

[52] Yang C-C, Hua M-S, Tu Y-K, Huang S-J. Early clinical characteristics of patients with persistent post-concussion symptoms: a prospective study. Brain Inj 2009;23(4):299–306. Available from: https://doi.org/10.1080/02699050902788543.

[53] Ganti L, Khalid H, Patel PS, Daneshvar Y, Bodhit AN, Peters KR. Who gets post-concussion syndrome? An emergency department-based prospective analysis. Int J Emerg Med 2014;7(1):31.

[54] Meehan III WP, Mannix RC, Stracciolini A, Elbin RJ, Collins MW. Symptom severity predicts prolonged recovery after sport-related concussion, but age and amnesia do not. J Pediatric 2013;163(3):721–5.

[55] Lau B, Lovell MR, Collins MW, Pardini J. Neurocognitive and symptom predictors of recovery in high school athletes. Clin J Sport Med 2009;19(3):216–21.

[56] Graves AB, White E, Koepsell TD, Reifler BV, Van Belle G, Larson EB, et al. The association between head trauma and Alzheimer's disease. Am J Epidemiol 1990;131(3):491–501.
Guskiewicz KM, Marshall SW, Bailes J, McCrea M, Cantu RC, Randolph C, et al. Association between recurrent concussion and late-life cognitive impairment in retired professional football players. Neurosurgery 2005;57(4):719–26 Mayeux et al., 1995.

[57] Baugh CM, Stamm JM, Riley DO, Gavett BE, Shenton ME, Lin A, et al. Chronic traumatic encephalopathy: neurodegeneration following repetitive concussive and subconcussive brain trauma. Brain Imag Behav 2012;6(2):244–54. Available from: https://doi.org/10.1007/s11682-012-9164-5.

[58] McKee AC, Cantu RC, Nowinski CJ, Hedley-Whyte ET, Gavett BE, Budson AE, et al. Chronic traumatic encephalopathy in athletes: progressive tauopathy after repetitive head injury. J Neuropathol Exp Neurol 2009;68(7):709–35. Available from: https://doi.org/10.1097/NEN.0b013e3181a9d503.

[59] Omalu BI, DeKosky ST, Minster RL, Kamboh MI, Hamilton RL, Wecht CH. Chronic traumatic encephalopathy in a national football league player. Neurosurgery 2005;57(1):128–34. Available from: https://doi.org/10.1227/01.NEU.0000163407.92769.ED.

[60] Stern RA, Riley DO, Daneshvar DH, Nowinski CJ, Cantu RC, McKee AC. Long-term consequences of repetitive brain trauma: chronic traumatic encephalopathy. PM&R 2011;3(10):S460–7. Available from: https://doi.org/10.1016/J.PMRJ.2011.08.008.

[61] Kahan BC, Jairath V, Doré CJ, Morris TP. The risks and rewards of covariate adjustment in randomized trials: an assessment of 12 outcomes from 8 studies. Trials 2014;15(1):139. Available from: https://doi.org/10.1186/1745-6215-15-139.

[62] Steyerberg EW, Mushkudiani N, Perel P, Butcher I, Lu J, McHugh GS, et al. Predicting outcome after traumatic brain injury: development and international validation of prognostic scores based on admission characteristics. PLoS Med 2008;5(8):e165. Available from: https://doi.org/10.1371/journal.pmed.0050165.

[63] Pitas RE, Boyles JK, Lee SH, Foss D, Mahley RW. Astrocytes synthesize apolipoprotein E and metabolize apolipoprotein E-containing lipoproteins. Biochim Biophys Acta—Lipids Lipid Metab 1987;917(1):148–61. Available from: https://doi.org/10.1016/0005-2760(87)90295-5.

[64] Müller K, Ingebrigtsen T, Wilsgaard T, Wikran G, Fagerheim T, Romner B, et al. Prediction of time trends in recovery of cognitive function after mild head injury. Neurosurgery 2009;64(4):698–704. Available from: https://doi.org/10.1227/01.NEU.0000340978.42892.78.

[65] Ferguson SC, Deary IJ, Evans JC, Ellard S, Hattersley AT, Frier BM. Apolipoprotein-E influences aspects of intellectual ability in type 1 diabetes. Diabetes 2003;52(1):145–8. Available from: https://doi.org/10.2337/diabetes.52.1.145.

[66] MacLullich AMJ, Seckl JR, Starr JM, Deary IJ. The biology of intelligence: from association to mechanism. Intelligence 1998;26(2):63–73. Available from: https://doi.org/10.1016/S0160-2896(99)80053-1.

[67] Zhou W, Xu DI, Peng X, Zhang Q, Jia J, Crutcher KA. Meta-analysis of APOE4 allele and outcome after traumatic brain injury. J Neurotrauma 2008;25:279–90. Available from: https://doi.org/10.1089/neu.2007.0489.

[68] Heitger MH, Jones RD, Dalrymple-Alford JC, Frampton CM, Ardagh MW, Anderson TJ. Mild head injury—a close relationship between motor function at 1 week post-injury and overall recovery at 3 and 6 months. J Neurol Sci 2007;253(1–2):34–47.

[69] Mayer AR, Ling J, Mannell MV, Gasparovic C, Phillips JP, Doezema D, et al. A prospective diffusion tensor imaging study in mild traumatic brain injury. Neurology 2010;74(8):643—50. Available from: https://doi.org/10.1212/WNL.0B013E3181D0CCDD.

[70] Matsushita M, Hosoda K, Naitoh Y, Yamashita H, Kohmura E. Utility of diffusion tensor imaging in the acute stage of mild to moderate traumatic brain injury for detecting white matter lesions and predicting long-term cognitive function in adults. J Neurosurg 2011;115(1):130—9. Available from: https://doi.org/10.3171/2011.2.JNS101547.

[71] Messé A, Caplain S, Paradot G, Garrigue D, Mineo J-F, Soto Ares G, et al. Diffusion tensor imaging and white matter lesions at the subacute stage in mild traumatic brain injury with persistent neurobehavioral impairment. Hum Brain Mapp 2011;32(6):999—1011. Available from: https://doi.org/10.1002/hbm.21092.

[72] de Kruijk JR, Leffers P, Menheere PPCA, Meerhoff S, Rutten J, Rwijnstra A. Prediction of post-traumatic complaints after mild traumatic brain injury: early symptoms and biochemical markers. J Neurol Neurosug Psychiat 2002;73(6):727—32. Available from: https://doi.org/10.1136/jnnp.73.6.727.

[73] Zetterberg H, Blennow K. Fluid markers of traumatic brain injury. Mol Cell Neurosci 2015;66(Pt B):99—102. Available from: https://doi.org/10.1016/j.mcn.2015.02.003.

[74] Yamazaki Y, Yada K, Morii S, Kitahara T, Ohwada T. Diagnostic significance of serum neuron-specific enolase and myelin basic protein assay in patients with acute head injury. Surg Neurol 1995;43(3):267—70 discussion 270-261.

[75] Lucke-Wold BP, Turner RC, Logsdon AF, Bailes JE, Huber JD, Rosen CL. Linking traumatic brain injury to chronic traumatic encephalopathy: identification of potential mechanisms leading to neurofibrillary tangle development. J Neurotrauma 2014;31(13):1129—38. Available from: https://doi.org/10.1089/neu.2013.3303.

[76] Ross SA, Cunningham RT, Johnston CF, Rowlands BJ. Neuron-specific enolase as an aid to outcome prediction in head injury. Br J Neurosurg 1996;10(5):471—6.

[77] Papa L, Akinyi L, Liu MC, Pineda JA, Tepas III. JJ, Oli MW, et al. Ubiquitin C-terminal hydrolase is a novel biomarker in humans for severe traumatic brain injury. Crit Care Med 2010;38(1):138—44. Available from: https://doi.org/10.1097/CCM.0b013e3181b788ab.

[78] Ost M, Nylen K, Csajbok L, Ohrfelt AO, Tullberg M, Wikkelso C, et al. Initial CSF total tau correlates with 1-year outcome in patients with traumatic brain injury. Neurology 2006;67(9):1600—4. Available from: https://doi.org/10.1212/01.wnl.0000242732.06714.0f.

[79] Siman R, Shahim P, Tegner Y, Blennow K, Zetterberg H, Smith DH. Serum SNTF increases in concussed professional ice hockey players and relates to the severity of postconcussion symptoms. J Neurotrauma 2015;32(17):1294—300. Available from: https://doi.org/10.1089/neu.2014.3698.

Regulatory considerations for diagnostics and biomarkers of traumatic brain injury

Lakshman Ramamurthy

DxDevice Strategies LLC (formerly CDRH, USFDA), Rockville, MD, United States

3.1 Background

The US Food and Drug Administration (FDA) recently marked the passing of over four decades following the establishment of the medical device amendments to the Food Drug & Cosmetic Act (FDCA).[1] The Medical Device Amendment (MDA) of 1976 established a risk-based classification system that categorizes all medical devices including diagnostics into three classes according to their complexity and the degree of risk posed to patients. The original law established several key postmarket requirements: registration of establishments and listing of devices with the FDA, Good Manufacturing Practices (GMPs), and reporting of adverse events involving medical devices. In 2016 the 40-year anniversary coincided with the passage of the 21st Century Cures Act[2] that demonstrates a continually evolving[3] regulatory framework, including expanded application of the "least burdensome" provisions to encourage innovation, codifying the designation of breakthrough device, allowing for priority reviews and streamlining processes for exempting devices from premarket notification, or expediting the review of medical devices through the introduction of new pilot programs.

---

[1] https://www.govinfo.gov/content/pkg/STATUTE-90/pdf/STATUTE-90-Pg539.pdf

[2] https://www.congress.gov/bill/114th-congress/house-bill/34/text

[3] https://www.fda.gov/medical-devices/overview-device-regulation/history-medical-device-regulation-oversight-united-states

3.2 Risk-based classification of medical devices

3.2.1 Class I—Low-risk devices

Class I medical devices are those products deemed to be low-risk, and while they must be registered with FDA, they are not required to undergo premarket review and as such are subject to the least amount of regulatory control. Devices on the class I exemption list include enzyme controls, tonometers, stethoscopes, irrigating dental syringes, finger cots, protective restraints for patients and general controls and reagents used in various diagnostic tests. The Agency continually reviews the list based on whether they are still actively marketed and if the risk posed to the patients have shown to be reduced, and as recently as 2016, an additional 70 devices were added to the Class I exempt list.

3.2.2 Class II—Moderate-risk devices—premarket notification—510(k) program

Most medical devices and diagnostics fall in the Class II category, and manufacturers of such devices are required to notify the FDA prior to marketing those devices via a 510(k) submission (premarket notification [PMN]). More than 80% of devices are reviewed through this pathway. The 510(k) application requires the manufacturer to demonstrate that its device is "substantially equivalent" in terms of its intended use, safety, and effectiveness to an already legally marketed "predicate" medical device in the United States. There are different kinds of 510(k) submissions, and these are categorized as Traditional, Special, and Abbreviated 510(k)s. The user fees are the same for all three different types of submissions, but the review time and the data requirement vary for each of them. The majority of device manufacturers would file a traditional 510(k) while the other two categories are allowed under specific conditions. A manufacturer should use the guidance[4] provided by the FDA in determining if the device is eligible to be reviewed as a traditional 510(k) submission. While the basic content requirements apply to all 510(k)s, the type of data and information necessary to establish substantial equivalence varies by the type of device and the differences between the new device and the predicate device. The FDA review time for a traditional 510(k) is 90 days. This time can extend beyond that based on if the agency requests additional information as part of its review and the time taken by the manufacturer to respond to such information requests. The FDA regularly issues many device-specific guidance documents[5] that clarify the type of data that should be included in 510(k)s for particular device types. When a manufacturer is unsure of what information to include within a 510(k) submission, the manufacturer may contact the FDA and submit a presubmission request to seek additional feedback, including study design, statistical plan, etc., to ensure that their regulatory application contains the appropriate data elements. Generally speaking, the 510(k) paradigm and evidentiary threshold has evolved and continually changed over the years and has been the subject of much debate and peer

[4] https://www.fda.gov/media/82395/download

[5] https://www.fda.gov/medical-devices/device-advice-comprehensive-regulatory-assistance/guidance-documents-medical-devices-and-radiation-emitting-products

review, including one by the Institute of Medicine on whether this regulatory framework is sufficient to ensure safety and and effectiveness ensuring public health.[6] Some policy makers and patients have expressed concern about the ability of the 510(k) process to ensure that medical devices on the market are safe and effective. Other policy makers and patients, as well as the medical device industry, have asserted that the process has become too burdensome and time-consuming and that it is delaying important new innovations from entering the market. The following sections will discuss the various types of 510(k) submissions.

3.2.3 Special 510(k)

The Special 510(k) Program, is typically submitted in response to an iterative change in a previously cleared device, and was limited to the review of changes that did not alter or affect the device's intended use nor alter the device's fundamental scientific technology. Under this approach, Special 510(k)s that included modifications to the indications for use or any labeling change that affected the device's intended use and/or modifications that had the potential to alter the fundamental scientific technology of the device compared to the manufacturer's own legally marketed predicate device were routinely converted to Traditional 510(k)s. However, by virtue of a new guidance issued in September 2019,[7] the FDA claims to be attempting to improve the efficiency of 510(k) reviews and has issued a new pilot program for all devices submitted after October 2018 that will allow certain changes to the indications for use that may be made. Through publication of this guidance document, the FDA has also clarified the types of changes to technological characteristics that are appropriate for review as a Special 510(k). For certain device changes, the FDA has concluded that design control procedures can produce reliable results that can form the basis for a substantially equivalent (SE) determination without compromising the statutory and regulatory criteria for SE. For instance, if a manufacturer modifies an in vitro diagnostic (IVD), the manufacturer's design inputs should include any relevant clinical and laboratory standards recognized by FDA. This may reduce the time and resource required to generate analytical and clinical data when an iterative improvement is made on the device. This has a significant impact as the review time for a Special 510(k)[8] is only 30 days and is expected to shorten the time to market for a device. While this does provide a time-efficient pathway for market authorization, the sponsor should carefully consider if their device is eligible for the Special 510 (k) pathway as per the new guidance and gain concurrence with the agency ahead of time as the conversion of a Special 510(k) to a Traditional 510(k) may cause added delay to the overall review of the device, and require the generation of new reports containing analytical and clinical data.

[6] http://www.nationalacademies.org/hmd/Reports/2011/Medical-Devices-and-the-Publics-Health-The-FDA-510k-Clearance-Process-at-35-Years.aspx

[7] https://www.fda.gov/media/116418/download

[8] https://www.fda.gov/media/132151/download

3.2.4 Abbreviated 510(k)

Another type of 510(k) submission allows the sponsor to provide the rationale that its review can rely on an FDA guidance document(s) or is subject to special controls published by the FDA. If found valid, the manufacturer may be eligible for an abbreviated 510 (k) and would have to simply provide a summary report that describes how the guidance (s) was used to demonstrate substantial equivalence and/or how the device complies with the special control(s). These reports will be expected to summarize the device description, the manufacturer's device design requirements, risk management information, and a description of test methods used to address performance characteristics. If a sponsor is not sure if their device is eligible for this pathway, they may request a brief meeting or teleconference with the agency and discuss if the reliance on a special control is sufficient for clearance of the iterative improvement of their device.

3.2.5 Class III—High-risk devices—premarket approval

Class III is reserved for devices deemed high risk and they are subject to a premarket approval application (PMA) process, like that for new drugs. By statute, under Section 515 of the FDCA, the PMA process is reserved for medical devices that "support or sustain human life, are of substantial importance in preventing impairment of human health, or which present a potential, unreasonable risk of illness or injury." They represent about 10% of all the medical devices regulated by the FDA, in contrast to 43% that are classified as Class II moderate risk. Examples of high-risk devices include implantable pacemakers and breast implants, and almost all companion diagnostics that may direct pharmaceutical patient treatment are also categorized as Class III.

PMA is the most involved process that a medical device manufacturer typically pursues. The FDA's PMA process is typically long and expensive. Manufacturers are usually required to undertake randomized controlled clinical trials that can cost millions of dollars and require years to complete.[9] In addition, the FDA charges manufacturers a "user fee" of over $320,000 to review a PMA application.[10] PMA application is expected to have several key administrative elements, but good science and scientific writing is a key to the approval of PMA application. The FDA will refuse to file a PMA application and will not proceed with the in-depth review of scientific and clinical data if it lacks the key administrative elements. If a PMA application lacks valid clinical information and scientific analysis on sound scientific reasoning, it could impact the FDA's review and approval. PMA applications that are incomplete, inaccurate, inconsistent, omit critical information, and/or poorly organized have resulted in delays in approval or denial of those applications. Manufacturers typically perform a quality control audit of a PMA application before sending it to the FDA to assure that it is scientifically sound and presented in a well-organized format. The review of a PMA by the FDA will comprise a cross-disciplinary team including a lead reviewer, statistician, medical officer, software reviewer (if the device contains

[9] CDG White Paper, Keeping study costs under control, http://clinicaldevice.typepad.com/ cdg_whitepapers/budgets-costs/; August 5, 2010

[10] https://www.fda.gov/industry/fda-user-fee-programs/medical-device-user-fee-amendments-mdufa

TABLE 3.1   Comparison of 510(k), de novo, and premarket approval.

Requirements	510(k)	De Novo	Premarket approval
Regulatory standard	Substantial equivalence to a legally marketed predicate	Safety & efficacy (no predicate)	Safety & efficacy, high-risk device
Examples	Most devices, diagnostics	Novel devices	Implantables, companion diagnostics and novel devices
Clinical study design	Clinical study seldom required	Clinical study often required	Large randomized control trials
Special controls or guidance	No; guidance for Abbreviated 510(k)	Yes	No
User fees	~ $10,000	~ $96,000	~ $320,000
Statutory review time frame	90 days; 30 days for Special 510(k)	150 days	180 days

software components), and a reviewer that will ascertain if the device follows GMP. When a manufacturer submits a PMA, it will often trigger a premarket inspection by FDA auditors to certify whether the manufacturer's processes comply with the requirements of Quality System Regulation (QSR) as described in the Code of Federal Regulations 21 CFR Part 820. Such GMP audits will lead to findings that may result in either no actions, voluntary actions, or official actions indicated.[11] The latter means significant violations or discrepancies have been noted that have to be addressed before the PMA can proceed or be favorably reviewed. The experts from the FDA and other industry bodies, including the Regulatory Affairs Professional Society (RAPS), hold workshops to educate and inform new manufacturers on the Quality System audit procedures. Since most PMAs require clinical studies to be performed, the agency will also often perform a bioresearch monitoring (BIMO) audit where the agency's inspectors will audit the clinical sites or the manufacturing sites to ensure that records accurately reflect how the studies were conducted, ensure data integrity, and that no results were mistakenly obtained or manipulated to support the PMA. Poorly kept records, evidence or suspicion of data manipulation can lead to delays in review and, in extreme circumstances, place a manufacturer on a data integrity hold. This is indicative of the high evidentiary bar and costs associated with the requirement of a PMA for a device. Manufacturers are often very discouraged to learn that their device is classified as high-risk and requires a PMA, which can be associated with a high-risk or a novel device with no legally cleared predicate. The FDA has been sensitive to this perceived obstacle to innovation and in response to industry feedback has aggressively pursued making alternatives like the 510(k) and de novo regulatory pathways more accessible for novel devices, as evidenced in the recent devices cleared for traumatic brain injury (TBI). Table 3.1 below lists the standard regulatory pathways for Class II and III products and the alternative de novo pathway.

[11] https://www.fda.gov/media/94076/download

TABLE 3.2   Requirements for the humanitarian device exemption pathway.

Requirements	Humanitarian device exemption
Standard	Safety & probable benefit
Population	<8000 patients per year
Clinical study design	Clinical study often useful but not absolutely required
IRB approval after market	Yes
Selling price	Limited profit allowed
Statutory review time frame	75 days

3.3 Non-standard regulatory pathways

3.3.1 Humanitarian use devices for rare disorders

In the case of rare diseases, where only a few patients are afflicted, the collection of clinical evidence can be challenging. To serve such patients, and to encourage sponsors to innovate in these clinically unmet areas the FDA, via the Orphan Drug Act of 1984, has provided the humanitarian device exemption (HDE) pathway.[12] This pathway is accessible for interventions for diseases afflicting fewer than 200,000 patients in the United States. There are specific prohibitions on profit-making with the initial HDE approval, but if sponsors can provide sufficient rationale, they may be able to submit a supplement that will allow them to maintain humanitarian use device (HUD) status while generating a profit. More recently, the 21st Century Cures Act (Pub. L. No. 114–255) broadens the HUD/HDE program by increasing the population estimate requirement from "fewer than 4000" to "not more than 8000." This increase should hopefully allow the HUD/HDE pathway to facilitate a greater number of devices to market for the treatment or diagnosis of rare diseases or conditions. The HUD/HDE pathway has been used by manufacturers due to the fact that clinical trials for HDE devices were relatively small compared to those for PMA devices; most were open-label, single-arm trials. This is also a pathway that allows manufacturers to bring a device to market early while they generate more data for a broader regulatory authorization. Table 3.2 lists the elements of HDE regulatory pathway.

3.3.2 De novo 510(k)

CDRH's de novo process provides a pathway for a new medical device for which there is no legally marketed predicate device. This is particularly beneficial to a manufacturer who has a novel innovative device that can be classified as moderate risk but there are no devices available to which they can demonstrate substantial equivalence. Such a device is first automatically classified in Class III, and then reclassified as a Class II with an

---

[12] https://pdfs.semanticscholar.org/3316/14ef8ffa1d46d14c0c97bb83bb70447ad720.pdf

accompanying special controls guidance document. The granting of de novo status for a medical device is a step-by-step process. According to the FDA there are two options for how a manufacturer can go about obtaining a de novo designation.

- Option 1: After receiving a high-level not SE (NSE) determination (that is, no predicate, new intended use, or different technological characteristics that raise different questions of safety and effectiveness) in response to a 510(k) submission.
- Option 2: Upon the requester's determination that there is no legally marketed device upon which to base a determination of substantial equivalence (therefore without first submitting a 510(k) and receiving a high-level NSE determination).

The current lack of a de novo-specific regulation puts the de novo program at somewhat of a disadvantage compared to the 510(k) and PMA review pathways, therefore the CDRH has been actively working with Congress in proposing a new rule to address this issue. According to the FDA, if the manufacturer demonstrates that the relevant criteria of the FD&C Act are met, the agency will grant the de novo request, in which case the specific device and device type is classified in class I or class II. The granting of the de novo request allows the device to be marketed immediately, creating a classification regulation for devices of this type, and permits the device to serve as a predicate device for future iterations of a similar application. Once classified, the FDA subsequently will publish a notice in the Federal Register announcing the classification and the controls necessary to provide reasonable assurance of safety and effectiveness.

The first examples of a software-based and biomarker-based tests for TBI were both authorized through the de novo process as no legally marketed predicates were available. The FDA reviewed the Banyan BTI IVD chemiluminescent enzyme-linked immunosorbent assay (ELISA) initially as a de novo device, and classified it as a Class II device under the generic name "brain trauma assessment test," creating a new product code QAT and requiring special controls. The impact of this classification is such that future devices, with similar intended use and technological properties, may now be automatically classified as Class II devices as long as they demonstrate substantial equivalence to the Banyan BTI predicate and meet the requirements of the special controls' guidance accompanying this classification. We will study these cases in more detail as we explore this topic further later in this chapter.

3.3.3 Use of real-world data in device clearance/approvals—a new initiative

Although clinical trials represent the most rigorous approach to PMA, manufacturers sometimes have difficulty recruiting patients to participate in clinical trials due to the potential risks and uncertainty about whether those who participate will actually receive the treatment or device in question. The latest user fee authorization, FDA Reauthorization Act of 2017 (FDARA),[13] therefore has codified the use of real-world evidence (RWE) as an alternative to randomized controlled trials and requires that priority be given to "devices and device types for which the collection and analysis of RWE regarding a device's safety and effectiveness is likely to advance public health." Additionally, the new law also states

[13] https://www.congress.gov/bill/115th-congress/house-bill/2430/text

that the FDA review process considers the use of "...electronic health data including claims data, patient survey data, or any other data..." as deemed appropriate. This continual evolution of the regulatory agency is intended to cope with and support technological advancements in medical devices and diagnostics and to aid speedier access of these devices to patients.

As a direct result of the passage of the 21st Century Cures Act in 2016, and in incorporating the RWE framework, the FDA has been actively participating in a multistakeholder partnership that includes public and private entities in the creation of National Evaluation System for Health Technology (NEST). The stated mission of this partnership is to accelerate the development and translation of new and safe health technologies leveraging real-world data (RWD). RWD/RWE includes a variety of sources of data, such as electronic health records, claims, billing data, pharmacy data, wearables, and mobile technology. The claims and billing data is expected to contain outcome data, which allows one to study the clinical impact of the device intervention. The founding NEST network collaborators include over 195 hospitals and 3942 outpatient clinics across the United States who will coordinate to improve evidence generation for medical devices to inform decisions across the total product life cycle, including marketing authorization, postmarket surveillance, payer coverage and reimbursement, clinical practice, and patient choice.

In this first expansive collaborative effort, the test cases, selected after a thorough review process from topics proposed by the medical device industry, are designed to explore the feasibility of generating RWE in preparation for regulatory submissions. These medical devices will span disease areas from cardiology, to vascular, orthopedic, surgical, and dermatological areas. The technologies include both lower-risk devices designated through the 510(k) pathway and higher-risk devices requiring a PMA. According to FDA, seven of the studies will use retrospective data already collected by the health systems, whereas one will require prospective data collection.[14] An important by-product is that while there are significant opportunities for increasing the quality and quantity of evidence for medical devices using RWD, concerns about the study validity when using RWD/RWE is intended to appropriately focus on two areas: the quality of the source data and the appropriateness of the analysis methods. The taskforce under the aegis of this partnership will generate methods, and lessons learnt that can be applicable to future regulatory review of medical devices. The advent of such methods coincides with our ability to generate massive amounts of clinical use data and our ability to store, modify, and analyze such data, as long as considerations are taken to protect patient-specific private information.

3.3.4 Oversight of laboratory developed tests

No discussion of device and diagnostic regulation can be complete without tracing the backstory on LDT regulation and how it continues to evolve. Historically, the FDA did not intend to regulate all diagnostic devices similarly. In fact, acceding to the need of certain diagnostic tests to address emergent conditions in local communities, the agency traditionally allowed local enforcement of such tests and assays. These were often referred to as "home-brew" tests and were typically developed in community or hospital laboratories

[14] https://ascpt.onlinelibrary.wiley.com/doi/full/10.1002/cpt.1380

under the direction of or reviewed by an experienced pathologist or laboratory director. The rationale behind the FDA ceding control was mainly that these "laboratory-developed tests" had reduced exposure and the risk was localized, manageable, and therefore mitigated. However, over the years, as the laboratory industry expanded and the advent of the internet revolution shrunk the world allowing for greater access to markets, major test manufacturers and reference laboratories continued to use the LDT provision to reach a larger public than originally perceived by the FDA as manageable or risk-mitigated. The agency fears the public health danger posed by what it has termed "problematic LDTs."[15] Importantly, the LDT enforcement discretion and the non-level playing field incentivized hospital and reference laboratories to avoid the expensive processes required to get a 510 (k) or PMA approval and has encouraged an alternative marketing pathway. Separately, Clinical Laboratory Improvement Amendments Act (CLIA) is administered by CMS, which sets the standards for operation of the laboratories that use LDTs as well as FDA-approved tests. This has led to much confusion and this came to a head in the marketing of direct-to-consumer genetic tests, from manufacturers like 23andMe and others. In 2010 the FDA, recognizing that the complexity of these LDTs was increasing, announced that the agency was developing a guidance to actively regulate LDTs under a risk-based framework.[16]

The guidance intended to inform industry as to how LDTs would be regulated by the FDA and the requirements necessary to ensure patient safety. In response to criticism from laboratories that the tests already complied with existing CLIA regulations, the agency asserted that accuracy and validity demonstration are outside the realm of CLIA regulation. In addition, the FDA stated that they wanted to ensure that the accuracy and clinical validity of LDTs were established before they were used in clinical decision-making. A draft guidance was sent to the Office of Management and Budget (OMB) by the FDA where it sat for several years with no clear data on when it was to be released. In the summer of 2013 at the American Society of Clinical Oncology, the FDA Commissioner Margaret Hamburg, expressed concerns that, "...LDT's have become more sophisticated and complex. Results from these tests are rapidly becoming a staple of medical decision-making..." and the FDA "...is working to make sure that the accuracy and clinical validity of high-risks tests are established before they come to market."[17]

Soon after, on July 2, 2014, five US senators jointly wrote a letter to the OMB asking the Office to release the FDA guidance on LDTs for public comment and feedback. In this letter, they stated that "...for years this draft guidance has languished at OMB causing continued unpredictability and uncertainty for industry, clinicians, patients and the general public." They further stated, "...Because these more advanced LDTs are a staple of clinical decision-making and are being used to diagnose, high-risk, and relatively common

---

[15] https://www.fda.gov/media/102367/download

[16] Food and Drug Administration. FDA/CDRH public meeting: oversight of Laboratory Developed Tests (LDTs), http://www.fda.gov/medicaldevices/newsevents/workshopsconferences/ucm212830.htm; 2010.

[17] Turna R. After long silence on LDT regulation, FDA commish revives thorny topic at ASCO. GenomeWeb, http://www.genomeweb.com/after-long-silence-ldt-regulation-fda-commish-revives-thorny-topicasco; 2013.

disease, it is imperative that they perform as they are expected. Incorrect results mean that patients either will not seek out the care and therapy that is needed or will be subject to treatments that do not work or are harmful."[18] This continues to be an evolving framework and most recently Commissioner Scott Gottlieb was quoted at a major conference saying, "This is now a mature industry. This is not an industry where FDA can continue to just exercise enforcement discretion because it's a mom-and-pop industry and it's a bunch of small operators. This is a vast industry and we are not going to be able to step away from it in the long run. I think the right way to approach is through legislation."[19] His comment was soon followed by the introduction in Congress of the "Verifying Accurate Leading-edge IVCT Development Act" (VALID) act in December 2018 where IVCT refers to in vitro clinical tests, and, recognizing the growing divergence between the two, defines a broader category that includes IVDs and LDTs.[20] According to the summary of the bill, introduced in December 2018, "...the draft legislation would establish a risk-based approach to IVCT regulation, prioritizing FDA resources for the highest-risk tests that expose patients to serious or irreversible harm. The legislation also would establish a precertification program for lower-risk tests that are not otherwise required to go through premarket review. High-risk tests, such as novel tests, would be required to undergo premarket review to verify analytical and clinical validity. FDA could require that any test undergo premarket review after providing the developer an opportunity to address issues identified by the agency." The FDA has welcomed this legislative measure and has commented favorably on this approach stating, "The current paradigm for clinical testing leads to questions about the accuracy and reliability of certain diagnostic tests. The disparity can create disincentives for manufacturers to invest in the development of innovative tests that meet FDA's standard of evidence for clinical validity when they have to compete with LDTs that aren't being FDA-reviewed. It inhibits coverage decisions by payors. It's generating increasing uncertainty in the marketplace. And ultimately, it could limit patient access to effective treatments."[21] While various public agencies and private payers may come to their decisions independently, in a value-based environment, it is becoming increasingly evident that robust evidence of a test's performance and the claims made in the label are critical to ensure therapeutic validity and quality patient care.

3.4 Evolving European regulatory framework

While we have been discussing the FDA's premarket review and risk-based classification, particularly Class II and III devices, and how they have been constantly evolving

[18] Senator Ed Markey, Letter to Office of Management and Budget, http://www.markey.senate.gov/imo/media/doc/2014-07-02_Deese_LDTs.pdf; July 2, 2014

[19] https://medcitynews.com/2017/09/fdas-scott-gottlieb-ldts-no-longer-mom-pop-industry-need-legislative-approach/

[20] https://www.360dx.com/sites/default/files/valid_act_discussion_draft_12.6.18.pdf

[21] https://www.fda.gov/news-events/fda-voices-perspectives-fda-leadership-and-experts/fda-proposes-new-steps-advance-clinical-testing-deliver-new-cures

over these four decades, they vary sharply from the prevailing European requirements for diagnostics and medical devices. The current European regulatory framework for diagnostic devices is enshrined in the IVD Medical Devices Directive (IVDD) 98/79/EC which was published in 1998 and has since been the governing document for companies seeking to market diagnostic devices in the European Economic Area. The directives require that manufacturers meet specific international standards, demonstrate conformity with those standards, perform technical evaluations and assemble the results in a dossier, and optionally send this package to an authorized notifying body (NB), which then enables the manufacturer to affix a Conformité Européene (CE) mark on the product prior to marketing. As part of this regulatory regime, there are two methods for market entry: self-certification (about 80% of products) or NB approval (about 20% of products). Products subject to NB approval are limited to a series of specific products identified under Annex II, Lists A and B, and largely encompass diagnostic products that are used in blood banking, devices for self-testing, and certain infectious diseases. It is worth noting that CE marking is only obligatory for products for which EU specifications exist and require the affixing of CE marking.

However, in 2017, the European parliament and the Council of the European Union decided to do away with IVDD and resolved to implement new regulations for medical devices and IVDs declaring[22] that, "Directive 98/79/EC of the European Parliament and of the Council constitutes the Union regulatory framework for IVD medical devices. However, a fundamental revision of that Directive is needed to establish a robust, transparent, predictable and sustainable regulatory framework for IVD medical devices which ensures a high level of safety and health whilst supporting innovation." And thus the Council of the EU, representing 27 member states in Europe, jointly agreed to introduce IVD Regulations (IVDR) which will be fully implemented in 2022, and has the following key elements:

(1) Classification system: the IVDR introduces a risk-based classification system for IVDs quite like the US FDA. IVDs will now be classified into four different classes based on risk from class A (low) to class D (high). This will mean that regulation and assessment for each class of device can be tailored accordingly. (2) Changes to conformity assessment procedures: IVDs will now be subject to independent review and conformity assessment based on the classification of the device. Classes B, C, and D IVDs will all require assessment and certification by a notified body for medical devices (appropriately designated for IVDs) prior to being placed on the market. This represents a significant change in the system today where many IVDs are self-declared devices rather than being assessed by a notified body. (3) Performance evaluation and clinical data requirements: the requirements for performance evaluation of IVDs are defined in much greater detail in the new regulations. Specific requirements are also defined in relation to the use of clinical data for IVDs and the conduct of clinical performance studies. (4) Changes to requirements for "in-house" manufacturing of IVDs: under the existing legislation IVDs, which are manufactured within a healthcare institution and for use within that health institution—a la laboratory developed tests (LDTs)—are exempted from the directive. Such tests may be developed due to the lack of a commercially available alternative, e.g., for rare diseases. The new regulation places

---

[22] http://www.ce-mark.com/IVD%20Regulation.pdf

requirements on "in-house" or home-brew IVDs and the healthcare institutions which manufacture them and allows the introduction of additional requirements at national level by individual member states. This ensures the in-house LDTs are localized and are not used as an avenue to large-scale marketing of IVDs, not unlike the evolving LDT oversight and regulatory landscape in the United States.

3.5 Elements of Food and Drug Administration review and regulation—case study of two traumatic brain injury-related devices

3.5.1 Case study 1: ImPACT and ImPACT pediatric

The first case study for our discussion will focus on The Immediate Post-Concussion Assessment and Cognitive Testing (ImPACT) and ImPACT Pediatric, which, in 2016, were the first medical devices permitted for marketing that are intended to assess cognitive function following a possible concussion. They are part of the medical evaluation workup that doctors perform to assess signs and symptoms of a head injury and not intended to diagnose concussions or determine appropriate treatments. According to the FDA, the devices are intended to "test cognitive skills such as word memory, reaction time and word recognition, all of which could be affected by a head injury. The results are compared to an age-matched control database or to a patient's preinjury baseline scores, if available."[23] ImPACT software is designed to run on a desktop or laptop and is intended for those aged 12–59, while the ImPACT Pediatric runs on an iPad and is designed for children aged 5–11. The software is authorized to be used by licensed healthcare professionals where they alone should perform the test analysis and interpret the results. As the manufacturer, healthcare providers can administer the ImPACT Quick Test in 5–7 minutes, using an iPad. The FDA reviewed the ImPACT device through its de novo classification process, where to support this marketing authorization the manufacturer submitted over 250 peer-reviewed articles, of which half were independently conducted clinical research studies.

ImPACT's design is based on the traditional neurocognitive testing standards as defined by the American Academy of Clinical Neuropsychology and the National Academy of Neuropsychology. These organizations released a position paper with recommendations on appropriate standards and conventions for computerized neuropsychological assessment devices. In addition, the FDA hosted a workshop cosponsored by three clinical professional societies—Academy of Neurology, American Epilepsy Society, and National Academy of Neuropsychology—to discuss issues related to the validation and labeling of devices used to assess seizures, cognitive function, TBI, and concussion. The FDA concluded that these studies and peer consultation provided valid scientific evidence to support the safety and effectiveness of the ImPACT and ImPACT Pediatric devices. The specific evidentiary studies cited by the agency in its decision summary included the following.[24]

[23] https://www.fda.gov/news-events/press-announcements/fda-allows-marketing-first-kind-computerized-cognitive-tests-help-assess-cognitive-skills-after-head

[24] https://www.accessdata.fda.gov/cdrh_docs/reviews/DEN150037.pdf

3.5.1.1 *Test battery validity*

To demonstrate clinical validity the manufacturer provided published studies in support of the ImPACT battery of tests. The four studies reported results from over 250 students and athletes where the results obtained from ImPACT were compared to traditional neuropsychological scores including the Symbol Digit Modalities Test (SDMT). The sponsor provided information on the standardization of the ImPACT test battery and the development of the normative database. Standardization was accomplished through participation of test subjects from high schools and colleges from around the country that are representative of the intended use population. Older adults were drawn from adult athlete populations or were coaches, school administrators, and nurses. Although not keyed specifically to the US Census, the sample was inclusive of minorities at a rate that reflected the composition of the school systems involved. The standardization sample consisted of 17,013 individuals who underwent baseline ImPACT testing.

3.5.1.2 *Reliability*

The sponsor also provided five published studies, which assessed the reliability of the ImPACT test battery using different intervals between assessments ranging from 30 days to 2 years between tests. The ImPACT software calculates a relative change index (RCI), which provides information regarding if a change in the ImPACT score from baseline to postinjury is a change that is not due to either practice effects or the result of measurement error. The RCI method for interpreting change on neurocognitive tests is a method for determining change. This method relies on the standard error of the difference score. For developing the normative database for the ImPACT Pediatric test, the subjects were 915 children between the ages of 5 and 12 years. Here again, the validity of the test battery was demonstrated using results from 83 children, while the RCI and its reliability was demonstrated by results from 100 children between the ages of 5 and 12 years. The FDA concluded that the research publications analyzed the scientific value of the ImPACT devices including the devices' validity, reliability, and ability to detect evidence of cognitive dysfunction that might be associated with a concussive head injury.

The ImPACT software presented the first of its kind medical device to serve the diagnostic needs of possible concussion caused by force or trauma.

3.5.2 Case study 2: Banyan brain trauma indicator

Three years after ImPACT was cleared by the FDA, the de novo and subsequent Class II classification of the Banyan BTI biomarker-based test, also intended for diagnosing TBI, was quite different from how ImPACT was reviewed.[25] In early 2018 the FDA permitted marketing of the first blood test to evaluate mild TBI (mTBI), as part of its Breakthrough Devices program. In authorizing this test, FDA Commissioner Scott Gottlieb, MD said, "A blood-testing option for the evaluation of mTBI/concussion not only provides healthcare professionals with a new tool, but also sets the stage for a more modernized

---

[25] https://www.fda.gov/news-events/press-announcements/fda-authorizes-marketing-first-blood-test-aid-evaluation-concussion-adults

standard of care for testing of suspected cases. In addition, availability of a blood test for mTBI/concussion will likely reduce the CT scans performed on patients with concussion each year, potentially saving our healthcare system the cost of often unnecessary neuroimaging tests."

The Brain Trauma Indicator (BTI) measures levels of proteins, known as UCH-L1 and GFAP, that are released from the brain into blood and measured within 12 hours of head injury. Levels of these blood proteins after mTBI/concussion can help predict which patients may have intracranial lesions visible by CT scan and which won't. Being able to predict if patients have a low probability of intracranial lesions can help healthcare professionals in their management of patients and the decision to perform a CT scan. Test results can be available within 3–4 hours. The FDA evaluated data from a multicenter, prospective clinical study of 1947 individual blood samples from adults with suspected mTBI/concussion and reviewed the product's performance by comparing mTBI/concussion blood tests results with CT scan results. BTI was able to predict the presence of intracranial lesions on a CT scan 97.5% of the time and those who did not have intracranial lesions on a CT scan 99.6% of the time.

In its review[26] of BTI, via the de novo pathway, the FDA concluded that the test can reliably predict the absence of intracranial lesions and that healthcare professionals can incorporate this tool into the standard of care for patients to rule out the need for a CT scan in at least one third of patients who are suspected of having mTBI.

The Banyan BTI consists of two kits, one for the ubiquitin C-terminal hydrolase-L1 (UCH-L1) assay components and one for glial fibrillary acidic protein (GFAP) assay components. Each kit is packaged individually in a box and consists of the following: 96-well microtiter strip plate, each well coated with mouse monoclonal UCH-L1 antibody or mouse monoclonal GFAP capture antibody; and calibrators and controls that will allow the end user to ensure the reliable and accurate performance of the kit. Unlike ImPACT, the Banyan BTI is a traditional biomarker-based assay and the FDA required the submission of detailed analytical and clinical validation studies. The analytical validation studies were performed following guidelines provided by Clinical Laboratory Standards Institute (CLSI), and included results from precision studies, linearity studies, interference testing, method comparison studies, limit of detection studies, stability studies, and establishment of reference intervals. Following acceptance of the device via the de novo pathway, the BTI was granted a classification of Class II and a new product code was created that represented brain assessment tests. Subsequent tests that have the same intended use will be classified into this product code and will be reviewed by the 510(k) regulatory pathway.

Precision is the variability of the device when used over an indefinitely long period and to some degree several sources of variability contribute to this long-term precision. The CLSI guideline EP-05[27] describes the studies that assess performance of the device including precision within-run, between-run, between-day, and within-laboratory. For the BTI studies, as described by the FDA,[28] two separate panels, consisting of five human sera

[26] https://www.accessdata.fda.gov/cdrh_docs/reviews/DEN170045.pdf

[27] https://clsi.org/standards/products/method-evaluation/documents/ep05/

[28] https://www.accessdata.fda.gov/cdrh_docs/reviews/DEN170045.pdf

samples each with levels of UCH-Ll or GFAP that cover the measuring range of the respective kits, were tested at one site, using one instrument and one reagent lot, over the course of 20 days. The panel members were made of pooled human sera from healthy volunteers. Higher panel members were spiked with one or more positive clinical specimens (i.e., sera containing high level of endogenous UCH-Ll or GFAP) from subjects with a severe TBI or with the recombinant UCH-Ll or purified native GFAP protein. Each panel member was tested each day with two runs per day and two replicate measurements per sample per run for a total of 80 replicates per sample. Results showed the standard deviation across measurements and percent coefficient of variance demonstrating limited variability and reliable precision. Due to the semi-quantitative or qualitative nature of the test, studies were also performed where the levels of UCH-L1 or GFAP were either above or below a cutoff value and qualitative precision was assessed, that is, number of positive or negative calls. 180 samples were tested and almost 100% of the assessments were accurate.

In addition to the qualitative nature of the test, the BTI is also expected to report a quantitative result. For any diagnostic test that is expected to report such a value, the FDA also requires studies that assess linearity. The primary objective of such a study, according to CLSI EP-06, is to determine the concentration(s) where a method is not linear and the extent of the nonlinearity at that level. The basic data collection requires multiple measurements from five to nine samples with varying concentrations, which are known relative to one another by dilution ratios or by formulation, although there is no requirement for the sample concentrations to be equidistant; and there is no requirement for the assumed values to be obtained by dilution. The BTI studies assessed 11 samples with varying concentrations for each UCH-L1 and GFAP and percent recovery ranged from 87% to 100%, demonstrating that the assay is able to perform reliably across a range of concentrations of the analyte. In addition to precision and linearity, BTI assay also demonstrates traceability.[29] In addition, the regulatory review of any biomarker-based assay kit requires the demonstration of kit stability—both open kit and closed kit stability. Another important requirement of the studies that a sponsor submits as part of the device review is to demonstrate how the assay performs as it relates to stability of a labile sample. In this case, the sponsor included studies with nine serum samples spanning the measuring range of each kit (two close to the cutoff, two low, and five high values for UCH-L1 and one close to the cutoff, two low, and six high values for GFAP) tested in five replicates to determine sample storage and freeze/thaw stability. Studies showed that, for reliable results, samples should not be subjected to more than five freeze/thaw cycles. Additional studies included limit of quantitation (LoQ), which measures the lowest amount of analyte that the assay can reproducibly detect. Serum samples that contain lower than the LoQ will report a negative or "not detectable" result. Analytical specificity was studied by spiking positive samples with over 25 substances that could possibly interfere with the assay performance, including prescription pain killers, blood thinners, and other components that may be found in the serum of a normal person or a person with a TBI.[30]

---

[29] http://clinchem.aaccjnls.org/content/55/6/1067

[30] Page 16, https://www.accessdata.fda.gov/cdrh_docs/reviews/DEN170045.pdf

To assess clinical sensitivity, the Banyan BTI result was compared to the consensus head CT scan result for each patient. Of the 1947 evaluable subjects, 120 had positive CT scan results. Of the 120 subjects with positive CT scan results, 117 had a positive Banyan BTI result (sensitivity = 97.5%). The remaining three CT scan positive subjects had negative results from the Banyan BTI test. The rate of false negative (FN) results was 2.5% (3/120). None of the five subjects identified with a lesion requiring surgical intervention had a FN result suggesting that Banyan BTI correctly classified all these five CT-positive subjects as assay positive. The negative predictive value (NPV) of the assay was 99.6% (666/669). The potential benefit of the assay would be a reduction in unnecessary CT scans by approximately one third (36.5% or 666 of 1827 subjects had true negative assay results). The FDA concluded that the assay provides clinicians with an additional assessment tool for a heterogeneously presenting condition with a high NPV. The device displays a high sensitivity for detection of intracranial bleeds with little risk of adverse events or subject burden. Therefore the benefits appear to outweigh the probable risk in light of the special controls established for this device and in combination with general controls.

3.6 User fees and their impact on Food and Drug Administration

In summary, over these past four decades the US FDA has continually evolved the medical device regulatory framework. In doing so it has attempted to keep up with technological innovations, ranging from assay-based to software-based diagnostic devices. It can be said without argument that this has been aided by the active involvement of industry and academia. The next generation of devices already challenging this framework include advances in the use of artificial intelligence and machine learning. While there will always be tension between whether there is excessive regulation or whether the user fees have the unintended consequence of too much influence by industry, overall, the FDA has maintained its reputation in ensuring the safety and effectiveness standard.

As mentioned earlier, device user fees were first established in 2002 by the Medical Device User Fee and Modernization Act (MDUFMA). Premarket review by FDA—both PMA and 510(k)—requires the payment of a user fee. As of 2011,[31] the FDA evaluated more than 4000 510(k) notifications and about 40 original PMA applications each year. User fees have been renewed every 5 years after that, in 2007 with the Medical Device User Fee Amendments to the FDA Amendments Act (MDUFA II), in 2012 with the Medical Device User Fee Amendments to the FDA Safety and Innovation Act (MDUFA III), and in 2017 with the Medical Device User Fee Amendments to the FDA Reauthorization Act (MDUFA IV). MDUFA IV will be in place from October 1, 2017 to September 30, 2022. Each of these renewals has meant that the FDA and industry renegotiate the FDA's review practices and the regulations that guide the agency. With every quinquennial renewal, a larger proportion of the FDA budget relies on user fees and proportionally less of the congressionally appropriated budget, essentially ceding the

[31] U.S. Congress, Senate Special Committee on Aging, A Delicate Balance: FDA and the Reform of the Medical Device Approval Process, Testimony of William Maisel, Deputy Center Director for Science, FDA/CDRH, 112th Congress, 1st session, April 13, 2011.

authority of regulating medical devices from the electorate to industry. While user fees have certainly aided in the hiring of more personnel, and expanding the resources of the agency, it can be argued whether that is the responsibility of the government and the exchequer, instead of the industry. This makes for an interesting policy discussion in the wake of the changes in the device and diagnostic regulatory regime in Europe. During the beginning of his tenure in 2011 as the Director of the Center for Devices and Radiological Health, when questioned during a congressional testimony on why the FDA device review took longer than the European review process, Dr. Jeff Shuren invited much criticism and trans-Atlantic spat for famously saying, "we don't use our people as guinea pigs in the US."[32] Recent developments, however, demonstrate that Europe has changed course and is introducing a tighter risk-based framework and requiring stricter oversight by independent review bodies and standards more like the FDA. While there is no fear of this happening anytime soon, from a policy development point of view, it would certainly be interesting and counterintuitive if the regulatory pendulum both in Europe and the United States began to swing in opposite directions.

[32] https://www.reuters.com/article/health-devices/rpt-update-1-guinea-pig-remark-spurs-us-eu-device-spat-idUSN2427308720110225?pageNumber = 1

Pathophysiology of TBI

Peripheral markers of TBI and blood – brain barrier disruption

Jolewis Washington[1], Robert M. Murcko[2] and Damir Janigro[1,3]

[1]FloTBI Inc., Cleveland, OH, United States [2]The Ohio State University, Columbus, OH, United States [3]Case Western Reserve University, Cleveland, OH, United States

4.1 Introduction

Several excellent review articles are available to describe the relevance, nature and limitations of biomarkers in general [1], or specifically for TBI biomarkers [2]. Here we will first give a compendium of the best-known biomarkers, and we will then attempt to present answers and challenges to questions that arose during the review of the literature.

The term "biomarker," a combination of "biological and marker," refers to a broad and heterogeneous family of objective indications of medical state as seen from the caretaker's point of view (i.e., outside the patient). A necessary virtue of biomarkers is the fact that they can be measured accurately and reproducibly. Medical symptoms, which are signs and subjective determinations by the patients are, by definition, not biomarkers, and thus do not need to be accurate or reproducible. For this review, we will greatly narrow the definition of biomarker, to encompass signs of neurological diseases that can be measured in body fluids of affected (or at risk) individuals. This intentionally excludes imaging biomarkers (MRI, CT, etc.) which are the clinical standards for diagnosis and prognosis of TBI. A recent review describing the relationship between body fluid biomarkers and imaging findings can be found online [3].

4.2 Biomarkers' properties

Biomarkers which can be sampled from peripheral fluids belong to three broad families:

1. Protein markers. These are most widely used and studied. An FDA-approved protein panel has been proposed as a diagnostic means acutely after TBI [4]. See also commentaries [5,6].

2. Nucleic acids. This is a dishomogenous family including nuclear or circulating DNA/RNA and the more recently discovered miRNA [7].
3. Vesicular biomarkers [8]. These consist of cellular fragments containing variable amounts of the biomarkers listed above.

Biomarkers can also be categorized by their origin. We propose four different classes depending on the site of initial release. Biomarkers can be:

1. Intracellular/nuclear. In this case their presence in peripheral fluids requires either necrotic/apoptotic cell degeneration, or vesicular release.
2. Extracellular, soluble protein or nucleic acids. In the majority of known TBI markers, glial cells, neurons, and cerebrospinal fluid are their primary source but these can often easily gain access to peripheral fluids [7].
3. Originating from the CNS.
4. Originated outside the CNS. In the case of cellular, genomic DNA, this is not an important differentiation because every cell contains the same DNA (with exception somatic mutations, mosaicisms, etc.).

4.2.1 Nucleic acids as biomarkers

Nucleic acids have been identified as biomarkers for traumatic injuries and, more in general, inflammation; thus circulating nuclear biomarkers can potentially be used as diagnostic tools for trauma/TBI patients [7]. The following section provides an analysis based on current research and pharmacodynamic considerations (see [9,10] and Fig. 4.1)

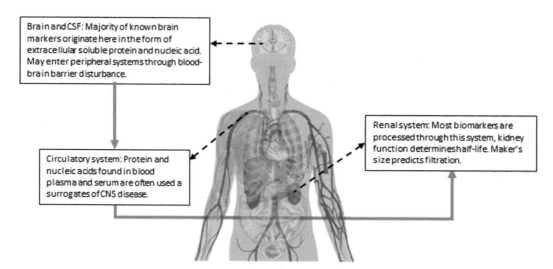

FIGURE 4.1   TBI Biomarkers throughout the body, brain and peripheral systems. Note the involvement of kidney filtration, a predictor of biomarkers' half-life [9,10]. Also note that for brain-derived markers, the volemia of the circulatory district is several-fold bigger than the volume of extracellular and ventricular CNS space. Also note that the BBB controls the passage of brain signals into peripheral blood.

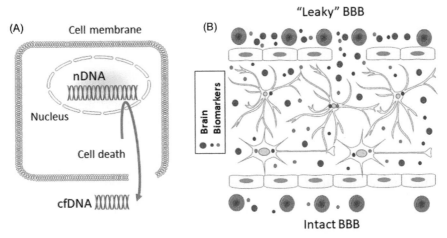

FIGURE 4.2   A) Cell death and the release of cfDNA. B) "Leaky" BBB vs Intact BBB. Note that biodistribution of intracellular markers is precluded by the cell membrane and that in an analogous fashion extravasation from brain to blood is similarly controlled by a dual membrane layer in endothelial cells.

to determine whether nucleic acids show potential as biomarkers or diagnostic tools for brain injuries and their sequelae.

The most studied nucleic acid in diagnostics is DNA. There are two forms of DNA that are found in circulation, cell-free or "floating" (cfDNA) and nuclear, genomic DNA (nDNA). The two convey different significance, inasmuch as cfDNA is an indicator of cell death or damage, whereas nDNA has genetic or mutation-related implications (Fig. 4.2). The latter, not surprisingly, has been found useful in the diagnosis of tumors and diseases associated with a genetic predisposition.

4.2.1.1 Genetics of posttraumatic events

In the case of TBI, a significant impact of genetic background on severity and outcome has been found (and excellently reviewed in [11]). The genes involved in the pathology of TBI belong to two broad categories: pathways that control and predict the extent of the injury (e.g., genes encoding inflammatory factors, cytokines and their receptors or antagonists, apoptosis/necrosis genes) and those that affect neuronal plasticity (e.g., brain-derived neurotrophic factor, BDNF). An additional genetic marker of TBI is Apolipoprotein e (apoE, protein; *APOE*, gene), the most studied gene with respect to outcome after neurotrauma [12,13]. ApoE is the major apolipoprotein produced in the central nervous system where it is synthesized by astrocytes, pericytes, and microglia [7]. The effects of apoE are multiple, and involve neurons and glial cells. Neurons primarily express apoE receptors, while glia are the physiological cell type involved in release into the extracellular milieu. See [14–16] for detailed mechanisms of action. Relevant to this review, APOE also impacts the functional integrity of the blood–brain barrier (BBB), which has been shown to underlie the onset of posttraumatic sequelae including early onset dementia [17–19]. APOE is therefore one of the several etiologic players in posttraumatic BBB failure [20–22].

Human apoE is a 34 kDa, 299 amino acid protein, and has three common isoforms, designated apoE2, E3, and E4, which differ by single amino acid changes (cysteine and arginine) at residues 112 and 158. Variants of *APOE* have been shown to predict certain forms of familiar dementias [15] as well as a spectrum of neuroinflammatory diseases (e.g., multiple sclerosis [15]). This, of course, generated interest in the field of TBI, where dementia is a well-known delayed consequence and a clearly defined neuroinflammatory component. A breakthrough study by Mayeux et al [23]. reported that individuals with an APOE4 allele and history of TBI had a 10-fold increased risk of developing Alzheimer's disease relative to a twofold increase of risk for those with APOE4 in the absence of injury, whereas TBI in the absence of APOE4 did not increase risk over a general population. The field of *APOE* is rapidly evolving and a summary of its state-of-the-art is well beyond the scope of this chapter. It helps however to underscore that genetic factors may have a profound effect on posttraumatic brain injury sequelae [17−19].

Another example of increase post-TBI risk beyond cognitive decline is posttraumatic epilepsy (PTE [24,25]). After TBI there is an increased risk of developing epilepsy. When compared to patients with no brain injury, the relative risk (RR) of epilepsy has been found to be two times higher after mild TBI (RR 2.22, 95% CI 2.07−2.38) and seven times higher after severe brain injury (RR 7.40, 95% CI 6.16−8.89) [24]. One mechanism that has emerged as having potentially prognostic importance after TBI is systemic or brain inflammation leading to BBB disruption [26]. In the field of PTE, most genetic associations examined have been single-nucleotide polymorphisms (SNPs), a common variation within a population that can be defined as a variation of a single nucleotide, adenine (A), guanine (G), thymine (T), or cytosine (C), between individuals. A recent finding shows that a SNP of IL-1β influences the probability of PTE after TBI [27]. More specifically, the *rs1143634* polymorphism favored development of PTE by affecting the CSF-to-serum ratio of this cytokine. The TT variant in *rs1143634* protected from PTE. Similar dual effects of SNPs were found for *GAD1* and *A1AR*, encoding the glutamic acid decarboxylase gene and the gene for adenosine A1 receptor, respectively [24]. All these genes, and in particular IL1-B [28], are involved in the regulation of BBB permeability, while IL-1B is directly linked to ictogenesis [29].

In conclusion, there is therefore convincing evidence that these genomic variations and polymorphisms act simultaneously and perhaps synergistically in brain and BBB cells.

4.2.1.2 Cell death and cfDNA are posttraumatic events

One of the immediate effects of traumatic brain injury is cell death. In the case of TBI without polytrauma, the main cellular degeneration occurs in the CNS; after either penetrating brain injuries and concomitant polytrauma, cell death is more pronounced and not limited to the CNS. Thus cfDNA will be either primarily derived from brain cells or of mixed CNS/peripheral origin. We will only focus on isolated CNS trauma without other lesions (e.g., closed head injury). Even when in the presence of specific CNS trauma, there are several considerations to be made as to the significance of cfDNA and its association with other biomarkers.

In the early phase after trauma, damage-associated molecular patterns (DAMPs [7]) are released and give rise to sterile systemic inflammatory response. This type of response is not specific for TBI, but rather common in a variety of neurological diseases [7]. As shown in Fig. 4.3, there is a significant overlap between DAMP, markers of BBB integrity, and

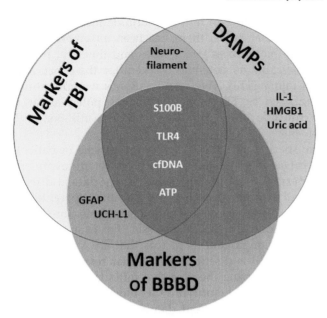

FIGURE 4.3 Venn diagram comparison between Markers of BBBD, markers of TBI, and DAMPs. *ATP*, Adenosine trisphosphate; *cfDNA*, cell-free DNA; *GFAP*, Glial fibrillary acidic protein; *HMGB1*, High mobility group box 1; *Il-1*, Interleukin 1beta; *TRL4*, Toll-like receptor 4; *UCHL-1*, Ubiquitin carboxy-terminal hydrolase L1.

biomarkers of TBI. For this reason, they will be here presented together remaining aware that DAMPS are not a homogenous molecular family.

The mammalian immune system relies on the close collaboration of the innate and adaptive immune systems aiming at fast detection of pathogens or threats to body homeostasis. Recognition of pathogen-derived molecules is carried by receptors such as Receptor for Advanced Glycation End Products (RAGE) and toll-like receptor 4 TLR4. The same receptors are efficient. An interesting aspect of DAMPs is that in addition to their diagnostic value, they also bear etiologic significance. While the downstream effects of, for example, S100B and toll-like receptor 4 (TLR4) are not fully elucidated, both share a proinflammatory action as detectors of misplaced or altered self-molecules that signal tissue damage and cell death. S100B is a ligand for RAGE (and possibly TRL4), while TRL4 binds lipopolysaccharide (LPS) and High mobility group protein B1 (HMGB1). Interestingly, HMGB1 is released by an active transport from the nucleus or by passive diffusion in cell death, in analogy to what is shown in Fig. 4.2 for nucleic acids. There are scarce data on whether astrocytic proteins have an active release mechanism, but GFAP or S100B are both present in cerebrospinal fluid (CSF) under resting conditions, and massively released after glial injury or death. From the diagnostic point of view this is important because distinct plateau levels may be reached when only available extracellular markers are measured, or after loss of plasma membrane integrity and release of much more abundant intracellular/cytoskeletal GFAP or S100B. This has been predicted [30,31] and later confirmed by [32,33].

4.2.1.3 MicroRNAs as biomarkers

MicroRNAs (miRs) are short (<30 nucleotides) noncoding, single-stranded RNAs that are crucial in cell expression. They act at the posttranscriptional level to regulate protein synthesis. Many of these RNAs are found circulating in human biofluids including blood plasma and cerebrospinal fluid (CSF). In recent years, there has been an emergence of using these endogenous RNA molecules as biomarkers for diseases and illnesses. In fact, these molecules are currently being investigated as potential markers for the concerning neurological disorder of traumatic brain injury (TBI). Twelve microRNAs were identified that had the highest potential of being used as TBI biomarker. These potential target RNAs were miR-151, miR-16, miR-195, miR-20a, miR-21, miR-30, miR-320, miR-362 miR-451, miR-486, miR-505, and miR-92a [34–36].

Studies have identified many of these specific microRNAs in serum/plasma of patients with TBI. Researchers believe this is because an estimated 70% of all miRs are expressed in the brain, spinal cord, or peripheral nerves. Experiments using patient data and miRs are promising but limited due to the small sample size. The future of miRs' potential as an indicator of the diagnosis, severity, and prognosis of TBI is questionable. Interest in miRs stems from the role they have in controlling cellular processes. For example, miR-21 and miR-16 regulate apoptosis and target angiogenesis factors that are known to be critical to BBB maintenance [34]. When the BBB is disrupted, a cellular response causes these, along with other miRs, to respond, supporting the idea that miRs facilitate neurogenesis and acute repair responses following TBI. Quantifying this biochemical response into a specific concentration that is consistent with patient data has been identified as the next step.

Although data has shown promise in miRs usage in TBI, their most predominant usage has been with other illnesses (see Table 4.1). All of these targets had a dysfunction associated with them other than TBI, a detrimental issue in biomarkers discovery because of nonspecificity. Many of these RNA targets appear to be more selective for various types of cancer detection rather than TBI. miR-30 and miR-92a were the least specific, being a target marker for five or more conditions. MicroRNAs have not shown substantial evidence to

TABLE 4.1   Microrna marker usage for illness/injury other than TBI.

MicroRNA (MIR)	Disease/Illness	Ref.
MIR-151	Papillary thyroid carcinomas (PTC)	[37]
MIR-16	Various cancers, chronic kidney disease (CKD),	[38]
MIR-195	Osteosarcoma, breast cancer, diabetes	[39]
MIR-20A	Various cancers	[40]
MIR-21	Kidney fibrosis, various cancers, cardiac disease	[41]
MIR-30	Lymphoma, cardiovascular disease, renal disease, various cancers, tuberculosis, osteoarthritis	[36]
MIR-320	Prostate cancer, Waldenström macroglobulinemia	[42]
MIR-362	Melanoma, acute myeloid leukemia (AML)	[43]
MIR-92A	Mercury poisoning, colorectal cancer, leukemia, primary CNS lymphoma (PCNSL), atherosclerosis	[44–47]

support their ability to be selective and specific enough to be a strong biomarker for the diagnosis of traumatic brain injury.

4.2.1.3.1 BBB, protein markers, and TBI

BBB breakdown has often been documented in patients with TBI, but the role of this pathology in neurological dysfunction has only recently been explored [48–50]. Animal studies have demonstrated that BBB breakdown is involved in the initiation of transcriptional changes in the neurovascular network that ultimately lead to delayed neuronal dysfunction and degeneration. Brain imaging data have confirmed the high incidence of BBB breakdown in patients with TBI and suggest that such pathology could be used as a biomarker in the clinic. The recently provided [48] clinical evidence for involvement of BBB breakdown in mTBI highlights the need for future basic and clinical studies (Tables 4.2 and 4.3).

As stated above, an important clinical feature of mild traumatic brain injury, is the rapid disruption of the BBB that has been recognized by radiologic (e.g., MRI [48–50]) and laboratory findings, such as the albumin quotient (see below and [72]). Concussions, or traumatic brain injury in general, are thus associated with a rapid loss of cerebrovascular (BBB) integrity followed (or not) by the development of brain damage [73,74]. It is therefore significant to detect early BBB changes to predict development of postconcussion brain damage. S100B and GFAP have emerged as candidate peripheral biomarkers of BBB permeability and acutely posttraumatic changes. Elevation of S100B serum levels reflect the presence of a damaged BBB and may predict or rule out brain injury [75,76]. Most importantly, S100B increases also after a mTBI characterized by CT changes consistent with intracranial events. In studies where S100B serum levels were compared with CT-based diagnosis of mTBI, a

TABLE 4.2 Putative or proven markers of BBB permeability.

Marker	Role in BBB dysfunction	Presumed cellular/organ origin	Sample origin	Levels in CNS/blood	Refs.
GFAP	Reporter of BBB function	Astrocytes. No extracranial sources reported in humans	Venipuncture	10–50-fold higher in CNS	[51–55]
S100B	Reporter of BBB function	Astrocytes, perhaps extracranial sources	Venipuncture, but can be measured in urine or saliva	10–50-fold higher in CNS	[53–58]
P-tau	None known; linked to BBBD	Axons; specific phosphorylation sites in CNS	Venipuncture	Virtual absence from normal serum/plasma	[59,60]
MMP-9	Causative role in BBBD	Nonspecific/inflammatory cells	Venipuncture	Increases at time of increased BBB permeability	[61]
VEGF	Causative role in BBBD	Nonspecific/inflammatory cells	Venipuncture	Increases at time of increased BBB permeability	[62–64]

TABLE 4.3　Peripheral markers as predictors of brain imaging findings.

Marker	Imaging modality	Main findings	Predictive value of marker vs. imaging	Disease condition	References
S100B	CT with contrast	Normal levels predict normal findings	>90% negative predictive value for intracranial lesions (epidural, subdural hematomas, etc.)	TBI Stroke	[53–58]
S100B	Gd-MRI	Excellent correlation with normal findings	>90% negative predictive value for abnormal extravasation of Gd	Brain tumors Brain metastases Meningioma	[51,52]
	FLAIR	Excellent correlation with normal findings	Good NPV with FLAIR	Seizure disorders Animal models	[54,55,65]
GFAP	CT with contrast	Excellent correlation with normal findings	Good negative predictive value for abnormal extravasation of Gd;	TBI	[51,66]
Autoreactive IgGs against S100B and GFAP	DTI	Correlation with white matter changes (FA & MD)	NA	Postconcussion syndrome, acute and chronic	[62–64,67,68]
	Gd-MRI	Correlation with white matter changes (by Gd)	Good negative predictive value for small vessel disease	Aging, risk of secondary brain metastases	[69–71]

negative predictive value of >95% was reported [30,77−79]. In a recent study [66] the negative predictive value of S100B was compared with GFAP and UCHL-1.

An important feature of S100B is its excellent negative predictive value for sequelae of BBB disruption or traumatic brain injury [66,75,80]. In contrast, other markers are more geared toward a good positive predictive value. For the marker UCHL-1 with a total of 1138 TBI cases and 1373 controls there was a significant increase in serum UCH-L1 levels in patients with TBI compared to controls (weighted mean difference, 0.96; 95% CI 0.31−1.61; $P = .004$) [81]. Two independent meta-analyses for S100B in TBI concluded that "Low serum S100B levels accurately predict normal CT findings after mTBI and that S100B sampling within 3 hours of injury should be considered when no focal neurological deficit, or significant extracerebral injury is present." These studies recommend a cutoff for omitting CT [82,83]. There is therefore an opportunity to produce a test with high negative predictive value as a point-of-care device so that many unnecessary scans can be avoided, and separately, a laboratory-based positive predictive value test to diagnose complications after TBI. A recent paper describes the validation of S100B NPV in TBI in some detail [80].

Bazarian and colleagues confirmed that serum S100B is a marker of BBB function, at least when taken acutely after TBI [75]. Assessment of BBB status is not routine in clinical practice because available techniques are invasive. The gold-standard measure, the cerebrospinal fluid (CSF)-serum albumin quotient (QA), requires the measurement of albumin in CSF and serum collected contemporaneously. Accurate, less invasive techniques are necessary. The objective of this study was to evaluate the relationship between QA and serum concentrations of S100B. Nine subjects with severe traumatic brain injury (TBI; Glasgow Coma Scale (GCS) score 8) and 11 subjects with nontraumatic headache who had CSF collected by ventriculostomy or lumbar puncture (LP) were enrolled. Serum and CSF were collected at the time of LP for headache subjects and at 12, 24, and 48 h after ventriculostomy for TBI subjects. The QA was calculated for all time points at which paired CSF and serum samples were available. Pearson's correlation coefficient and area under the receiver operating characteristic (ROC) curve were used to determine a statistically significant linear correlation between serum S100B and QA was present (r2 0.432, $P < 0.02$). ROC analysis demonstrated a significant relationship between QA and serum S100B concentrations.

4.3 Conclusions

Sequelae of TBI are followed by or associated with BBB disruption, providing a window to the brain "biomarker bank." Markers of BBB dysfunction are nonspecific and may carry limited significance when searching for specific posttraumatic sequelae such as epileptogenesis. However, understanding BBB status at a time of markers' measurements is crucial because if the BBB is at that moment not permeable to a specific marker, a false negative interpretation may occur.

Acknowledgments

RM wishes to thank Dr. Liang Guo and Dr. Marcia Bockbrader, for showing him the endless possibilities of neuroscience.

Reference

[1] Strimbu K, Tavel JA. What are biomarkers? Curr Opin HIV AIDS 2010;5(6):463–6.

[2] Mondello S., Sorinola A., Czeiter E. et al. Blood-Based Protein Biomarkers for the Management of Traumatic Brain Injuries in Adults Presenting with Mild Head Injury to Emergency Departments: A Living Systematic Review and Meta-Analysis. J Neurotrauma 2017.

[3] Zhang J., Puvenna V., Janigro D. Biomarkers of Traumatic Brain Injury and Their Relationship to Pathology. 2016.

[4] Bazarian JJ, Biberthaler P, Welch RD, et al. Serum GFAP and UCH-L1 for prediction of absence of intracranial injuries on head CT (ALERT-TBI): a multicentre observational study. Lancet Neurol 2018;17(9):782–9.

[5] Maas AIR, Lingsma HF. ALERT-TBI study on biomarkers for TBI: has science suffered? Lancet Neurol 2018;17 (9):737–8.

[6] Posti JP, Takata K, Tenovuo O. TBIcare Investigator's response to "Raising the Bar for Traumatic Brain Injury Biomarker Research: Methods Make a Difference" by Papa and Wang. J Neurotrauma 2019; neu.2017.5209.

[7] Holtzman DM, Herz J, Bu G. Apolipoprotein E and apolipoprotein E receptors: normal biology and roles in Alzheimer disease. Cold Spring Harb Perspect Med 2012;2(3):a006312.

[8] Ramirez SH, Andrews AM, Paul D, Pachter JS. Extracellular vesicles: mediators and biomarkers of pathology along CNS barriers. Fluids Barriers CNS 2018;15(1):19.

[9] Dadas A, Janigro D. The Role and Diagnostic Significance of Cellular Barriers after Concussive Head Trauma. Concussion 2018;3(1):CNC53. Available from: https://doi.org/10.2217/cnc-2017-0019.

[10] Dadas A, Washington J, Marchi N, Janigro D. Improving the clinical management of traumatic brain injury through the pharmacokinetic modeling of peripheral blood biomarkers. Fluids Barriers CNS 2016;13(1):21.

[11] Bennet ER-RKLD. Genetic Influences in Traumatic Brain Injury. Translational Research in Traumatic Brain Injury. Boca Raton, FL: CRC Press/Taylor and Francis Group; 2016. Available from: https://www.ncbi.nlm.nih.gov/books/NBK326717/.

[12] Chamelian L, Reis M, Feinstein A. Six-month recovery from mild to moderate Traumatic Brain Injury: the role of APOE-epsilon4 allele. Brain 2004;127(Pt 12):2621–8.

[13] Zhou W, Xu D, Peng X, Zhang Q, Jia J, Crutcher KA. Meta-analysis of APOE4 allele and outcome after traumatic brain injury. J Neurotrauma 2008;25(4):279–90.

[14] Arranz AM, De SB. The role of astroglia in Alzheimer's disease: pathophysiology and clinical implications. Lancet Neurol 2019;18(4):406–14.

[15] Verghese PB, Castellano JM, Holtzman DM. Apolipoprotein E in Alzheimer's disease and other neurological disorders. Lancet Neurol 2011;10(3):241–52.

[16] Mahley RW, Huang Y. Apolipoprotein e sets the stage: response to injury triggers neuropathology. Neuron 2012;76(5):871–85.

[17] Main BS, Villapol S, Sloley SS, et al. Apolipoprotein E4 impairs spontaneous blood brain barrier repair following traumatic brain injury. Mol Neurodegener 2018;13(1):17.

[18] Shi Y, Holtzman DM. Interplay between innate immunity and Alzheimer disease: APOE and TREM2 in the spotlight. Nat Rev Immunol 2018;18(12):759–72.

[19] Ma Q, Zhao Z, Sagare AP, et al. Blood-brain barrier-associated pericytes internalize and clear aggregated amyloid-beta42 by LRP1-dependent apolipoprotein E isoform-specific mechanism. Mol Neurodegener 2018;13(1):57.

[20] Tagge CA, Fisher AM, Minaeva OV, et al. Concussion, microvascular injury, and early tauopathy in young athletes after impact head injury and an impact concussion mouse model. Brain 2018;141(2):422–58.

[21] Ruber T, David B, Luchters G, et al. Evidence for peri-ictal blood-brain barrier dysfunction in patients with epilepsy. Brain 2018;141(10):2952–65.

[22] Ivens S, Gabriel S, Greenberg G, Friedman A, Shelef I. Blood-brain barrier breakdown as a novel mechanism underlying cerebral hyperperfusion syndrome. J Neurol 2010;257(4):615–20.

[23] Mayeux R, Ottman R, Maestre G, et al. Synergistic effects of traumatic head injury and apolipoprotein-epsilon 4 in patients with Alzheimer's disease. Neurology 1995;45(3 Pt 1):555–7.

[24] Cotter D, Kelso A, Neligan A. Genetic biomarkers of posttraumatic epilepsy: A systematic review. Seizure 2017;46:53–8.

[25] Wilson L, Stewart W, Dams-O'Connor K, et al. The chronic and evolving neurological consequences of traumatic brain injury. Lancet Neurol 2017;16(10):813–25.

[26] Dadas A, Janigro D. Breakdown of blood brain barrier as a mechanism of post-traumatic epilepsy. Neurobiol Dis 2018.

[27] Diamond ML, Ritter AC, Failla MD, et al. IL-1beta associations with posttraumatic epilepsy development: A genetics and biomarker cohort study. Epilepsia 2014.

[28] Argaw AT, Zhang Y, Snyder BJ, et al. IL-1beta regulates blood-brain barrier permeability via reactivation of the hypoxia-angiogenesis program. J Immunol 2006;177(8):5574–84.

[29] Marchi N, Fan QY, Ghosh C, et al. Antagonism of peripheral inflammation reduces the severity of status epilepticus. Neurobiol Dis 2009;33(2):171–81.

[30] Marchi N, Cavaglia M, Bhudia S, Hallene K, Janigro D. Peripheral markers of blood-brain barrier damage. Clinica Chimica Acta 2004;342(1-2):1–12.

[31] Marchi N, Rasmussen PA, Kapural M, Fazio V, Cavaglia M, Janigro D. Peripheral markers of brain damage and blood-brain barrier dysfunction. Restorative Neurology and Neuroscience 2003;21(3-4):109–21.

[32] Lee JY, Lee CY, Kim HR, Lee CH, Kim HW, Kim JH. A Role of Serum-Based Neuronal and Glial Markers as Potential Predictors for Distinguishing Severity and Related Outcomes in Traumatic Brain Injury. J Korean Neurosurg Soc 2015;58(2):93–100.

[33] Thelin EP, Nelson DW, Bellander BM. Secondary peaks of S100B in serum relate to subsequent radiological pathology in traumatic brain injury. Neurocrit Care 2014;20(2):217–29.

[34] Atif H, Hicks SD. A Review of MicroRNA Biomarkers in Traumatic Brain Injury. J Exp Neurosci 2019;13 1179069519832286.

[35] Di Pietro V, Yakoub KM, Scarpa U, Di Pietro C, Belli A. MicroRNA Signature of Traumatic Brain Injury: From the Biomarker Discovery to the Point-of-Care. Frontiers in neurology 2018;9:429.

[36] Mao L., Liu S., Hu L. et al. miR-30 Family: A Promising Regulator in Development and Disease. Biomed Res Int 2018;2018:9623412.

[37] McNally ME, Collins A, Wojcik SE, et al. Concomitant dysregulation of microRNAs miR-151-3p and miR-126 correlates with improved survival in resected cholangiocarcinoma. HPB (Oxford) 2013;15(4):260—4.

[38] Lange T, Stracke S, Rettig R, et al. Identification of miR-16 as an endogenous reference gene for the normalization of urinary exosomal miRNA expression data from CKD patients. Plos One 2017;12(8):e0183435.

[39] Cai H, Zhao H, Tang J, Wu H. Serum miR-195 is a diagnostic and prognostic marker for osteosarcoma. Journal of Surgical Research 2015;194(2):505—10.

[40] Huang D, Peng Y, Ma K, et al. MiR-20a, a novel promising biomarker to predict prognosis in human cancer: a meta-analysis. BMC Cancer 2018;18(1):1189.

[41] Glowacki F, Savary Gg, Gnemmi V, et al. Increased circulating miR-21 levels are associated with kidney fibrosis. Plos One 2013;8(2):e58014.

[42] Lieb V, Weigelt K, Scheinost L, et al. Serum levels of miR-320 family members are associated with clinical parameters and diagnosis in prostate cancer patients. Oncotarget 2017;9(12):10402—16.

[43] Ma QL, Wang JH, Yang M, Wang HP, Jin J. MiR-362-5p as a novel prognostic predictor of cytogenetically normal acute myeloid leukemia. J Transl Med 2018;16(1):68.

[44] Ding E, Guo J, Bai Y, et al. MiR-92a and miR-486 are potential diagnostic biomarkers for mercury poisoning and jointly sustain NF- + ¦B activity in mercury toxicity. Sci Rep 2017;7(1):15980.

[45] Huang Y, Tang S, Ji-yan C, et al. Circulating miR-92a expression level in patients with essential hypertension: a potential marker of atherosclerosis. Journal Of Human Hypertension 2016;31:200.

[46] Wu CW, Ng SSM, Dong YJ, et al. Detection of miR-92a and miR-21 in stool samples as potential screening biomarkers for colorectal cancer and polyps. Gut 2012;61(5):739.

[47] Schee K., Boye K., Abrahamsen T.W., Fodstad + , Flatmark K.

[48] Weissberg I, Veksler R, Kamintsky L, et al. Imaging blood-brain barrier dysfunction in football players. JAMA Neurol 2014;71(11):1453—5.

[49] Tomkins O, Feintuch A, Benifla M, Cohen A, Friedman A, Shelef I. Blood-brain barrier breakdown following traumatic brain injury: a possible role in posttraumatic epilepsy. Cardiovasc Psychiatry Neurol 2011;2011 765923.

[50] Shlosberg D, Benifla M, Kaufer D, Friedman A. Blood-brain barrier breakdown as a therapeutic target in traumatic brain injury. Nature Reviews Neurology 2010;6(7):393—403.

[51] Takala RS, Posti JP, Runtti H, et al. Glial Fibrillary Acidic Protein and Ubiquitin C-Terminal Hydrolase-L1 as Outcome Predictors in Traumatic Brain Injury. World Neurosurg 2016;87:8—20.

[52] Mondello S, Kobeissy F, Vestri A, Hayes RL, Kochanek PM, Berger RP. Serum Concentrations of Ubiquitin C-Terminal Hydrolase-L1 and Glial Fibrillary Acidic Protein after Pediatric Traumatic Brain Injury. Sci Rep 2016;6:28203.

[53] Marchi N, Granata T, Janigro D. Inflammatory pathways of seizure disorders. Trends Neurosci 2014;37 (2):55—65.

[54] Marchi N, Granata T, Alexopoulos A, Janigro D. The blood-brain barrier hypothesis in drug resistant epilepsy. Brain 2012;135(Pt 4):e211.

[55] Marchi N, Granata T, Ghosh C, Janigro D. Blood-brain barrier dysfunction and epilepsy: pathophysiologic role and therapeutic approaches. Epilepsia 2012;53(11):1877—86.

[56] Bargerstock E, Puvenna V, Iffland P, et al. Is peripheral immunity regulated by blood-brain barrier permeability changes? Plos One 2014;9(7):e101477.

[57] Pham N, Fazio V, Cucullo L, et al. Extracranial Sources of S100B Do Not Affect Serum Levels. Plos One 2010;5(9):e12691.

[58] Kanner AA, Marchi N, Fazio V, et al. Serum S100beta: a noninvasive marker of blood-brain barrier function and brain lesions. Cancer 2003;97(11):2806—13.

[59] Puvenna V, Engeler M, Banjara M, et al. Is phosphorylated tau unique to chronic traumatic encephalopathy? Phosphorylated tau in epileptic brain and chronic traumatic encephalopathy. Brain Res 2015.

[60] Shahim P, Tegner Y, Wilson DH, et al. Blood Biomarkers for Brain Injury in Concussed Professional Ice Hockey Players. JAMA Neurol 2014.

[61] Kazmierski R, Michalak S, Wencel-Warot A, Nowinski WL. Serum tight-junction proteins predict hemorrhagic transformation in ischemic stroke patients. Neurology 2012;79(16):1677—85.

[62] Kauvar L.M., Janigro D. DIAGNOSTIC MARKER FOR TREATMENT OF CEREBRAL ISCHEMIA. 9-17-2015. US Patent 20,150,258,193. Ref Type: Generic

[63] Kanazawa M, Igarashi H, Kawamura K, et al. Inhibition of VEGF signaling pathway attenuates hemorrhage after tPA treatment. J Cereb Blood Flow Metab 2011;31(6):1461—74.

[64] Kim H, Lee JM, Park JS, et al. Dexamethasone coordinately regulates angiopoietin-1 and VEGF: a mechanism of glucocorticoid-induced stabilization of blood-brain barrier. Biochem Biophys Res Commun 2008;372(1):243—8.

[65] Marchi N, Granata T, Freri E, et al. Efficacy of Anti-Inflammatory Therapy in a Model of Acute Seizures and in a Population of Pediatric Drug Resistant Epileptics. Plos One 2011;6:3.

[66] Welch RD, Ayaz SI, Lewis LM, et al. Ability of Serum Glial Fibrillary Acidic Protein, Ubiquitin C-Terminal Hydrolase-L1, and S100B to Differentiate Normal and Abnormal Head Computed Tomography Findings in Patients with Suspected Mild or Moderate Traumatic Brain Injury. J Neurotrauma 2015.

[67] Marchi N, Bazarian JJ, Puvenna V, et al. Consequences of repeated blood-brain barrier disruption in football players. Plos One 2013;8(3):e56805.

[68] Bazarian JJ, Zhu T, Zhong J, et al. Persistent, Long-term Cerebral White Matter Changes after Sports-Related Repetitive Head Impacts. Plos One 2014;9(4):e94734.

[69] Brennan C, Achey R, Wathen C, Janigro D. Imaging as Means to Study Cerebrovascular. Pathophysiology. *Brian Mapping: An Encyclopedic Reference.* Elsevier; 2014.

[70] Mazzone P, Tierney W, Hossain M, Puvenna V, Janigro D, Cucullo L. Pathophysiological Impact of Cigarette Smoke Exposure on the Cerebrovascular System with a Focus on the Blood-brain Barrier: Expanding the Awareness of Smoking Toxicity in an Underappreciated Area. International Journal of Environmental Research and Public Health 2010;7(12):4111—26.

[71] Vogelbaum MA, Masaryk T, Mazzone P, et al. S100beta as a predictor of brain metastases: brain versus cerebrovascular damage. Cancer 2005;104(4):817—24.

[72] Blyth B, Farahvar A, He H, et al. Elevated Serum Ubiquitin Carboxy-terminal Hydrolase L1 is Associated with Abnormal Blood Brain Barrier Function after Traumatic Brain Injury. J Neurotrauma 2011;28(12):2453—62.

[73] Masel BE, DeWitt DS. Traumatic brain injury: a disease process, not an event. J Neurotrauma 2010;27(8):1529—40.

[74] Menon DK, Schwab K, Wright DW, Maas AI. Demographics and Clinical Assessment Working Group of the International. Position statement: definition of traumatic brain injury. Arch Phys Med Rehabil 2010;91(11):1637—40.

[75] Blyth BJ, Farahvar A, Gee C, et al. Validation of Serum Markers for Blood-Brain Barrier Disruption in Traumatic Brain Injury. J Neurotrauma 2009;26(9):1497—507.

[76] Ruan S, Noyes K, Bazarian JJ. The Economic Impact of S-100B as a Pre-Head CT Screening Test on Emergency Department Management of Adult Patients with Mild Traumatic Brain Injury. J Neurotrauma 2009;26(10):1655—64.

[77] Biberthaler P, Mussack T, Wiedemann E, et al. Evaluation of S-100b as a specific marker for neuronal damage due to minor head trauma. World J Surg 2001;25(1):93—7.

[78] Biberthaler P, Mussack T, Wiedemann E, et al. Rapid identification of high-risk patients after minor head trauma (MHT) by assessment of S-100B: ascertainment of a cut-off level. Eur J Med Res 2002;7(4):164—70.

[79] Biberthaler P, Mussack T, Kanz KG, et al. Identification of high-risk patients after minor craniocerebral trauma. Measurement of nerve tissue protein S100. Unfallchirurg 2004;107(3):197—202.

[80] Unden L, Calcagnile O, Unden J, Reinstrup P, Bazarian J. Validation of the Scandinavian guidelines for initial management of minimal, mild and moderate traumatic brain injury in adults. BMC Med 2015;13:292.

[81] Li J, Yu C, Sun Y, Li Y. Serum ubiquitin C-terminal hydrolase L1 as a biomarker for traumatic brain injury: a systematic review and meta-analysis. Am J Emerg Med 2015;33(9):1191—6.

[82] Heidari K, Vafaee A, Rastekenari AM, et al. S100B protein as a screening tool for computed tomography findings after mild traumatic brain injury: Systematic review and meta-analysis. Brain Inj 2015;1—12.

[83] Unden J, Romner B. Can low serum levels of S100B predict normal CT findings after minor head injury in adults?: an evidence-based review and meta-analysis. J Head Trauma Rehabil 2010;25(4):228—40.

The role of autoimmunity after traumatic brain injury

Mahasweta Das[1,2], Shyam S. Mohapatra[2,3] and Subhra Mohapatra[1,2]

[1]Department of Molecular Medicine, College of Medicine, University of South Florida, Tampa, FL, United States [2]James A. Haley VA Hospital, Tampa, FL, United States [3]Department of Internal Medicine, College of Medicine, University of South Florida, Tampa, FL, United States

5.1 Introduction

Traumatic brain injury (TBI) is a leading cause of death and disability affecting both children and adults and poses a significant social burden. TBI is frequently related to motor vehicle accidents, sports, and war field injuries. However, falls and physical abuse are common causes as well. According to National Center for Injury Prevention and Control's 2015 report to Congress, in the United States 3.2–5.3 million people live with TBI [1]. Based on a 2010 report the approximate annual financial burden of TBI was estimated as $76.5 billion [2]. As a measurement of severity of TBI, a Glasgow Coma Scale (GCS) value of ≥ 14 is considered mild TBI, 9–13 is considered moderate TBI, and ≤ 8 is considered severe TBI [3]. Among the leading causes of TBI falls (40% of total) comes first, especially in children and elderly people. It is followed by blunt trauma (sports, war field) comprising 15%, and road accidents comprising 14% of all reported head trauma. Assaults or abuse-related head traumas are also reported. Some sports activities like boxing, soccer, hockey, martial arts, and also high-speed games like cycling, motor racing, horse riding, skiing, and skating are often associated with repetitive mild TBI or concussion, with a cumulative effect later in life [4].

TBI is not a single pathophysiological event, rather it is considered a multimodal disease process [5]. The primary insult mechanically damages the brain cells, both neurons and glia, and compromises the blood–brain barrier (BBB). The secondary injury evolves over time—from minutes to years after the primary injury—and involves cellular, molecular, and functional events. This causes endogenous neurochemical changes and gives rise to systemic or local neuroinflammatory events which ultimately lead to secondary brain cell death or survival, plasticity, tissue damage or atrophy [6–8]. Secondary injury may also cause changes in cellular calcium homeostasis, glutamate excitotoxicity, mitochondrial dysfunction, free radical generation, systemic and neuroinflammation, increased lipid peroxidation, apoptosis, and diffuse axonal injury [9,10]. In addition, the damaged and dying cells release proteins and fragments of proteins into the cerebrospinal fluid (CSF) and blood. The displaced cell debris, proteins, and their breakdown products (BDP), although of self-origin, are recognized by the immune cells as foreign materials and antibodies are developed against these antigens. The antibodies developed against self-antigens are the autoantibodies (aAbs) which, depending on their subtypes, can be maintained for years in the bloodstream [11] and target-specific brain cells causing further damage. Studies have shown the involvement of brain-directed autoimmunity in different neurological disorders, including Alzheimer's disease (AD) [12], multiple sclerosis (MS) [13], stroke, epilepsy [14,15], spinal cord injury (SCI) [16–19], and TBI [20]. Patients with MS develop aAb against circulating myelin basic protein (MBP) [13], a central nervous system (CNS) protein that has been implicated in white matter injury following TBI. The development of antipituitary antibodies (APA) has been reported by researchers [21,22]. Throughout the years, researchers have discovered novel biomarkers in the diagnosis, management, and therapy of CNS trauma including TBI. Certain proteins, their BDPs and microRNAs (miRNA), have traditionally been considered as biomarkers of TBI. Neuron-specific enolase (NSE), glial calcium-binding protein (S100B), glial fibrillary acidic protein (GFAP), MBP, ubiquitin carboxyl hydrolase-like 1 (UCH-L1), neurofilament proteins, and αII-spectrin BDPs (SBDPs) [11,23–25] have been identified as biomarkers in human body fluids after TBI, although most investigators have focused on MBP, S100B, and glutamate receptors in human patients [13,20,26,27]. Recently, increasing interest has been observed in investigating the role of aAbs as biomarkers of CNS trauma, neurodegenerative disorders, stroke, neuropsychiatric diseases, and neurotoxicity. The importance of these new classes of biomarkers lies in the fact that while autoantigens like cellular proteins and their BDPs may serve as biomarkers for acute injury, the aAbs developed against these antigens will last for a long time in the biofluids and represent long-lasting, chronic, signature biomarkers associated with the advanced or chronic status of the injury. Due to their specificity, aAbs may be regarded as important biomarkers of disease processes as well. Here we will discuss the mechanism of development of aAbs following TBI, the role of different immune cells, potential targets, and the pathophysiological consequences. In this discussion we will also bring in the context of SCI-induced autoimmunity because of the mechanistic similarities with that of TBI-induced autoimmunity.

5.2 Traumatic brain injury may induce autoimmune disorders

Brain-directed autoimmunity has been reported in autoimmune diseases like MS, AD, stroke, epilepsy [11,12,14], and pituitary disorders [22,28,29]. For a long period of time physicians have speculated that TBI may be responsible for the onset or aggravation of MS, an autoimmune disease in which aAbs are directed against CNS antigen MBP [13].

Like infection, head and neck trauma (for example, cervical cord hyperextension—hyperflexion) may unmask or even worsen MS symptoms in genetically predisposed patients [30]. TBI enhances the production of proinflammatory cytokines and nitric oxide triggering MS symptoms [30]. MBP may be produced after TBI as the myelinated nerve fibers are damaged. Both TBI and MS share similar pathologies including demyelination, gliosis, and axonal loss.

Increases in the incidence of neurodegenerative conditions like AD and other forms of dementias as a result of head trauma have also been reported [31,32]. AD is the most common form of neurodegenerative disorders in modern society. It accounts for 50%—60% of all dementia [33]. TBI and AD share many overlapping pathologies and possible clinical links. For example, the nucleotide-binding domain leucine-rich repeats (NLR) family of pattern recognition receptors (PRRs) can be activated by TBI-induced tissue damage and can form multiprotein complexes called inflammasomes. NLRP3 inflammasomes have been detected in neurons, astrocytes, and microglia in the cortex after TBI [34] and also demonstrated to be associated with CNS inflammatory disorders like AD [35], indicating TBI as a risk factor for AD. In a study involving 2719 subjects with mild cognitive impairment (MCI) with or without a history of TBI, LoBue et al. observed a history of TBI was not associated with progression from MCI to AD but suggested that TBI might reduce the threshold for the onset of MCI and certain neurodegenerative conditions [36]. Head trauma can lead to overexpression of β-amyloid precursor protein which may accumulate in the brain in a similar way to that observed in AD patients [37]. Research data have shown that people with a history of TBI are more prone to the development of AD pathologies due to altered brain vasculature [38].

TBI-induced pituitary dysfunction is a common occurrence [39] and was first described 95 years ago [40]. Pituitary dysfunction resulting from mild or moderate TBI may be self-recovering; however, adrenocorticotropic hormone (ACTH) and GH deficiency may be persistent in severe TBI patients [39]. Mild repetitive head trauma is often associated with hypopituitarism—the inability of the pituitary to provide sufficient hormones in the body to maintain homeostasis. Eight percent to 57% of children [3,41] and 11%—69% of adults [42,43] suffer from TBI-induced hypopituitarism. Oftentimes it may remain unrecognized because of its nonspecific disease manifestations, the underestimated health risks associated with it, and the lack of physicians' awareness [43,44]. In addition to these, symptoms like attention deficits, depression, sleep abnormalities, impulsive disorders, and cognitive disorders are seen in TBI patients with or without neuroendocrine changes [39], which make the diagnosis more difficult. In a study involving more than 1000 adult patients, Schneider et al. observed that 27.5% of TBI patients suffered from hypopituitarism [45] with male patients in their 30s being typically affected [46]. Total pituitary dysfunction has been found to be permanent while partial dysfunction evolves over time and the symptoms may manifest in a few days to years after injury, resolving or worsening over time [43,44,46]. In children the major complications associated with TBI-induced pituitary dysfunction involve hyperprolactinemia and growth hormone (GH) deficiency which are often resolved in a year postinjury [41,47]. Due to its anatomical location the anterior pituitary is most vulnerable to primary mechanical insult [42,48]. The hypothalamopituitary structure has a unique vasculature and microanatomy with specialized anterior pituitary cells producing different hormones. Because of the anatomical location and structure, the

GH-producing cells of the anterior pituitary are the most vulnerable to traumatic insults and GH deficiency (GHD) is the most common pituitary dysfunction observed after TBI [40]. Secondary insults including hypotension, hypoxia, elevated intracranial pressure, edema, hemorrhage, and metabolites may also contribute to the hypothalamic–pituitary axis (HPA) damage [48].

The concept of autoimmunity in the development of hypopituitarism was first proposed by Goudie and Pinkerton in 1962 [49]. The association of TBI and hypopituitarism has been gaining attention since then and has been reported by several authors. Recently guidelines for appropriate screening and treatment have been developed [42–44]. As a major possible mechanism of TBI-induced hypopituitarism, persistent neuroinflammation and autoimmunity have been proposed, especially in genetically predisposed patients [40]. Persistent neuroinflammation including the increase of IL 1β and GFAP in the cortex, hypothalamus, and pituitary, leading to secondary neurodegeneration in experimental animals, could be responsible for HPA dysfunction [50]. Tanriverdi et al. showed the involvement of APA in TBI-induced pituitary dysfunction in human subjects. They conducted a study to investigate the role of APAs in the development of post-TBI pituitary insufficiency in a cohort of patients who completed 3 years of follow-up. 44.8% of TBI patients showed serum APA compared to 0% in normal, age-matched controls. They observed significant association between APA level and TBI-induced pituitary dysfunction [22]. These observations were verified by subsequent studies [22,51]. In a 5-year follow-up study patients who were suffering from persistent pituitary deficiency were diagnosed with strong APA positivity and the patients who recovered had no antibody developed [51]. In a recent study among 61 boxers suffering from mild repetitive head trauma, Tanriverdi et al. assessed the HPA axis function and autoimmunity. Antihypothalamic antibody (AHA) and APA were found in 23.1% and 22.9% of boxers, respectively, but not in the healthy, age-matched controls. Eleven of the 61 boxers showed symptoms of hypopituitarism, two with ACTH deficiency, six with GH deficiency, three with both. Six of the boxers were AHA positive and three were APA positive [21]. These results show that TBI-associated hypopituitarism is a frequent phenomenon. It mostly affects the GH axis and suggests the involvement of HPA autoimmunity in its pathogenesis. The presence of AHA and APA at high titers is the risk factor for the onset and persistence of TBI-induced hypopituitarism, in which chronic neuroinflammation plays a major role [4].

5.3 How the immune system responds to traumatic brain injury? Role of innate and adaptive immune responses

Traditionally it has been believed that only innate immune response is responsible for TBI-induced immune response and inflammation, but recent studies have shown that adaptive responses may also play significant roles. During early neuroinflammatory response following TBI, the primary injury causes the release of cytokines and chemokines, resulting in local and systemic immune response, the main objective of which is to limit the spread of damage and restore homeostasis [52–55].

5.3.1 Innate immune response to traumatic brain injury: role of cytokines and chemokines

Cytokines, released by a variety of cells including microglia, macrophages, T and B cells, endothelial, and mast cells [56,57], are mediators of cellular immune response and antibody synthesis and can be pro- or antiinflammatory in function [9]. Several investigators have reported that TNF α, IL1-β, and IL18 are some of the major cytokines involved in the development of inflammatory reactions in the brain. IL1 receptors are primarily present on microglia and astrocytes but their presence on the infiltrating immune cells has also been reported [58,59]. Binding of IL1-β with IL1 receptors activates the release of other cytokines including TNFα, IL18, and more IL1-β [59] and initiates the proinflammatory reactions that are potentially damaging to the brain tissues [52−54,60−62]. TNFα is especially important in triggering cytokine production including IL1-β and IL6, chemokine production, and also activation of the transcription factors of the nuclear factor kappa B (NFκB) family [53,63,64], and thus modulates the inflammation in neuronal and nonneuronal tissues. On the other hand, IL18 when binding with IL18 receptors activates a neuroinflammatory cascade which plays an important role in delayed neuroinflammation and neuronal injury [52,65].

Chemokines are small ($\leq$10 kDa), chemoattractant proteins that cause the migration of immune cells and their interaction with target cells. In the CNS, astrocytes and microglia have been reported to synthesize and release chemokines. Macrophages, granulocytes, dendritic cells (DCs), mast cells, and natural killer (NK) cells also produce chemokines [66−68]. Following TBI chemokines attract the immune cells to the site of damage [69,70]. For example, CXC chemokines activate the migration of lymphocytes to the injury sites [71]. CCL chemokines, like CCL2, CCL3, CCL5, CCL7, CCL8, CCL13, CCL17, and CCL22, attract monocytes and macrophages to the brain following injury [72−74]. CCL1, CCL2, CCL17, and CCL22 are also involved in the recruitment of T cells [73]. It has also been observed that CCL20 is expressed locally and systemically following TBI in an experimental rat model of lateral fluid percussion injury and plays an important role in neurodegeneration [75,76]. This chemokine has also been implicated in aggravating neuroinflammation and attracting Th17 cells following SCI [77].

Cytokines and chemokines are also involved in activating PRRs which identify danger-associated molecular patterns (DAMPs) of cellular stress or damage. This identification elicits responses that help in evoking the defense mechanism to reduce cellular loss or damage [78,79]. For example, cytoplasmic NLRs, also known as nucleotide oligomerization domain (NOD)−like receptors [80], help in regulating inflammation, apoptosis, and innate immune response [81,82] by forming multiprotein "inflammasomes" complexes (NLRP3) after TBI [34]. NLRP3 inflammasomes have been reported to be expressed in neurons and glial cells, especially in astrocytes and microglia, and are associated with IL1-β and IL18 pathways [34,35,81].

Thus cytokines and chemokines play vital roles in immune cell migration to the injury site and mounting innate immune response.

5.3.2 Innate immune response after traumatic brain injury: role of immune cells

Immune cells migrate to the injury site after TBI [69,83,84]. It has been shown that peripheral inflammation may also influence TBI outcome [75,85,86]. After TBI, immune cells in the spleen increase in number and exit the spleen to contribute to cerebral inflammation [85,87,88]. Macrophages, granulocytes, DCs, and NK cells coordinate the innate immune response [9]. In the early phase of TBI, neutrophils and macrophages infiltrate the brain [89,90] and phagocytose the damaged cellular materials [84,91], release free radicals, secrete lysosomal enzymes, cause microvascular occlusion, increase vascular permeability [92–94], and cause BBB breakdown [91,95]. DCs, on the other hand, play an important role in antigen presentation. On contact with the damaged cellular components in the brain DCs get activated and process the antigenic materials. The DCs then travel to lymph nodes, present antigens and evoke systemic immune response [9]. T cells then get activated, migrate toward the brain and accumulate at the injury site, which negatively affects the TBI outcome [84,96,97]. Both resident microglia and infiltrating peripheral macrophages have been observed in high numbers in the injury sites, especially in the cortex [91,98,99]. It has been shown that soluble factors from other cells in the microenvironment of the traumatized brain may influence the macrophages and cause the polarization. Verma et al. have shown that damaged endothelial cells secrete cytokines such as TNFα, TGFβ, IL6, IL25, and IFN-γ, which can affect microglia to macrophage polarization [100], whereas infiltrating T cells can influence macrophage to microglia polarization [101]. Microglial phenotypic shift is of special interest since M2 to M1 polarization has been correlated to impaired basal neurogenesis [100] and functional recovery [102,103]. Peripheral, infiltrating T cells may also get activated by direct contact with antigen-presenting DCs, macrophages and resident microglia [104,105] and the T cell recognition of the presented antigens is the hallmark event in transitioning from innate to adaptive immune response after TBI. Steady increase in the number and types of T cells in the injury site suggests the transition from innate to adaptive immune response [9]. Gelderblom et al. showed that γδ-T cells respond faster than αβ-T cells in an early phase of TBI [106]. The γδ-T cells along with CD4 + and CD8 + T helper-1 cells (T$_H$-1) may cause cytotoxicity and proinflammatory actions [107,108], although there are some suggestions that T cells could be neuroprotective which will be discussed later. The immune cells also play an important role in the transition to adaptive immune response after TBI.

5.3.3 Adaptive immunity after traumatic brain injury

After TBI, once the antigens are processed and presented by professional antigen-presenting cells (APC), T cells recognize the presented antigen and mount the adaptive immune response. Although there are not many studies pointing to this direction, a few studies indicate the switch from innate to adaptive immune response after TBI in rodents [85] and in humans [109]. The cell-mediated adaptive immune response may be carried out by resident brain cells or infiltrating immune cells gaining access through the compromised BBB or chemotactic signals [9]. In most of the cases TBIs are nonpenetrating which causes damage of the tissues and therefore the antigens that are presented to the T cells to evoke adaptive immune response are self-antigens. And thus TBI induces autoimmunity, the mechanisms of which are discussed in detail below.

5.4 Mechanism of autoimmunity development after traumatic brain injury

5.4.1 Autoantigens and autoantibodies

Under normal physiological conditions the immune system is tolerant of the body's own or self-molecules. Natural antibodies that recognize the body's own molecules (self-antigens) are called aAbs and these antibodies provide the body with the first line of defense against pathogens, serve housekeeping functions, and maintain homeostasis [110]. Under normal physiological conditions B lymphocytes produce low amounts of antibodies against self-antigens including a variety of serum proteins, cell surface structures, and intracellular structures [111]. These are encoded by unmutated V(D)J genes [110]. These can be IgG, IgM, or IgA classes of antibodies, have moderate affinity to self-antigens, provide the first line of defense, and are responsible for the homeostasis of the immune system. On the other hand, somatically mutated IgG aAbs indicate pathologic processes. These aAbs are highly specific and may serve as biomarkers of disease processes [110]. aAbs may bind a specific tissue and injure a particular organ (organ-specific aAb) or may bind with circulating or free antigens causing systemic autoimmune disorders [110]. Studies on target-specific autoimmune disorders, such as myasthenia gravis (MG), indicate that development of aAbs is stimulated by inflammation in the target organs [110]. Modifications including phosphorylation, oxidation, and cleavage of these self-antigen molecules give rise to neoepitopes which may also be recognized by the immune cells. As the BBB is disrupted following TBI, the release of these molecules in the peripheral circulation is facilitated. The circulating aAgs are then recognized and treated by the immune cells as foreign antigens and evoke the systemic production of both IgM and IgG isoforms of aAbs. The aAbs produced in the serum may penetrate the BBB and affect the CNS functions [15]. Brain-specific aAbs have been proposed by several authors and their contributions in the development of brain pathologies have been debated. In subsets of TBI patients, these circulating aAbs have been shown to recognize a range of brain proteins, including glial proteins like GFAP, S100B, and peroxiredoxin, and neuroreceptors such as glutamate receptor subunits NR1 and MBP from oligodendrocytes [112]. Recently, Davies and Skoda have shown that TBI or SCI patients developed a number of brain-directed aAbs targeting a number of CNS self-antigens including GM1 gangliosides, myelin-associated glycoprotein, alpha-amino-3-hydroxy-5-methyl-4-isoxazolepropionic acid (AMPA), N-methyl-D-aspartate (NMDA) glutamate receptors, and beta-III-tubulin and nuclear antigens [113–115]. Later on, data presented by Marchi [116] and Zhang [11] on TBI and Ankeney and Popovich [16] on SCI strongly suggest that the antibrain immune reactivity poses a potential threat to brain tissue integrity [117] (Fig. 5.1).

GFAP is one of the major targets of brain-directed autoimmunity. It is a monomeric, intermediate filament protein encoded by the GFAP gene. It is specific to brain tissues and is expressed in the cytoskeleton of astrocytes, the most abundant cell type in the CNS [118]. GFAP aAb (anti-GFAP-IgG) has been correlated to autoimmune astrocytopathy [119]. Under physiological condition it has not been detected in the CSF or peripheral circulation. However, the death of astrocytes due to traumatic events in the brain releases GFAP in the peripheral circulation and can evoke the production of the antibody. Thus it

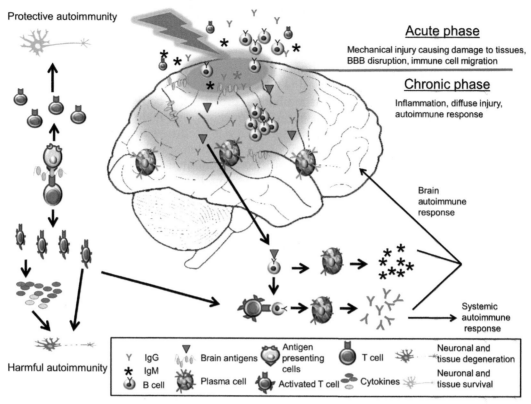

FIGURE 5.1   Schematic representation of development and consequences of autoimmunity in the brain. Following TBI in the acute phase, neurons and other tissues degenerate, BBB disrupts, immune cells migrate to the injury site. In the chronic phase diffuse axonal injury occurs, B cells aggregate and elicit autoimmune responses. Cellular degeneration releases autoantigens which are presented by APCs and T cells are activated. The autoimmunity can be harmful or protective. Th1 and Th17 cells may release cytokines which destroy the neurons and other tissues. On the other hand, Th2 cells produce IL4 and CD4 + cells produce BDNF which are neuroprotective. B cells presenting autoantigens react with activated T cells and produce plasma cells. Plasma cells release autoantibodies which can be brain directed causing further cellular damage in the brain and chronic neuroinflammation in the brain or elicit systemic autoimmune responses.

can be used as a biomarker in the detection of TBI [120]. Investigators have also established the correlation between serum GFAP levels, pathological changes of the brain and clinical outcomes in patients suffering from TBI [121]. It has a greater prognostic value compared to other TBI biomarkers like NSE and S100B protein [122]. In a study, serum levels of aAbs from 53 patients with severe TBI were compared with age-matched healthy controls. TBI patients developed aAbs directed mainly against GFAP and its BDPs. GFAP aAbs of IgG subtype developed at day 7 post TBI in 67% of the patients and possibly could remain up to 6 months after injury. The aAb developed in the TBI patients caused glial cytotoxicity. Thus TBI aAb was potentially pathogenic during the recovery phase after TBI [11]. The mechanistic role of the anti-GFAP aAbs is still not clear. An increased level of GFAP aAb indicates more severe injury, although the presence of this aAb in 16% of apparently normal patients indicates a nonpathogenic role of this aAb [11]. Regardless of its beneficial or pathogenic role, anti-GFAP aAb can potentially serve as a biomarker for TBI in humans [11], which has been described in detail later in this chapter.

S100B is an astroglial protein. BBB disruption following TBI may cause leakage of this protein in the serum resulting in a surge in the serum protein level and evoke aAb development. A study conducted by Marchi et al. [116] among American football players having repeated TBI or concussions (rTBI) showed an increase in serum S100B protein and serum aAb correlated with neurological changes as detected by diffusion tensor imaging (DTI). These changes were linked with BBB disruption and the future risk of cognitive deficits. A high level of aAb to S100B was observed in the first days of severe TBI in children. This along with low levels of aAb to NR2-subtype of glutamate receptors indicated a failure of the compensatory-adaptive immunological mechanism and the presence of a highly permeable BBB associated with poor prognosis in children with severe TBI [123]. Sorokina et al. [124] correlated S100B protein and serum aAB to the severity and outcomes of TBI. In patients with complete recovery, moderate or high level of disability, S100B level in serum did not depend on the severity of the brain damage. In these patients the elevated levels of S100B went back to normal level in 2–3 days after injury. On the other hand, increase in aAb in these groups started 3–5 days post injury depending on the severity of the damage. They also observed that in the patients who developed a vegetative state or died the serum S100B protein level was low and aAB to S100B was elevated [124].

Enolase is a glycolytic enzyme and plasminogen binding protein playing multiple roles in growth control, hypoxia, immune tolerance, and ischemia [125–128]. It can stimulate IgG production [129] and take part in immune reactions. Following injury it increases and activates the endothelial cells [130]. Its function in promoting pathologies in injury, infection, transplantation, or autoimmunity depends on the inflammatory signals it receives [125,127,131]. Although it is expressed in tissues throughout the body, its isoforms are tissue specific. Enolase 2 or γ enolase is the NSE isoform found in neurons. Following injury it is secreted in the blood or CSF, increasing its level in the biofluid, and may serve as an indicator of the severity of spinal cord or brain injury [129,132]. It is potentially damaging to the neurons and elevated levels cause neurotoxicity, neuronal apoptosis, and evoke neuroinflammation.

MBP with its several splice variants is an important protein for myelination of the nerve fibers. MBP has been extensively studied in the demyelinating disease of MS. Studies have shown the role of aAb against MBP in the development of MS [133]. Axonal injury is a key feature of TBI in which the integrity of the myelin sheath is compromised. Increased CSF concentration of MBP after severe TBI in children has been shown by Su et al. [134]. In a rat model of TBI Liu et al. have reported that the 21.5- and 18.5-kDa MBP isoforms degraded into N-terminal fragments of 10 and 8 kDa in the ipsilateral hippocampus and cortex after controlled cortical impact induced TBI [135]. In another study by Ngankam et al., CSF of 100 TBI patients was assessed for MBP and phospholipids (PL) aAbs on the first, 10th, and 21st days postinjury. Interestingly, aAbs against MBP and PL were elevated in TBI groups. MBP aAbs were shown to correlate with the GCS in the first days and the level of recovery on the 21st day. PL aAbs were correlated to the severity of vascular complications of trauma [136].

Peroxiredoxin 6 (PRDX6), an antioxidant enzyme, could be a target for aAbs following TBI. This enzyme is expressed in the perivascular space and contained within the astrocytic foot processes of rats and highly expressed in human cerebral cortex and platelets [137]. An immunosorbent electrochemiluminescent assay has shown that circulating level of this enzyme increases fourfold following TBI in humans. In addition, proteolytic fragments of ubiquitin D-terminal hydrolase-L-1 (UCH-L1), a highly specific neuronal protein and essential component of ubiquitin protease system, have been observed after TBI [138–140].

5.4.2 Role of B and T cells in traumatic brain injury-induced autoimmunity

In classical neurodegenerative diseases like AD and MS, inflammation as well as immune regulation plays an important role in the disease development process. But in the case of TBI how the brain affects the immune system and how the immune system reacts to TBI is not fully known. However, recent research data shows that T and B cells play key roles in brain injury and repair [141–143]. Also, in traumatic SCI, the role of aAbs in exacerbating tissue damage and impairing neurological recovery has been shown [141,142].

Traditionally it has been believed that CNS is an immune-privileged site. However, under physiological conditions the spaces of the CNS drained by CSF, such as the perivascular, leptomeningeal, and ventricular spaces, can be accessed by activated cells of the adaptive immune system in the absence of neuroinflammation in their search for cognate antigens. Bone marrow-derived macrophages and DCs have been observed in these spaces to present CNS antigens [144]. In the case of CNS pathologies like MS, stroke, trauma, etc., immune cells migrate to the CNS. The BBB is disrupted and allows the migrating bone marrow-derived macrophages to invade the brain in support of resident microglia. Likewise, under physiological conditions T lymphocytes are not found in the brain parenchyma, but are instead located in the meninges. Kivisakk et al. [145] and Schlager et al. [146], using intravital two-photon microscopy, showed that T cells enter the meninges and CSF through blood vessels in the pia mater and arachnoid space, collectively called leptomeninges, the blood vessels in the dura mater, and the choroid plexus [145,146]. The cells exit the meninges through the meningeal lymphatic vessels to the deep cervical lymph nodes [147–149]. TBI leads to the development of inflammatory cascades that cause the activation and migration of immune cells to the site of injury [150,151] and the release of cytokines and chemokines. Injury to CNS leads to global immunological changes in the body [109], including changes in the spleen, deep cervical lymph nodes, meningeal compartments, including CSF, and the injury site [75,86,152–156]. Following injury, the injured tissue releases cytokines such as interleukin 33 (IL33), ATP, and HMGB1. These molecules activate the glial cells and recruit granulocytes and monocytes to the injury site [153,157]. It has been shown that mice lacking IL33 or HMGB1 fail to recruit monocytes and show worse injury outcome [158].

In the case of infections, the invading "nonself" pathogens are recognized by mature B cell receptors and coreceptors and presented to T cells. T-cell recognition and subsequent proliferation and cytokine release initiate an inflammatory reaction cascade in an attempt to remove the antigen from the body. But, when the antigens originate from the host body proteins, which are nonpathogenic and of "self" origin, autoreactive immune cells recognize them and an autoimmune response is elicited. During development most of the highly autoreactive lymphocytes are deleted from the body by a negative selection mechanism in the thymus. The surviving lymphocytes undergo positive selection in which they are exposed to "subthreshold" stimulation with self-antigens and this process helps increase the lymphocyte sensitivity to pathogenic antigens [159]. When the self-antigenic stimulation crosses the threshold, the autoreactive cells cause pathological damage to organs. It has been reported that T-dependent and T-independent self-antigens caused by traumatic injuries of the CNS elicit adaptive immune responses causing functional consequences [141,142,160]. After injury the autoantigens drain into peripheral lymphatic system which might activate naïve neuroantigen-reactive lymphocytes. In addition, in SCI patients B cell responses are enhanced and IgM- and IgG-secreting cells in bone marrow and spleen increase postinjury [142]. Approximately 50%−60% of TBI or SCI patients produce aAbs against several neuroantigens including myelin-associated glycoprotein, GM1 gangliosides, AMPA and NMDA glutamate receptors, β-III-tubulin, and nuclear antigens [113,114].

5.4.2.1 B cells and autoantibody production

A hallmark event in the posttraumatic immune reaction cascade, besides the activation of neutrophils and T lymphocytes [161−165], is the activation of B cells. When the B cells are activated in the presence of their cognate antigens they start differentiating into antibody secreting plasma cells [166,167]. B cells can also act as APCs [167,168]. These activated B cells make their way to secondary lymphoid tissues, bone marrow, and CNS [166,167]. It has been a long time since a study by Prochazka et al. revealed the higher levels of antibodies against gangliosides and PL in sera from humans suffering from TBI [169]. Rudehill et al. analyzed the expression pattern of antibrain immunity after TBI in experimental animals. They used serum collected from control rat or rat undergone experimental TBI incubated with rat brains to detect autoreactive IgG and IgM antibodies. They used antirat IgG and IgM antibodies to identify tissue-bound aAbs. Immunohistochemistry with rat serum was used to detect antineuronal and antiastrocytic antibodies. The aAbs were identified in the serum but not in the brain tissues 2 weeks postinjury, indicating the reformation of BBB prevented the chronic passage of the aAbs to the brain parenchyma. They identified antibrain-reactive B cells but not T cells and observed the appearance of antineuronal antibodies early in the inflammatory sequels indicating the potential of B cells in causing delayed neurodegeneration following TBI [117]. Fig. 5.1 shows a schematic representation of autoimmunity development after TBI.

5.4.2.2 T cells and traumatic brain injury-induced autoimmunity

Although not fully understood, most of the research data indicate that the net outcome of the spontaneous T cell response to injury is that neuroprotective. T cells seem to help in the recovery phase after TBI [147]. Following TBI T cells are recruited from the bloodstream starting at day 1 post injury and reach their peak around days 4−10 post injury [152]. Chemokine signaling and upregulated adhesion molecules on the vascular endothelium [170] initiate the recruitment. Activated integrins on the T cell surface facilitate the binding and extravasation [171]. Adhesion molecules are tissue specific. For example, T cell extravasation and homing to the CNS and meninges is facilitated by binding of very late antigen 4 (VLA4) to vascular cell adhesion molecule 1 (VCAM1) [172]. T cell homing in the meninges is antigen dependent [173], although not much information is available regarding the antigen specificity of the T cells [171]. Investigators have suggested that the beneficial effect of T cells are mediated by autoreactive T cell-specific brain antigens [174–178]. In optic nerve crush and SCI models investigators have found MBP-specific T cell accumulation in the injury site limiting the secondary neurodegeneration [176,179,180].

The normal T cell repertoire of the body contains self-reacting lymphocytes, including antimyelin lymphocytes [181,182], which under normal circumstances remain under control, but after TBI the systemic release of myelin protein may break the tolerance causing proliferation and expansion of the T cells [20]. These antimyelin T cells may be involved in mediating cerebral inflammation [183] and could promote repair. Cox et al. [20] have shown that in mice autoreactive T cell responses against myelin antigens are associated with improved neuronal survival and functional recovery [20]. Other studies have demonstrated that systemic autoreactive T cells including T helper type 1 (Th1) cells reduce neuronal cell death in murine models [184,185]. Similar responses were observed in humans after TBI where a T-cell expansion recognizing the myelin protein was observed after TBI [20]. In stroke model also T cell autoimmune responses have been implicated in both worsening or improving the recovery [186]. MBP-responsiveness of Th1 cells indicated worsening [187,188], whereas reactivity to neural antigens was associated with improvement [189]. A recent study by Walsh et al. has pointed to an antigen-independent mechanism of T cell action after trauma. Although the beneficial response was found not to be completely dependent on T cell receptor (TCR)—major histocompatibility complex II (MHC II) interaction, it was dependent on myeloid differentiation primary response protein 88 (MYD88) and T cell-derived IL-4 [152], thus indicating multiple mechanisms, antigen dependent or independent, of T cell action after injury.

Type 1 immunity characterized by intense phagocytic activity is mediated by Th1 lymphocytes which secrete interleukin (IL)-2, interferon-gamma (IFNγ), and lymphotoxin-α. On the other hand, type 2 immunity is characterized by high antibody titers where Th2 cells secrete IL-4, IL-5, IL-9, IL-10, and IL-13. Type 1 and type 2 immunities are not strictly cell-mediated. These are also humoral immunity because Th1 cells stimulate moderate levels of antibody production and Th2 cells suppress phagocytic activities [190]. Proinflammatory Th1-mediated responses are generally considered harmful to the host. However, in a landmark study, Moalem et al. [174] reported that pathogenic Th1 cells exerted protective effect at the trauma site in the CNS as the rat was developing EAE at the same time [174]. When autoreactive T cells were injected in subpathogenic number into naïve animals, macrophages were recruited and activated simultaneously with the neuroprotective effect of Th1 cells. This observation indicates that Th1 cells were probably responsible for the recruitment and activation of macrophages, which is an essential step in the development of autoimmune disorders [191,192]. Contradictory reports also exist. Rapalino et al. observed that implanted macrophages promoted tissue repair [193]. Thus whether the type 1 autoimmune response is beneficial or harmful to the host remains debatable. Initially all investigators believed that type 2 autoimmune responses were Th1 mediated [194]. Subsequently it has been observed that autoreactive Th2 cells may also induce pathology on their own [195,196].

5.5 Autoantibodies as putative biomarkers

aAbs developed against a distinct antigen may have potentially beneficial or harmful consequences in the disease process. They may be protective or pathogenic, but they might serve as important biomarkers in the diagnosis of the diseases. As mentioned earlier, while aAgs may serve as biomarkers of the acute injury, aAbs represent potential biomarkers for chronic, long-lasting injury phases. aAbs can be correlated to several disease activities, disease or injury-related symptoms years before the onset of the symptoms, and also to the severity of the diseases [115]. aAbs are also valuable indicators of therapeutic response to biologic drugs, side effects, diagnosis, and management of organ-specific or nonorgan-specific disorders [115,197]. Table 5.1 lists aAbs related to TBI and other neurodegenerative conditions.

Studies conducted by Marchi et al. [116] on American football players and Zhang et al. [11] on human patients show the real utility of aAbs as potential biomarkers. In 2013 Marchi et al. published their study on American college football players. Football players experiencing repeated concussions had elevated serum levels of astrocytic S100B protein and aAb-S100B. Marchi et al. hypothesized that BBB disruption was coupled with S100B protein in blood which led to elevated aAb-S100B. Sixty-seven players were evaluated before and after the game and the number of repeated hits was recorded for each player and compared. Using DTI white matter damage was identified and this data was correlated with serum levels of S100B pre- and postseason. The evaluation was conducted at 6-month intervals. The data was then correlated with functional and cognitive assessments. Abnormal cognitive changes were associated with white matter damage (as observed with DTI) and elevated serum S100B levels. They also observed that increased aAb-S100B was correlated to repeated concussion and BBB disruption [116]. Soon after this study, Zhang et al. published their observation on human TBI serum sample analysis. They performed a systematic analysis of human TBI serum samples to identify aAb responses to brain-specific antigens. They observed that human aAbs were immunoreactive to a cluster of proteins. This cluster of proteins of 38—50 kDa was identified as GFAP and their BDPs, belonging to the IgG subtype, and it increased at 7—10 days post injury. They translated this result into rats and showed that human TBI aAbs were colocalized in the injured rat

TABLE 5.1   TBI-induced autoantibodies, their location, and potential targets.

Autoantibody	Biofluid compartment	Target	References
Antineurofilament	Serum, CSF	Axonal protein	[198—201]
Antineuronal antibody	Serum	Neurons	[202,203]
Antimyelin basic protein	Serum	Myelin	[26]
Antiglial fibrillary acidic protein	Serum	Glial protein	[11,204,205]
Antiacetylcholine receptor	Serum	Acetylcholine receptor	[11,201,206]
Antispectrin	Serum, CSF, Saliva	Spectrin (αII spectrin)	[25,201,206—208]
Anti-S100B	Serum	S100 family	[116,209]
Antienolase (neuron-specific enolase)	Serum, CSF	Enolase	[177,210,211]

brain following TBI. They further observed that these aAbs were colocalized in the primary culture indicating the possibility of the entry of the aAbs into the astrocytes compromising their survival. The in vitro study indicated that calpain was responsible for yielding 38 kDa GFAP-BDP by fragmenting GFAP. A neuroproteomic analysis was conducted on 53 severe TBI patients and age-matched healthy controls. Serum samples were collected on 0−10 days post injury. Sixty-seven percent of TBI patients showed, on an average, 3.77-fold increase in anti-GFAP antibodies on 0−1 days (early) to 7−10 days (late) post injury. A 6-month follow-up showed that these increased levels of anti-GFAP antibody were negatively correlated to GCS score, indicating that TBI patients with higher levels of anti-GFAP antibody had worse outcome. Thus aAb-GFAP represents an excellent potential biomarker with the potential to be used in monitoring and assessing the status of injured brain long after TBI [11].

In addition to the abovementioned studies, Ngankam et al. found aAb against MBP in CSF of TBI patients which was correlated to GCS to show the recovery on the 21st day [136]. Sorokina et al. found aAb against α7 subunit of acetylcholine receptor in children with craniocerebral trauma and correlated the trauma severity with antibody titer [115]. S100β protein and aAb levels were assessed in children with varied severity and outcome. The maximum levels were identified in children with fatal outcome and in groups with complete recovery, moderate or high disability; S100β did not depend on the degree of brain damage. The S100β protein levels went up the first day and then declined. On the other hand, S100β aAbs were elevated at days 3 and 5 [124].

These studies clearly demonstrate the potential of aAbs as biomarkers in TBI. The properties of different aAbs are shown in Table 5.1.

5.6 Conclusion

TBI is a combination of complex pathophysiological events with the potential to cause several short- and long-term detrimental consequences. TBI evokes a complex brain−immune system interaction. In this complex mechanism following TBI, aAbs are produced causing further damage to the brain tissues. It is also possible that in this process memory T cells are produced and reactivation of these cells by injury or other neuroinflammatory stimulus might reopen the BBB to initiate another sequelae of inflammatory cascades leading to posttraumatic autoimmune disorders. Thus TBI-induced aAbs provide a new area of investigation as putative biomarkers. The importance of cognate proteins as short-term biomarkers and their corresponding aAbs as long-term biomarkers should be appreciated.

References

[1] Centers for Disease Control and Prevention, C., Report to congress on traumatic brain injury in the United States: epidemiology and rehabilitation. National Center for Injury Prevention and Control; Division of Unintentional Injury Prevention. Atlanta, GA; 2015.
[2] National Center for Injury Prevention and Control, C., Rates of TBI-related emergency dartment visits, hospitalizations, and deaths—United States, 2001−2010; 2016.

[3] Personnier C, et al. Prevalence of pituitary dysfunction after severe traumatic brain injury in children and adolescents: a large prospective study. J Clin Endocrinol Metab 2014;99(6):2052−60.

[4] Guaraldi F, et al. Hypothalamic-pituitary autoimmunity and traumatic brain injury. J Clin Med 2015;4 (5):1025−35.

[5] Masel BE, DeWitt DS. Traumatic brain injury: a disease process, not an event. J Neurotrauma 2010;27 (8):1529−40.

[6] Thompson HJ, et al. Lateral fluid percussion brain injury: a 15-year review and evaluation. J Neurotrauma 2005;22(1):42−75.

[7] Bramlett HM, Dietrich WD. Progressive damage after brain and spinal cord injury: pathomechanisms and treatment strategies. Prog Brain Res 2007;161:125−41.

[8] Marklund N, et al. Evaluation of pharmacological treatment strategies in traumatic brain injury. Curr Pharm Des 2006;12(13):1645−80.

[9] Nizamutdinov D, Shapiro LA. Overview of traumatic brain injury: an immunological context. Brain Sci 2017;7(1).

[10] Povlishock JT, Christman CW. The pathobiology of traumatically induced axonal injury in animals and humans: a review of current thoughts. J Neurotrauma 1995;12(4):555−64.

[11] Zhang Z, et al. Human traumatic brain injury induces autoantibody response against glial fibrillary acidic protein and its breakdown products. PLoS One 2014;9(3):e92698.

[12] Colasanti T, Rosano BC, Malorni G, Ortona W. E., Autoantibodies in patients with Alzheimer's disease: pathogenetic role and potential use as biomarkers of disease progression. Autoimmun Rev 2010;12:807−11.

[13] Ponomarenko NA, et al. Catalytic activity of autoantibodies toward myelin basic protein correlates with the scores on the multiple sclerosis expanded disability status scale. Immunol Lett 2006;103(1):45−50.

[14] Dambinova SA, et al. Blood test detecting autoantibodies to N-methyl-D-aspartate neuroreceptors for evaluation of patients with transient ischemic attack and stroke. Clin Chem 2003;49(10):1752−62.

[15] Lang B, Dale RC, Vincent A. New autoantibody mediated disorders of the central nervous system. Curr Opin Neurol 2003;16(3):351−7.

[16] Ankeny DP, Popovich G. B cells and autoantibodies: complex roles in CNS injury. Trends Immunol 2010;31 (9):332−8.

[17] Popovich G, Stokes BT, Whitacre CC. Concept of autoimmunity following spinal cord injury: possible roles for T lymphocytes in the traumatized central nervous system. J Neurosci Res 1996;45(4):349−63.

[18] Schwartz M, Hauben E. T cell-based therapeutic vaccination for spinal cord injury. Prog Brain Res 2002;137:401−6.

[19] Hauben E, Nevo U, Yoles E, Moalem G, Agranov E, Mor F, et al. Autoimmune T cells as potential neuroprotective therapy for spinal cord injury. Lancet 2000;355(9200):286−7.

[20] Cox AL, et al. An investigation of auto-reactivity after head injury. J Neuroimmunol 2006;174(1−2):180−6.

[21] Tanriverdi F, et al. Investigation of antihypothalamus and antipituitary antibodies in amateur boxers: is chronic repetitive head trauma-induced pituitary dysfunction associated with autoimmunity? Eur J Endocrinol 2010;162(5):861−7.

[22] Tanriverdi F, et al. Antipituitary antibodies after traumatic brain injury: is head trauma-induced pituitary dysfunction associated with autoimmunity? Eur J Endocrinol 2008;159(1):7−13.

[23] Anderson KJ, et al. The phosphorylated axonal form of the neurofilament subunit NF-H (pNF-H) as a blood biomarker of traumatic brain injury. J Neurotrauma 2008;25(9):1079−85.

[24] Brophy GM, et al. Biokinetic analysis of ubiquitin C-terminal hydrolase-L1 (UCH-L1) in severe traumatic brain injury patient biofluids. J Neurotrauma 2011;28(6):861−70.

[25] Brophy GM, et al. alphaII-Spectrin breakdown product cerebrospinal fluid exposure metrics suggest differences in cellular injury mechanisms after severe traumatic brain injury. J Neurotrauma 2009;26(4):471−9.

[26] Hedegaard CJ, et al. Autoantibodies to myelin basic protein (MBP) in healthy individuals and in patients with multiple sclerosis: a role in regulating cytokine responses to MBP. Immunology 2009;128(1 Suppl.): e451−61.

[27] Goryunova AV, et al. Glutamate receptor autoantibody concentrations in children with chronic post-traumatic headache. Neurosci Behav Physiol 2007;37(8):761−4.

[28] Tanriverdi F, Kelestimur F. Neuroendocrine disturbances after brain damage: an important and often undiagnosed disorder. J Clin Med 2015;4(5):847−57.

[29] Tanriverdi F, et al. Pituitary dysfunction after traumatic brain injury: a clinical and pathophysiological approach. Endocr Rev. 2015;36(3):305−42.

[30] Chaudhuri A, Behan O. Acute cervical hyperextension-hyperflexion injury may precipitate and/or exacerbate symptomatic multiple sclerosis. Eur J Neurol 2001;8(6):659−64.

[31] Rugbjerg K, et al. Risk of Parkinson's disease after hospital contact for head injury: population based case-control study. BMJ 2008;337:a2494.

[32] Nemetz N, et al. Traumatic brain injury and time to onset of Alzheimer's disease: a population-based study. Am J Epidemiol 1999;149(1):32−40.

[33] Andersen OM, et al. Molecular dissection of the interaction between amyloid precursor protein and its neuronal trafficking receptor SorLA/LR11. Biochemistry 2006;45(8):2618−28.

[34] Liu HD, et al. Expression of the NLRP3 inflammasome in cerebral cortex after traumatic brain injury in a rat model. Neurochem Res 2013;38(10):72−2083.

[35] Martinon F, Burns K, Tschopp J. The inflammasome: a molecular platform triggering activation of inflammatory caspases and processing of proIL-beta. Mol Cell 2002;10(2):417−26.

[36] LoBue C, et al. Traumatic brain injury history and progression from mild cognitive impairment to Alzheimer disease. Neuropsychology 2018;32(4):401−9.

[37] Graham DI, et al. Altered beta-APP metabolism after head injury and its relationship to the aetiology of Alzheimer's disease. Acta Neurochir Suppl 1996;66:96−102.

[38] Franzblau M, et al. Vascular damage: a persisting pathology common to Alzheimer's disease and traumatic brain injury. Med Hypotheses 2013;81(5):842−5.

[39] Kelestimur F. Growth hormone deficiency after traumatic brain injury in adults: when to test and how to treat? Pediatr Endocrinol Rev 2009;6(Suppl. 4):534−9.

[40] Karaca Z, et al. GH and pituitary hormone alterations after traumatic brain injury. Prog Mol Biol Transl Sci 2016;138:167−91.

[41] Auble BA, et al. Hypopituitarism in pediatric survivors of inflicted traumatic brain injury. J Neurotrauma 2014;31(4):321−6.

[42] Richmond E, Rogol AD. Traumatic brain injury: endocrine consequences in children and adults. Endocrine 2014;45(1):3−8.

[43] Gasco V, et al. Hypopituitarism following brain injury: when does it occur and how best to test? Pituitary 2012;15(1):20−4.

[44] Ghigo E, et al. Consensus guidelines on screening for hypopituitarism following traumatic brain injury. Brain Inj 2005;19(9):711−24.

[45] Schneider HJ, et al. Prevalence of anterior pituitary insufficiency 3 and 12 months after traumatic brain injury. Eur J Endocrinol 2006;154(2):259−65.

[46] Benvenga S, et al. Clinical review 113: hypopituitarism secondary to head trauma. J Clin Endocrinol Metab 2000;85(4):1353−61.

[47] Ulutabanca H, et al. Prospective investigation of anterior pituitary function in the acute phase and 12 months after pediatric traumatic brain injury. Childs Nerv Syst 2014;30(6):1021−8.

[48] Dubourg J, Messerer M. Sports-related chronic repetitive head trauma as a cause of pituitary dysfunction. Neurosurg Focus 2011;31(5):E2.

[49] Goudie RB, Pinkerton H. Anterior hypophysitis and Hashimoto's disease in a young woman. J Pathol Bacteriol 1962;83:584−5.

[50] Kasturi BS, Stein DG. Traumatic brain injury causes long-term reduction in serum growth hormone and persistent astrocytosis in the cortico-hypothalamo-pituitary axis of adult male rats. J Neurotrauma 2009;26(8):1315−24.

[51] Tanriverdi F, et al. A five year prospective investigation of anterior pituitary function after traumatic brain injury: is hypopituitarism long-term after head trauma associated with autoimmunity? J Neurotrauma 2013;30(16):1426−33.

[52] Yatsiv I, et al. Elevated intracranial IL-18 in humans and mice after traumatic brain injury and evidence of neuroprotective effects of IL-18−binding protein after experimental closed head injury. J Cereb Blood Flow Metab 2002;22(8):971−8.

[53] Minami M, Kuraishi Y, Satoh M. Effects of kainic acid on messenger RNA levels of IL-1 beta, IL-6, TNF alpha and LIF in the rat brain. Biochem Biophys Res Commun 1991;176(2):593−8.

[54] Liu T, et al. Tumor necrosis factor-alpha expression in ischemic neurons. Stroke 1994;25(7):1481—8.

[55] Chizzolini C, Dayer JM, Miossec P. Cytokines in chronic rheumatic diseases: is everything lack of homeostatic balance? Arthritis Res Ther 2009;11(5):246.

[56] Iwasaki A, Medzhitov R. Regulation of adaptive immunity by the innate immune system. Science 2010;327 (5963):291—5.

[57] Zhang JM, An J. Cytokines, inflammation, and pain. Int Anesthesiol Clin 2007;45(2):27—37.

[58] Dinarello CA. Immunological and inflammatory functions of the interleukin-1 family. Annu Rev Immunol 2009;27:519—50.

[59] Garlanda C, Dinarello CA, Mantovani A. The interleukin-1 family: back to the future. Immunity 2013;39 (6):1003—18.

[60] Dinarello CA. Blocking IL-1 in systemic inflammation. J Exp Med 2005;201(9):1355—9.

[61] Dinarello CA. Interleukin 1 and interleukin 18 as mediators of inflammation and the aging process. Am J Clin Nutr 2006;83(2):447S—55S.

[62] Lu KT, et al. Extracellular signal-regulated kinase-mediated IL-1-induced cortical neuron damage during traumatic brain injury. Neurosci Lett 2005;386(1):40—5.

[63] Grilli M, Memo M. Nuclear factor-kappaB/Rel proteins: a point of convergence of signalling pathways relevant in neuronal function and dysfunction. Biochem Pharmacol 1999;57(1):1—7.

[64] Baeuerle A, Baltimore D. NF-kappa B: ten years after. Cell 1996;87(1):13—20.

[65] Sims JE, Smith DE. The IL-1 family: regulators of immunity. Nat Rev Immunol 2010;10(2):89—102.

[66] Kamimura D, et al. The gateway theory: bridging neural and immune interactions in the CNS. Front Neurosci 2004;7:204.

[67] Gyoneva S, Ransohoff RM. Inflammatory reaction after traumatic brain injury: therapeutic potential of targeting cell-cell communication by chemokines. Trends Pharmacol Sci 2015;36(7):471—80.

[68] Choi SS, et al. Human astrocytes: secretome profiles of cytokines and chemokines. PLoS One 2014;9(4): e92325.

[69] Helmy A, et al. The cytokine response to human traumatic brain injury: temporal profiles and evidence for cerebral parenchymal production. J Cereb Blood Flow Metab 2011;31(2):658—70.

[70] Helmy A, et al. Principal component analysis of the cytokine and chemokine response to human traumatic brain injury. PLoS One 2012;7(6):e39677.

[71] Ono SJ, et al. Chemokines: roles in leukocyte development, trafficking, and effector function. J Allergy Clin Immunol 2003;111(6):1185—99.

[72] Proudfoot AE, et al. Glycosaminoglycan binding and oligomerization are essential for the in vivo activity of certain chemokines. Proc Natl Acad Sci U S A 2003;100(4):1885—90.

[73] Mantovani A, et al. The chemokine system in diverse forms of macrophage activation and polarization. Trends Immunol 2004;25(12):677—86.

[74] Shi C, Pamer EG. Monocyte recruitment during infection and inflammation. Nat Rev Immunol 2011;11 (11):762—74.

[75] Das M, et al. Lateral fluid percussion injury of the brain induces CCL20 inflammatory chemokine expression in rats. J Neuroinflammation 2011;8:148.

[76] Leonardo CC, et al. CCL20 is associated with neurodegeneration following experimental traumatic brain injury and promotes cellular toxicity in vitro. Transl Stroke Res 2012;3(3):357—63.

[77] Hu J, et al. C-C motif chemokine ligand 20 regulates neuroinflammation following spinal cord injury via Th17 cell recruitment. J Neuroinflammation 2016;13(1):162.

[78] Tang D, et al. PAMPs and DAMPs: signal 0s that spur autophagy and immunity. Immunol Rev 2012;249 (1):158—75.

[79] Sansonetti J. The innate signaling of dangers and the dangers of innate signaling. Nat Immunol 2006;7 (12):1237—42.

[80] Trinchieri G, Sher A. Cooperation of Toll-like receptor signals in innate immune defence. Nat Rev Immunol 2007;7(3):179—90.

[81] Ting JP, et al. The NLR gene family: a standard nomenclature. Immunity 2008;28(3):285—7.

[82] Strober W, et al. Signalling pathways and molecular interactions of NOD1 and NOD2. Nat Rev Immunol 2006;6(1):9—20.

[83] Trahanas DM, et al. Differential activation of infiltrating monocyte-derived cells after mild and severe traumatic brain injury. Shock 2015;43(3):255–60.

[84] Rhodes J. Peripheral immune cells in the pathology of traumatic brain injury? Curr Opin Crit Care 2011;17 (2):122–30.

[85] Tobin RP, et al. Traumatic brain injury causes selective, CD74-dependent peripheral lymphocyte activation that exacerbates neurodegeneration. Acta Neuropathol Commun 2014;2:143.

[86] Das M, Mohapatra S, Mohapatra SS. New perspectives on central and peripheral immune responses to acute traumatic brain injury. J Neuroinflammation 2012;9:236.

[87] Schwartz M, Deczkowska A. Neurological disease as a failure of brain-immune crosstalk: the multiple faces of neuroinflammation. Trends Immunol 2016;37(10):668–79.

[88] Schwartz M. Helping the body to cure itself: immune modulation by therapeutic vaccination for spinal cord injury. J Spinal Cord Med 2003;26(Supppl. 1):S6–10.

[89] Foley LM, et al. Magnetic resonance imaging assessment of macrophage accumulation in mouse brain after experimental traumatic brain injury. J Neurotrauma 2009;26(9):1509–19.

[90] Kenne E, et al. Neutrophil depletion reduces edema formation and tissue loss following traumatic brain injury in mice. J Neuroinflammation 2012;9:17.

[91] Soares HD, et al. Inflammatory leukocytic recruitment and diffuse neuronal degeneration are separate pathological processes resulting from traumatic brain injury. J Neurosci 1995;15(12):8223–33.

[92] Harlan JM. Leukocyte-endothelial interactions. Blood 1985;65(3):513–25.

[93] Kochanek M, Hallenbeck JM. Polymorphonuclear leukocytes and monocytes/macrophages in the pathogenesis of cerebral ischemia and stroke. Stroke 1992;23(9):1367–79.

[94] Lucchesi BR, Mullane KM. Leukocytes and ischemia-induced myocardial injury. Annu Rev Pharmacol Toxicol 1986;26:201–24.

[95] Burke-Gaffney A, Keenan AK. Modulation of human endothelial cell permeability by combinations of the cytokines interleukin-1 alpha/beta, tumor necrosis factor-alpha and interferon-gamma. Immunopharmacology 1993;25(1):1–9.

[96] Zindler E, Zipp F. Neuronal injury in chronic CNS inflammation. Best Pract Res Clin Anaesthesiol 2010;24 (4):551–62.

[97] Herz J, Zipp F, Siffrin V. Neurodegeneration in autoimmune CNS inflammation. Exp Neurol 2010;225 (1):9–17.

[98] Jin X, et al. Temporal changes in cell marker expression and cellular infiltration in a controlled cortical impact model in adult male C57BL/6 mice. PLoS One 2012;7(7):e41892.

[99] Mukherjee S, et al. Early TBI-induced cytokine alterations are similarly detected by two distinct methods of multiplex assay. Front Mol Neurosci 2011;4:21.

[100] Verma S, et al. Release of cytokines by brain endothelial cells: a polarized response to lipopolysaccharide. Brain Behav Immun 2006;20(5):449–55.

[101] Biswas SK, Mantovani A. Macrophage plasticity and interaction with lymphocyte subsets: cancer as a paradigm. Nat Immunol 2010;11(10):889–96.

[102] Hu X, et al. Microglia/macrophage polarization dynamics reveal novel mechanism of injury expansion after focal cerebral ischemia. Stroke 2012;43(11):3063–70.

[103] Roughton K, et al. Lipopolysaccharide-induced inflammation aggravates irradiation-induced injury to the young mouse brain. Dev Neurosci 2013;35(5):406–15.

[104] Ni K, O'Neill HC. The role of dendritic cells in T cell activation. Immunol Cell Biol 1997;75(3):223–30.

[105] Pozzi LA, Maciaszek JW, Rock KL. Both dendritic cells and macrophages can stimulate naive CD8 T cells in vivo to proliferate, develop effector function, and differentiate into memory cells. J Immunol 2005;175 (4):2071–81.

[106] Gelderblom M, Arunachalam P, Magnus T. gammadelta T cells as early sensors of tissue damage and mediators of secondary neurodegeneration. Front Cell Neurosci 2014;8:368.

[107] Sobottka B, et al. Collateral bystander damage by myelin-directed CD8 + T cells causes axonal loss. Am J Pathol 2009;175(3):1160–6.

[108] Melzer N, Meuth SG, Wiendl H. CD8 + T cells and neuronal damage: direct and collateral mechanisms of cytotoxicity and impaired electrical excitability. FASEB J 2009;23(11):3659–73.

[109] Hazeldine J, Lord JM, Belli A. Traumatic brain injury and peripheral immune suppression: primer and prospectus. Front Neurol 2015;6:235.

[110] Elkon K, Casali P. Nature and functions of autoantibodies. Nat Clin Pract Rheumatol 2008;4(9):491−8.

[111] Coutinho A, Kazatchkine MD, Avrameas S. Natural autoantibodies. Curr Opin Immunol 1995;7(6):812−18.

[112] Tan Zhihui TZ, Weissman AS, Jaalouk E, Rathore DS, Romo P, Shi Y, et al. Autoimmunity and traumatic brain injury. Curr Phys Med Rehabil Rep 2017;5(1):22−9.

[113] Davies AL, Hayes KC, Dekaban GA. Clinical correlates of elevated serum concentrations of cytokines and autoantibodies in patients with spinal cord injury. Arch Phys Med Rehabil 2007;88(11):1384−93.

[114] Skoda D, et al. Antibody formation against beta-tubulin class III in response to brain trauma. Brain Res Bull 2006;68(4):213−16.

[115] Kobeissy F, Moshourab RA. Autoantibodies in CNS trauma and neuropsychiatric disorders: a new generation of biomarkers. In: Kobeissy FH, editor. Brain Neurotrauma: Molecular, Neuropsychological, and Rehabilitation Aspects. Boca Raton (FL): CRC Press/Taylor & Francis; 2015: Chapter 29. Available from: https://www.ncbi.nlm.nih.gov/books/NBK299208/

[116] Marchi N, et al. Consequences of repeated blood-brain barrier disruption in football players. PLoS One 2013;8(3):e56805.

[117] Rudehill S, et al. Autoreactive antibodies against neurons and basal lamina found in serum following experimental brain contusion in rats. Acta Neurochir (Wien) 2006;148(2):199−205 discussion 205.

[118] Middeldorp J, Hol EM. GFAP in health and disease. Prog Neurobiol 2011;93(3):421−43.

[119] Flanagan EP, et al. Glial fibrillary acidic protein immunoglobulin G as biomarker of autoimmune astrocytopathy: analysis of 102 patients. Ann Neurol 2017;81(2):298−309.

[120] Schiff L, et al. A literature review of the feasibility of glial fibrillary acidic protein as a biomarker for stroke and traumatic brain injury. Mol Diagn Ther 2012;16(2):79−92.

[121] Nylen K, et al. Increased serum-GFAP in patients with severe traumatic brain injury is related to outcome. J Neurol Sci 2006;240(1−2):85−91.

[122] Honda M, et al. Serum glial fibrillary acidic protein is a highly specific biomarker for traumatic brain injury in humans compared with S-100B and neuron-specific enolase. J Trauma 2010;69(1):104−9.

[123] Pinelis VG, et al. Biomarkers in children with traumatic brain injury. Zh Nevrol Psikhiatr Im S S Korsakova 2015;115(8):66−72.

[124] Sorokina EG, et al. S100B protein and autoantibodies to S100B protein in diagnostics of brain damage in craniocerebral trauma in children. Zh Nevrol Psikhiatr Im S S Korsakova 2010;110(8):30−5.

[125] Pancholi V. Multifunctional alpha-enolase: its role in diseases. Cell Mol Life Sci 2001;58(7):902−20.

[126] Diaz-Ramos A, et al. alpha-Enolase, a multifunctional protein: its role on pathophysiological situations. J Biomed Biotechnol 2012;2012:156795.

[127] Fan SS, et al. Decreased expression of alpha-enolase inhibits the proliferation of hypoxia-induced rheumatoid arthritis fibroblasts-like synoviocytes. Mod Rheumatol 2015;25(5):701−7.

[128] Fukano K, Kimura K. Measurement of enolase activity in cell lysates. Meth Enzymol 2014;542:115−24.

[129] Vermeulen N, et al. Anti-alpha-enolase antibodies in patients with inflammatory Bowel disease. Clin Chem 2008;54(3):534−41.

[130] Bock A, et al. alpha-enolase causes proinflammatory activation of pulmonary microvascular endothelial cells and primes neutrophils through plasmin activation of protease-activated receptor 2. Shock 2015;44 (2):137−42.

[131] Shi J, et al. Upregulation of alpha-enolase in acute rejection of cardiac transplant in rat model: implications for the secretion of interleukin-17. Pediatr Transpl 2014;18(6):575−85.

[132] Berger RP, et al. Neuron-specific enolase and S100B in cerebrospinal fluid after severe traumatic brain injury in infants and children. Pediatrics 2002;109(2):E31.

[133] Berger T, et al. Antimyelin antibodies as a predictor of clinically definite multiple sclerosis after a first demyelinating event. N Engl J Med 2003;349(2):139−45.

[134] Su E, et al. Increased CSF concentrations of myelin basic protein after TBI in infants and children: absence of significant effect of therapeutic hypothermia. Neurocrit Care 2012;17(3):401−7.

[135] Liu MC, et al. Extensive degradation of myelin basic protein isoforms by calpain following traumatic brain injury. J Neurochem 2006;98(3):700−12.

[136] Ngankam, L. et al. *Immunological markers of severity outcome of traumatic brain injury.* Zh Nevrol Psikhiatr Im S S Korsakova, 2011, **111**(7): p. 61–5.

[137] Buonora JE, et al. Autoimmune profiling peveals peroxiredoxin 6 as a candidate traumatic brain injury biomarker. J Neurotrauma 2015;32(22):1805–14.

[138] Posti JP, et al. The levels of glial fibrillary acidic protein and ubiquitin C-terminal hydrolase-L1 during the first week after a traumatic brain injury: correlations with clinical and imaging findings. Neurosurgery 2016;79(3):456–64.

[139] Mondello S, et al. CSF and plasma amyloid-beta temporal profiles and relationships with neurological status and mortality after severe traumatic brain injury. Sci Rep 2014;4:6446.

[140] Yan EB, et al. Post-traumatic hypoxia is associated with prolonged cerebral cytokine production, higher serum biomarker levels, and poor outcome in patients with severe traumatic brain injury. J Neurotrauma 2014;31(7):618–29.

[141] Ankeny DP, Guan Z, Popovich G. B cells produce pathogenic antibodies and impair recovery after spinal cord injury in mice. J Clin Invest 2009;119(10):2990–9.

[142] Ankeny DP, et al. Spinal cord injury triggers systemic autoimmunity: evidence for chronic B lymphocyte activation and lupus-like autoantibody synthesis. J Neurochem 2006;99(4):1073–87.

[143] Popovich G, Longbrake EE. Can the immune system be harnessed to repair the CNS? Nat Rev Neurosci 2008;9(6):481–93.

[144] Ousman SS, Kubes P. Immune surveillance in the central nervous system. Nat Neurosci 2012;15 (8):1096–101.

[145] Kivisakk P, et al. Human cerebrospinal fluid central memory CD4 + T cells: evidence for trafficking through choroid plexus and meninges via P-selectin. Proc Natl Acad Sci U S A 2003;100(14):8389–94.

[146] Schlager C, et al. Effector T-cell trafficking between the leptomeninges and the cerebrospinal fluid. Nature 2016;530(7590):349–53.

[147] Kipnis J. Multifaceted interactions between adaptive immunity and the central nervous system. Science 2016;353(6301):766–71.

[148] Aspelund A, et al. A dural lymphatic vascular system that drains brain interstitial fluid and macromolecules. J Exp Med 2015;212(7):991–9.

[149] Louveau A, et al. Structural and functional features of central nervous system lymphatic vessels. Nature 2015;523(7560):337–41.

[150] Holmin S, et al. Intracerebral inflammatory response to experimental brain contusion. Acta Neurochir (Wien) 1995;132(1–3):110–19.

[151] Holmin S, et al. Intracerebral inflammation after human brain contusion. Neurosurgery 1998;42(2):291–8 discussion 298–299.

[152] Walsh JT, et al. MHCII-independent CD4 + T cells protect injured CNS neurons via IL-4. J Clin Invest 2015;125(2):699–714.

[153] Gadani SP, et al. The glia-derived alarmin IL-33 orchestrates the immune response and promotes recovery following CNS injury. Neuron 2015;85(4):703–9.

[154] Walsh JT, et al. Regulatory T cells in central nervous system injury: a double-edged sword. J Immunol 2014;193(10):5013–22.

[155] Roth TL, et al. Transcranial amelioration of inflammation and cell death after brain injury. Nature 2014;505 (7482):223–8.

[156] Russo MV, McGavern DB. Immune Surveillance of the CNS following Infection and Injury. Trends Immunol 2015;36(10):637–50.

[157] Gadani SP, et al. Dealing with danger in the CNS: the response of the immune system to injury. Neuron 2015;87(1):47–62.

[158] Schmitz J, et al. IL-33, an interleukin-1-like cytokine that signals via the IL-1 receptor-related protein ST2 and induces T helper type 2-associated cytokines. Immunity 2005;23(5):479–90.

[159] Stefanova I, Dorfman JR, Germain RN. Self-recognition promotes the foreign antigen sensitivity of naive T lymphocytes. Nature 2002;420(6914):429–34.

[160] Schwartz M, Kipnis J. Protective autoimmunity: regulation and prospects for vaccination after brain and spinal cord injuries. Trends Mol Med 2001;7(6):252–8.

[161] Blight AR. Remyelination, revascularization, and recovery of function in experimental spinal cord injury. Adv Neurol 1993;59:91−104.

[162] Blight AR. Effects of silica on the outcome from experimental spinal cord injury: implication of macrophages in secondary tissue damage. Neuroscience 1994;60(1):263−73.

[163] Fleming JC, et al. The cellular inflammatory response in human spinal cords after injury. Brain 2006;129(Pt 12):3249−69.

[164] Kigerl KA, McGaughy VM, Popovich G. Comparative analysis of lesion development and intraspinal inflammation in four strains of mice following spinal contusion injury. J Comp Neurol 2006;494(4):578−94.

[165] Popovich G, et al. Depletion of hematogenous macrophages promotes partial hindlimb recovery and neuroanatomical repair after experimental spinal cord injury. Exp Neurol 1999;158(2):351−65.

[166] Dalakas MC. B cells as therapeutic targets in autoimmune neurological disorders. Nat Clin Pract Neurol 2008;4(10):557−67.

[167] Dalakas MC. Invited article: inhibition of B cell functions: implications for neurology. Neurology 2008;70 (23):2252−60.

[168] Waubant E. Spotlight on anti-CD20. Int MS J 2008;15(1):19−25.

[169] Prochazka M, Voltnerova M, Stefan J. Studies of immunologic reactions after brain injury. II. Antibodies bratissue lipids blunt head injury man. Int Surg 1971;55(5):322−6.

[170] Engelhardt B, Ransohoff RM. Capture, crawl, cross: the T cell code to breach the blood-brain barriers. Trends Immunol 2012;33(12):579−89.

[171] Filiano AJ, Gadani SP, Kipnis J. How and why do T cells and their derived cytokines affect the injured and healthy brain? Nat Rev Neurosci 2017;18(6):375−84.

[172] Yednock TA, et al. Prevention of experimental autoimmune encephalomyelitis by antibodies against alpha 4 beta 1 integrin. Nature 1992;356(6364):63−6.

[173] Radjavi A, et al. Dynamics of the meningeal CD4(+) T-cell repertoire are defined by the cervical lymph nodes and facilitate cognitive task performance in mice. Mol Psychiatry 2014;19(5):531−3.

[174] Moalem G, et al. Autoimmune T cells protect neurons from secondary degeneration after central nervous system axotomy. Nat Med 1999;5(1):49−55.

[175] Kipnis J, et al. Neuronal survival after CNS insult is determined by a genetically encoded autoimmune response. J Neurosci 2001;21(13):4564−71.

[176] Kipnis J, et al. T cell immunity to copolymer 1 confers neuroprotection on the damaged optic nerve: possible therapy for optic neuropathies. Proc Natl Acad Sci U S A 2000;97(13):7446−51.

[177] Haque A, et al. Neuron specific enolase: a promising therapeutic target in acute spinal cord injury. Metab Brain Dis 2016;31(3):487−95.

[178] Yoles E, et al. Protective autoimmunity is a physiological response to CNS trauma. J Neurosci 2001;21 (11):3740−8.

[179] Hauben E, et al. Passive or active immunization with myelin basic protein promotes recovery from spinal cord contusion. J Neurosci 2000;20(17):6421−30.

[180] Moalem G, et al. Autoimmune T cells retard the loss of function in injured rat optic nerves. J Neuroimmunol 2000;106(1−2):189−97.

[181] Mein LE, et al. Encephalitogenic potential of myelin basic protein-specific T cells isolated from normal rhesus macaques. Am J Pathol 1997;150(2):445−53.

[182] Pette M, et al. Myelin basic protein-specific T lymphocyte lines from MS patients and healthy individuals. Neurology 1990;40(11):1770−6.

[183] Fee D, et al. Activated/effector CD4 + T cells exacerbate acute damage in the central nervous system following traumatic injury. J Neuroimmunol 2003;136(1−2):54−66.

[184] Ibarra A, Hauben E, Butovsky O, Schwartz M. The therapeutic window after spinal cord injury can accommodate T cell-based vaccination and methylprednisolone in rats. Eur J Neurosci 2004;19(11):2984−90.

[185] Kipnis J, et al. Neuroprotective autoimmunity: naturally occurring CD4 + CD25 + regulatory T cells suppress the ability to withstand injury to the central nervous system. Proc Natl Acad Sci U S A 2002;99 (24):15620−5.

[186] Urra X, et al. Antigen-specific immune reactions to ischemic stroke. Front Cell Neurosci 2014;8:278.

[187] Becker KJ, et al. Autoimmune responses to the brain after stroke are associated with worse outcome. Stroke 2011;42(10):2763−9.

[188] Zierath D, et al. CNS immune responses following experimental stroke. Neurocrit Care 2010;12(2):274–84.

[189] Planas AM, et al. Brain-derived antigens in lymphoid tissue of patients with acute stroke. J Immunol 2012;188(5):2156–63.

[190] Spellberg B, Edwards Jr. JE. Type 1/Type 2 immunity in infectious diseases. Clin Infect Dis 2001;32 (1):76–102.

[191] Brosnan JV, et al. Disease patterns in experimental allergic neuritis (EAN) in the Lewis rat. Is EAN a good model for the Guillain-Barre syndrome? J Neurol Sci 1988;88(1–3):261–76.

[192] Hinrichs DJ, Wegmann KW, Dietsch GN. Transfer of experimental allergic encephalomyelitis to bone marrow chimeras. Endothelial cells are not a restricting element. J Exp Med 1987;166(6):1906–11.

[193] Rapalino O, et al. Implantation of stimulated homologous macrophages results in partial recovery of paraplegic rats. Nat Med 1998;4(7):814–21.

[194] Rocken M, Racke M, Shevach EM. IL-4–induced immune deviation as antigen-specific therapy for inflammatory autoimmune disease. Immunol Today 1996;17(5):225–31.

[195] Lafaille JJ, et al. Myelin basic protein-specific T helper 2 (Th2) cells cause experimental autoimmune encephalomyelitis in immunodeficient hosts rather than protect them from the disease. J Exp Med 1997;186 (2):307–12.

[196] Hofstetter HH, et al. Autoreactive T cells promote post-traumatic healing in the central nervous system. J Neuroimmunol 2003;134(1–2):25–34.

[197] Tron F. Autoantibodies as biomarkers. Presse Med 2014;43(1):57–65.

[198] Abou-Donia MB, et al. Autoantibodies to nervous system-specific proteins are elevated in sera of flight crew members: biomarkers for nervous system injury. J Toxicol Env Health A 2013;76(6):363–80.

[199] Fialova L, et al. Serum and cerebrospinal fluid heavy neurofilaments and antibodies against them in early multiple sclerosis. J Neuroimmunol 2013;259(1–2):81–7.

[200] Fialova L, et al. Serum and cerebrospinal fluid light neurofilaments and antibodies against them in clinically isolated syndrome and multiple sclerosis. J Neuroimmunol 2013;262(1–2):113–20.

[201] Jones AL, et al. Elevated levels of autoantibodies targeting the M1 muscarinic acetylcholine receptor and neurofilament medium in sera from subgroups of patients with schizophrenia. J Neuroimmunol 2014;269 (1–2):68–75.

[202] Darnell RB, Furneaux HM, Posner JB. Antiserum from a patient with cerebellar degeneration identifies a novel protein in Purkinje cells, cortical neurons, and neuroectodermal tumors. J Neurosci 1991;11 (5):1224–30.

[203] Ekizoglu E, et al. Investigation of neuronal autoantibodies in two different focal epilepsy syndromes. Epilepsia 2014;55(3):414–22.

[204] El-Fawal HA, et al. Neuroimmunotoxicology: humoral assessment of neurotoxicity and autoimmune mechanisms. Env Health Perspect 1999;107(Suppl. 5):767–75.

[205] Storoni M, Petzold A, Plant GT. The use of serum glial fibrillary acidic protein measurements in the diagnosis of neuromyelitis optica spectrum optic neuritis. PLoS One 2011;6(8):e23489.

[206] Sorokina EG, et al. Autoantibodies to alpha7-subunit of neuronal acetylcholine receptor in children with traumatic brain injury. Zh Nevrol Psikhiatr Im S S Korsakova 2011;111(4):56–60.

[207] Chen S, et al. Role of alpha-II-spectrin breakdown products in the prediction of the severity and clinical outcome of acute traumatic brain injury. Exp Ther Med 2016;11(5):2049–53.

[208] Wang YZ, et al. Delivery of an miR155 inhibitor by anti-CD20 single-chain antibody into B cells reduces the acetylcholine receptor-specific autoantibodies and ameliorates experimental autoimmune myasthenia gravis. Clin Exp Immunol 2014;176(2):207–21.

[209] Mecocci P, et al. Serum anti-GFAP and anti-S100 autoantibodies in brain aging, Alzheimer's disease and vascular dementia. J Neuroimmunol 1995;57(1–2):165–70.

[210] Wang KK, et al. An update on diagnostic and prognostic biomarkers for traumatic brain injury. Expert Rev Mol Diagn 2018;18(2):165–80.

[211] Forooghian F, et al. Enolase and arrestin are novel nonmyelin autoantigens in multiple sclerosis. J Clin Immunol 2007;27(4):388–96.

Traumatic brain injury: glial fibrillary acidic protein posttranslational modification

Justyna Fert-Bober[1], Rakhi Pandey[1], Victoria J. Dardov[1], Timothy E. Van Meter[2], Donna J. Edmonds[2] and Jennifer E. Van Eyk[1]

[1]The Advanced Clinical Biosystems Research Institute, The Smidt Heart Institute, Cedars Sinai Medical Center, Los Angeles, CA, United States [2]ImmunArray, Richmond, VA, United Kingdom

Abbreviations

AD	Alzheimer's disease
ECL-ELISA	enhanced chemiluminescence immunosorbent assay
GFAP	glial fibrillary acidic protein
IF	intermediate filaments
PADs	peptidylarginine deiminases
PTM	posttranslational modification
SNPs	single-nucleotide polymorphisms
TBI	traumatic brain injury

6.1 Introduction

Traumatic brain injury (TBI) is caused by sudden and violent trauma to the brain, which could include vehicle accidents, falls, sport-related injuries, and acts of violence. It is characterized as a direct, mechanical compression-induced tissue injury and can be associated with hemorrhage and contusion at the site of impact. This results in a series of biochemical processes, like inflammatory and cytotoxic processes, which can then result in secondary brain injury [1]. This can evolve into a series of medical complications including

Biomarkers for Traumatic Brain Injury
DOI: https://doi.org/10.1016/B978-0-12-816346-7.00006-3

posttraumatic hydrocephalus, hypertension, and endocrine complications. TBI is also considered a risk factor for the development of dementia-like symptoms including Alzheimer's disease (AD). Furthermore, it is challenging to accurately phenotype the injury and to determine an early diagnosis of mild injury [2,3]. One significant obstacle is the limited knowledge about the complex cellular cascades following initial injury. The complex cascades include (1) cellular inflammatory responses following TBI [4]; (2) neuronal damage or death caused by excitotoxicity [5]; (3) apoptosis or necrosis [6]; and (4) prolonged disruption of cellular calcium homeostasis [7]. Although our understanding of these mechanisms has increased significantly in recent years it is not yet clear how specific alterations in these cellular networks arise, and how the downstream effects on protein PTMs occur and play a role. Understanding these mechanistic details is key for both the development of accurate biomarkers as well as to find therapeutic interventions, especially for long-term TBI-associated effects. To address this need, mass spectrometry (MS)-based proteomics has been one method of choice for analysis of tissue and biofluids after TBI. Recent advancement in instrument sensitivity and postanalysis methodology for posttranslational events, including phosphorylation, glycosylation, and oxidation/reduction, allows more detailed study of the dynamic regulation of many brain-specific proteoforms. In this chapter, we will review the known cellular processes related to citrullination in the brain, with a focus on the intermediate filament protein, glial fibrillary acidic protein (GFAP). GFAP has a number of single-nucleotide polymorphisms (SNP) and other PTMs, at least some of which have been shown to alter its biological function [8].

6.2 The protein posttranslational modification, citrullination

Citrullination is a posttranslational conversion of the arginine side chain, peptidylarginine, to peptidylcitrulline. Specifically, the guanidine group of the arginine side chain is converted to an ureido group, which is also known as deimination or citrullination. This conversion results in a mass increase of 0.98 Da, a loss of positive charge per conversion, and the release of ammonia. This leads to an overall decrease in positive charge, which can lead to potential changes in protein conformation and function [9]. Protein citrullination is catalyzed by a family of calcium-binding enzymes, the peptidylarginine deiminases (PAD). Five PAD isoenzymes have been identified so far, PAD1−4 and 6, with uniport accession numbers of Q9ULC6, Q9Y2J8, Q9ULW8, Q9UM07, and Q6TGC4, respectively [10,11]. All of the PAD isoforms are located at a single cluster spanning a region of about 355 kb in length on chromosome 1p36.1 [12] and mouse chromosome 4E1 with intron and exon boundaries well conserved throughout evolution [13]. The PAD2 protein is considered to be the main central nervous system isoform [14], with predominant expression in the retina and optic nerve [15]. PAD3 and PAD4 are also detected in neural tissue [16]. PAD1 is detected throughout the epidermis with an increased involvement in the late stages of epidermal differentiation [17]. PAD6 is localized to eggs, ovary, and the early embryo [18]. Not surprisingly, upregulation of PAD isoforms, particularly PAD2 and PAD4, or an increase in their catalytic activity has been associated with neurodegenerative and immunopathological conditions such as rheumatoid arthritis (RA), AD [19,20], and multiple sclerosis [21−23].

6.3 Role of citrullination in the polymerization of glial fibrillary acidic protein

Acute TBI pathophysiologic, involves several coincidence processes, including (1) ischemia and brain tissue reperfusion, (2) cell necrosis and apoptosis, (3) cellular inflammatory responses, and (4) increases in membrane permeability, including destabilization of intracellular calcium and sodium concentration [24]. This shift in ionic balance can cause excitotoxicity in neurons, and activates several damaging intracellular cascades in a variety of cell types, including activation of the PAD enzymes which could result in citrullination [25]. Several studies show an increase of global citrullinated proteins, including the intermediate filament proteins GFAP and vimentin, in reactive gliosis following TBI [25–27].

Along with microtubules and microfilaments, intermediate filaments (IF) make up the cytoskeleton of most eukaryotic cells. IF proteins are subdivided into six classes based on sequence homology [28]. GFAP, along with vimentin, desmin, and peripherin, are classified as type III IF proteins. Type III IF proteins facilitate integration of cell structure and function and allow for resilience to mechanical strain. Some IFs are specialized for specific cell types, like desmin for cardiac myocytes and GFAP for astrocytes. There are ten different isoforms of GFAP based on differential splicing of the gene, each with sublocalization within astrocytes and their IF assembly network [29]. Although GFAP is alternatively spliced, the major splice variant termed α-GFAP is expressed at the highest levels in astrocytes of the central nervous system. GFAP is also a target for SNPs, more precisely 76 single-nucleotide mutations have been reported so far [29]. Most SNPs are found in coding regions of the gene (L47; C79; H79; E223, H239; A244, R258, C289; D295, and R416), some are found in the promoter regions. All identified SNPs result in gain-function mutations with a redout of GFAP protein deposits known as Rosenthal fibers in Alexander disease, a primary genetic disorder of astrocytes [30,31] (see Fig. 6.1 for details).

GFAP gene activation and protein translation plays a critical role in astrogliosis following CNS injuries and in neurodegeneration [32]. A major hallmark of reactive gliosis is the overabundance of the soluble tetrameric precursors of GFAP, which, along with vimentin, copolymerize into long filamentous forms that create an elaborate cytoskeleton network [33]. In addition to many SNPs, GFAP is also subject to several PTMs, including phosphorylation, acetylation, and citrullination. Six lysine residues in GFAP, with the ability to be acetylated, have been reported [34]. The residues are located across the whole protein in the four highly conserved α-helical coiled-coil domains (CC1a, CC1b, CC2a, CC2b). The most apparent effect of lysine acetylation is the inhibition of proteasome-mediated protein degradation [35], and accumulation of insoluble protein aggregates in astrocytes [36]. Under normal conditions, at least four amino acid residues in the head domain of GFAP have been shown to be phosphorylated in vitro by protein kinases, such as protein kinase A, protein kinase C, Ca^{2+}/calmodulin-dependent protein kinase II, Rho kinase, and Cdc2 kinase [37–39] (Fig. 6.1 for more details). Studies by Inagaki and colleagues have shown that phosphorylation of these residues (Thr-7, Ser-8, Ser-13, and Ser-34 on the head and Ser-389 on the tail) plays a role in structural plasticity of astrocytic processes and that it can protect GFAP against degradation [40,41]. Interestingly, although the head domain of GFAP is highly polymorphic among species, amino acid residues that undergo phosphorylation are conserved, thus implying the physiological importance of phosphorylation of GFAP proteins. It has been suggested that citrullination may affect the formation of

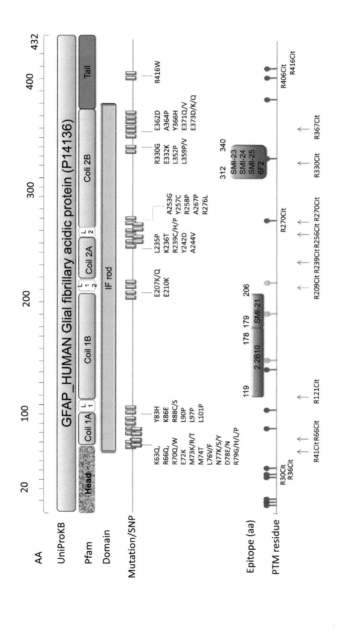

FIGURE 6.1 Schematic representation of the molecular architecture of GFAP with the linear structure, functional domains, and key modifications. GFAP comprises a central α-helical rod, flanked by the N-terminal head and C-terminal tail domains. The presentation emphasizes the modular construction of the protein and distribution of mutations in the GFAP gene based on the Uniprot database. The GFAP domains containing the epitopes (blue areas, amino acid (aa) sequence) recognized by indicated GFAP antibodies were shown elsewhere (https://doi.org/10.1371/journal.pone.0180694). The posttranslational modified residues include acetylation (marked in orange: K89,K153,K189,K259,K331), citrullination (Cit; marked in red: R30,R36,R270,E406,R416), and phosphorylation (marked in green: T7,S8,S13,S17,S38,S289).

filaments by blocking phosphorylation sites located on the head domain of GFAP [42]. Based on our own in vitro investigation, we support these findings. We show that citrullination of GFAP decreases its ability to polymerize and bind (Fig. 6.2, unpublished data). We used an ultracentrifugation cosedimentation assay to probe the effect of citrullination on GFAP filamentation. The assay determines whether GFAP stays at polymerized filament form and binds to a protein of interest (pellet) or exists in monomer form in supernatant. In our experiment a protein of interest is first incubated with GFAP in solution. Then, differential centrifugation was used to sediment the GFAP filaments, and the pelleted material was analyzed by sodium dodecyl sulfate polyacrylamide gel electrophoresis (SDS-PAGE). Interestingly, our cosedimentation assay shows that citrullination of GFAP protein in vitro alters its binding to αB-crystallin (also known as HspB5), a well-known GFAP binding partner [43,44], which can also be citrullinated. In contrast, citrullination of αB-crystallin does not affect its binding with GFAP (Fig. 6.2). This implies that citrullination could disrupt GFAP's ability to polymerize and to bind to binding partners within the cell, disrupting its cellular function. This also implies that citrullination of only certain proteins affects their function; citrullinated GFAP was unable to polymerize or bind αB-crystallin, but citrullinated αB-crystallin was able to bind to itself and GFAP with little change compared to wild-type αB-crystallin. αB-crystallin is a well-characterized member of the small heat shock protein family responsible for clearance of misfolded proteins. If citrullination of GFAP affects its binding to this chaperone, consequently there could be lack of clearance of the aggregated form of GFAP. Wizeman et al. have shown an increase in global protein citrullination and GFAP citrullination over a period of 1–7 days after retinal injury, supporting this hypothesis [26]. Notably, β-actin, vimentin, and other cytoskeletal proteins were identified to be deiminated in acute central nervous system damage and to exhibit neuroprotective effects, shown using pharmacological pan-PAD inhibition (Cl-amidine), described in several models of spinal cord injury [16,21,45].

6.4 Citrullination of glial fibrillary acidic protein as a hallmark mechanism in the pathogenesis of traumatic brain injury

Following acute structural disintegration of brain tissue, there is excitotoxic calcium overload [46]. It could lead to activation of the PAD enzymes followed by citrullination of highly abundant brain proteins, including GFAP, dynamin-1, tubulins, and syntaxin-binding protein 1, among others [24]. Most of the citrullinated proteins are cytoskeletal components, or function in cell–cell signaling or synaptic transmission. Several groups have shown that protein degradation fragments were citrullinated, for example, citrullinated GFAP, and were released from intracellular compartments into the bloodstream, where they can be measured [47]. The magnitude of GFAP elevation is correlated to lesion size, injury severity, and clinical outcomes [48–50]. Clinical studies also indicate that GFAP can be used as a good predictive biomarker and have demonstrated significant discrimination of injury severity [51]. For example, GFAP levels were significantly elevated in mild TBI patients with intracranial lesions compared to those without, and could predict which patients required neurosurgery [52]. However, further validation studies in concussion cohorts with longitudinal measures are warranted, especially when different GFAP

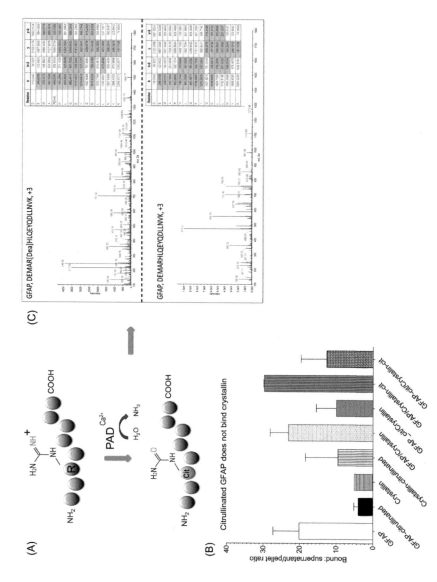

FIGURE 6.2 GFAP oligomerization after citrullination. (A) Citrullination schema. (B) Cosedimentation assays of GFAP with binding partner αB-crystallin. Citrullinated GFAP or GFAP in native form were mixed with a fixed amount of αB-crystallin or citrullinated αB-crystallin, incubated for 1 h, and then centrifuged at high speed to pellet the cytoskeletal polymer and associated protein. A sample of the pellets and supernatant were separated on a 10% polyacrylamide gel and stained with Coomassie. The experiment was repeated three times. The gels were then scanned and densitometry analysis was performed. The results of independent experiments were plotted on a graph with Prism software. The citrullination of GFAP decrease its polymerization and decrease GFAP binding to αB-crystallin. (C) Representative mass spectrometry spectrum of GFAP peptide, with citrullinated arginine residue (*top*) and nonmodified arginine residue (*bottom*).

isoforms control intermediate filament network dynamics and underlie isoform-specific functions [53,54]. Importantly, almost all the studies rely on the antibody-GFAP capture and detection in a sandwich ELISA. Fig. 6.1 presents a panel of commonly used anti-GFAP antibodies with defined epitopes located within the regions extending across the rod domain of GFAP [55]. This location of GFAP is also where there are SNPs and reported PTMs. To date in the literature, it has been reported that GFAP has five citrullinated residues [56]. Two of these sites are located in the head domain (R30Cit, R36Cit), one residue located in the central rod region (R270Cit) and two in the protein tail (R406 and R416Cit). Fig. 6.1 shows the citrullinated residues and epitopes of the current antibodies used in ELISA studies for measuring GFAP protein in the biofluid samples. As mentioned above, the conversion of the arginine side chain to a neutral group alters the overall charge and hydrogen bonding capabilities of this amino acid, which can fundamentally alter its structural interactions with other proteins, including antibodies. At the level of intact proteins, citrullination can increase protein antigenicity by eliciting changes in the primary, secondary, and tertiary structures of proteins. This may mean that citrullination and other PTMs could alter antigen processing, antigen presentation, and the binding of the antibodies to any of the circulating GFAP that has modification near or within the binding site of the antibodies being used. Additionally, citrullination can change the presentation of the native epitopes for nonmodified forms of proteins. Therefore new antibodies against citrullinated forms of proteins, or new methodology for measurement of citrullinated form of GFAP are needed as currently available antibodies are not specific enough to detect posttranslational modified GFAP. Measuring the immune recognition of citrullinated proteins with new antibodies could therefore be relevant to disease risk and progression [57].

6.5 Citrullination: method of detection

It is important to gain insight into the mechanism of citrullination itself and the activity of the PAD enzymes in complex biological samples. Gaining additional information about the substrate specificity, cell localization, specific regulation of each PAD isoform, and the functional effects of the modified proteins individually and as a network within the cell, would allow us to better understand the pathophysiological protein network, and could to be used for development of new diagnostic and prognostic tools. Several methods for the detection of PAD activity and the assessment of the protein citrullination have been described over the years. However, lack of the specificity of these methods can give false-positive results [53–55]. MS-based proteomics remains the only method for identifying the exact site of citrullination. It relies on a monoisotopic mass difference of +0.984016 [56], and loss of positive charge [57,58]. However, this small change, combined with the low abundance of citrullinated proteins, is easily confused with a deamidation event or a ^{13}C isotope. Therefore the correct identification of citrullinated peptides from MS data by automated search engines remains difficult, and caution must be taken when interpreting citrullinated spectra [56,59]. Our laboratories recently applied a complete proteomic workflow to robustly enrich, detect, and localize citrullinated residues in complex biological samples [58]. We used this workflow to confirm and expand identification of citrullinated proteins in serum samples obtained from healthy and TBI patients. Serum was collected

TABLE 6.1   GFAP level detected in human patient based on enhanced chemiluminescence immunosorbent assay (ECL-ELISA) performed by ImmunArray.

Patient status	ECL_ELISA (ng/mL)
Healthy	0.23
Healthy	4
Healthy	0.24
Healthy	0.44
TBI	2.36
TBI	16.3
TBI	2.26
TBI	24.6
TBI	18.1
TBI	27.7
TBI	2.69
TBI	26.4
TBI	3.03
TBI	2.95

TBI, traumatic brain injury.

from patients who were generally healthy, with no history of prior TBI or major disease; and from patients that sustained a TBI and met the American College of Emergency Physicians for CT scan eligibility, and or the American Congress for Rehabilitative Medicine criteria for symptom-based diagnosis of mild TBI (samples provide by ImmunArray). The patients' samples were interrogated for GFAP protein by an enhanced chemiluminescence immunosorbent assay (ECL-ELISA; MesoScale Discovery Quickplex 120 instrument, performed at ImmunArray, Inc., Richmond VA) method which captures the GFAP protein on an antibody-coated surface, followed by detection with a different anti-GFAP monoclonal antibody targeting a second independent epitope. The assay sensitivity range was determined to be 0.2–30 ng/mL. Ranges of protein concentration detected by this assay in healthy control and TBI patients are shown in Table 6.1. Note that the range of GFAP concentration based on immunoassay in healthy controls overlaps that observed in the TBI patients, even though the average concentration is higher in mild TBI (mTBI) patients compared to controls (Table 6.1). This data is echoed in several published studies that evaluate GFAP in mTBI (and reviewed in another chapter of this book).

To determine more specific information about how the TBI event can change the amount or repertoire of citrullination, new methods using MS were devised. Fig. 6.3 presents the MS-based workflow for a GFAP immunocapture method, including immunoprecipitation using anti-GFAP antibody (Dako, Clone 6F2), followed by LysC digestion and MS detection of GFAP. This method, followed by bioinformatics analysis customized to

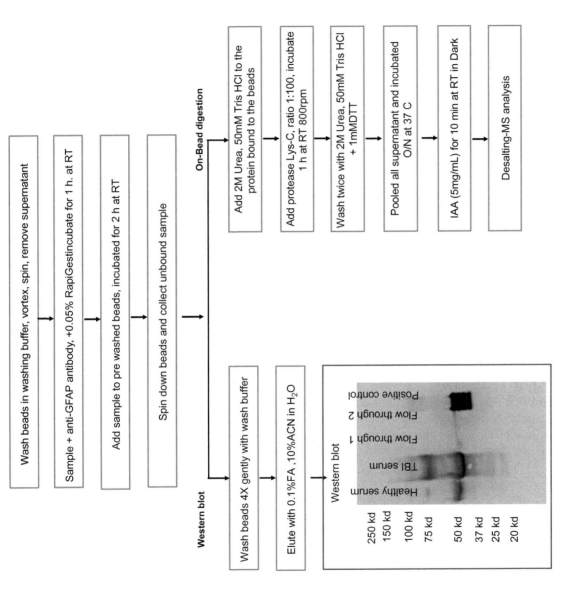

FIGURE 6.3 Schematic of the proteomic workflow for immunoprecipitation of GFAP protein from serum samples. The GFAP fragments in the serum fractions from ten individual TBI and three non-TBI, healthy controls were immunoprecipitated with the anti-GFAP antibody, and analyzed by Western blotting and MS. Western blotting with recombinant GFAP as positive control was used as a control for the inputted proteins.

reduce false-positive results and increase accuracy on citrullination detection, was performed using the same patient samples run previously by ECL-ELISA. LysC was used as the proteolytic enzyme instead of the traditional trypsin proteases that selectively cleave after positively charged residues. This additionally improved the accuracy of citrullination detection, since citrullination is known to eliminate tryptic sites, resulting in larger peptides that are harder to detect and sequence [56]. Using the refined method, both the total amount of the GFAP and each of its citrullinated forms were measured. In addition to GFAP protein, we identified 667 serum proteins as a result of minimum washes during immunoprecipitation steps. Of the 667 serum proteins detected, there were 112 citrullinated residues; of these, 10 of the citrullinated peptides showed significant difference between the healthy and TBI groups and include GFAP, vimentin, syntaxin-binding protein 1, heat shock 70 kDa protein 4, carbonic anhydrase 2, kynurenine–oxoglutarate transaminase 3, peroxiredoxin-1, endoplasmic reticulum chaperone BiP, Ras-related protein Rab-7a, and fumarate hydratase. All of these proteins have been previously described as proteins associated with neurological disease [59–62]. Furthermore, we were able to detect 10 potentially citrullinated residues in GFAP protein, with R367 shown to be statistically different between healthy controls and TBI. A correlation between the ECL-ELISA and MS was also performed, as presented in Fig. 6.4C. Overall, the GFAP amount measured by the MS and ECL-ELISA were consistently higher in TBI samples. However, we did not find a strong correlation between ECL-ELISA and MS values. One explanation could be that the GFAP is susceptible to proteolysis, both in vivo and in vitro. The proteases responsible for GFAP proteolysis include calpains and caspases [63]. Zhang et al. found that GFAP fragments between 25 and 35 kDa (it is not known what amino acid sequences these fragments are composed of) can be detected by immunoblotting of both mouse and human samples. These fragments, 25 and 35 kDa, could potentially affect the digestion efficiency and may not be useful for absolute quantification by MS. On the other hand, the monoclonal antibody utilized in the ECL-ELISA binds to a single peptide fragment of GFAP, and may bind differently to GFAP isoforms, yielding underestimated concentrations, particularly in individuals with different severity of TBI. Results presented in Fig. 6.4D from our study suggest that identification of citrullinated forms of GFAP, and perhaps one particular residue, might be a better marker of the specific disease than total GFAP levels, as GFAP levels are consistently elevated in cerebrospinal fluid and blood of patients with AD [19,64], amyotrophic lateral sclerosis [34], or intracerebral hemorrhage [47].

6.6 Conclusion and future research

A major problem facing therapeutic research is the identification of suitable biomarkers that reflect key pathways of disease, and that could be responsive to drugs or other types of treatment. As illustrated in Fig. 6.5, novel biomarkers of TBI should focus on detection of very early stages after injury (hyper acute and acute TBI), which will allow for implementation of treatments at an earlier point in the pathogenic cascade and could assist in the selection of patients at greater risk for adverse outcome or secondary injury, such as midline shifts or hemorrhage. In addition, biomarkers monitoring treatment efficacy, especially at the level of neuronal integrity, should be of great use [65]. To precisely measure

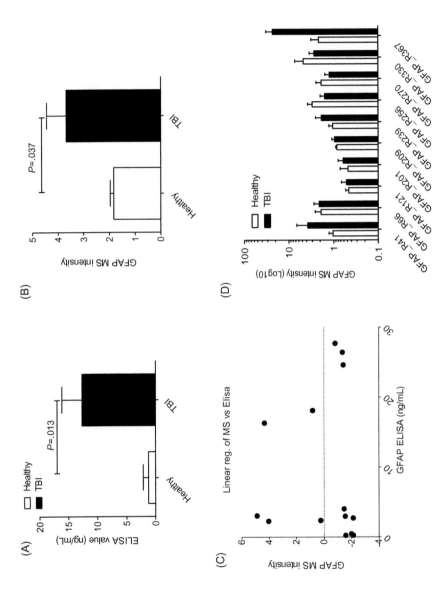

FIGURE 6.4 GFAP protein in human serum samples of TBI and healthy controls when measured by (A) ECL-ELISA assay and mass spectrometry (B). Data presented as means ± 1 S.D. (n = 4 and 10, healthy and TBI respectively). (One-way ANOVA with post hoc Bonferroni t-test; *P < .05). (C) Correlation of monoclonal ECL-ELISA with LC-MS/MS measures of GFAP protein identified in healthy and TBI patient. (D) Potential citrullinated residues in GFAP protein in serum samples.

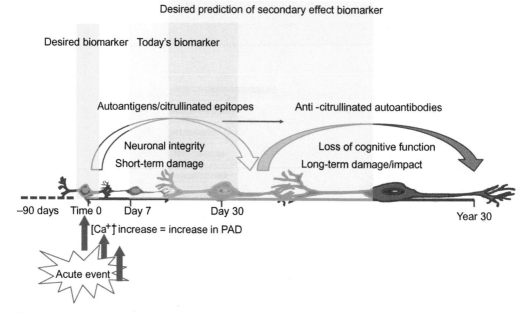

FIGURE 6.5 A schematic overview of the current state of biomarkers of the brain after TBI injury. Circulating disease-induced proteins can be detected in plasma of individuals with acute and traumatic brain injury. Some of these altered proteins cause autoantibodies that will go on to attack the brain and cause secondary effects, including dementia-like symptoms or even Alzheimer's disease development.

the very early stages of disease, it may be worthwhile to develop isoform-specific PAD activity assays, since TBI triggers calcium influx. Furthermore, the identification of biomarkers that reflect key pathways for chronic effects of TBI and that could predict the susceptibility and onset of neurodegenerative changes such as those associated with chronic traumatic encephalitis, or other forms of dementia. [65].

There is a growing literature on how PTMs are involved in the generation of neoantigens [65]. These neoantigens trigger activation of autoreactive T and B cells and induce an autoimmune response. The sequence of events connects environmental changes and autoimmunity and therefore can be used as a unique disease-specific marker. Well-described examples of citrullinated epitopes, like fibrin, fibrinogen, α-enolase, and vimentin, come from RA studies [57]. Interestingly, antibodies to citrullinated proteins, anti-CCP2 antibodies of both the IgG and IgA isotypes, have been found in the sera several years before the clinical symptoms of RA appear [66]. Emerging data support the relevance of citrullinated epitopes in other autoimmune diseases, including type 1 diabetes [67] and multiple sclerosis [68], whose susceptible HLA haplotypes also preferentially present citrullinated peptides. In respect to TBI, the above studies suggest that tissue- and disease-specific citrullinated proteins offer the possibility to increase the sensitivity and specificity of biomarker assays for diagnosis and prognosis. Therefore characterization of T-cell and antibody responses to TBI-specific citrullinated self-antigens, as well as PAD activity assays, may lead to improvements in risk stratification of TBI patient subgroups and allow for monitoring of therapeutic interventions in clinical trials.

References

[1] Dash HH, Chavali S. Management of traumatic brain injury patients. Korean J Anesthesiol 2018;71(1):12−21.

[2] Hoge CW, et al. Mild traumatic brain injury in U.S. soldiers returning from Iraq. N Engl J Med 2008;358 (5):453−63.

[3] Prince C, Bruhns ME. Evaluation and treatment of mild traumatic brain injury: the role of neuropsychology. Brain Sci 2017;7(8):105.

[4] Corrigan F, Mander KA, Leonard AV, Vink R. Neurogenic inflammation after traumatic brain injury and its potentiation of classical inflammation. J Neuroinflamm 2016;13(1):264.

[5] Walker K, Tesco G. Molecular mechanisms of cognitive dysfunction following traumatic brain injury. Front Aging Neurosci 2013;5(29).

[6] Fujikawa DG. The role of excitotoxic programmed necrosis in acute brain injury. Comput Struct Biotechnol J 2015;13:212−21.

[7] Floyd CL, Gorin FA, Lyeth BG. Mechanical strain injury increases intracellular sodium and reverses $Na + / Ca2 +$ exchange in cortical astrocytes. Glia 2005;51(1):35−46.

[8] Middeldorp J, Hol EM. GFAP in health and disease. Prog Neurobiol 2011;93(3):421−43.

[9] Gyorgy B, Toth E, Tarcsa E, Falus A, Buzas EI. Citrullination: a posttranslational modification in health and disease. Int J Biochem Cell Biol 2006;38(10):1662−77.

[10] Arita K, et al. Structural basis for $Ca(2 +)$-induced activation of human PAD4. Nat Struct Mol Biol 2004;11 (8):777−83.

[11] Darrah E, Rosen A, Giles JT, Andrade F. Peptidylarginine deiminase 2, 3 and 4 have distinct specificities against cellular substrates: novel insights into autoantigen selection in rheumatoid arthritis. Ann Rheum Dis 2012;71(1):92−8.

[12] Guerrin M, et al. cDNA cloning, gene organization and expression analysis of human peptidylarginine deiminase type I. Biochem J 2003;370(1):167−74.

[13] Chavanas S, et al. Comparative analysis of the mouse and human peptidylarginine deiminase gene clusters reveals highly conserved non-coding segments and a new human gene, PADI6. Gene 2004;330:19−27.

[14] Wood DD, et al. Myelin localization of peptidylarginine deiminases 2 and 4: comparison of PAD2 and PAD4 activities. Lab Invest 2008;88:354.

[15] Bhattacharya SK, Bhat MB, Takahara H. Modulation of peptidyl arginine deiminase 2 and implication for neurodegeneration. Curr Eye Res 2006;31(12):1063−71.

[16] Lange S, et al. Protein deiminases: new players in the developmentally regulated loss of neural regenerative ability. Dev Biol 2011;355(2):205−14.

[17] Dong S, et al. Crucial roles of MZF1 and Sp1 in the transcriptional regulation of the peptidylarginine deiminase type I gene (PADI1) in human keratinocytes. J Invest Dermatol 2008;128(3):549−57.

[18] Bicker KL, Thompson PR. The protein arginine deiminases: structure, function, inhibition, and disease. Biopolymers 2013;99(2):155−63.

[19] Ishigami A, et al. Mass spectrometric identification of citrullination sites and immunohistochemical detection of citrullinated glial fibrillary acidic protein in Alzheimer's disease brains. J Neurosci Res 2015;93 (11):1664−74.

[20] Gallart-Palau X, Serra A, Lee BST, Guo X, Sze SK. Brain ureido degenerative protein modifications are associated with neuroinflammation and proteinopathy in Alzheimer's disease with cerebrovascular disease. J Neuroinflammation 2017;14(1):175.

[21] Tejeda EJC, et al. Noncovalent Protein Arginine Deiminase (PAD) Inhibitors are efficacious in animal models of multiple sclerosis. J Med Chem 2017;60(21):8876−87.

[22] Tu R, Grover HM, Kotra LP. Peptidyl arginine deiminases and neurodegenerative Diseases. Curr Med Chem 2016;23(2):104−14.

[23] Yang L, Tan D, Piao H. Myelin basic protein citrullination in multiple sclerosis: a potential therapeutic target for the pathology. Neurochem Res 2016;41(8):1845−56.

[24] Sun DA, et al. Traumatic brain injury causes a long-lasting calcium $(Ca2 +)$-plateau of elevated intracellular Ca levels and altered $Ca2 +$ homeostatic mechanisms in hippocampal neurons surviving brain injury. Eur J Neurosci 2008;27(7):1659−72.

[25] Lazarus R, et al. Protein citrullination: a proposed mechanism for pathology in traumatic brain injury. Front Neurol 2015;6:204.

[26] Wizeman JW, Nicholas AP, Ishigami A, Mohan R. Citrullination of glial intermediate filaments is an early response in retinal injury. Mol Vis 2016;22:1137—55.

[27] Algeciras ME, Bhattacharya SK, Takahara H. Mechanical stretching elevates peptidyl arginine deiminase 2 expression in astrocytes. Curr Eye Res 2008;33(11):994—1001.

[28] Szeverenyi I, et al. The human intermediate filament database: comprehensive information on a gene family involved in many human diseases. Hum Mutat 2008;29(3):351—60.

[29] Yang Z, Wang KKW. Glial fibrillary acidic protein: from intermediate filament assembly and gliosis to neuro-biomarker. Trends Neurosci 2015;38(6):364—74.

[30] Jany Paige L, Hagemann Tracy L, Messing A. GFAP expression as an indicator of disease severity in mouse models of Alexander disease. ASN Neuro 2013;5(2):e00109.

[31] Quinlan RA, Brenner M, Goldman JE, Messing A. GFAP and its role in Alexander disease. Exp Cell Res 2007;313(10):2077—87.

[32] Brenner M. Role of GFAP in CNS injuries. Neurosci Lett 2014;565:7—13.

[33] Pekny M, et al. Abnormal reaction to central nervous system injury in mice lacking glial fibrillary acidic protein and vimentin. J Cell Biol 1999;145(3):503—14.

[34] Liu D, et al. Proteomic analysis reveals differentially regulated protein acetylation in human amyotrophic lateral sclerosis spinal cord. PLoS One 2013;8(12):e80779.

[35] Nakamura S, Roth JA, Mukhopadhyay T. Multiple lysine mutations in the C-terminal domain of p53 interfere with MDM2-dependent protein degradation and ubiquitination. Mol Cell Biol 2000;20(24):9391—8.

[36] Bruijn LI, et al. ALS-linked SOD1 mutant G85R mediates damage to astrocytes and promotes rapidly progressive disease with SOD1-containing inclusions. Neuron 1997;18(2):327—38.

[37] Takemura M, Gomi H, Colucci-Guyon E, Itohara S. Protective role of phosphorylation in turnover of glial fibrillary acidic protein in mice. J Neurosci 2002;22(16):6972—9.

[38] Herskowitz JH, et al. Phosphoproteomic analysis reveals site-specific changes in GFAP and NDRG2 phosphorylation in frontotemporal lobar degeneration. J Proteome Res 2010;9(12):6368—79.

[39] Anonymous. Control of the phosphorylation of the astrocyte marker glial fibrillary acidic protein (GFAP) in the immature rat hippocampus by glutamate and calcium ions: possible key factor in astrocytic plasticity. Braz J Med Biol Res 1997;30:325—38.

[40] Inagaki M, Nakamura Y, Takeda M, Nishimura T, Inagaki N. Glial fibrillary acidic protein: dynamic property and regulation by phosphorylation. Brain Pathol 1994;4(3):239—43.

[41] Inagaki M, et al. Phosphorylation sites linked to glial filament disassembly in vitro locate in a non-alpha-helical head domain. J Biol Chem 1990;265(8):4722—9.

[42] Inagaki M, Takahara H, Nishi Y, Sugawara K, Sato C. Ca2 + -dependent deimination-induced disassembly of intermediate filaments involves specific modification of the amino-terminal head domain. J Biol Chem 1989;264(30):18119—27.

[43] Shimizu M, Tanaka M, Atomi Y. Small heat shock protein alphaB-crystallin controls shape and adhesion of glioma and myoblast cells in the absence of stress. PLoS One 2016;11(12):e0168136.

[44] Tang G, Perng MD, Wilk S, Quinlan R, Goldman JE. Oligomers of mutant glial fibrillary acidic protein (GFAP) Inhibit the proteasome system in alexander disease astrocytes, and the small heat shock protein alphaB-crystallin reverses the inhibition. J Biol Chem 2010;285(14):10527—37.

[45] Lange S, et al. Peptidylarginine deiminases: novel drug targets for prevention of neuronal damage following hypoxic ischemic insult (HI) in neonates. J Neurochem 2014;130(4):555—62.

[46] Lee JM, Grabb MC, Zipfel GJ, Choi DW. Brain tissue responses to ischemia. J Clin Invest 2000;106(6):723—31.

[47] Mayer CA, et al. Blood levels of glial fibrillary acidic protein (GFAP) in patients with neurological diseases. PLoS One 2013;8(4):e62101.

[48] Yates D. Traumatic brain injury: serum levels of GFAP and S100B predict outcomes in TBI. Nat Rev Neurol 2011;7:63.

[49] Diaz-Arrastia R, et al. Acute biomarkers of traumatic brain injury: relationship between plasma levels of ubiquitin C-terminal hydrolase-L1 and glial fibrillary acidic protein. J Neurotrauma 2014;31(1):19—25.

[50] Posti JP, et al. The levels of glial fibrillary acidic protein and ubiquitin C-terminal hydrolase-L1 during the first week after a traumatic brain injury: correlations with clinical and imaging findings. Neurosurgery 2016;79(3):456—64.

[51] McMahon PJ, et al. Measurement of the glial fibrillary acidic protein and its breakdown products GFAP-BDP biomarker for the detection of traumatic brain injury compared to computed tomography and magnetic resonance imaging. J Neurotrauma 2015;32(8):527—33.

[52] Papa L, et al. GFAP out-performs S100beta in detecting traumatic intracranial lesions on computed tomography in trauma patients with mild traumatic brain injury and those with extracranial lesions. J Neurotrauma 2014;31(22):1815—22.

[53] Perng MD, et al. Glial fibrillary acidic protein filaments can tolerate the incorporation of assembly-compromised GFAP-delta, but with consequences for filament organization and alphaB-crystallin association. Mol Biol Cell 2008;19(10):4521—33.

[54] Moeton M, et al. GFAP isoforms control intermediate filament network dynamics, cell morphology, and focal adhesions. Cell Mol Life Sci 2016;73(21):4101—20.

[55] Lin N-H, Messing A, Perng M-D. Characterization of a panel of monoclonal antibodies recognizing specific epitopes on GFAP. PLoS One 2017;12(7):e0180694.

[56] Jin Z, et al. Identification and characterization of citrulline-modified brain proteins by combining HCD and CID fragmentation. Proteomics 2013;13(17):2682—91.

[57] Nguyen H, James EA. Immune recognition of citrullinated epitopes. Immunology 2016;149(2):131—8.

[58] Fert-Bober J, et al. Citrullination of myofilament proteins in heart failure. Cardiovasc Res 2015;108(2):232—42.

[59] Yu P, et al. Biochemical and phenotypic abnormalities in kynurenine aminotransferase II-deficient mice. Mol Cell Biol 2004;24(16):6919—30.

[60] Saito K, et al. Kynurenine pathway enzymes in brain: responses to ischemic brain injury versus systemic immune activation. J Neurochem 1993;61(6):2061—70.

[61] Jian B, et al. Activation of endoplasmic reticulum stress response following trauma-hemorrhage. Biochim Biophys Acta 2008;1782(11):621—6.

[62] Guo F, Hua Y, Wang J, Keep RF, Xi G. Inhibition of carbonic anhydrase reduces brain injury after intracerebral hemorrhage. Transl Stroke Res 2012;3(1):130—7.

[63] Zhang Z, et al. Human traumatic brain injury induces autoantibody response against glial fibrillary acidic protein and its breakdown products. PLoS One 2014;9(3):e92698.

[64] Jany PL, et al. CSF and blood levels of GFAP in Alexander sisease. eNeuro 2015;2(5).

[65] Karsdal MA, et al. Novel combinations of Post-Translational Modification (PTM) neo-epitopes provide tissue-specific biochemical markers—are they the cause or the consequence of the disease? Clin Biochem 2010;43(10):793—804.

[66] Kokkonen H, et al. Antibodies of IgG, IgA and IgM isotypes against cyclic citrullinated peptide precede the development of rheumatoid arthritis. Arthritis Res Ther 2011;13(1):R13.

[67] Roep BO, Kracht MJL, van Lummel M, Zaldumbide A. A roadmap of the generation of neoantigens as targets of the immune system in type 1 diabetes. Curr Opin Immunol 2016;43:67—73.

[68] Bradford CM, et al. Localisation of citrullinated proteins in normal appearing white matter and lesions in the central nervous system in multiple sclerosis. J Neuroimmunol 2014;273(1):85—95.

TBI biomarkers in medical practice

Economics of traumatic brain injury biomarkers

Clara E. Dismuke-Greer

Health Economics Resource Center (HERC), Ci2i, VA Palo Alto Health Care System, Palo Alto, CA, United States

7.1 Introduction

Traumatic brain injury (TBI) is the leading cause of death and disability among all trauma-related injuries globally [1]. The global incidence of all-cause all-severity TBI has been estimated to be 939 per 100,000 population, resulting in an estimated 69 million individuals exposed to TBI each year [2]. Mild TBI affects about 740 per 100,000 individuals, approximately 55.9 million each year worldwide [2]. Severe TBI has been estimated to affect about 73 per 100,000, approximately 5.48 million individuals each year worldwide [2].

7.1.1 Traumatic brain injury biomarkers

As of this writing, one blood biomarker (Banyan Brain Trauma Indicator) has been approved by the US Food and Drug Administration (FDA) for evaluating mild TBI (concussion) in adults in the United States [3]. The FDA News Release states that prior to the blood biomarker, the standard of care in US adults with a possible head injury was examination using the Glasgow Coma Scale (GCS) and a computed tomography (CT) scan of the head [3]. The GCS assesses responses in three domains: eye (score range 1−4), motor (score range 1−6), and verbal (score range 1−5) for a total score range from 3−15 [4,5]. Mild TBI has been defined as GCS 13−15, moderate as GCS 9−12, and severe as GCS 3−8 [4,5]. However, the GCS does not distinguish between the different pathoanatomical subsets of TBI [5]. The CT scan is the most frequently used imaging modality in diagnosing TBI [5]. Scanning time is relatively quick, and processing of the images is instantaneous [5]. However, a CT scan is not a very sensitive diagnostic tool as only 5% of patients suspected of having a mild TBI will have abnormal findings on their CT [5].

95

The FDA states that the availability of a blood test for mild TBI (concussion) will aid healthcare providers to determine the necessity of CT scans for individuals suspected of having mild TBI (concussion) while preventing unnecessary neuroimaging and the radiation exposure and healthcare costs associated with it [3].

The Brain Trauma Indicator (BTI) is a blood biomarker for TBI, developed by Banyan Biomarkers Inc., in partnership with the Department of Defense US Army Medical Research and Materiel Command [3,6]. The BTI assesses the measurable levels of ubiquitin C-terminal hydrolase-L1 (UCH-L1) and glial fibrillary acidic (GFAP) proteins released from the brain into the blood after a head injury [6]. The levels of UCH-L1 and GFAP proteins after mTBI (concussion) can aid in the prediction of the probability that intracranial legions will be visible on head CT in individuals who have sustained head trauma [3]. If performed within 12 hours of injury, the test is almost 100% accurate, taking about 3−4 hours to perform [3,6]. The test predicted intracranial lesions with 97.5% accuracy and absence of intracranial lesions with 99.6% accuracy in individuals with head trauma [6].

The BTI was approved by the FDA based on results from the prospective, multicenter ALERT-TBI clinical trial which enrolled 1947 individuals with suspected mild TBI/concussion at 24 clinical sites [7]. The researchers state that the results of this study support the potential for the blood test to indicate whether or not a CT was necessary for individuals with head trauma [7]. They add that routine use of the blood test in US hospital emergency departments could reduce the number of CT scans by as much as 35% [7]. As of this writing, there is no public pricing information for the BTI [8]. Worldwide, there is one additional serum biomarker being used in Europe to aid in the diagnosis of mild TBI (concussion) in adults. S100B is listed in the *Scandinavian Guidelines* for triage of individuals with head trauma into CT imaging [7,9]. All traumatic cerebral injuries have been shown to increase S100B in serum, and S100B has been shown to have the ability to distinguish between injury severity in individuals with head trauma [10]. A meta-analysis on S100B and mild TBI, which examined 2466 individuals from 12 studies, found that the pooled negative predictive value (NPV) was more than 99%, with a sensitivity of 97%, using a cutoff value of 0.10 µg/L for S100B detecting CT-visual brain pathology [9,11]. If the concentration of S100B is less than 0.10 µg/L within 6 hours of head trauma and the individual does not have extra cranial trauma or other risk factors, then healthcare providers should consider not performing a CT [10].

A pediatric study of S100B measurement in 446 French children found that S100B identified children correctly for bad versus good clinical evaluation with 100% sensitivity and 36% specificity [12]. Bad clinical evaluation included vomiting, facial paralysis, movement disorders, vertigo, photo motor reflex disorder, seizure, progressive headache, or behavior change over 24 hours [12]. A good clinical evaluation included the absence of any of these symptoms over 24 hours [12]. S100B measurement was also found to correctly identify CT findings with a sensitivity of 100% and specificity of 33% [12].

There are additional biomarkers being tested for acute and chronic TBI. GFAP, UCH-L1, and S100B are acute-phase biomarkers [5]. For the chronic stages of TBI, tau and phosphorylated tau are under examination as markers of neurodegeneration for in vivo detection of neurodegenerative disorders which are possible long-term sequelae of TBI such as Alzheimer's disease (AD) and chronic traumatic encephalopathy (CTE) [5].

7.1.2 Economic evaluations of traumatic brain injury biomarkers

It is important to have some notion of costs for identifying TBI. In addition to a potential reduction in radiation, cost reductions exist in the Swedish health system for the S100B biomarker [13]. The average cost for S100B analysis was 21 Euros ($24.34), and the average cost for a noncontrast cranial CT was 130 Euros ($150.66) [13,14]. This represents significant potential savings in healthcare costs as well as a reduction in radiation from the use of S100B in individuals with head trauma.

Currently, in the United States, the Banyan BTI is the only FDA-approved blood biomarker indicated for use in adults with head trauma. As the price is yet undetermined for the BTI, there is a limitation in estimating the cost-effectiveness of the test. However, the standard process of cost-effectiveness evaluation requires that the new intervention be evaluated against the usual current standard of care for the targeted disease [15].

Economic evaluations of the relative costs and benefits of TBI interventions provide information to support health providers and policy makers as well as other stakeholders in their decision-making regarding the allocation of limited healthcare resources to achieve the most optimal clinical health results for their patients with TBI [16]. For example, a review of 24 TBI economic evaluation studies reported the results of the high-quality studies as determined by the authors [16]. They reported that a policy of CT scanning for injury inflicted (by another person) in asymptomatic infants seen in the emergency department was less costly in the unexplained scalp-bruising scenario, with $3880 saved for each severe or fatal TBI averted, but cost $72,744 per case averted in the life-threatening event scenario [16,17]. From a societal perspective which incorporates the costs of child protective services, the CT scan strategy cost $132,701 per case averted for bruising, and $209,328 per case averted for life-threatening event [16,17].

7.1.3 Current traumatic brain injury standard of care: computed tomography and magnetic resonance imaging

Though CT is currently the primary imaging mechanism for individuals with head trauma, CT is relatively insensitive since fewer than 5% of individuals with suspected TBI are seen as having CT abnormalities [5]. Standard clinical magnetic resonance imaging (MRI) has a higher sensitivity for parenchymal lesions, especially in the posterior fossa, brain stem, and superficial cortical areas [5]. MRI is generally considered to be superior to CT 48–72 hours postinjury [18]. CT is better for detecting anatomical pathology and early bleeds, but MRI's ability to detect hematomas improves over time [18]. MRI is superior to CT in detecting axonal injury, subtle neuronal damage, and small areas of contusion, with studies showing that CT has missed about 10%–20% of abnormalities detected by MRI [18]. MRI is generally more sensitive than CT for detecting neuronal damage. Individuals whose brains show widespread MRI abnormalities or brain stem injuries commonly fail to achieve significant neurological recovery, even in the presence of normal CT scans [18].

For prognosis and rehabilitation guidance, MRI has been used to detect white matter abnormalities and provides better information [18]. Functional MRI, which is generally not readily available in healthcare facilities, can detect persistent changes in brain activation patterns of individuals with mild TBI [18]. Other imaging modalities which are promising but not readily available in healthcare facilities are single-photon emission computed tomography (SPECT) and (positron emission tomography [PET]). SPECT can detect abnormalities in cerebral blood flow and may be better than CT or MRI in determining long-term prognosis [18]. PET measures the cerebral metabolism of various substrates and may help distinguish reversible from irreversible lesions for therapeutic interventions to reduce further damage [18]. PET can also detect confounding neuropsychiatric conditions such as depression or substance abuse [18]. PET and SPECT have also been successful in measuring cerebral blood flow improvements due to hyperbaric oxygen and hyperventilation therapy in individuals diagnosed with TBI [18].

7.1.4 Creating benchmark cost data for traumatic brain injury biomarkers

Though we are unable to conduct a cost-effectiveness analysis of the FDA-approved BTI blood biomarker, we have conducted an analysis of the cost of two imaging modalities used in the standard of care for individuals with head trauma, in a relevant population which is especially vulnerable to TBI, due to military service and subsequent high-risk activities. We have examined the per unit as well as the associated inpatient, outpatient, pharmacy, and total costs of CT and MRI over a 14-year period (2000–2014) in veterans using Veterans Health Administration (VHA) medical centers and community-based outpatient clinics (CBOCs). The results of this study can provide benchmark information by which BTI and other blood biomarkers developed for TBI diagnosis and management can be compared, for future economic evaluations and cost-effectiveness analyses.

7.2 Methods

7.2.1 Procedures

As shown in Fig. 7.1, 79,276 veterans were identified with a TBI diagnosis from VA Informatics and Computing Infrastructure (VINCI) inpatient and outpatient patient treatment file (PTF) databases between January 1, 2000, and December 31, 2010, with information on utilization and cost by VA clinic stop codes. Diagnosis and TBI severity were determined by International Classification of Diseases, Ninth Revision (ICD-9) codes for TBI, postconcussive syndrome, and TBI-related late effects, according to the Military Health System and Defense Health Agency TBI DoD Standard Surveillance Case Definition for TBI Adapted for AFHSB Use [19].

Utilization and cost of CT and MRI were determined based on the VA clinic stop codes 150 and 151 [20]. Health Economics Resource Center (HERC) files were linked to PTF files using a scrambled social security number to identify VHA annual costs per veteran from FY2000–2014. Comorbidities were obtained by applying the Elixhauser enhanced algorithm to the PTFs [21]. All study procedures followed a protocol approved by the local Institutional Review Board and VA Research and Development Committee.

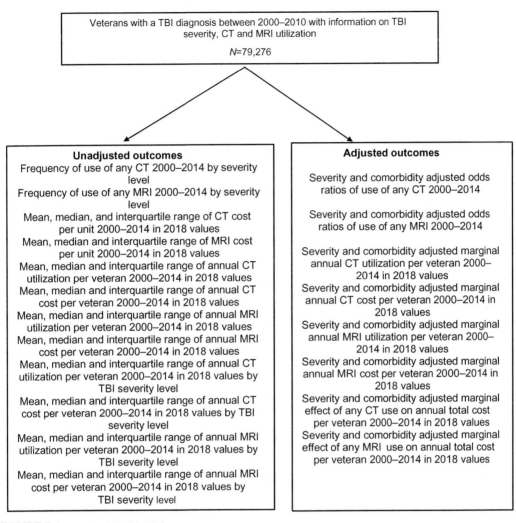

FIGURE 7.1   Study CONSORT diagram.

7.2.2 Measurements

7.2.2.1 Clinically diagnosed traumatic brain injury

Veterans with VHA clinician-confirmed diagnoses of TBI were included in the current study. Veterans with clinically diagnosed TBI were identified based on having an ICD-9 code for TBI in an inpatient hospitalization or outpatient encounter of 310.2, 850.xx, 851.xx, 852.xx, 853.xx, 854.xx, 800.xx, 801.xx, 803.xx, 804.xx, 950.1x, 907.0, 959.01, and V15.xx, according to Military Health System and The Defense Health Agency guidelines [19]. TBI severity was also classified according to the Military Health System and the Defense Health Agency guidelines as mild, moderate/severe/penetrating, or unknown based on

ICD-9 codes and the guidelines [19]. When a veteran had more than one TBI ICD-9 code, the highest level of TBI severity recorded for that veteran in ICD-9 was used. Severity status was classified as mild and higher severity TBI (moderate, severe, penetrating).

7.2.2.2 CT and MRI utilization and costs

CT and MRI utilization was identified using the VA clinic stop codes and by counting the number of occurrences of those codes per veteran. CT and MRI costs were estimated using the HERC outpatient cost files, whereby CT and MRI costs were identified based on their associated clinic stop codes [22]. The sum of utilization and costs per veteran by CT and MRI were estimated over the time span the veteran was included in the study.

7.2.2.3 Veterans Health Administration health services costs

Annual per veteran total, inpatient, outpatient, and pharmaceutical costs were obtained from HERC files for FY2000−2014 [23]. These costs are estimated by HERC using actual cost data from VA facilities and estimates provided by Medicare. HERC inpatient costs consist of acute hospital care, inpatient nonacute care, and long-term care. Acute hospital care cost estimates are based on relative value units (RVUs) from Medicare. VA RVUs are based on the relationship between cost-adjusted charges, diagnosis, and length of stay. The RVUs reflect the effect of diagnosis on the relative quantity of resources used in a hospital stay. HERC acute hospital care cost estimates reflect the effect of diagnosis on resource use and are based on the assumptions that RVUs such as Diagnosis Related Group (DRG) weights and length of stay, based on non-VA costs, reflect the relative costs of VA hospital stays, and all stays with the same characteristics have the same cost.

Inpatient nonacute care estimates are based on the cost of inpatient stays in rehabilitation, domiciliary, psychiatric, substance abuse, and intermediate medicine treatment units. HERC finds the average cost of a day of stay, and applies it to estimate the cost of care. HERC makes the assumption that every day of stay has the same cost.

Long-term care cost estimates between FY1998 and FY2000 were based on incorporating the relative values for resource utilization from Medicare Resource Utilization Groups (RUGs). VA undertakes a biannual assessment to assign every long-term care patient to a RUG. HERC used these data to assess cost while assuming the cost of long-term care is proportionate to the RUG relative value. Since FY2001, HERC has calculated costs based on an average daily rate.

Outpatient Visit Costs are estimated using the relative values of all Current Procedures and Terminology (CPT) codes assigned to the visit. HERC uses the relative values from the Medicare Resource-Based Relative Value System (RBRVS), which is used to reimburse providers for services provided to Medicare patients. HERC assigns every VA visit to one of 12 categories of outpatient care. For each category, HERC finds a specific factor to convert the relative value to a VA cost estimate. HERC assumes that the resources used to provide VA outpatient care are proportionate to the relative values assigned in the Medicare reimbursement.

Outpatient Pharmacy costs are estimated by HERC from the Managerial Cost Accounting (MCA) national extracts from VA facilities which include estimates of all prescriptions dispensed to an individual on a given day.

7.2.2.4 Comorbid conditions

The 31 Elixhauser comorbidities were measured as binary indicators based on ICD codes identified as congestive heart failure, cardiac arrhythmias, valvular disease, pulmonary circulation disorders, peripheral vascular disorders, uncomplicated hypertension, complicated hypertension, paralysis, other neurological disorders, chronic pulmonary disease, uncomplicated diabetes, complicated diabetes, hypothyroidism, renal failure, liver disease, peptic ulcer disease excluding bleeding, AIDS/HIV, lymphoma, metastatic cancer, solid tumor without metastasis, rheumatoid arthritis/collagen vascular diseases, coagulopathy, obesity, weight loss, fluid and electrolyte disorders, blood loss anemia, deficiency anemia, alcohol abuse, drug abuse, depression, and psychoses [21].

7.2.3 Analysis

A series of preliminary analyses were conducted. First, the unadjusted percentage of veterans using CT and MRI was calculated by severity status. Second, the unadjusted mean, median, and interquartile range of cost per unit of CT and MRI were estimated by TBI severity status. Third, the unadjusted mean, median, and interquartile range of annual CT and MRI utilization were estimated by TBI severity status. Fourth, the mean, median, and interquartile range of the annual per veteran cost of CT and MRI were estimated by TBI severity status. Because it was not possible to distinguish CT and MRI utilization based on reason for the CT or MRI, it is essential to adjust for comorbidities other than TBI that a veteran may have. To achieve this, Elixhauser comorbidity as well as TBI severity-adjusted models were estimated. First, a logit model of the likelihood a veteran received a CT was estimated adjusting for TBI severity and the 31 Elixhauser comorbidities. Similarly, a logit model of the likelihood that a veteran received an MRI was estimated by TBI severity, adjusting for the Elixhauser comorbidities. Second, annual CT and annual MRI utilization models by TBI severity were estimated using generalized linear models (GLM), and assuming a Poisson family, due to the count nature of utilization. As with the logit models, adjustments were made for Elixhauser comorbidities [21]. Third, annual CT and MRI cost per veteran models by TBI severity were estimated, using GLM models assuming a Gaussian family and identity link [24]. As with the utilization models, the CT and MRI cost models were adjusted for Elixhauser comorbidities [21].

Fourth, total annual VHA cost by any CT and any MRI use was estimated to examine the independent marginal impact of any CT and any MRI use on total VHA annual cost per veteran. Similar to the annual CT and MRI cost per veteran models, a GLM model assuming a Gaussian family and identity link was used, adjusting for Elixhauser comorbidities as well as TBI severity [21,24]. Finally, the impact of any CT and any MRI use on annual inpatient, outpatient, and pharmacy VHA costs per veteran was estimated, using seemingly unrelated regression (SUR), which allows for correlation between cost categories [25]. This approach was used as decisions regarding inpatient, outpatient, and pharmaceutical health services are likely to be coordinated by providers within the VHA. Similar to the annual total VHA cost per veteran model, TBI severity and Elixhauser comorbidities were adjusted for [21]. All costs were converted to 2018 dollar values using the US Department of Labor Consumer Price Index (CPI) Inflation Calculator [26].

Predicted mean annual VHA cost burden per veteran of any CT and any MRI use was estimated. All analyses were performed using STATA version 15.0 in VINCI. Statistical significance was determined at $P < .05$.

7.3 Results

Table 7.1 shows the unadjusted frequency of utilization of any CT or MRI by veterans diagnosed with TBI by TBI severity. Approximately 84.78% of all veterans with TBI, 75.63% of mild TBI severity veterans, and 88.10% of higher TBI severity veterans had some CT utilization. Approximately 61.29% of all veterans with TBI, 70.29% of mild TBI severity veterans, and 58.02% of higher TBI severity veterans had some MRI utilization.

Table 7.1 also shows the mean, median, and interquartile per unit cost of CT and MRI in 2018 value by TBI severity. For all TBI severity, the mean ($468), median ($422), and

TABLE 7.1 Unadjusted per unit and per veteran utilization and costs of CT and MRI 2000−14 in 2018 value by TBI severity level.

	CT			MRI		
Variables	All severity	Mild TBI (n = 21,283)	Higher severity TBI (n = 58,443)	All severity	Mild TBI (n = 21,283)	Higher severity TBI (n = 58,443)
Any use of imaging	67,588 (84.78%)	16,097 (75.63%)	51,491 (88.10%)	48,868 (61.29%)	14,959 (70.29%)	33,909 (58.02%)
Cost per unit						
Mean	$468	$460	$470	$732	$692	$750
Median	$422	$410	$425	$639	$595	$655
25 Percentile	$315	$309	$319	$532	$530	$534
75 Percentile	$554	$551	$556	$833	$795	$843
Annual utilization per veteran						
Mean	0.84	0.43	0.99	0.39	0.35	0.40
Median	0.5	0.25	0.64	0.21	0.20	0.21
25 Percentile	0.2	0.06	0.30	0	0	0
75 Percentile	1.125	0.53	1.33	0.54	0.46	0.60
Annual cost per veteran						
Mean	$409	$205	$484	$288	$240	$305
Median	$221	$100	$289	$136	$131	$138
25 Percentile	$77	$20	$113	$0	$0	$0
75 Percentile	$516	$244	$615	$393	$315	$425

CT, Computed tomography; *MRI*, magnetic resonance imaging; *TBI*, Traumatic brain injury.

interquartile range ($315–554) cost per unit was lower for CT than the mean ($732), median ($639), and interquartile range ($542–833) for MRI. The mean ($470), median ($425), and interquartile range ($319–556) cost per unit for CT in higher TBI severity veterans was higher than the mean ($460), median ($410), and interquartile range ($309–551) for mild severity TBI veterans. Similarly, the mean ($750), median ($655), and interquartile range ($534–843) per unit MRI cost for higher TBI severity veterans was higher than the mean ($692), median ($595), and interquartile range ($530–795) cost per unit for MRI for mild TBI severity veterans.

Finally, Table 7.1 shows the annual utilization of CT and MRI per veteran diagnosed with TBI, by TBI severity. The mean (0.84), median (0.5), and interquartile range (0.2–1.125) annual utilization of CT for all TBI severity veterans was more than twice (0.84) that of mean (0.39), median (0.20), and interquartile range (0–0.46) MRI utilization. Higher severity TBI veterans had twice the mean (0.99), median (0.64), and interquartile range (0.30–1.33) CT utilization than the mean (0.43), median (0.25), and interquartile range (0.06–0.53) utilization for mild TBI severity veterans. Higher severity TBI veterans had higher (but not twice) the mean (0.40), median (0.21), and interquartile range (0–60) MRI utilization than the mean (0.35), median (0.20), and interquartile range (0–0.46) mild TBI severity MRI utilization.

Table 7.2 shows the odds ratios and corresponding 95% confidence intervals (CI) of higher TBI severity relative to mild TBI severity, as well as the odds ratios and 95% CI of all 31 Elixhauser comorbidities in predicting the likelihood of any CT and MRI utilization by veterans diagnosed with TBI. The comorbidity-adjusted odds ratio (1.43; 95% CI 1.37:1.49) of higher severity TBI relative to mild TBI was significantly ($P < .05$) greater than 1, which suggested that the likelihood of any CT utilization was increased by TBI severity. However, the reverse was found for MRI, where the odds ratio (0.68; 95% CI 0.66:0.71) was significantly less than 1, which suggested that the likelihood of any MRI utilization was decreased by TBI severity.

Table 7.3 contains the comorbidity-adjusted marginal effects of higher TBI severity relative to mild TBI severity on the annual number and cost of CT and MRIs utilized per veteran, along with the 95% CI. The significant comorbidity-adjusted marginal effect of higher TBI severity, relative to mild TBI severity, was 0.42 (95% CI 0.410:0.437) CT scans at a marginal cost of $171 (95% CI $164:$177) per year per veteran for CT use. The significant comorbidity-adjusted marginal effect of higher TBI severity, relative to mild TBI severity, was 0.09 (95% CI 0.083:0.102) MRIs at a marginal cost of $78 (95% CI $72:$84) per veteran per year.

Table 7.4 shows the comorbidity and TBI severity-adjusted marginal effects of any CT and or MRI use on annual total, inpatient, outpatient, and pharmacy VHA cost per veteran.

The significant marginal effect of any CT use was $1775 (95% CI $1514:$2035) on annual total cost, $1646 (95% CI $1529:$1763) on annual outpatient cost, and $373 (95% CI $315: $431) on annual pharmacy cost per veteran. Any CT use did not have a significant comorbidity-adjusted marginal effect on annual inpatient cost per veteran.

The significant marginal effect of any MRI use was $851 (95% CI $582:$1120) on annual total cost, − $1522 (95% CI − $1742: − $1302) on annual inpatient cost, $1983 (95% CI $1899:$2067) on annual outpatient cost, and $389 (95% CI $348:$431) on pharmacy cost per veteran.

TABLE 7.2 Odds ratios from logit models of any CT and MRI relative to no CT or MRI use per veteran.

Variables	CT Odds ratio	CT 95% CI	MRI Odds ratio	MRI 95% CI
Severity				
Mild (reference)				
Higher severity	1.43*	1.37:1.49	0.68*	0.66:0.71
Comorbidities				
Congestive heart failure	1.31*	1.14:1.50	0.60*	0.56:0.62
Cardiac arrhythmias	1.54*	1.43:1.65	0.91*	
Valvular disease	1.23*	1.06:1.42	0.99	0.93:1.05
Pulmonary circulation disorder	1.36*	1.08:1.70	0.95	0.88:1.03
Peripheral vascular disorder	1.70*	1.52:1.90	0.96	0.92:1.01
Hypertension uncomplicated	1.57*	1.49:1.64	0.90*	0.87:0.94
Hypertension complicated	1.10	0.91:1.33	1.14*	1.06:1.23
Diabetes complicated	1.15*	1.01:1.31	1.06	0.97:1.12
Diabetes uncomplicated	1.24*	1.14:1.35	0.89*	0.85:0.93
Paralysis	1.14*	1.01:1.29	0.96	0.90:1.02
Other neurological disorder	1.20*	1.13:1.28	1.13*	1.09:1.17
Chronic pulmonary disease	1.66*	1.57:1.76	1.01	0.98:1.05
Thyroid	1.23*	1.11:1.36	0.98	0.93:1.03
Renal failure	1.22	0.96:1.30	0.91*	0.85:0.97
Liver disease	1.80*	1.63:1.98	0.98	0.95:1.04
HIV/AIDS	1.41	0.98:2.01	1.66	0.98:1.39
Lymphoma	1.38	0.98:1.93	1.14	0.98:1.31
Metastatic cancer	1.58*	1.15:2.16	1.20*	1.09:1.32
Tumor without metastasis	2.10*	1.88:2.33	0.96	0.92:1.01
Rheumatoid arthritis	1.42*	1.26:1.60	1.52*	1.43:1.62
Coagulopathy	1.39*	1.18:1.63	0.85*	0.80:0.91
Fluid electrolyte disorders	2.04*	1.87:2.23	0.80*	0.77:0.83
Blood loss anemia	2.11*	1.23:3.62	0.83*	0.73:0.95
Deficiency anemia	1.42*	1.25:1.62	1.01	0.96:1.07
Alcohol abuse	1.09*	1.04:1.15	0.88*	0.85:0.91
Drug abuse	1.39*	1.31:1.48	1.11*	1.06:1.15
Psychoses	1.27*	1.19:1.35	0.91*	0.88:0.95
Depression	0.64*	0.61:0.67	1.95*	1.89:2.02
Obesity	1.06*	1.01:1.12	1.40*	1.35:1.45
Weight loss	1.77*	1.58:1.97	0.85*	0.81:0.89
Peptic ulcer disease	1.61*	1.39:1.87	1.13*	1.05:1.20

Note: * indicates significant at $P < 0.05$.
CT, Computed tomography; *MRI*, magnetic resonance imaging.

TABLE 7.3 Severity and comorbidity-adjusted annual CT and MRI utilization and costs per veteran 2000−2014 in 2018 values.

	CT		MRI	
Variables	**Number (95% CI)**	**Cost (95% CI)**	**Number (95% CI)**	**Cost (95% CI)**
Severity				
Mild (reference)				
Higher severity	**0.42* (0.410:0.437)**	**$171* (164:177)**	**0.09* (0.083:0.102)**	**$78* (72:84)**
Comorbidities				
Congestive heart failure	− 0.02* (−0.040: − 0.001)	−$23* (−40: − 5)	− 0.12* (−0.141: − .104)	−$78* (−90:67)
Cardiac arrhythmias	0.09* (0.079:0.110)	$47* (36:58)	− 0.01* (−0.026: − .003)	−$9* (−18:0)
Valvular disease	0.02* (0.001:0.043)	$8 (−10:27)	0.00 (−0.016:0.021)	$5 (−8:18)
Pulmonary circulation disorder	0.11* (0.089:0.141)	$109* (80:138)	0.01 (−0.012:0.037)	$14 (−5:33)
Peripheral vascular disorder	0.10* (0.091:0.125)	$103* (87:119)	− 0.02* (−0.034: − 0.005)	$0 (−10:10)
Hypertension uncomplicated	0.075* (0.059:0.092)	$12* (4:21)	− 0.06* (−0.071: − 0.051)	−$37* (−44: − 29)
Hypertension complicated	− 0.00 (−0.027:0.027)	−$11 (−35;13)	0.02 (−0.004:0.044)	$13 (−3:30)
Diabetes complicated	− 0.00 (−0.029:0.015)	−$21* (−39: − 3)	0.01 (−0.007:0.030)	$6 (−6:19)
Diabetes uncomplicated	0.02* (0.003:0.041)	411 (−2:24)	− 0.05* (−0.064: − 0.035)	−$32* (−42:22)
Paralysis	0.05* (0.029:0.075)	414 (−5:33)	0.04* (0.021:0.057)	$63* (46:81)
Other neurological disorder	0.123* (0.109:0.138)	$36* (26:47)	0.06* (0.048:0.069)	$72* (63:81)
Chronic pulmonary disease	0.13* (0.120:0.148)	$63* (54:72)	− 0.00 (−0.013:0.006)	−$1 (−8:6)
Thyroid	0.01 (−0.011:0.028)	−$5 (−21:10)	− 0.01 (−0.026:0.005)	$3 (−9:16)
Renal failure	− 0.00 (−0.030:0.019)	−$25* (−46:4)	− 0.03* (−0.051: − 0.008)	−$16* (−30: − 1)
Liver disease	− 0.14* (0.119:0.155)	$118* (103:133)	− 0.00 (−0.017:0.011)	$3 (−8:1)
HIV/AIDS	0.019 (−0.045:0.084)	$0 (−44:45)	0.01 (−0.038:0.062)	$26 (−13:65)
Lymphoma	0.297* (0.257:0.337)	$559* (463:653)	0.06* (0.023:0.099)	$82* (40:124)
Metastatic cancer	0.32* (0.294:0.349)	$584* (523:644)	0.13* (0.105:0.158)	$167* (132:203)
Tumor without metastasis	0.235* (0.218:0.252)	$219* (203:235)	0.02* (0.002:0.031)	$37* (26:48)

(Continued)

III. TBI biomarkers in medical practice

TABLE 7.3　(Continued)

Variables	CT		MRI	
	Number (95% CI)	Cost (95% CI)	Number (95% CI)	Cost (95% CI)
Rheumatoid arthritis	0.09* (0.073:0.119)	$57* (39:75)	0.12* (0.101:0.134)	$97 (82:112)
Coagulopathy	0.12* (0.095:0.137)	$116* (93:139)	−0.02* (−0.042: −0.003)	−$8 (−23:7)
Fluid electrolyte disorders	0.22* (0.203:0.234)	$132* (119:145)	−0.036* (−0.049: −0.024)	−$23 (−32:14)
Blood loss anemia	0.00 (−0.040:0.044)	$10 (−35:56)	−0.06* (−0.102: −0.012)	−$44* (−69: −19)
Deficiency anemia	0.05* (0.029:0.068)	$41* (23:59)	−0.00 (−0.022:0.011)	$3 (−9:15)
Alcohol abuse	−0.01 (−0.025:0.006)	−$10* (−19: −1)	−0.05* (−0.057: −0.035)	−$38* (−46: −30)
Drug abuse	0.07* (0.050:0.084)	$25* (15:35)	0.01 (−0.001:0.021)	$6 (−3:14)
Psychoses	0.04* (0.027:0.057)	$6 (−5:16)	−0.02* (−0.030: −0.008)	−$7 (−16:1)
Depression	−0.06* (−0.074: −0.044)	−$16* (−25:7)	0.17* (0.163:0.187)	$108* (101:115)
Obesity	−0.03* (−0.040: −0.011)	−$6 (−14:2)	0.05* (0.045:0.064)	$37* (30:44)
Weight loss	0.08* (0.064:0.099)	−$78* (62:94)	−0.03* (−0.050: −0.020)	−$18* (−29: −7)
Peptic ulcer disease	0.07* (0.048:0.095)	$63* (42:84)	0.01 (−0.011:0.028)	$5 (−8:18)

CT, Computed tomography; *MRI*, magnetic resonance imaging.

Table 7.5 shows the comorbidity-adjusted predicted annual mean CT and MRI cost per veteran as well as the comorbidity-adjusted predicted mean annual total, inpatient, outpatient, and pharmacy cost per veteran by any CT and any MRI use. Veterans with mild TBI severity were predicted to have annual mean CT cost of $284 (95% CI $279:$289) and MRI cost of $230 ($225:$235) per veteran per year. Veterans with higher TBI severity were predicted to have annual mean CT cost of $455 (95% CI $451:$459) and MRI cost of $309 ($305:$313) per veteran per year.

Veterans with TBI and no CT use had a predicted annual mean total cost of $13,237 (95% CI $12,981 to $13,494), inpatient cost of $6686 (95% CI $6408:$6963), outpatient cost of $5259 (95% CI $5153:$5365), and pharmacy cost of $1292 ($1240:$1344). Veterans diagnosed with TBI and any CT use had a predicted annual mean total cost of $15,012 (95% CI $14,895:$15,129), inpatient cost of $6441 (95% CI $6331:$6550), outpatient cost of $6906 (95% CI $6864:$6947), and pharmacy cost of $1665 (95% CI $1645:$1686).

Veterans diagnosed with TBI and no MRI use had a predicted annual mean total cost of $14,220 (95% CI $14,003:$14,438), inpatient cost of $7411 (95% CI $7244:$7578), outpatient cost of $5439 (95% CI $5375:$5503), and pharmacy cost of $1370 (95% CI $1338:$1401). Veterans diagnosed with TBI and any MRI use had a predicted annual mean total cost of $15,072 ($14,934:$15,210), inpatient cost of $5889 (95% CI $5758:$6019), outpatient cost of $7423 (95% CI $7373:$7473), and pharmacy cost of $1759 (95% CI $1735:$1784).

TABLE 7.4 Severity and comorbidity-adjusted marginal effect of any CT and MRI use on total VHA cost per veteran 2000−2014 in 2018 values.

Variables	Total cost (95% CI)	Inpatient cost (95% CI)	Outpatient cost (95% CI)	Pharmacy cost (95% CI)
Any CT	$1775* (1514:2035)	−$245 (−551:61)	$1646* (1529:1763)	$373* (315:431)
Any MRI	$851* (582:1120)	−$1522* (−1742: − 1302)	$1983* (1899:2067)	$389* (348:431)
Severity				
Mild (reference)				
Higher severity	$19 (−185:223)	$393* (160:626)	−$390* (−479:301)	$16 (−27:60)
Comorbidities				
Congestive heart failure	$2815* (2250:3380)	$2012* (1645:2380)	$663* (523:804)	$138* (69:208)
Cardiac arrhythmias	$1758* (1403:2114)	$1095* (835:1355)	$606* (507:706)	$56* (7:19)
Valvular disease	$1462* (835:2088)	$1083* (685:1481)	$434* (282:586)	−$56 (−130:19)
Pulmonary circulation disorder	$3973* (3051:4894)	$2821* (2291:3351)	$845* (643:1048)	$306* (206;406)
Peripheral vascular disorder	1816* (1355:2277)	$1372* (1056:1688)	$311* (191:432)	$132* (72:191)
Hypertension uncomplicated	−$620* (−875: − 365)	−$531* (−770: − 293)	−$261* (−352: − 170)	$173* (128:218)
Hypertension complicated	$2497* (1722:3272)	$1558* (1050:2066)	$893* (699:1087)	$46 (−49:141)
Diabetes complicated	$2191* (1592:2790)	$730* (328:1133)	$958* (804:1111)	$502* (426:578)
Diabetes uncomplicated	$1221* (763:1679)	$672* (352:991)	$235* (113:357)	$314* (253:374)
Paralysis	$8449* (7564:9334)	$7309* (6890:7728)	$431* (271:591)	$708* (630:787)
Other neurological disorder	$3500* (3154:3845)	$2919* (2671:3167)	$188 (94:283)	$392* (345:438)
Chronic pulmonary disease	$837* (564:1111)	$224 (−3:451)	$256* (169:342)	$357* (314:400)
Thyroid	$657* (162:1152)	$127 (−221:477)	$245* (112:379)	$283* (217:349)
Renal failure	$1149* (478:1820)	$461* (8.5:914)	$530* (357:703)	$157* (72:243)
Liver disease	$2602* (2138:3067)	$2197* (1875:2519)	$312* (189:435)	$92* (31:153)
HIV/AIDS	$7445 (5658:9231)	$606 (−548:1760)	$1661* (1220:2102)	$314* (253:374)
Lymphoma	$4790* (3357:6222)	$1079* (170:1987)	$2382* (2035:2729)	$5177* (4960:5395)
Metastatic cancer	$6175* (5080:7269)	$4109* (3469:4749)	$1474* (1230:1719)	$590* (469:711)
Tumor without metastasis	$1470* (1048:1893)	$284 (−29:598)	$961* (841:1081)	$225* (166:284)
Rheumatoid arthritis	$1442* (876:2007)	−$33 (−452:385)	$954* (794:1114)	$521* (442:600)

(Continued)

III. TBI biomarkers in medical practice

TABLE 7.4　(Continued)

Variables	Total cost (95% CI)	Inpatient cost (95% CI)	Outpatient cost (95% CI)	Pharmacy cost (95% CI)
Any CT	**$1775* (1514:2035)**	**−$245 (−551:61)**	**$1646* (1529:1763)**	**$373* (315:431)**
Any MRI	**$851* (582:1120)**	**−$1522* (−1742: − 1302)**	**$1983* (1899:2067)**	**$389* (348:431)**
Coagulopathy	$4475* (3783:5168)	$3374* (2960:3788)	$789* (631:947)	$311* (233:389)
Fluid electrolyte disorders	$5987* (5592:6383)	$5105* (4828:5381)	$690* (584:796)	$192* (140:244)
Blood loss anemia	$3838* (2323:5354)	$3229* (2353:4105)	$541* (207:876)	$67 (−97:232)
Deficiency anemia	$3587* (2973:4201)	$2455* (2095:2816)	$835* (698:973)	$295* (227:363)
Alcohol abuse	$2202* (1921:2483)	$1820* (1573:2068)	$547* (453:642)	−166* (−213: − 119)
Drug abuse	$3884* (3563:4773)	$2282* (2017:2547)	$1429* (1328:1530)	$172* (122:222)
Psychoses	$4409* (4045:4773)	$2989* (2735:3243)	$928* (831:1026)	$491* (443:539)
Depression	$2975* (2708:3241)	$735* (495:975)	$1862* (1770:1953)	$378* (332:423)
Obesity	$1096* (841:1352)	−$402* (−627: − 177)	$1194* (1108:1280)	$304* (262:347)
Weight loss	$2833* (2309:3357)	$2291* (1968:2614)	$281* (158:405)	$260* (199:321)
Peptic ulcer disease	$1224* (576:1872)	$923 (487:1358)	$217* (51:384)	$83* (1.26:1.65)

CT, Computed tomography; MRI, magnetic resonance imaging; VHA, Veterans Health Administration.

TABLE 7.5　Severity and comorbidity-adjusted predicted mean annual CT, MRI, and total VHA cost per veteran 2000−2014 in 2018 values.

Variables	CT cost	MRI cost	Total cost	Inpatient cost	Outpatient cost	Pharmacy cost
Severity						
Mild	$284* (279:289)	$230* (225:235)				
Higher severity	$455* (451:459)	$309* (305:313)				
Any CT use						
No			$13,237* (12,981:13,494)	$6686* (6408:6963)	$5259* (5153:5365)	$1292* (1240:1344)
Yes			$15,012* (14,895:15,129)	$6441* (6331:6550)	$6906* (6864:6947)	$1665* (1645:1686)
Any MRI use						
No			$14,220* (14,003:14,438)	**$7411* (7244:7578)**	$5439* (5375:5503)	$1370* (1338:1401)
Yes			$15,072* (14,934:15,210)	**$5889* (5758:6019)**	$7423* (7373:7473)	$1759* (1735:1784)

CT, Computed tomography; MRI, magnetic resonance imaging; VHA, Veterans Health Administration.

7.4 Discussion

The results of this study have provided important benchmark costs, against which new TBI biomarkers can be compared as their pricing becomes available. The only biomarker currently in use in Sweden, has been shown to cost approximately US$25 [13,14]. If individuals, providers, insurers, and policy makers wish to compare per unit cost of a new biomarker against the standard of care of CT and MRI use, then the mean 2018 dollar value per unit cost of CT has been shown to be approximately $468, with a range of $460 for mild TBI severity to $470 for higher TBI severity, in a large cohort of TBI diagnosed veterans.

The mean 2018 value per unit cost of MRI has been shown to be approximately $732, with a range of $692 for mild TBI severity to $750 for higher TBI severity, in the same cohort.

Interestingly, the unadjusted frequency of any CT use is higher among veterans with higher TBI severity, but the unadjusted frequency of any MRI use is higher among veterans with mild TBI severity. It is possible that this is due to providers, when facing an absence of findings on CT, but symptoms which could be associated with TBI, choose to perform MRI exams.

This result is reinforced in the comorbidity-adjusted logit models, which showed that higher TBI severity is associated with a much lower likelihood of any MRI use. Finally, the exciting result that any MRI use was associated with a significant marginal reduction in annual inpatient cost of $1522 per veteran suggests that MRI use is being used in TBI diagnosis and management to reduce inpatient hospital care and cost. This is consistent with the literature stating that CT is better for detecting anatomical pathology and early bleeds, while MRI's ability to detect hematomas improves over time [18]. Also, MRI is superior to CT in detecting axonal injury, indirect neuronal damage, and small areas of contusion. In fact, some studies have shown that CT has missed about 10%−20% of abnormalities detected by MRI [18]. In addition, MRI is generally more sensitive than CT for detecting neuronal damage, with individuals whose brains show widespread MRI abnormalities or brain stem injuries, regularly failing to achieve significant neurological recovery, even in the presence of normal CT scans [18].

Finally, for prognosis and rehabilitation guidance, MRI has been used to detect white matter abnormalities and provide better information [18].

7.4.1 Study limitations

Our study cohort was based on all Veterans with an ICD-9 code for TBI between 2000 and 2010 using VHA inpatient, outpatient, and pharmaceutical services and having available information on VHA use by clinic stop codes. Our severity findings with such a high proportion of moderate/severe/penetrating severity relative to mild was different from the Defense and Veterans Brain Injury Center (DVBIC) which reports 85.15% of military TBIs were mild since 2000, representing the Operation Enduring Freedom/Operation Iraqi Freedom (OEF/OIF) cohort [27].

It is important to note that in the cohort used for this study, only about a third of veterans were OEF/OIF. Thus it is possible that only those veterans whose TBI is more apparent are documented in the VHA, especially among pre-OEF/OIF veterans. It is also possible that there is variation in clinician assignment of TBI diagnoses and severity between VA medical centers and clinics. Therefore the conclusions of this study may not reflect the experience of OEF/OIF veterans, only those who have used VHA inpatient, outpatient, and pharmacy services.

Another limitation of the study is that clinic stop codes ascertained CT and MRI utilization. The reason for the CT and MRI use was not known, which is why it was essential to adjust for comorbidities. The cost information is limited to internal VHA inpatient, outpatient, and pharmaceutical costs. It did not include fee-basis costs which are VA payments to providers outside of the VA. Also, FY 2000 costs began on October 1, 1999, so for veterans who had FY2000 costs, these would include last quarter 1999 costs as well.

7.4.2 Implications for policy and practice

Despite the limitations, the findings of this study provide a benchmark of per unit pricing and annual marginal total, inpatient, outpatient, and pharmacy cost per veteran associated with CT and MRI use. An exciting finding was that MRI use was associated with a significant reduction in annual inpatient costs per veteran, even though its cost per unit was higher than CT. These findings that MRI use is associated with a reduction in inpatient costs that are approximately twice the MRI's per unit cost, suggests that MRI may be much more cost-effective than has been previously documented in the literature, especially for mild TBI diagnosis and management.

7.4.3 Directions for future research

The ideal would have been to be able to compare pricing and cost impact of the new blood biomarker. The S100B biomarker has a per unit cost of about $25 in Sweden [12,13]. However, the marginal impact of S100B biomarker on long-term inpatient, outpatient, and pharmacy costs are not yet known. When the pricing has become available, and the technology has begun to spread through the VA system, a study comparing similar per unit, per veteran, and the marginal impact on total, inpatient, outpatient, and pharmacy VA cost will be illuminating.

This study has served to provide important benchmark information by which new TBI biomarkers could be compared in the future. The results are especially relevant, given the finding that, although having a higher per unit cost than CT, any MRI use has been shown to reduce inpatient costs in veterans by approximately double the MRI's per unit cost in veterans diagnosed with TBI.

Acknowledgments

This material is based upon work supported by the US Army Medical Research and Material Command and from the US Department of Veterans Affairs Chronic Effects of Neurotrauma Consortium under Award No. W81XWH-13-2-0095. The US Army Medical Research Acquisition Activity, 820 Chandler Street, Fort Detrick MD

21702-5014 is the awarding and administering acquisition office. Any opinions, findings, conclusions, or recommendations expressed in this publication are those of the author(s) and do not necessarily reflect the views of the US Government, or the US Department of Veterans Affairs, and no official endorsement should be inferred.

This work was also supported by the Health Economics Resource Center (HERC), Ci2i, VA Palo Alto Health Care System. The authors report no conflicts of interest. The views, opinions, and or/findings contained in this article are those of the authors and should not be construed as an official Veterans Affairs or Department of Defense position, policy, or decision unless so designated by other official documentation. A special thanks for Boyd Davis, PhD for linguistic review.

References

[1] Rubiano AM, Carney N, Chesnut R, Puyana JC. Global neurotrauma research challenges and opportunities. Nature 2015;527:S193−7.

[2] Dewan MC, Rattani A, Gupta S, Baticulon RE, Hung Y-C, Punchak M, et al. Estimating the global incidence of traumatic brain injury. J Neurosurg 2018;Apr 27:1−18. Available from: https://doi.org/10.3171/2017.10.JNS17352 [Epub ahead of print].

[3] Food and Drug Administration. FDA authorizes marketing of first blood test to aid in the evaluation of concussion in adults, <https://www.fda.gov/newsevents/newsroom/pressannouncements/ucm596531.htm>; February 14, 2018 [accessed 29.08.18].

[4] Teasdale G, Jennett B. Assessment of coma and impaired consciousness: a practical scale. Lancet 1974;2:81−4.

[5] The Lancet Neurology Commission. Traumatic brain injury: integrated approaches to improve prevention, clinical care, and research. Lancet Neurol 2017;16:987−1048.

[6] Samson K. FDA approves first blood test for brain bleeds after mild TBI/concussion. Neurol Today 2018; March 22.

[7] Bazarian JJ, Biberthaler P, Welch RD, Lewis LM, Barzo P, Bogner-Flatz V, et al. Serum GFAP and UCH1-L1 in prediction of absence of intracranial injuries on head CT (ALERT-TBI): a multi-center observational study. Lancet Neurol 2018;7(9):782−9.

[8] Communication, Dr. Yingling. Banyan biomarkers; August 15, 2018.

[9] Unden J, Ingebrigtsen T, Romner B, Scandinavian Neurotrauma C. Scandinavian guidelines for initial management of minimal, mild and moderate head injuries in adults: an evidence and consensus-based update. BMC Med 2013;11:50.

[10] Thelin EP, Nelson DW, Bellander B-M. A review of the clinical utility of serum S100B protein levels in the assessment of traumatic brain injury. Acta Neurochir 2017;159:209−25.

[11] Unden L, Calcagnile O, Unden J, Reinstrup P, Bazarian J. Validation of the Scandinavian guidelines for initial management of minimal, mild, and moderate brain injury in adults. BMC Med 2015;13:292.

[12] Bouvier D, Fournier M, Dauphin J-B, Amat F, Ughetto S, Labbe A, et al. Serum S100B determination in the management of pediatric mild traumatic brain injury. Clin Chem 2012;57(7):1116−22.

[13] Calcagnile O, Anell A, Unden J. The addition of S100B to guidelines for management of mild head injury is potentially cost saving. BMC Neurol 2016;16:200.

[14] OANDA Currency Converter. <https://www.oanda.com/currency/converter> [accessed 29.08.18].

[15] Sanders GD, Neumann PJ, Basu A, Brock DW, Feeny D, Krahn M, et al. Recommendations for conduct, methodological practices, and reporting of cost-effectiveness analyses: second panel on cost-effectiveness in health and medicine. JAMA 2016;316(10):1093−103.

[16] Alali AS, Burton K, Fowler RA, Naimark DMJ, Scales DC, Mainprize TG, et al. Economic evaluations in the diagnosis and management of traumatic brain injury: a systematic review and analysis of quality. Value Health 2015;18:721−34.

[17] Campbell KA, Berger RP, Ettaro I, Roberts MS. Cost-effectiveness of head computed tomography in infants with possible inflicted traumatic brain injury. Pediatrics 2007;120:295−304.

[18] Lee B, Newberg A. Neuroimaging in traumatic brain imaging. J Am Soc Exp NueroTher 2005;2:372−83.

[19] Military Health System and the Defense Health Agency Traumatic Brain Injury (TBI) DoD Standard Surveillance Case Definition for TBI Adapted for AFHSB Use. AFHSB surveillance case definitions FINAL April 2016. Military Health System and the Defense Health Agency, <https://health.mil/Military-Health-

Topics/Health-Readiness/Armed-Forces-Health-Surveillance-Branch/Epidemiology-and-Analysis/Surveillance-Case-Definitions>; 2016. [accessed 29.08.18].

[20] VA Information Resource Center. VIReC VHA Managerial Cost Accounting (MCA) historical stop codes. Hines, IL: VA Information Resource Center; 2018.

[21] Quan H, Sundararajan V, Halfon P, Fong A, Burnand B, Luthi JC, et al. Coding algorithms for defining comorbidities in ICD-9-CM and ICD-10 administrative data. Med Care 2005;43(11):1130–9.

[22] VA Health Economics Resource Center. Outpatient cost files, <http://vaww.herc.research.va.gov/include/page.asp?id = outpatient> [accessed 29.08.18].

[23] VA Health Economics Resource Center. Average cost, <http://vaww.herc.research.va.gov/include/page.asp?id = average-cost> [accessed 29.08.18].

[24] Polgreen LA, Brooks JM. Estimating incremental costs with skew: a cautionary note. Appl Health Econ Health Policy 2012;10(5):319–29.

[25] Willan AR, Briggs AH, Hoch JS. Regression methods for covariate adjustment and subgroup analysis for non-censored cost-effectiveness data. Health Econ 2004;13:461–75.

[26] US Department of Labor Consumer Price Index (CPI) Inflation Calculator. <https://www.bls.gov/data/inflation_calculator.htm> [accessed 29.08.18].

[27] Defense and Veterans Brain Injury Center (DVBIC). DoD worldwide numbers for TBI, <http://dvbic.dcoe.mil/dod-worldwide-numbers-tbi> [accessed 29.08.18].

Electrophysiology monitoring

James W.G. Thompson[1], *Barry Kosofsky*[2], *Elvisha Dhamala*[2]
and Ryan Duggan[2]

[1]Evoke Neuroscience, Inc., New York, NY, United States [2]Weill Cornell Medicine, New York, NY, United States

8.1 Introduction

Traumatic brain injury (TBI) can be induced by a direct or indirect insult that results in sudden acceleration, deceleration, and/or rotation of the head. TBI has multiple possible causes, including motor vehicle accidents, falls, collisions in sports and recreation, or physical assault, and can be classified by the mechanism of injury, clinical severity, or the characterization of physical injury. However, the heterogeneity of the disease has made the determination of TBI pathophysiology elusive and therefore the ability to predict prognosis and clinical outcomes, guide rehabilitation protocols, or track recovery beyond symptom resolution has been limited.

One consistency in the understanding of brain injury lies in the agreement that there is an interruption of neural function, with electrical, chemical, and morphological disruption, as a result of trauma exerted on the skull [1−4]. However, beyond that commonality, the multitude of symptoms present at the time of injury, and in many cases the prolonged nature of symptoms even in the absence of similar immediate injury characteristics, is forcing the conclusion that TBI is an injury that is unique across individuals with multiple underlying pathophysiological affects that can occur across multiple body systems.

In order to overcome these shortcomings currently plaguing TBI care, medicine must move beyond simple symptom-based diagnoses and clinical care to more advanced processes utilizing multimodal assessment tools that provide direct measurement of the pathophysiology of TBI. As Shaw [5] stated, "the almost instantaneous onset of a concussive state following the blow, its striking reversibility, the seeming absence of any necessary structural change in brain substance plus the inconsistency of any neuropathology which may occur are all compatible with the conception of concussion as fundamentally a physiological disturbance." [5] As such, electrophysiology is one of the only currently available tools that directly reflects real-time neurological function through the measurement of the moment-to-moment electrical discharges of firing neurons. Tools such as

Biomarkers for Traumatic Brain Injury
DOI: https://doi.org/10.1016/B978-0-12-816346-7.00008-7

electroencephalography (EEG), event-related potentials (ERPs), and the electrocardiogram (ECG) are reliable, valid, and clinically available tools that have decades of research and clinical support for their use in evaluating the negative effects of TBI on nervous system function and have a unique ability to help determine the pathophysiology of TBI for diagnostic use as well as ascertaining underlying causes of protracted recovery in people suffering postconcussion syndrome (PCS). This chapter focuses on ERPs and ANS metrics that have demonstrated utility in assessment, prognosis, and recovery tracking for individuals suffering TBI.

8.2 The autonomic nervous system

The autonomic nervous system, or ANS, which along with the somatic nervous system makes up the peripheral nervous system, helps regulate activity in the body through excitatory and inhibitory control processes. These functions are accomplished through two pathways: the excitatory sympathetic nervous system, and the inhibitory parasympathetic nervous system. The interaction between these two systems serves to maintain homeostasis in the body by regulating autonomic bodily functions and the functioning of internal organs [6]. The ANS is also crucial in mobilizing to external stimuli in several ways: in response to outside stressors or threats, the sympathetic nervous system increases blood pressure and heart rate, inhibits activity unnecessary to respond to the threat, such as the functioning of the digestive system and urinary tracts, and shunts blood to more important skeletal muscles via vasoconstriction [7]. (This is commonly referred to as the "fight or flight" response). The parasympathetic system, by contrast, maintains bodily functions at rest and restores homeostasis once a threat has past, reducing heart rate to its resting level and counteracting changes induced by the sympathetic nervous system [8].

Although the ANS acts upon the peripheral nervous system there is significant interplay between the brain and the ANS. The central autonomic network (CAN) is a complex network in the central nervous system (CNS) involving multiple regions of the brain, including the prefrontal cortex, amygdala, hypothalamus, and brainstem [8]. In particular, the frontal lobes play a large role influencing vagus nerve function while the amygdala is believed to exert a large amount of influence over autonomic, endocrine, and cardiovascular responses [9–12]. One critical function performed by the ANS via inputs from the CAN is the regulation of cardiovascular activity through both the sympathetic and parasympathetic systems. The excitatory sympathetic nervous system increases activity by releasing the catecholamine norepinephrine into the bloodstream, causing blood vessel constriction (and thus increased blood pressure), increased heart rate, and other physiological changes that prepare the body for increased activity or response to an external stressor [13]. The inhibitory parasympathetic system, by contrast, communicates with the cardiovascular system via the vagus nerve (cranial nerve X). This comparatively more direct innervation, when activated, serves to conserve energy under resting conditions, for example through decreasing heart rate and blood pressure by releasing acetylcholine [14]. The ANS is additionally involved in multiple other processes that maintain homeostasis including, but not limited to, innervation of cardiac muscle and smooth muscle, the activity of most tissues and organ systems in the body, regulation of blood pressure, focusing of the eyes, and thermoregulation. Due to the importance of the CAN, which comprises multiple brain regions, and the significant role of the vagus nerve in regulating autonomic function in the body, brain and vagal dysfunction can have a variety of significant downstream effects. One of the most significant of which is the cardiovascular and autoregulatory impairment that is found in concussion [15,16].

The involvement of the ANS in cardiovascular regulation also includes control of cerebral blood flow (CBF) through the baroreceptor reflex. This feedback system responds to changes in arterial pressure, prompting the ANS to increase or decrease blood pressure, heart rate, and other automatic physiological processes by both sympathetic and parasympathetic signaling pathways to the heart in order to maintain equilibrium in CBF [15]. This process is crucial to maintaining cognitive and neurological functioning, as the brain's high metabolic demands require a responsive autoregulatory system to maintain and modify cerebral perfusion [17].

Based on this well-established role of the ANS in cardiovascular regulation and cerebral autoregulation, measurements of heart rate and related cardiac rhythmicity have emerged as prominent biomarkers of autonomic function [18]. One such metric involves the short-term variability in heart rate, which measures the change in duration between heartbeats over a specified period of time. This is known as heart rate variability (HRV), which refers to both the beat-to-beat variation in instantaneous heart rate as well as changes in the interval between R peaks in the cardiac QRS complex (called the "R-R interval").

An increasing volume of literature has shown the validity of using HRV as a biological correlate of autonomic activity as well as an indicator of autonomic and cardiovascular health, and as such a marker for ANS dysfunction following TBI [19]. For example, studies have shown a correlation between increased cardiovascular fitness and higher HRV, suggesting a link between this metric and overall physical health [19,20]. Other studies have indicated a link between low HRV and increased mortality rates and risk of heart attack in humans [21]. Because heart rate depends not only on this parasympathetic-vagal regulation, but also on hormonal sympathetic input, HRV measurements represent a function of the interaction between both branches of the ANS [22,23].

Various HRV analysis methods have been developed, falling into the broad categories of time domain and frequency domain methods [18]. Among time domain analysis of changes over time, the most commonly used methods are average R-R interval and a measurement calculated from the mean R-R interval called the standard deviation of the normal-to-normal interval (SDNN) [18,19]. Further derivation of HRV can be conducted to calculate measurements such as RMSSD (the square root of the mean squared differences between successive R-R intervals) [10].

Frequency domain methods of analysis are used to understand the power spectrum, or spectral density, of an HRV recording, as well as the distribution of the frequency segments, which represent the effects of different autonomic pathways on HRV. The HRV frequency spectrum is divided into three bands, very low frequency (VLF), low frequency (LF), and high frequency (HF), with the distribution of power between these bands reflecting the distribution of power and amount of influence the sympathetic and parasympathetic systems play in regulating cardiovascular activity, also known as sympathovagal balance, and cardiac autonomic regulation [17,20,24−27]. This relationship has led to the understanding that HRV measurement is a strong marker of autonomic health and, as such, an invaluable tool in the assessment and management of autonomic dysfunction in TBI. A breakdown of the two cardiac function domains can be seen in Table 8.1 [19].

TABLE 8.1   Cardiac autonomic function can be assessed in two domains: time and frequency.

Outcome	Measurement	Description
Heart rate (HR)	Beats per minute (bpm)	Mean number of heartbeats per minute
Heart rate variability: time domain measures		
Mean RR interval (R-R)	Milliseconds (ms)	The average time interval between consecutive heartbeats, as measured from R-wave to R-wave [10]
SDNN	Milliseconds (ms)	Standard deviation of all R-R intervals [10]
RMSSD	Milliseconds (ms)	The square root of the mean of the sum of the squares of differences between adjacent R-R intervals [10]
NN50	Count	The number of pairs of R-R intervals differing by more than 50 ms in a recording [10]
pNN50	Percentage (%)	The number of pairs of R-R intervals differing by more than 50 ms in a recording, divided by the total number of R-R intervals [10]
Heart rate variability: frequency domain measures		
Total power	Milliseconds squared (ms^2)	The variance of all R-R interval [10]
LF	Milliseconds squared (ms^2)	Power in the low frequency range (i.e., 0.04–0.15 Hz) [10]
LFnu	Normalized units (nu)	Power in the low frequency range divided by the difference between total power and very low frequency (i.e., ≤ 0.04 Hz), multiplied by 100 [10]
HF	Milliseconds squared (ms^2)	Power in the high frequency range (i.e., 0.15–0.4 Hz) [10]
HFnu	Normalized units (nu)	Power in the high frequency range divided by the difference between total power and very low frequency (i.e., ≤ 0.04 Hz), multiplied by 100 [10]
LF:HF	Not applicable	The ratio of LF power to HF power [10]
Heart rate variability: other measures		
Approximate entropy (ApEn)	Not applicable	The likelihood of regularity in the signal with more regularity yielding smaller values and less regularity yielding larger values [28]
QT interval variability index (QTVI)	Not applicable	The proportion of the respective variances of QT and R-R intervals normalized to their means [29]
Coefficient variation of R-R		

Time domain measurements assess change in HRV over time, while frequency domain measures use power spectral analysis to analyze the frequency distribution of HRV.

8.2.1 Effect of traumatic brain injury on the autonomic nervous system

The physiology of the ANS facilitates communication between the CNS and the cardio-vascular system, but this connection also makes the ANS vulnerable to disruption after traumatic injury. TBI can impair cognitive function and nervous system activity in a variety of ways depending on the specific characteristics of the injury. More systematic dysfunction can result from the postinjury neuroinflammatory response or catecholamine release seen in TBI [30]. Both the initial injury and this secondary response can cause cardiovascular and ANS dysfunction, as well as impaired communication between the two systems. It is also possible for autonomic dysfunction to be caused by the force of impact in close proximity to the brainstem and the medulla, as well as from diffuse axonal injury in which the neural connections in cerebral white matter are lesioned by the shearing forces caused by acceleration and deceleration during TBI [30]. However, the ANS can be disrupted even in the absence of a direct impact on these areas, suggesting that autonomic function is mediated by multiple parallel pathways and is thus vulnerable to disruption at many points in these lines of communication.

It has been established that the biomechanical force of TBI disrupts homeostasis down to the cellular level, causing damage to the integrity of cellular structures and triggering an "energy crisis" as an imbalance between supply and demand overwhelms the nervous system [13]. This is caused by the brain's reaction to the acute perturbation of equilibrium, which involves the initial period of hypermetabolic activity followed by a metabolic depression as energy is depleted and CBF decreases, causing cerebral energy demand to outstrip supply [17]. This uncoupling of supply and demand, which leads to dysfunction in cerebral autoregulation, is thought to be one of the underlying cause of the symptoms of postconcussive syndrome (PCS), such as headache, dizziness, fatigue, and sleep problems [31,32].

During the acute period, the sympathetic nervous system enters into a hyperactive phase in which increasing amounts of catecholamines are released into the bloodstream [30,33]. This stress response-induced increase in circulating dopamine, epinephrine, and norepinephrine causes increased blood pressure and tachycardia. The amount of increased circulation and severity of the response is more pronounced in more severe TBI than in mild TBI (mTBI), suggesting that there is a gradient of catecholamine response that corresponds with injury severity [33,34]. This sympathetic hyperactivity, which has been found in patients with mTBI as well as more severe injuries, has been associated with increased long-term cardiovascular risk as well as a potential increase in mortality [25,26]. In some cases the massively increased peripheral catecholamine release can cause persistent cardiovascular dysfunction, which along with other long-term changes can significantly reduce the patient quality of life [35].

Beyond the purely acute, relatively localized changes instigated by TBI, the neuroinflammatory response can lead to more systemic, chronic impairment in systems mediated by the ANS. Following injury, both human and animal models demonstrate a sharp acute increase in cytokine activity, specifically an upregulation of interleukin-1α, a cytokine involved in inflammatory response regulation, as well as a slower increase in expression of the similarly proinflammatory IL-1β [36]. This inflammatory response is thought to play a neuroprotective role in the acute postinjury period, as IL-1β promotes the release of other proinflammatory factors that have a downstream neurotrophic effect in recovery from injury. The amount of cytokines released is dependent on severity of injury, however, and chronically higher concentrations in the postacute period have been associated with neurotoxicity and prolonged dysfunction [36,37].

TBI has also been shown to increase the permeability of the blood−brain barrier (BBB), which can allow the inflammatory response of the CNS to spread to the level of systemic dysfunction as proinflammatory cytokines pass through the BBB into the bloodstream [30].

The vagus nerve, which receives input from, and is responsible for the regulation of the immune system, also responds to proinflammatory signals by subsequently attenuating the neuroinflammatory response and reducing the release of cytokines like IL-1β before their effects become neurotoxic [38,39]. However, postinjury autonomic dysfunction can include impairment of the vagal signaling pathway, a disruption that would also prevent the ANS response to TBI-induced neuroinflammation, leading to further systemic dysfunction [30,40].

Additionally, the neuroinflammatory response of the CNS to TBI has been shown to result in increased intracranial pressure, disrupting autonomic pathways in the brainstem, specifically those of the sympathetic nervous system [30]. The mechanism by which this acute swelling directly impairs the CAN is unclear, though it has been proposed that the inflammation causes autonomic dysfunction through direct herniation of cortical, brainstem, and medullary CAN nuclei in more severe TBI [29]. The breakdown in cerebral autoregulation after TBI, in which the brain experiences a hypermetabolic increase in cerebral blood flow and volume, can subsequently cause an increase in intracranial pressure [28,41]. Recent research in animal models of TBI has indicated that increases and decreases in intracranial pressure are significantly correlated with corresponding changes in muscle and renal sympathetic nerve activity [42]. Although more research is needed to confirm this relatively novel line of inquiry, it appears plausible that postinjury increases in intracranial pressure play an additional role in autonomic dysfunction after TBI.

One of the most significant overall effects of the systemic destabilization of equilibrium following TBI is the disruption of ANS regulation of cardiovascular activity. Patients with mTBI show characteristic cerebrovascular dysregulation: reduction in parasympathetic activity and an increase in sympathetic activity [17]. Another study found that patients with a history of mTBI had significantly elevated heart rates and reduced HRV after moving from a supine to a standing position [43]. This phenomenon has also been observed in patients with severe TBI and consequent dysautonomia, indicating an uncoupling between the cardiovascular system and the ANS [44]. Research findings of Baguley et al. are shown in Table 8.2 and demonstrate significant prolonged negative effects in multiple HRV parameters for TBI subjects [44]. A more comprehensive review of the literature has confirmed a similar pattern across all levels of injury severity, showing a consistent reduction in parasympathetic activity and more variability in the presence and severity of postinjury sympathetic dysfunction, in studies of athletes and the general population [15]. Research has established that patients with a history of mTBI also demonstrated an impaired baroreflex when subjected to the Valsalva maneuver, a standardized test of forced breathing against a closed airway, which measures changes in blood pressure and other cardiovascular metrics [11,45]. This research found that patients with mTBI had lower HRV at rest compared to control subjects, and took longer to return to their resting levels following increases induced by the Valsalva maneuver, indicating a link between head injury, impaired autonomic regulation, and the baroreflex [11].

8.2.2 Autonomic nervous system biomarkers in traumatic brain injury

As the 2017 Concussion in Sport Group consensus statement notes, despite the immense body of research into the causes, progression of symptoms, and treatment of TBI,

TABLE 8.2   Comparing characteristics of subjects with TBI and age-matched controls.

	Control, M (SD)	TBI group, M (SD)	p	Normative values (12), M (SD)
Demographics				
N	16	16		
Age at injury (years)	31.5 (9.5)	32.0 (12.0)		
M:F	9:7	13:3		
Injury mode				
MVA		8		
Assault		4		
Fall		2		
Sport		2		
Days postinjury		81 (58)		
HRV data				
Heart rate (bpm)	67.6 (12.1)	89.5 (11.0)	0.000	—
Total power (ms^2)	4065 (4082)	1656 (1237)	0.037	3466 (1018)
VLF power (ms^2)	1695 (1423)	1191 (1034)	0.262	—
LF power (ms^2)	1304 (1484)	189 (152)	0.009	1170 (416)
HF power (ms^2)	1019 (1588)	203 (397)	0.063	975 (203)
SDNN (ms)	60.2 (26.9)	40.6 (16.4)	0.018	141 (39)
LF/HF ratio	1.8 (0.9)	3.7 (3.0)	0.029	1.5 − 2.0
LF/HF$_{mod}$ ratio	0.8 (0.9)	2.5 (3.4)	0.070	—

bpm, Beats per minute; *MVA*, motor vehicle accident related injury.
Data comparison table from Baguley et al (2006). Subjects with concussion had significantly higher heart rates (in beats per minute or bpm). Spectral analysis of HRV showed lower total power in TBI subjects, as well as significantly lower low-frequency power, and a significantly elevated low-frequency/high-frequency ratio.

an objective, widely applicable biomarker has yet to be developed [46]. In the absence of such a universal diagnostic tool, physicians have relied on a combination of neurocognitive testing and symptom evaluation to diagnosis TBI and mitigate PCS [46]. Similarly, the variable etiology of postconcussive autonomic dysfunction complicates diagnosis and treatment. Autonomic regulation of the cardiovascular system is vulnerable to disruption at multiple points, with the potential for different causes and mechanisms of prolonged dysfunction.

Due to the strong body of evidence linking TBI and autonomic dysfunction, HRV has shown promise as a barometer of autonomic health in TBI patients. Diagnosis and treatment of TBI is currently based around clinical evaluation and subjective measures including self-report inventories of PCS symptom severity. Since these questionnaires are not objective measures, they are insufficient to serve as a basis for concussion management [16]. Additionally, while both symptom inventories and neuropsychological testing have clinical utility in assessing concussion severity and the progress of recovery, in the case of athletes, there may be an incentive to minimize the extent of their impairment or of injury severity in order to more quickly return to play [47]. Considering the limitations of existing assessment tools the development of useful biomarkers is of particular importance in the field and is the subject of much ongoing research. As a result of the demonstrated connection between TBI and autonomic and cardiovascular dysfunction, it is necessary to develop more objective biomarkers of concussion that include ANS measures.

Specifically pertaining to TBI, exercise tolerance has been demonstrated to be a correlated biomarker of recovery from PCS, with both symptom resolution and improved HRV being outcome measures of this biomarker [48]. Dr. John Leddy and his colleagues at the University at Buffalo have developed a protocol using these biomarkers called the Buffalo Concussion Treadmill Test. The test consists of a graded exercise cardiac stress test in which concussed patients exercised until the onset or exacerbation of PCS symptoms [49]. This test, which was validated with a randomized controlled trial of adolescent concussion patients, also demonstrated the ability to assess recovery from concussion in the acute period; participants were retested two weeks after the initial test, and 80% were found to have returned to normal exercise tolerance levels [49]. On this basis, the authors suggested that the Buffalo Exercise Protocol could serve as an objective way to assess both the severity of concussion and track the progress of recovery.

To this end, a growing body of research suggests that autonomic recovery following TBI may not match the physiological timeline of recovery as measured by resolution of symptoms [32]. Although 80%–90% of postconcussive symptoms resolve within 10 days, autonomic abnormalities such as reduced CBF, itself indicative of impaired cerebral autoregulation, can persist for 30 days or more [32,47]. Further longitudinal research assessing changes in HRV in athletes during a sit-to-stand test at multiple time points, including after return to play, has confirmed that altered HRV persists even after subjects were asymptomatic [32,50,51]. Research conducted by Wright et al., recorded beat-by-beat arterial blood pressure (BP) and middle cerebral artery blood velocity (MCAv) during five minutes of repetitive squat–stand maneuvers [32]. This activity induced BP oscillations at 0.05 and 0.10 Hz (20- and 10s cycles, respectively) and the BP–MCAv relationship was quantified using transfer function analysis to estimate coherence (correlation), gain (amplitude ratio), and phase (timing offset). Their findings demonstrated that 0.10 Hz phase was significantly reduced following an acute concussion, and compared to preseason was reduced by 23% at 72 h, and by 18% at 2 weeks post injury, indicating impaired autoregulatory functioning [32]. Recovery to preseason values did not occur until 1 month post injury (Fig. 8.1), indicating physiologic dysfunction persisting beyond clinical recovery in many cases [32]. Thus even when the majority of symptoms are no longer present, ongoing autoregulatory deficits can persist and may be connected to more persistent PCS symptoms or likelihood of secondary injury. Further evidence to demonstrate the need for taxing the ANS in order to properly assess the functionality of the ANS control system is provided by many other research studies, including research by J.P. Abaji et al. who found that, while high-frequency HRV was significantly reduced in concussed athletes during isometric handgrip tests, it did not differ significantly at rest [50].

Additional research has demonstrated significant differences in cardiovascular activity at rest, but these differences resolved within one day of the injury, further providing

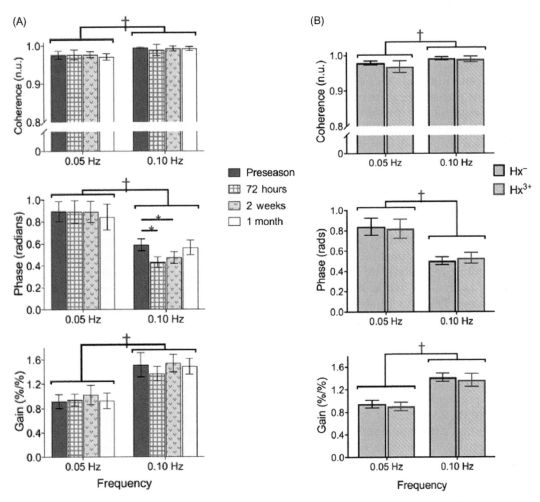

FIGURE 8.1 Results of transfer function analysis in Wright et al. (2018), showing coherence (the proportion of output signal explained by the input), phase (the timing offset between input and output), and gain (the ratio of amplitudes of inputs and outputs). Measures were taken during squat-stand maneuvers assessed at (A) preseason and each post-concussion time point; (B) preseason in athletes with zero and three or more previous concussions. † represents significant main effect of frequency (p all < 0.01), * denotes significant simple effect of time (p all < 0.01). Data is presented as mean $\pm$ SE.

evidence of the necessity of exertion and ANS system challenges to more fully tease out residual ANS dysfunction that may not be readily apparent under resting clinical conditions but which may negatively affect injured individuals during day-to-day activities or sports [52]. One must note that many studies have methodological limitations, such as small sample sizes, homogeneous samples, and potential biases that limit their applicability [19]. Therefore, although ANS disruption is a now known effect of TBI, further research is needed to fully understand the development of autonomic dysfunction after concussion, as well as whether the sympathetic and parasympathetic systems are differentially affected.

In the search for autonomic and electrophysiological biomarkers of concussion, HRV has emerged as a promising candidate [17]. As has been previously discussed, the general link between HRV and ANS activity is well-established. The ability of HRV to serve as a quantifiable physiological correlate of autonomic function demonstrates its potential utility in the assessment and treatment of TBI and managing persisting PCS symptoms. Recent studies of mTBI have additionally demonstrated a link between ANS dysfunction and certain PCS symptoms, especially dizziness, that had previously been attributed to vestibular injury [53]. In a retrospective review, these researchers found that performing the tilt-table test, a procedure used to diagnose autonomic or cardiovascular dysfunction, upon patients with concussion and PCS, led to significant dysfunctional autonomic response including tachycardia and blood pressure instability [53]. In addition to strengthening the proposed link between autonomic dysfunction and PCS, these and similar studies have provided further evidence of the utility of HRV as a clinical metric of concussion symptom severity. Another test of ANS function that may be able to bridge the gap between physiological and autonomic recovery is the cold pressor test, in which a patient's hand is immersed in a bath of cold water while measurements of heart rate and blood pressure are taken [54,55]. In non-TBI individuals exposure to the water at near-freezing temperatures causes activation of the sympathetic nervous system and excitatory pathways and a corresponding depression of parasympathetic activity [55].

Building off the evidence that patients with TBI show reduced HRV in aerobic exercise, but not isometric handgrip exercise, researchers investigating the cold pressor test as an exercise-independent diagnostic tool measured HRV in concussed patients and controls [54]. This preliminary research found that participants with TBI had a blunted sympathetic response to the cold pressor test compared to healthy control participants, as well as a relatively normal parasympathetic response, expressed as RMSSD [54]. While these findings are preliminary and require further investigation, the cold pressor test may represent an additional use of HRV as a biomarker of autonomic dysfunction after mTBI.

8.2.3 Autonomic nervous system biomarkers in traumatic brain injury rehabilitation

Since the changes in HRV caused by TBI are well-established and understood, they can be used alongside standard treatment protocols to track recovery from injury, and better assess an individual's readiness to return to activity. In cases where PCS symptom resolution precedes autonomic return to baseline after TBI, a common occurrence, HRV measurement would serve as a more accurate metric of recovery than simply assessing symptoms with a graded exercise protocol [51]. Treatment plans designed with HRV as an outcome measure would therefore reduce the risks associated with premature return to play, such as increased PCS symptom severity, delayed recovery, and greater risk of repeated injury [56].

Targeting HRV as a specific focus of treatment would also be beneficial for its own sake, as there is a large body of research documenting the association of cardiovascular-autonomic uncoupling with increased mortality rates with the effect increasingly pronounced in more severe TBI [25,43]. Furthermore, reduced HRV in particular has been shown to be a predictor of postinjury mortality in severe TBI, with one study also finding a strong association between cardiac uncoupling and increased inflammatory response postinjury [57]. A promising line of treatment that directly addresses cardiovascular dysregulation is the use of beta-blockers against TBI-induced sympathetic hyperactivity. As one comprehensive retrospective review notes, beta-adrenergic antagonists appeared to significantly reduce mortality in TBI patients regardless of the specific medication used during hospital admission [25]. More recent research comparing the relative benefits of different beta-blockers has shown that propranolol more significantly decreased mortality than any other type of beta-blocker in a population of TBI patients receiving inpatient care postinjury [58]. These findings indicate that in TBI patients with severe persistent autonomic dysfunction beta-blockers could provide an essential supplemental therapy in recovery following injury.

In cases of less severe persistent sympathetic hyperactivity, HRV biofeedback training has demonstrated utility as a method of restoring balanced ANS activity [59]. An example of this training is the protocol developed by Dr. Paul Lehrer and colleagues which involves determining the resonance frequency of a patient's cardiovascular system and training them to breathe at this rate in order to maximize their HRV [60]. This protocol stipulates two daily 20-minute sessions of "resonance breathing" over the course of weeks or months, along with five to ten clinical follow-up visits over the same timeline [60]. Studies of long-term biofeedback protocols indicate that such training can significantly increase both HRV and the low-frequency/high-frequency power ratio measurement of cardiovascular health [61,62]. Another benefit of biofeedback is the strengthening of the baroreflex that occurs over time, an improvement that correlates with increased HRV [61,63]. There is also preliminary evidence that HRV biofeedback can strengthen vagal tone, restoring the resting predominance of parasympathetic activity over sympathetic activity, suggesting that this therapy could effectively address sympathetic hyperactivity following TBI [63].

There has been a significant amount of research into genetic contributions to HRV. For example, the Framingham Heart Study determined that genetic contributions ranged from 13% to 23% of variation in heart rate variance, with the highest contribution attributed to the low-frequency/high-frequency ratio [64]. Research into brain-derived neurotrophic factor (BDNF), another relevant genetic influence, has proved a promising line of investigation into the link between autonomic and cardiac biomarkers [65]. A single-nucleotide polymorphism (SNP) of the BDNF gene called Val66Met, which has been shown to cause reduced BDNF expression in humans and animal models, has also been connected to mental dysfunction in humans [66,67]. Prospective studies of active-duty American soldiers found that those with the BDNF Met/Met genotype had a significantly greater risk of concussion than soldiers with other genotypes [68,69]. The same polymorphism has also been suggested to influence autonomic function in healthy individuals, with participants in one study with the Met/Met genotype demonstrating significantly reduced HRV compared to other genotypes [67]. This group also demonstrated a significantly increased low-frequency/high-frequency power ratio, suggesting an altered balance between sympathetic and parasympathetic influence on cardiac activity [67].

Studies of gene expression in mice have also shown that BDNF levels are generally reduced in those with the Met/Met genotype compared to Val/Val [70,71]. These findings further suggest that BDNF may have a neuroprotective role in TBI, and given the established connection between the BDNF Met/Met genotype and altered ANS regulation of cardiac activity, it is reasonable to suspect this gene is connected to TBI-induced autonomic dysfunction [67,72]. While investigators caution that small sample sizes and low statistical power limit the generalizability of these findings, understanding how BDNF affects the ANS before and after injury has informed the use of exercise as part of an autonomic-cardiovascular rehabilitative regimen following concussion. Research along these lines has found that aerobic exercise over time promotes BDNF expression in the brain and in serum, along with increased volume in the hippocampus, suggesting a neuroprotective role of increased BDNF secretion [49,73].

8.3 Event-related potentials

Many studies have shown that ERPs are an objective measure of cortical stimulus processing, and also a strong biomarker for use at multiple stages of TBI management [74]. ERPs are electrical field potentials generated by the brain during everyday activities and reflect changes of cognitive processes in a wide range of clinical disorders. This pattern of neuroelectric activation elicited in anticipation of, or in response to, a specific cognitive, sensory, or motor stimulus can be reliably measured using an electroencephalogram (EEG) [75]. An EEG recording collects information about thousands of simultaneous brain processes by recording the real-time electrical activity of active neurons. Therefore the response to a single stimulus of interest is not usually visible in the EEG recording of a single trial. To identify the brain's response to a single stimulus (i.e., sensory, motor, or cognitive), the recordings of many trials must be averaged to isolate the relevant waveform. ERPs in humans can be divided into two categories: (1) the early components (also known as "sensory" or "exogenous") that peak around the first 100 ms after stimulus presentation and largely depend on the physical parameters of the stimulus; and (2) the later components (also known as "cognitive" or "endogenous") that peak following the early components represent information processing [75].

Generally, there are five criteria that can be used to describe an ERP component: polarity, latency, duration, morphology, and topography [76]. The polarity refers to whether the voltage deflection is positive or negative, latency is the time delay, in milliseconds, between a given stimulus and the specific component, duration is the total time that the specific peak is observed, morphology describes the shape of the peak, and topography designates the general region of the brain in which the components are observed. Nomenclature of most ERP components includes the letter N (negative) or P (positive) indicating polarity and a number that either refers to the latency or the component's order in the waveform. For example, a positive peak that occurs around 300 ms and is the third peak observed after the stimulus is known as the P300 (based on polarity and latency) or P3 (based on polarity and order of the peak in the waveform) [77].

A significant advantage of ERP testing at all levels of TBI is their robustness in eliminating many of the confounding factors found in neuropsychological testing. The advantages inherent in neuropsychological testing, which include ease of administration, relatively short testing time (15–25 minutes), and low cost, are also shared beneficial characteristics of ERPs. In addition, ERPs also overcome some of the significant and well-known weaknesses of neuropsychological testing including practice effects and their reliance on best-effort, subject motivation, and honest reporting [78]. ERPs are objective, quantifiable measures of cognitive function that are not susceptible to internal factors, that elucidate specific cognitive processes and brain functions including processing speed, sustained attention, performance monitoring, inhibitory control, and cognitive flexibility [79]. Research utilizing the precise temporal resolution of ERPs demonstrates the differential sensitivity of ERP components to the effects of trauma. Qualitative disruption to early perceptual discrimination processes have a downstream effect on the speed of processing by delaying the transfer of information from stimulus processing to response selection [79]. These disruptions are reflected in the amplitudes and latencies of relevant ERP components and are discussed below.

8.3.1 Early event-related potential components

The early components of the ERPs, also known as sensory evoked potentials (SEPs), are the electrical potentials generated in sensory pathways at peripheral, spinal, subcortical, and cortical levels of the nervous systems. SEPs can be elicited from almost any nerve in a noninvasive means to assess somatosensory functioning [80]. Moreover, SEP recordings at different levels of the somatosensory pathways can be studied to assess the transmission of information from the periphery to the cortex. These recordings can be used to identify areas that have been damaged as a result of trauma or neurodegenerative diseases [81].

Several studies have looked at the correlates between TBI and SEPs with the findings showing strong utility for the clinical use of SEPs for diagnosis and prognosis for both positive and negative predictive outcomes in TBI patients [82–89].

8.3.2 Late event-related potential components

Over the past 30 years, the use of later stage or cognitive ERPs, has emerged as a technique to provide insight into the neural correlates underlying cognitive processes such as perception, memory, and action in TBI and as a tool for prognostic use in severe TBI [74,85–100].

The main benefits of using these cognitive ERPs lies in their temporal sensitivity, which allows the stimulus–response relationship to be parsed into its various component processes [78]. Moreover, ERPs are a direct quantitative measurement of neural function that cannot be manipulated by the subject [78]. The utility of cognitive ERPs in TBI is also underscored since in contrast to earlier components, cognitive ERPs are more strongly influenced by variation in subjects' cognitive processes, such as arousal and alertness, and personal salience of stimuli, thereby making them ideally suited for the known alterations in arousal and cognitive alertness seen in TBI [101].

8.3.3 P300 event-related potential component

The "oddball" paradigm is often used to elicit the P3 component of cognitive ERPs. In the single-stimulus task, the target is presented infrequently with no other stimuli. In the traditional two-stimulus oddball, the target is presented infrequently in a background of frequent standard stimuli. In the three-stimulus oddball, the target is presented infrequently in a background of frequently occurring distractor stimuli. The subject must respond to the target stimulus and not respond to any other stimuli. In each case, the target stimulus elicits a large positive-going potential, known as the P3, that increases in amplitude from the frontal to parietal electrodes and has a peak latency of 300–400 ms following stimulus onset. The major interpretation of the P3 amplitude is that it represents neural activity when the mental representation of a stimulus is updated [102]. After initial sensory processing of the stimulus presented, the stimulus is compared to the previous stimulus in working memory. If no differences are detected between the stimuli, the "schema" of the stimulus is maintained. However, if a new stimulus is detected, attentional resources are engaged to update the representation for the stimulus, leading to elicitation of the P3 [102].

The P3 potential can further be divided into the P3a and P3b subcomponents. The P3a component is typically elicited by an infrequent and uninstructed novel stimulus. It is localized in the frontocentral cortex and exhibits relatively short latency. The P3b component is elicited by an infrequently but instructed target stimulus and is localized in the parietal area [103].

The use of various stimuli over many trials has provided a basis for inferring what the P3a and P3b subcomponents represent. The P3a component is theorized to reflect the selection of stimulus information associated with attentional orienting to a change in the environment. It represents disengaging attentional focus from one aspect of the stimulus environment and reengaging attention towards another aspect of the environment [103]. The amplitude of the P3a represents the extent of attentional focus, with larger amplitudes indicating greater focal attention [103]. The P3b is believed to reflect processes associated with the allocation of attentional resources during cognitive tasks involved in updating working memory. The P3b amplitude is sensitive to the amount of attentional resources allocated toward a stimulus [103]. The P3b latency is sensitive to stimulus classification speed. It is therefore thought to reflect the time it takes to detect and evaluate a stimulus independent of the actions taken to respond to the stimulus [103]. For this reason the P3b component is uniquely qualified to be used in TBI evaluation since the physical response of the subject is not a factor in determining the level of function or dysfunction in a subject. In other words the P3b is a quantitative biomarker that cannot be manipulated or "faked" by a subject.

8.3.4 N2 event-related potential component

The N2 component is a small-negative going component of the ERP, which emerges just prior to the P3. With regards to the P3, a discernible N2 with a frontocentral maximum precedes the P3a and a separate N2 with a parietal maximum precedes the P3b. In response to an uninstructed, novel stimuli, a frontocentral N2 has been linked to mismatch of a stimulus from the preexisting mental template, suggesting it represents an increase in cognitive control over response inhibition. The N2 is also a known component in stimulus–response mapping as it relates to the P3 component [79]. In response to infrequent,

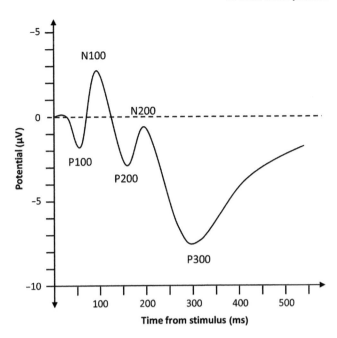

FIGURE 8.2 Schematic event-related potential (ERP) wave of an auditory oddball paradigm showing the typical designation of components.

target stimuli, the parietally occurring N2 has been associated with the amount of attention required to process the stimuli [103].

A schematic representation of ERP components in response to an auditory oddball paradigm stimuli is shown in Fig. 8.2 [104].

8.3.5 Event-related potentials as biomarkers in traumatic brain injury

8.3.5.1 *Moderate-to-severe traumatic brain injury*

SEPs have demonstrated a unique ability to predict both positive and negative outcomes in unresponsive and severe TBI patients. Hutchinson et al. studied 90 patients suffering severe TBI, recording SEPs within 3 days of injury, with a follow-up at 6 months [84]. Patients demonstrating the presence of bilateral SEPs had a favorable outcome while absence of one or both SEPs showed unfavorable outcomes [84]. This research showed the utility of SEPs for use in prediction of both favorable and unfavorable outcomes, making them highly valuable for clinical use in the early evaluation of severe TBI patients [84]. Research by J.D. Rollnik utilizing a large data sample of 803 brain-injured individuals supports these findings, whereby they demonstrated that the absence of SEP on one or both sides was associated with a poor outcome, with only 12.5% of such individuals recovering [99]. A literature review conducted by Carter and Butt reviewed research from as far back as 1980 that demonstrated significant support for the prognostic use of SEPs in TBI patients [105]. This review compared clinical examination (pupillary response, motor response, and the Glasgow Coma Scale), EEG, and computed tomography

(CT) to SEPs, confirming that in TBI patients, whether normal (positive outcomes) or bilaterally absent (negative outcomes), SEPs were the best single predictor of outcome. The authors concluded that "there is sufficient evidence for clinicians to use SEPs in the prediction of outcome after brain injury" [82,105]. Guerit followed up on work from over a decade earlier in which the combination of cortical function and brainstem conduction could be used in parallel to improve diagnosis and prognosis in TBI. The value of SEPs was unique in their ability to explain pathophysiology. Pattern 1 patients who showed no changes in SEPs and demonstrated good recovery. Pattern 2 patients, characterized by alterations of SEPs suggestive of midbrain dysfunction, generally recovered after a long vegetative period. Pattern 3 patients were characterized by alterations in SEPs suggestive of pontine involvement, generally had transtentorial herniation, and had poor outcomes. Pattern 4 patients had a full disappearance of all SEP activity and corresponded to brain death [83].

The most researched and clinically utilized ERP in TBI is the P3 component. This is likely due to the fact that TBI-related influences on the P3 ERP component appear to be disproportionately larger in response to tasks requiring greater amounts of cognitive engagement [106]. As previously discussed, the P3 component reflects neural inhibition. The amplitude of the P3 represents the suppression of extraneous neuronal activity during the engagement of focal attention (P3a) and the allocation of attentional resources toward working memory (P3b) [107]. Significant changes are found in the P3 component in patients with the absence of conscious mental activity [100].

Lew et al. combined SEPs with the P3 ERP and replicated the high predictive value of SEPs in patient outcomes. Specificity and positive predictive value of the finding of an absent SEP in predicting death or persistent vegetative state were as high as 100% [108]. Additionally, this research was unique in that it included cognitive P3 as an additional measure. The benefit of the P3 was that a normal P3 ERP showed a higher sensitivity and negative predictive value for prognosticating good outcomes than SEPs. This led the authors to conclude that SEPs continue to make reliable predictions of negative outcomes in TBI and the addition of the P3 can improve prediction of favorable outcomes and strengthen the overall prognosis [108].

There are multiple additional research papers supporting the use of the P3 ERP component in TBI prognosis. Yingling et al. used a tone-evoked P3 as a predictor of recovery from coma. Of the patients tested, 65% did not display a P300 response. Of those without P300 responses over 66% died within a week, while the remaining 34% survived but in a persistent vegetative state. In contrast, the patients with detectable P300 responses showed significant clinical improvement over the next several months. These findings lend further support for the use of the P3 response in predicting functional outcome of patients with severe TBI [109]. Cavinato's group looked at the ERP components in 34 patients in a vegetative state at 2—3 months and up to 1 year following a TBI. At the 1-year time point following injury, 26 of the patients had recovered consciousness while the other eight had not. Analysis of the data indicated that a detectable P3 response postinjury was a strong predictor of recovery of consciousness in these patients [89]. The ability of P3 to aid in prognosis was further supported in work by Zhang et al., who used P3 to assess higher-order cortical information processing in severe TBI. Results demonstrated a highly significant relationship between the presence of P3 and subsequent recovery, and the ability of

P3 to accurately characterize level of cognitive preservation and likelihood of recovery from disorders of consciousness following TBI [96].

Patients with TBI tend to have the most difficulty using flexible, novel approaches to solve new and complex problems, yet perform well on simple, automatic, or well-rehearsed tasks [92]. The susceptibility of the frontal cortex and its related circuitry via focal cortical contusions or diffuse white matter injury-disrupting dopaminergic input to the prefrontal cortex likely underlies TBI-related cognitive control deficit [93,110]. This has been supported by recent functional neuroimaging studies in mild and moderate-to-severe TBI [94,95,111,112]. As a result of the positive prognostic value of ERPs in severe TBI there continues to be a growing body of research in this area with ever-strengthening support for the use of ERPs in evaluating TBI patients. This work is of the utmost importance since prognostic uncertainty impedes accurate management decisions [94]. The ability of ERPs to assess brain function at higher levels than earlier SEPs is enhancing outcome prediction accuracy in coma patients [94,95].

8.3.5.2 Mild traumatic brain injury

Cognitive neuropsychological studies have long demonstrated slowing of reaction time and information processing speed in mTBI and more recent studies have suggested that this slowing occurs in conjunction with severity-dependent impairments in "executive" control [113–116]. A summary of some of the work looking at ERP and mTBIs was published in a paper by Broglio et al. in 2011 and can be found in Table 8.3 [74].

A study by Moore et al. looked at the influence of concussive and subconcussive impact on soccer players' neurophysiological and neuropsychological function. Athletes in the subconcussion and concussion groups exhibited similar amplitude reductions in the ERP measures of P3b and P3a relative to noncontact athletes, as shown in Fig. 8.3 [117].

Brooks et al. studied changes in P3b potentials in varsity football players associated with accumulated subconcussive head impacts. Head impacts were measured using an accelerometer adhered to the football helmet. Players were divided into three groups based on the position played: the small-skilled group consisted of wide receivers and defensive backs; the big-skilled group consisted of running backs, quarterbacks, and linebackers; and lastly the big-unskilled group consisted of offensive and defensive linemen. ERP components of the players were evaluated at baseline (preseason), midseason, and postseason. Players who experienced a high number of impacts showed significant decreases from baseline in P3b amplitude compared to low-impact players at midseason and postseason in the small-skilled and big-skilled groups, but not in the big-unskilled group. The significance of the findings from these studies on subconcussive impacts cannot be understated since these objective findings establish the negative effects of subconcussive impacts in contact athletes within a season of play. Athlete safety and training schedules should begin to reflect these now known negative effects of subconcussive impacts and should be taken as evidence that contact sport athletes require rest and recovery for their brain health as they do their physical health. Results are shown in Fig. 8.4 [118].

Broglio et al. studied the persistent effect of concussion on the neuroelectric indices of attention in athletes in 2009. Male and female athletes participating in organized ice hockey, soccer, judo, and track were studied using the oddball task. They found significant

TABLE 8.3 Summary of published ERP experiments.

Author	Sample population	Time from last injury	Method	Significant findings
Broglio et al. [103]	Intercollegiate and recreational athletes: Concussed ($m = 20$ years; $m = 1.7$ concussions); Controls ($m = 19.4$ years)	$m = 2.9$ years	Novelty oddball	Concussed participants had smaller N2 ($d = 2.89$), P3a ($d = 0.39$), and P3b ($d = 2.31$) amplitudes compared to controls.
De Beaumont et al. [91]	College football players: Controls ($m = 22.5$ years); 1 concussion ($m = 23$ years); 2 + concussions ($m = 23.5$ years, $m = 2.8$ concussions)	1 concussion $m = 4.7$ years; 2 + concussions $m = 2.6$ years	Visual search task	Participants suffering multiple concussions demonstrated smaller P3 amplitudes than participants with 1 concussion ($d \leq 2.71$)
De Beaumont et al. [91]	Concussed former athletes ($m = 61$ years), controls ($m = 59$ years)	$m = 34.7$ years	Auditory oddball	Concussed participants had longer P3a latencies ($d = 0.68$) and amplitude ($d = 0.39$), and P3b amplitudes ($d = 0.52$) compared to controls.
Broglio et al. [74]	Professional boxers ($n = 12$, $m = 28.1$ years), professional fencers ($n = 12$, $m = 26.3$ years), student-controls ($n = 12$, $m = 25.8$ years)	n/a	Go/No-Go	Boxers demonstrated suppressed P3b amplitude ($d \leq 3.7$) and increased latency ($d \leq 2.7$) during the No-Go task.
Broglio et al. [74]	Three groups of college athletes ($m = 21.5$: control, asymptomatic and symptomatic	Asymptomatic, $m = 9.75$ months; Symptomatic, $m = 1.7$ months	Visual oddball	Symptomatic participants demonstrated overall smaller P3 amplitudes compared to asymptomatic and control participants ($d = 1.02$)
Broglio et al. [74]	Contact athletes divided into groups by age [18–34 ($m = 25.5$) and 35–55 ($m = 42.4$)] and compared to controls	Age 18–34 ($m = 3.1$ years); 35–55 ($m = 3.13$ years)	Visual oddball tasks: word, shape, and number; Auditory oddball task	Concussed participants of all ages demonstrated longer P3 latencies during all visual oddball tasks ($d \leq 7.68$)
Broglio et al. [74]	High school Hockey players grouped by number of concussion: 0, 1, 2, or 3 +	All subjects were >6 months postinjury; 3 + group $m = 13.2$ months	Visual oddball task	3 + concussed participants demonstrated longer P3 latencies than control group ($d = 1.21$)
Broglio et al. [74]	Professional, semiprofessional and collegiate hockey and football players: control ($m = 22.0$ years); asymptomatic concussed ($m = 26.1$ years; $m = 3.5$ concussions); and symptomatic concussed ($m = 25.7$ years; $m = 5.1$ concussions)	Asymptomatic, $m = 5.3$ weeks; Symptomatic, $m = 15.1$ weeks	Auditory oddball	Symptomatic athletes demonstrated smaller P2 amplitude ($d = 0.74$) than controls; greater P3 amplitudes and longer P3 latencies were present in the concussed groups compared to the control group ($d = n/a$)

(Continued)

III. TBI biomarkers in medical practice

TABLE 8.3 (Continued)

Author	Sample population	Time from last injury	Method	Significant findings
Lavoie et al. [85]	Student athletes (18–26 years) grouped into control, asymptomatic (m concussion = 2.6), and symptomatic (m concussion = 3.2)	Asymptomatic (m = 9.9 months); Symptomatic (m = 1.7 months)	Modified visual oddball	Symptomatic participants demonstrated smaller P3 amplitude compared asymptomatic (d = 2.69) and controls (d = 1.72) participants
Broglio et al. [74]	Intercollegiate and recreational athletes: Concussed (m = 19.9 years; m = 1.7 concussions); Controls (m = 19.4 years)	m = 2.9 years	Modified flanker task	ERN (Ne) on error trials was smaller for concussed participants compared to controls (d = 3.11)
Broglio et al. [74]	Collegiate athletes: Concussed (m = 22.3 years) and Controls (n/a)	10–20 months	EEG during 25 and 50% maximum voluntary contraction (MVC) of the index finger	Concussed athletes had significantly smaller amplitudes during the 50% MVC for BP (d = 0.92–1.10), MP (d = 1.07–1.19) and MMP (d = 1.10–1.22)
Broglio et al. [74]	Collegiate athletes: Concussed (n/a)	Evaluations at baseline and days 3, 10, and 30 postconcussion	EEG taken during 3 static and 1 dynamic posture	Significant differences (BP, MP, and MMP) between baseline and postinjury days (d = n/a)
Broglio et al. [74]	Varsity high school athletes: 3 groups: Control (m = 22.1 years); Recent concussion (m = 22.6 years; m = 2.9 concussions); Late concussion (m = 22.9 years; m = 2.5 concussions);	Recent concussion m = 9.1 months; Late concussion m = 33.2 months	Auditory oddball	Recent concussed participants displayed smaller P3a (d = 1.41) and P3b (d = 1.16) amplitudes compared to controls. The Late concussion group displayed smaller P3a (d = 0.74) and P3b (d = 0.50) amplitudes compared to controls. Late concussion group participants also displayed large P3b amplitudes (d = 1.03), than those in the recent concussion group.

d, Cohen's d; n/a, data unavailable.
Effect sizes were calculated based on the values presented in the respective manuscripts as an estimate of concussion's impact on the various indices of brain function.

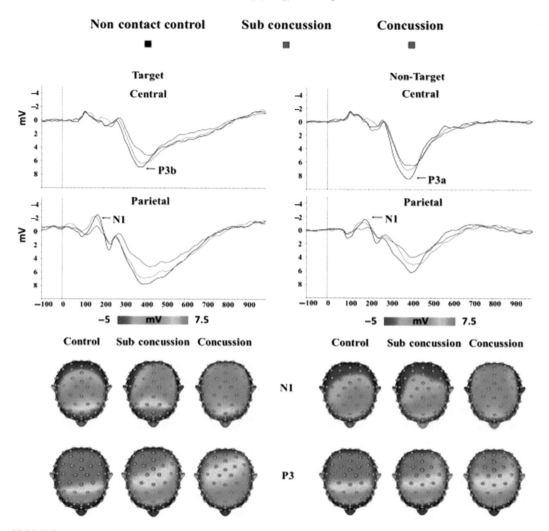

FIGURE 8.3 Graphical representation of ERP waveforms and topographic plots for the N1, P3a, and P3b components.

decrements in the N2 and P3b amplitudes of the stimulus-locked ERPs measured in athletes with a history of concussion relative to those without a history of concussion [103].

Duncan et al. evaluated survivors of head injury in visual and auditory discrimination tasks. In auditory tasks, survivors were found to have decreased amplitude and increased latency of N2 as well as increased latency of P3. The auditory N2 and P3 components also showed a strong correlation with duration of unconsciousness following injury. In contrast, in visual tasks, only a decreased amplitude of N2 compared to the controls was observed [119].

A study by Marc Lavoie's group looked at ERPs in three groups: (1) concussed athletes with symptoms up to 2 years after injury; (2) concussed athletes without symptoms up to

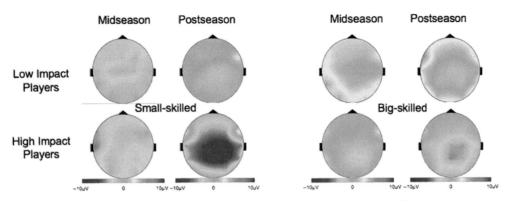

FIGURE 8.4   P3b amplitude differences from baseline at midseason and postseason. Low-impact players compared against high-low impact players amongst the small-skilled and big-skilled groups.

2 years after injury; and (3) athletes without a history of a concussion [85]. A visual oddball paradigm was used to elicit the P300 response. Symptomatic concussed athletes displayed longer reaction times than nonsymptomatic concussed athletes and athletes without a concussion history. The same symptomatic concussed athletes group also showed a more significant attenuation in the P300 amplitude in response to the rare target stimuli, as shown in Fig. 8.5 [85]. These results support the correlation between cognitive responses and the observed ERP components.

Solbakk and colleagues examined ERP components in patients with mild closed head injury, patients with verified frontal lobe damage, and healthy controls. The mTBI patients exhibited significantly longer reaction times to target stimuli in the ERP task accompanied with the most abnormal ERPs. The same mTBI group also exhibited significantly smaller N2 amplitudes compared to the other groups. The authors interpreted these results as evidence that the mild head injury patients were allocating the least amount of processing resources to the task compared to the other two groups [87].

Nandrajog et al. compared the amplitude and latency of the P300 component in mTBI patients and healthy controls in the immediate days (1−7 days) and months (2−3 months) following injury. They found that the latency of P300 was significantly prolonged in early (1−7 day period) mTBI patients compared to later (2−3 months period) TBI patients and healthy controls. Also, consistent with other research, the P300 amplitude was also significantly reduced in the early mTBI patients compared to healthy controls [120].

It is also important to note that some of the observed electrophysiological changes as a result of TBI show long-term effects on neurological function. A 2007 study by De Beaumont et al. looked at 47 university football players with a history of concussion. Athletes who had sustained a single concussion were studied an average of 59 months after injury, while athletes who had sustained multiple concussions were studied an average of 31 months after injury. The athletes who had sustained multiple concussions displayed significantly attenuated P3 compared to athletes with a single concussion or no concussion history even when using the time since latest concussion as a covariate [91]. A second study by the same group in 2009 looked at the effects of concussion on cognitive and motor function in retired athletes more than 30 years after the injury had been

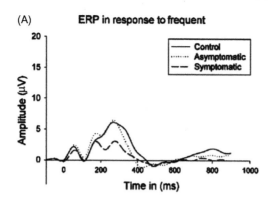

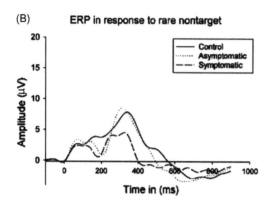

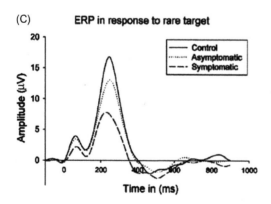

FIGURE 8.5 ERP waveforms comparing the responses of the three groups to the frequent (A), rare nontarget (B), and rare target (C) stimuli. Although the symptomatic group generally exhibited a reduced P300 amplitude compared to the other two groups, this difference became significant only in response to the rare target stimulus (C).

sustained. The P3a and P3b components showed significant increases in latency and attenuation of power in athletes with a prior history of concussion compared to those without a history. These results can be seen in Fig. 8.6 [121]. The finding that observed changes in

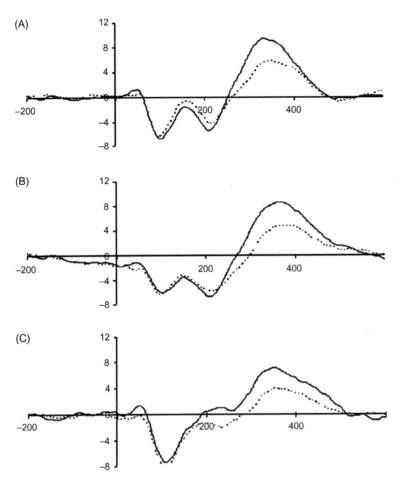

FIGURE 8.6 (A) Grand average P3b component evoked by target stimuli at parietal point. (B) Grand average P3b component evoked by target stimuli at central point. (C) Grand average P3a component evoked by deviant nontarget stimuli and recorded at frontal point. Continuous black trace represents group of former athletes with no prior concussion history. Dotted black trace represents group of former athletes with a history of sports concussion in early adulthood.

ERP components, particularly the P3, may be present more than 30 years after injury suggests that ERPs may be useful in determining the pathophysiology underlying negative effects of mTBI many years after the initial injury [121].

Bernstein also demonstrated the negative long-term effects of mTBI on neurological function in a study of information processing deficits following mTBI in students compared to healthy controls an average of 8 years following injury (range of 1−16.5 years). Reduced amplitude of the P300 ERP component on a set of easy and difficult attention tasks was observed in students with self-reported concussion. The same self-reported concussion group also performed more poorly than controls on cognitive tasks [90]. Similar to the previous study, these results support the correlation between cognitive performance and ERP components.

A 2014 study by Moore et al. evaluated the influence of mTBI incurred during early life on the cognitive control and neuroelectric function of young adults [122]. Decreased P3 amplitude during target detection within the oddball task and during the heterogeneous condition of the switch task was observed in the concussion group, compared to healthy controls. The concussion group also displayed increased N2 amplitude during the heterogeneous version for the switch task [122].

8.3.6 Event-related potentials as biomarkers in traumatic brain injury recovery

Medical advances over time have led to an increased number of survivors who have suffered from severe TBI. However, prior to the use of ERPs, there were very few reliable indicators that were able to predict and track eventual functional recovery for severe TBI patients [101,123,124]. Yet research studies over the last few decades have found success in the use of tone- and speech-evoked ERPs as a tool for predicting and evaluating functional recovery in this population and are useful when integrated into rehabilitation programs [108,109,125].

A case study by Pachalska et al. [126]. followed patient M. L-S, age 26, who suffered a brain injury in a skiing accident which resulted in a prolonged coma. In neuropsychological testing, M. L-S showed symptoms of frontal syndrome such as executive dysfunction and behavioral changes. The patient required the assistance of others to function in day-to-day life. Traditional rehabilitation programs were not successful and very little functional progress had been made. Over the course of the study completed by Pachalska et al., the patient was treated with two differentiated rehabilitation programs. Program A consisted of relative beta training, and behavioral training, while program B consisted of repetitive transcranial magnetic stimulation and behavioral training. The patient's ERPs were recorded at three time points to assess functional changes induced by the rehabilitation programs: (1) prior to rehabilitation programs; (2) after rehabilitation program A; and (3) after rehabilitation program B. These ERP recordings were then compared to the behavioral parameters measured in the Go/No-Go task at the same time points. At the first recording (prior to rehabilitation programs), the patient's performance (measured by the number of omission errors and the variance of the response) was significantly different from the norm. Following rehabilitation program A, there were no significant changes in the behavioral parameters. In contrast, substantial changes occurred after the rehabilitation program B. These observed behavioral changes paralleled the ERP results. The patient's ERPs differed from corresponding healthy controls at the initial time point and there were no visible changes that occurred after rehabilitation program A. However, statistically significant changes occurred after rehabilitation program B. Although the changes observed in both the behavioral parameters and ERPs following rehabilitation program B were more similar to the norm than prior to rehabilitation programs, they still remained significantly deviant from the norm [126]. This suggests that ERPs may be useful to not only predict functional outcomes but also evaluate the success of ongoing rehabilitation programs in severe TBI patients.

A case study by Faran et al. followed a 28-year-old man who was admitted to an intensive care unit in a comatose state after a severe car accident. Five days after the accident, he regained consciousness but maintained diminished gaze fixation and could not follow the simplest commands. He remained in a persistent vegetative state for 20 months following the incident. His cognitive abilities were evaluated at 3, 4, 6, 12, 18, and 28 months after the incident using cognitive auditory ERP tasks, including a semantic oddball and semantic congruence tasks. The semantic oddball task consisted of rare (Hebrew common words) and frequent (pronounceable nonwords) stimuli. Semantic congruence tasks consisted of: (1) pairs of strongly associated words (e.g., day—night) and pairs of unrelated words (e.g., fish—hand); and (2) simple sentences with a highly predictable word at the end and sentences with an unpredictable ending word. In the first two evaluations (at 3 and 4 months), cortical ERPs were undetectable. However, during the third examination (at 6 months), distinguishable P300 response in an oddball task and differentiated ERP responses in the word-pair task were observed, suggesting cortical processing of word meanings. The following two examinations (at 12 and 18 months) showed normal or close-to-normal responses in the semantic oddball and incongruent sentence conditions. However, clinical and neuropsychological examinations at these time points showed no behavioral improvements. About 20 months after the incident, after intensive physical and speech therapy, the patient began to articulate distinguishable sounds, followed by words. Soon after, he was able to recall details about his life and events preceding the crash. Two months later, he could recognize family and friends. At 28 months after the accident, the patient had fully recovered. In the case of this patient, the clinical improvement was preceded by an improvement in cognitive ERP data for more than a year. This suggests that ERP findings may be superior to clinical data as indices of consciousness awareness [127].

Onofrj et al. studied 10 patients with posttraumatic amnesia. ERPs, neuropsychological testing, and EEG were performed the day after trauma and at several following time points until patients had fully recovered. In all patients, P3 latencies the day after trauma were significantly longer than healthy controls. These P3 latencies decreased progressively during recovery, and these latency reductions correlated significantly with improvement of neuropsychological tests [128].

The preceding research studies and clinical case studies strongly demonstrate the significant role ERPs can play as an underlying metric for prognosis in TBI patients as well as for tracking injury recovery where clinical and behavioral testing may not be as sensitive or specific.

8.4 Conclusion

Over the past few decades there has been a significant increase in the use of electrophysiology in the diagnosis and prognosis of TBI. Although the ubiquitous use of electrophysiology in the clinical TBI setting has not yet been realized and further research as to the sensitivity of ANS and ERP biomarkers to identify TBI on an individual level still remains, the significant research and identification of reliable ANS and ERP biomarkers shows promise for the future. As demonstrated throughout this chapter, a number of promising biomarkers have been identified and successfully applied to aid clinicians in the differential diagnosis of the affected systems in TBI including the ANS and CNS. Additionally, clinicians are now able to effectively utilize objective testing tools that can aid treatment planning on a case-by-case basis. The importance of this personalized rehabilitation opportunity cannot be overstated since by its very nature TBI is an injury with a complex and distributed neuropathology that is unique between individuals [92]. In the cases of mTBI and concussion in particular, where structural imaging such as MRI and CT are negative, the acquisition of physiological data time-locked to specific behaviors and physical stressors offers a powerful approach to understanding the functional injury that TBI imparts on the nervous system and an otherwise unavailable means of assessing neuropathology.

References

[1] Denny-Brown D, Russell WR. Experimental cerebral concussion. Brain 1941;64(2–3):93–164.
[2] Gennarelli TA. The spectrum of traumatic axonal injury. Neuropathol Appl Neurobiol 1996;22(6):509–13.
[3] Gentry LR. Imaging of closed head injury. Radiology 1994;191(1):1–17.
[4] Kupina NC, Detloff MR, Bobrowski WF, Snyder BJ, Hall ED. Cytoskeletal protein degradation and neurodegeneration evolves differently in males and females following experimental head injury. Exp Neurol 2003;180(1):55–73.
[5] Shaw NA. The neurophysiology of concussion. Prog Neurobiol 2002;67(4):281–344.
[6] Lambert K, Kinsley C, Kinsley CH. Clinical neuroscience. Macmillan; 2004.
[7] Brown SP, Miller WC, Eason JM. Exercise physiology: basis of human movement in health and disease. Lippincott Williams & Wilkins; 2006.
[8] McCorry LK. Physiology of the autonomic nervous system. Am J Pharm Edu 2007;71(4):78.
[9] Bishop S, Dech R, Baker T, Butz M, Aravinthan K, Neary JP. Parasympathetic baroreflexes and heart rate variability during acute stage of sport concussion recovery. Brain Inj 2017;31(2):247–59.
[10] Conder RL, Conder AA. Heart rate variability interventions for concussion and rehabilitation. Front Psychol 2014;5:890.
[11] Hilz MJ, Liu M, Koehn J, et al. Valsalva maneuver unveils central baroreflex dysfunction with altered blood pressure control in persons with a history of mild traumatic brain injury. BMC Neurol 2016;16(1):61.
[12] Thayer JF, Lane RD. Claude Bernard and the heart–brain connection: further elaboration of a model of neurovisceral integration. Neurosci Biobehav Rev 2009;33(2):81–8.
[13] Giza CC, Hovda DA. The new neurometabolic cascade of concussion. Neurosurgery 2014;75(Suppl. 4): S24–33.
[14] Coote J. Myths and realities of the cardiac vagus. J Physiol 2013;591(17):4073–85.
[15] Pertab JL, Merkley TL, Cramond AJ, Cramond K, Paxton H, Wu T. Concussion and the autonomic nervous system: an introduction to the field and the results of a systematic review. NeuroRehabilitation 2018; (Preprint):1–31.
[16] Esterov D, Greenwald BD. Autonomic dysfunction after mild traumatic brain injury. Brain Sci 2017;7(8):100.
[17] Leddy JJ, Kozlowski K, Fung M, Pendergast DR, Willer B. Regulatory and autoregulatory physiological dysfunction as a primary characteristic of post concussion syndrome: implications for treatment. NeuroRehabilitation 2007;22(3):199–205.
[18] Heart rate variability: standards of measurement, physiological interpretation and clinical use. Task Force of the European Society of Cardiology and the North American Society of Pacing and Electrophysiology. Circulation 1996;93(5):1043–65.
[19] Blake TA, McKay CD, Meeuwisse WH, Emery CA. The impact of concussion on cardiac autonomic function: a systematic review. Brain Inj 2016;30(2):132–45.
[20] Sandercock GR, Bromley PD, Brodie DA. Effects of exercise on heart rate variability: inferences from meta-analysis. Med Sci Sports Exer 2005;37(3):433–9.
[21] Kleiger RE, Miller JP, Bigger Jr. JT, Moss AJ. Decreased heart rate variability and its association with increased mortality after acute myocardial infarction. Am J Cardiol 1987;59(4):256–62.
[22] Huston JM, Tracey KJ. The pulse of inflammation: heart rate variability, the cholinergic anti-inflammatory pathway and implications for therapy. J Int Med 2011;269(1):45–53.
[23] Sztajzel J. Heart rate variability: a noninvasive electrocardiographic method to measure the autonomic nervous system. Swiss Med 2004;134(35–36):514–22.
[24] Bootsma M, Swenne CA, Van Bolhuis HH, Chang PC, Cats VM, Bruschke A. Heart rate and heart rate variability as indexes of sympathovagal balance. Am J Physiol-Heart Circ Physiol 1994;266(4):H1565–71.

[25] Heffernan DS, Inaba K, Arbabi S, Cotton BA. Sympathetic hyperactivity after traumatic brain injury and the role of beta-blocker therapy. J Trauma Acute Care Sur 2010;69(6):1602−9.

[26] Hilz M, Koehn J, Ammon F, et al. Valsalva maneuver shows prolonged sympathetic outflow in patients with a history of mild traumatic brain injury. J Neuro Sci 2013;333:e688−9.

[27] Pagani M, Lucini D, Porta A. Sympathovagal balance from heart rate variability: time for a second round? Exp Physiol 2012;97(10):1141−2.

[28] Czosnyka M. Association between arterial and intracranial pressures. Brit J Neurosurg 2000;14(2):127−8.

[29] Mahoney EJ, Biffl WL, Harrington DT, Cioffi WG. Isolated brain injury as a cause of hypotension in the blunt trauma patient. J Trauma Acute Care Sur 2003;55(6):1065−9.

[30] Lim H, Smith M. Systemic complications after head injury: a clinical review. Anaesthesia 2007;62(5):474−82.

[31] Tan CO, Meehan WP, Iverson GL, Taylor JA. Cerebrovascular regulation, exercise, and mild traumatic brain injury. Neurology 2014;. Available from: https://doi.org/10.1212/WNL.0000000000000944.

[32] Wright AD, Smirl JD, Bryk K, Fraser S, Jakovac M, van Donkelaar P. Sport-related concussion alters indices of dynamic cerebral autoregulation. Front Neurol 2018;9:196.

[33] Hamill RW, Woolf PD, McDonald JV, Lee LA, Kelly M. Catecholamines predict outcome in traumatic brain injury. Ann Neurol 1987;21(5):438−43.

[34] Atkinson JL. The neglected prehospital phase of head injury: apnea and catecholamine surge. In: Paper presented at: Mayo Clinic Proceedings; 2000.

[35] Meyfroidt G, Baguley IJ, Menon DK. Paroxysmal sympathetic hyperactivity: the storm after acute brain injury. Lancet Neurol 2017;16(9):721−9.

[36] Patterson ZR, Holahan MR. Understanding the neuroinflammatory response following concussion to develop treatment strategies. Front Cell Neurosci 2012;6:58.

[37] Mayer CL, Huber BR, Peskind E. Traumatic brain injury, neuroinflammation, and post-traumatic headaches. Headache: J Head Face Pain 2013;53(9):1523−30.

[38] Borovikova LV, Ivanova S, Nardi D, et al. Role of vagus nerve signaling in CNI-1493-mediated suppression of acute inflammation. Auton Neurosci 2000;85(1−3):141−7.

[39] Czura C, Tracey K. Autonomic neural regulation of immunity. J Int Med 2005;257(2):156−66.

[40] La Fountaine MF, Heffernan KS, Gossett JD, Bauman WA, De Meersman RE. Transient suppression of heart rate complexity in concussed athletes. Auton Neurosci 2009;148(1−2):101−3.

[41] Smith M. Monitoring intracranial pressure in traumatic brain injury. Anesth Analg 2008;106(1):240−8.

[42] Schmidt EA, Despas F, Traon P-L, et al. Intracranial pressure is a determinant of sympathetic activity. Front Physiol 2018;9:11.

[43] Hilz MJ, DeFina PA, Anders S, et al. Frequency analysis unveils cardiac autonomic dysfunction after mild traumatic brain injury. J Neurotrauma 2011;28(9):1727−38.

[44] Baguley IJ, Heriseanu RE, Felmingham KL, Cameron ID. Dysautonomia and heart rate variability following severe traumatic brain injury. Brain Inj 2006;20(4):437−44.

[45] Porth C, Bamrah VS, Tristani F, Smith J. The valsalva maneuver: mechanisms and clinical implications. Heart Lung 1984;13(5):507−18.

[46] McCrory P, Meeuwisse W, Dvorak J, et al. Consensus statement on concussion in sport—the 5th international conference on concussion in sport held in Berlin, October 2016. Brit J Sports Med 2017;51(11):838−47.

[47] McCrory P, Meeuwisse WH, Aubry M, et al. Consensus statement on concussion in sport: the 4th International Conference on Concussion in Sport held in Zurich, November 2012. Brit J Sports Med 2013;47(5):250−8.

[48] Leddy J, Baker JG, Haider MN, Hinds A, Willer B. A physiological approach to prolonged recovery from sport-related concussion. J Athlet Train 2017;52(3):299−308.

[49] Leddy JJ, Willer B. Use of graded exercise testing in concussion and return-to-activity management. Curr Sports Med Rep 2013;12(6):370−6.

[50] Abaji JP, Curnier D, Moore RD, Ellemberg D. Persisting effects of concussion on heart rate variability during physical exertion. J Neurotrauma 2016;33(9):811−17.

[51] Senthinathan A, Mainwaring LM, Hutchison M. Heart rate variability of athletes across concussion recovery milestones: a preliminary study. Clin J Sport Med 2017;27(3):288−95.

[52] Dobson JL, Yarbrough MB, Perez J, Evans K, Buckley T. Sport-related concussion induces transient cardiovascular autonomic dysfunction. Am J Physiol-Reg I 2017;312(4):R575−84.

III. TBI biomarkers in medical practice

[53] Goodman B, Vargas B, Dodick D. Autonomic nervous system dysfunction in concussion (P01. 265). Neurology 2013;80(7 Suppl.):P01. 265−201.

[54] O'Leary MC, Sackett JR, Schlader ZJ, Leddy JJ, Johnson BD. Heart rate and heart rate variability during the cold pressor test in recently concussed patients. FASEB J 2017;31(Suppl. 1): 1077.1079-1077.

[55] Wirch JL, Wolfe LA, Weissgerber TL, Davies GA. Cold pressor test protocol to evaluate cardiac autonomic function. Appl Physiol Nutr Metab 2006;31(3):235−43.

[56] Kissick J, Johnston KM. Return to play after concussion: principles and practice. Clin J Sports Med 2005;15 (6):426−31.

[57] Norris PR, Ozdas A, Cao H, et al. Cardiac uncoupling and heart rate variability stratify ICU patients by mortality: a study of 2088 trauma patients. Ann Surg 2006;243(6):804.

[58] Schroeppel TJ, Sharpe JP, Magnotti LJ, et al. Traumatic brain injury and β-blockers: not all drugs are created equal. J Trauma Acute Care Surg 2014;76(2):504−9.

[59] Lagos L, Bottiglieri T, Vaschillo B, Vaschillo E. Heart rate variability biofeedback for postconcussion syndrome: implications for treatment. Biofeedback 2012;40(4):150−3.

[60] Lehrer P, Vaschillo B, Zucker T, et al. Protocol for heart rate variability biofeedback training. Biofeedback 2013;41(3):98−109.

[61] Lehrer PM, Vaschillo E, Vaschillo B, et al. Heart rate variability biofeedback increases baroreflex gain and peak expiratory flow. Psychosomat Med 2003;65(5):796−805.

[62] Steffen PR, Austin T, DeBarros A, Brown T. The impact of resonance frequency breathing on measures of heart rate variability, blood pressure, and mood. Front Public Health 2017;5:222.

[63] Lehrer PM, Gevirtz R. Heart rate variability biofeedback: how and why does it work? Front Psychol 2014;5:756.

[64] Singh J, Larson M, O'Donnell C, Tsuji H, Levy D. Heritability of heart rate variability: the Framingham heart study. J Am Coll Cardiol 1998;31(2SA) 169A.

[65] Panenka WJ, Gardner AJ, Dretsch MN, Crynen GC, Crawford FC, Iverson GL. Systematic review of genetic risk factors for sustaining a mild traumatic brain injury. J Neurotrauma 2017;34(13):2093−9.

[66] Notaras M, Hill R, Van Den Buuse M. The BDNF gene Val66Met polymorphism as a modifier of psychiatric disorder susceptibility: progress and controversy. Mol Psych 2015;20(8):916.

[67] Yang AC, Chen TJ, Tsai SJ, et al. BDNF Val66Met polymorphism alters sympathovagal balance in healthy subjects. Am J Med Genet Part B 2010;153(5):1024−30.

[68] Dretsch MN, Silverberg N, Gardner AJ, et al. Genetics and other risk factors for past concussions in active-duty soldiers. J Neurotrauma 2017;34(4):869−75.

[69] Dretsch MN, Williams K, Emmerich T, et al. Brain-derived neurotropic factor polymorphisms, traumatic stress, mild traumatic brain injury, and combat exposure contribute to postdeployment traumatic stress. Brain Behav 2016;6(1):e00392.

[70] Baj G, Carlino D, Gardossi L, Tongiorgi E. Toward a unified biological hypothesis for the BDNF Val66Met-associated memory deficits in humans: a model of impaired dendritic mRNA trafficking. Front Neurosci 2013;7:188.

[71] Mallei A, Baj G, Ieraci A, et al. Expression and dendritic trafficking of BDNF-6 splice variant are impaired in knock-in mice carrying human BDNF Val66Met polymorphism. Int J Neuropsychopharmacol 2015;18:12.

[72] Korley FK, Diaz-Arrastia R, Wu AH, et al. Circulating brain-derived neurotrophic factor has diagnostic and prognostic value in traumatic brain injury. J Neurotrauma 2016;33(2):215−25.

[73] Erickson KI, Miller DL, Roecklein KA. The aging hippocampus: interactions between exercise, depression, and BDNF. Neuroscientist 2012;18(1):82−97.

[74] Broglio SP, Moore RD, Hillman CH. A history of sport-related concussion on event-related brain potential correlates of cognition. Int J Psychophysiol 2011;82(1):16−23.

[75] Sur S, Sinha VK. Event-related potential: an overview. Ind Psychiatry J 2009;18(1):70−3.

[76] Kotchoubey B, Lang S, Mezger G, et al. Information processing in severe disorders of consciousness: vegetative state and minimally conscious state. Clin Neurophysiol 2005;116(10):2441−53.

[77] Key AP, Dove GO, Maguire MJ. Linking brainwaves to the brain: an ERP primer. Dev Neuropsychol 2005;27 (2):183−215.

[78] Ellemberg D, Henry LC, Macciocchi SN, Guskiewicz KM, Broglio SP. Advances in sport concussion assessment: from behavioral to brain imaging measures. J Neurotrauma 2009;26(12):2365−82.

[79] Dockree PM, Robertson IH. Electrophysiological markers of cognitive deficits in traumatic brain injury: a review. Int J Psychophysiol 2011;82(1):53–60.

[80] Mauguiere F, Allison T, Babiloni C, et al. Somatosensory evoked potentials. The International Federation of Clinical Neurophysiology. Electroencephalogr Clin Neurophysiol Suppl 1999;52:79–90.

[81] Passmore SR, Murphy B, Lee TD. The origin, and application of somatosensory evoked potentials as a neurophysiological technique to investigate neuroplasticity. J Can Chiropr Assoc 2014;58(2) 170–83.

[82] Carter BG, Butt W. A prospective study of outcome predictors after severe brain injury in children. Intensive Care Med 2005;31(6):840–5.

[83] Guerit JM. Evoked potentials in severe brain injury. Prog Brain Res 2005;150:415–26.

[84] Hutchinson DO, Frith RW, Shaw NA, Judson JA, Cant BR. A comparison between electroencephalography and somatosensory evoked potentials for outcome prediction following severe head injury. Electroencephalogr Clin Neurophysiol 1991;78(3):228–33.

[85] Lavoie ME, Dupuis F, Johnston KM, Leclerc S, Lassonde M. Visual p300 effects beyond symptoms in concussed college athletes. J Clin Exp Neuropsychol 2004;26(1):55–73.

[86] Mendez CV, Hurley RA, Lassonde M, Zhang L, Taber KH. Mild traumatic brain injury: neuroimaging of sports-related concussion. J Neuropsychiatry Clin Neurosci 2005;17(3):297–303.

[87] Solbakk AK, Reinvang I, Nielsen C, Sundet K. ERP indicators of disturbed attention in mild closed head injury: a frontal lobe syndrome? Psychophysiology 1999;36(6):802–17.

[88] Young GB, Wang JT, Connolly JF. Prognostic determination in anoxic-ischemic and traumatic encephalopathies. J Clin Neurophysiol 2004;21(5):379–90.

[89] Cavinato M, Freo U, Ori C, et al. Post-acute P300 predicts recovery of consciousness from traumatic vegetative state. Brain Inj 2009;23(12):973–80.

[90] Bernstein DM. Information processing difficulty long after self-reported concussion. J Int Neuropsychol Soc 2002;8(5):673–82.

[91] De Beaumont L, Brisson B, Lassonde M, Jolicoeur P. Long-term electrophysiological changes in athletes with a history of multiple concussions. Brain Inj 2007;21(6):631–44.

[92] Levine B, Katz DI, Dade L, Black SE. Novel approaches to the assessment of frontal damage and executive deficits in traumatic brain injury. In: Stuss DT, Knight RT, editors. Principles of frontal lobe function. New York: Oxford University Press; 2002: p. 448–65.

[93] Adams JH, Scott G, Parker LS, Graham DI, Doyle D. The contusion index: a quantitative approach to cerebral contusions in head injury. Neuropathol Appl Neurobiol 1980;6(4):319–24.

[94] Christodoulou C, DeLuca J, Ricker JH, et al. Functional magnetic resonance imaging of working memory impairment after traumatic brain injury. J Neurol Neurosurg Psychiatry 2001;71(2):161–8.

[95] McAllister TW, Saykin AJ, Flashman LA, et al. Brain activation during working memory 1 month after mild traumatic brain injury: a functional MRI study. Neurology 1999;53(6):1300–8.

[96] Zhang Y, Li R, Du J, Huo S, Hao J, Song W. Coherence in P300 as a predictor for the recovery from disorders of consciousness. Neurosci Lett 2017;653:332–6.

[97] Wang JT, Young GB, Connolly JF. Prognostic value of evoked responses and event-related brain potentials in coma. Can J Neurol Sci 2004;31(4):438–50.

[98] Morlet D, Fischer C. MMN and novelty P3 in coma and other altered states of consciousness: a review. Brain Topogr 2014;27(4):467–79.

[99] Rollnik JD. May clinical neurophysiology help to predict the recovery of neurological early rehabilitation patients? BMC Neurol 2015;15:239.

[100] Sharova EV, Oknina LB, Potapov AA, Zaitsev OS, Masherov EL, Kulikov MA. [The P300 component of the auditory evoked potential in the posttraumatic vegetative state]. Zh Vyssh Nerv Deiat Im I P Pavlova 1998;48(4):719–30.

[101] Lew HL, Poole JH, Castaneda A, Salerno RM, Gray M. Prognostic value of evoked and event-related potentials in moderate to severe brain injury. J Head Trauma Rehabil 2006;21(4):350–60.

[102] Polich J, Corey-Bloom J. Alzheimer's disease and P300: review and evaluation of task and modality. Curr Alzheimer Res 2005;2(5):515–25.

[103] Broglio SP, Pontifex MB, O'Connor P, Hillman CH. The persistent effects of concussion on neuroelectric indices of attention. J Neurotrauma 2009;26(9):1463–70.

[104] Olbrich S, Arns M. EEG biomarkers in major depressive disorder: discriminative power and prediction of treatment response. Int Rev Psychiatry 2013;25(5):604–18.

[105] Carter BG, Butt W. Are somatosensory evoked potentials the best predictor of outcome after severe brain injury? A systematic review. Intensive Care Med 2005;31(6):765–75.

[106] Parks AC, Moore RD, Wu CT, et al. The association between a history of concussion and variability in behavioral and neuroelectric indices of cognition. Int J Psychophysiol 2015;98(3 Pt 1):426–34.

[107] Polich J. Updating P300: an integrative theory of P3a and P3b. Clin Neurophysiol 2007;118(10):2128–48.

[108] Lew HL, Dikmen S, Slimp J, et al. Use of somatosensory-evoked potentials and cognitive event-related potentials in predicting outcomes of patients with severe traumatic brain injury. Am J Phys Med Rehabil 2003;82(1):53–61; quiz 62-54, 80.

[109] Yingling CD, Hosobuchi Y, Harrington M. P300 as a predictor of recovery from coma. Lancet 1990;336(8719):873.

[110] Adams JH, Graham DI, Murray LS, Scott G. Diffuse axonal injury due to nonmissile head injury in humans: an analysis of 45 cases. Ann Neurol 1982;12(6):557–63.

[111] McAllister TW, Sparling MB, Flashman LA, Guerin SJ, Mamourian AC, Saykin AJ. Differential working memory load effects after mild traumatic brain injury. Neuroimage 2001;14(5):1004–12.

[112] Perlstein WM, Cole MA, Demery JA, et al. Parametric manipulation of working memory load in traumatic brain injury: behavioral and neural correlates. J Int Neuropsychol Soc 2004;10(5):724–41.

[113] McDowell S, Whyte J, D'Esposito M. Working memory impairments in traumatic brain injury: evidence from a dual-task paradigm. Neuropsychologia 1997;35(10):1341–53.

[114] Polo MD, Newton P, Rogers D, Escera C, Butler S. ERPs and behavioural indices of long-term preattentive and attentive deficits after closed head injury. Neuropsychologia 2002;40(13):2350–9.

[115] Ponsford J, Kinsella G. Attentional deficits following closed-head injury. J Clin Exp Neuropsychol 1992;14(5):822–38.

[116] Rios M, Perianez JA, Munoz-Cespedes JM. Attentional control and slowness of information processing after severe traumatic brain injury. Brain Inj 2004;18(3):257–72.

[117] Moore RD, Lepine J, Ellemberg D. The independent influence of concussive and sub-concussive impacts on soccer players' neurophysiological and neuropsychological function. Int J Psychophysiol 2017;112:22–30.

[118] Brooks JST JW, Dickey JP. P3b event-related potentials show changes in varsity football players due to accumulated sub-concussive head impacts. In: Fifth annual symposium: research on the concussion spectrum of disorders, 2019.

[119] Duncan CC, Kosmidis MH, Mirsky AF. Event-related potential assessment of information processing after closed head injury. Psychophysiology 2003;40(1):45–59.

[120] Nandrajog P, Idris Z, Azlen WN, Liyana A, Abdullah JM. The use of event-related potential (P300) and neuropsychological testing to evaluate cognitive impairment in mild traumatic brain injury patients. Asian J Neurosurg 2017;12(3):447–53.

[121] De Beaumont L, Theoret H, Mongeon D, et al. Brain function decline in healthy retired athletes who sustained their last sports concussion in early adulthood. Brain 2009;132(Pt 3):695–708.

[122] Moore RD, Hillman CH, Broglio SP. The persistent influence of concussive injuries on cognitive control and neuroelectric function. J Athl Train 2014;49(1):24–35.

[123] Kraus JF, McArthur DL. Epidemiologic aspects of brain injury. Neurol Clin 1996;14(2):435–50.

[124] Ashley MJ, Persel CS, Clark MC, Krych DK. Long-term follow-up of post-acute traumatic brain injury rehabilitation: a statistical analysis to test for stability and predictability of outcome. Brain Inj 1997;11(9):677–90.

[125] Kane NM, Curry SH, Rowlands CA, et al. Event-related potentials—neurophysiological tools for predicting emergence and early outcome from traumatic coma. Intensive Care Med 1996;22(1):39–46.

[126] Pachalska M, Lukowicz M, Kropotov JD, Herman-Sucharska I, Talar J. Evaluation of differentiated neurotherapy programs for a patient after severe TBI and long term coma using event-related potentials. Med Sci Monit 2011;17(10):CS120–128.

[127] Faran S, Vatine JJ, Lazary A, Ohry A, Birbaumer N, Kotchoubey B. Late recovery from permanent traumatic vegetative state heralded by event-related potentials. J Neurol Neurosurg Psychiatry 2006;77(8):998–1000.

[128] Onofrj M, Curatola L, Malatesta G, Bazzano S, Colamartino P, Fulgente T. Reduction of P3 latency during outcome from post-traumatic amnesia. Acta Neurol Scand 1991;83(5):273–9.

Traumatic brain injury therapeutics

Peter Allfather[1], Imoigele P. Aisiku[1] and Claudia S. Robertson[2]

[1]Emergency Medicine and Pulmonary Critical Care, Brigham and Women's Hospital, Boston, MA, United States [2]Neurosurgery Department, Baylor College of Medicine, Houston, TX, United States

For patients who have suffered traumatic brain injury (TBI), a growing but limited number of treatment modalities exist across the spectrum of injury severity and clinical settings. A variety of scoring systems have been developed to help stratify the prognosis and severity of injury (IMPACT score, GCS, GOS, DRS, and Marshall CT classification [1]). The therapeutic approaches in the acute and rehabilitative phases vary dependent on the severity of brain injury. This chapter focuses on patients with severe TBI. At each stage in the treatment of TBI, from prehospital management to prolonged treatment in a dedicated neurocritical care unit, therapy is constrained by available resources, and the time frame in which the patient engages with a particular stage. However, there exists a common goal in the management of patients with TBI: the restoration of physiologic normality. Brain trauma, and the injuries and illnesses associated with it, put the body at substantial risk of abnormal physiology which can exacerbate brain injury, delay recovery, and monopolize limited resources. Care should be taken to avoid physiologic abnormalities associated with increased mortality and morbidity in TBI (i.e., hypoxemia, hypotension, hypercarbia, hypovolemia, and fever), as well as provide treatment interventions to improve brain function. As evidenced by the most recent Brain Trauma Foundation Guidelines [2], there is a limited number of therapeutic options with strong evidence to support their utilization. The focus here and the recommended therapeutics are supported by either expert consensus guidelines or medical evidence. An important concept to remember is that intracranial pressure, brain tissue oxygen, cerebral perfusion pressure, and other surrogate markers of brain dysfunction are important metrics and, while data exists to support therapeutics impacting these surrogate markers, the improvement of these markers does not correlate well with mortality and/or morbidity. This concept is critical to understanding TBI therapeutics, but in no way diminishes the current options available and hopefully allows the reader to place each treatment in perspective.

In the prehospital setting the initial steps in patients with suspected TBI are to restore systemic physiologic normality. Prehospital providers including paramedics, EMTs, and transport nurses are most constrained by an extremely resource limited setting where diagnostics are cursory and physical exam findings are the primary means of assessing injury and response to treatment. Airway protection is paramount to avoid hypoxemia, and early intubation for low GCS (<8) is encouraged. In contrast to the trauma literature supporting an approach of permissive hypotension in the traumatic nonhead injured patient, in an effort to avoid dislodging platelet plugs and disrupting early fibrin deposition [3], persistent hypotension is to be avoided in the severely head injured patient [4]. Cerebral blood flow (CBF) and the determinants of oxygen delivery may require vasopressor agents to target measurable surrogates of CBF including mean arterial pressure. Current guidelines recommend a MAP of 70 mmHg in the prehospital setting [5]. In the emergency department, patients with severe TBI should receive thorough, systematic, and time sensitive management without delay. Pharmacologic means of addressing elevated intracranial pressure (clinical or measured) are frequently employed and will be discussed further in this chapter. Early consultation with a neurosurgeon and neurocritical care physician is advised for consideration of possible surgical interventions and for eventual close monitoring in an ICU setting.

9.1 Airway and ventilator management

Airway and ventilator management is a mainstay of treatment in patients with TBI. Diminished consciousness, impaired respiratory drive, and an inability to protect airway patency results in the majority of patients with severe TBI being mechanically ventilated during their initial hospitalization. The need for tracheal intubation in patients with a significantly diminished GCS is well-established and is not contested in the contemporary TBI literature. Strategies for appropriately mechanically ventilating patients with TBI are subject of debate, however. The avoidance of hypoxemia and hypercarbia is critical to the successful management of patients with TBI. Cerebral autoregulation and blood flow have a more linear relationship with CO_2 when compared to oxygenation, therefore greater attention to CO_2 management is advised. Careful attention by clinicians treating patients in the emergency department and intensive care setting should focus on avoiding these adverse physiologic states. Targeting physiologically normal ranges of partial pressure for both carbon dioxide and oxygen is currently advised in the literature for the management of mechanically ventilated patients with TBI. In those particular patients who are experiencing cerebral herniation, a strategy for intentional hyperventilation to reduce the partial pressure of carbon dioxide has been proposed as a method of decreasing CBF, and by association decreasing intracranial pressure [6]. CBF is determined substantially by the partial pressure of carbon dioxide as it is a surrogate marker of the brain and metabolic demand. When $PaCO_2$ is artificially decreased through hyperventilation, there is a resultant decrease in CBF. While evidence exists describing harm associated with prolonged hyperventilation in severe TBI [7], there is no evidence to refute its usage as a temporizing measure prior to more definitive therapy for decreasing ICP such as pharmacologically or via decompressive surgical techniques. Typically, hyperventilation strategies are employed in the prehospital period, or in the emergency department en route to an emergent surgical decompression, after which ventilation goals transition to the maintenance of physiologic normality. The harm associated with prolonged use of hyperventilation is attributed to the fact that many patients with TBI have radiographic or histopathologic evidence of cerebral ischemia and thus prolonged strategies to reduce CBF to injured tissue with altered autoregulatory mechanisms may exacerbate and increase at-risk brain tissue ischemia [8].

9.2 Sedation and analgesia

In patients with severe TBI, significant levels of sedation and analgesia are required to prevent psychomotor agitation, decrease cerebral metabolic rate and demand, improve cerebral compliance, synchrony with mechanical ventilation, and to allow for invasive and painful procedures such as endotracheal or chest tubes, central lines, and intracranial pressure monitors or ventricular drainage devices [9,10]. There is significant evidence that an effective strategy for sedation and analgesia results in the lowering of intracranial pressure. The mechanism by which sedation achieves a reduction in ICP is not clearly defined and likely multifactorial. Proposed mechanisms involve decreased patient agitation and decreased intracranial metabolic demand [11]. Barbiturates, in particular, have a long history of use in TBI and have demonstrated reductions in ICP in this patient population. Their use is not routinely supported in high doses except for cases of refractory intracranial hypertension due to the significant side effect profile of barbiturates including systemic hypotension and their prolonged duration of action limiting the ability for intermittent neurological examination. A care plan must be taken by the clinician when implementing an appropriate strategy for sedation and analgesia that accounts for the potential adverse effects to hemodynamics while optimizing assessment of neurologic recovery. Many other commonly used analgesics and sedatives promote marked vasodilation which can, in turn, induce hypotension and subsequent tissue hypoperfusion. Current guidelines support the use of adequate sedation and analgesia with the concomitant understanding that there must be vigilant measurement of hemodynamics to ensure normotension. The mainstay of sedation/analgesia for patients with TBI is a combination of an intravenous sedative-hypnotic, such as propofol or a benzodiazepine, and an intravenous analgesic such as fentanyl, hydromorphone, or morphine administered as titrated continuous infusions.

Propofol is a widely utilized sedative-hypnotic which acts as a powerful stimulator of GABA receptors [12]. It is advantageous due to its short half-life which allows for rapid discontinuation of sedation for the purpose of intermittent neurological examination. Care must be taken however, as it is a potent vasodilatory agent that may cause systemic hypotension exceeding its concomitant reduction in intracranial pressure for a net decrease in cerebral perfusion pressure [10]. Propofol infusion syndrome is the most feared complication of its use, typically associated with administration at higher doses of the lipid emulsion, and can result in multiorgan failure and metabolic disarray. The syndrome is frequently marked by profound hypertriglyceridemia, metabolic acidosis, pancreatitis, and rhabdomyolysis with resultant hepatic, renal, and myocardial failure [13].

Dexmedetomidine is an alpha-2-agonist that is seeing more frequent use in TBI patients. It is advantageous as a sedative agent due to its frequent ability to provide adequate sedation without impairment in respiratory drive. Similar to propofol, it is rapidly cleared and may facilitate intermittent neurological examinations. It is a safe and effective sedative agent in neurosurgical patients, although a loading infusion should be avoided in this patient cohort due to an uncontrolled increase in systemic blood pressure which may have adverse effects on ICP or CBF [14]. Additionally, one study has suggested that while a loading infusion should be avoided, higher-dose maintenance infusion rates may result in a net increase in CPP with a concomitant decrease in ICP [15].

Ketamine is a dissociative anesthetic with associated analgesic properties that functions predominantly at the level of the NMDA-receptor [16]. Initially contraindicated in patients with traumatic brain injuries due to a theorized risk of ICP elevation [17], the use of ketamine has begun to gain favor in the neurocritical care setting. In numerous small trials ketamine has been safely used for neuroanesthesia in TBI patients [18], sedation in the ICU [19], and induction for intubation [20,21]. Another potential mechanism of action of ketamine's neuroprotective properties is its effects on the inflammatory response in TBI. The administration of ketamine resulting in the reduction in glutamate (an important mediator in the cerebral inflammatory cascade) concentrations in the brain has recently been confirmed with the use of magnetic resonance imaging [21]. Ketamine's antiinflammatory properties are further believed to act through its suppression of lipopolysaccharide-induced microglial activation and reducing inflammatory cytokines such as tumor necrosis factor and IL-6 [22]. These recent reports, although in small trials, may warrant reevaluating the use of ketamine in TBI patients.

9.3 Hyperosmolar therapy

In the history of TBI management, there have been numerous pharmacologic means by which clinicians have sought to reverse the injury patterns associated with brain trauma. Specifically, therapies have been trialed to reduce intracranial pressure by decreasing the volume of brain tissue through manipulation of the unique properties of the blood—brain barrier [23]. Hyperosmolar agents have long been used in the acute management of brain trauma via this mechanism, and persist today as a first-line therapy in the early stages of TBI. It is important to consider hyperosmolar therapy is ideally utilized when clinical signs of cerebral edema and herniation are present or when objective measures of ICP are in place. However, there is a paucity of evidence concerning its usage as prophylactic therapy [24]. There are several different pharmacologic hyperosmolar agents (mannitol, HTS, and 5% $NaHCO_3$), however, the two most widely utilized agents in the TBI population are mannitol and HTS [2,25]. The efficacy of ICP reduction between the agents is controversial, although slightly favors HTS [26], however, the impact on mortality or cognition is equal and controversial [2] Mannitol when dosed in a range from 1.0 g/kg to 1.5 g/kg of actual body weight, has been proven to reduce intracranial pressure [27]. Hypertonic saline utilizes a similar mechanism of action to mannitol with a potential advantage of being administered at a much smaller volume (important in patients for whom volume overload is disadvantageous) [28]. Neither therapy has robust mortality evidence to support their respective use in TBI, however, their use is supported by guidelines and expert consensus [29]. There is a long history of clinical practice utilizing mannitol in patients with TBI prior to formal ICP monitoring when there are convincing signs of rapid neurologic decompensation or herniation of brain tissue. Mannitol is a potent osmotic diuretic, and while it initially expands extracellular volume, there is an eventual risk of substantial fluid loss through osmotic diuresis. While the diuretic effect seen in mannitol administration is not observed with the use of hypertonic saline, this solution effects a substantial increase in serum sodium. Administration of hypertonic saline in patients with a significant chronic hyponatremia risks the development of central pontine myelinolysis, a devastating condition causing demyelination of brainstem nerve tissue, because of rapid osmotic shifts. Prolonged use of hyperosmolar agents for the management of elevated intracranial pressure in TBI is best performed in the intensive care setting, where vigilant monitoring of ICP, fluid balance, renal function, and serum electrolyte concentration can be assured.

9.4 External ventricular devices

Directly lowering the intracranial pressure (i.e., nonpharmacologically) may be achieved in a less invasive manner then decompressive craniectomy through the use of an external ventricular drain (EVD). Typically placed at the patient's bedside by a trained neurosurgeon either in the emergency department or intensive care setting, most modern EVD systems have the dual option of either measuring ICP or allowing for continuous or intermittent drainage of CSF to reduce intracranial pressure. The evidence to support the use of continuous CSF drainage is limited, though the practice is still widespread and endorsed in consensus guidelines. Contemporary evidence suggests that EVDs set to drain CSF continuously are capable of lowering ICP [30], however, there is no quality evidence that this decreased intracranial pressure is associated with a resultant decrease in mortality or morbidity in patients with TBI.

9.5 Decompressive craniectomy/craniotomy

In patients with SDH or EDH surgical evacuation of the hematoma via craniotomy or craniectomy is the mainstay of therapy, in the presence of neurol deficits or declining neurologic function. The superiority of one technique from a safety and efficacy perspective is unclear [31], however, surgical intervention is effective. Increasing cerebral edema in TBI results in both direct neuronal injury to brain tissue, as well as the secondary injuries stemming from a decrease in cerebral perfusion pressure and increasing brain tissue hypoxemia. In the presence of elevated ICP or refractory elevated ICP, surgical versus medical management remains controversial. Surgical intervention, that is, decompressive craniectomy involves the removal of a large section of the skull with the underlying dura opened [32]. The current recommendations support that when the surgical intervention is performed a sufficiently large DC should be done. Early bifrontal decompressive craniectomy is not supported by the results of the DECRA trial [33]. In the presence of persistent elevated ICP, rescue decompressive craniectomy, as published in the RESCUEicp trial [34], decreased mortality but increased patients in a vegetative state. Decompressive craniectomy, with relatively weak evidence, may be performed initially in the early phase of TBI as a primary means of addressing elevated intracranial pressure (with no mortality benefit), when associated with traumatic hemorrhagic clot and significant disability on exam, or secondarily after less invasive attempts at addressing intracranial hypertension have failed [2]. The role and timing of craniectomy for ICP management is controversial but remains a therapeutic option.

9.6 Therapeutic hypothermia

Over the years there have been many attempted therapies for TBI that have not borne positive results in the literature, and yet their use is still commonly discussed and warrants mentioning here. Therapeutic hypothermia has been utilized with significant success in the field post cardiac arrest management, and its clear neuroprotective benefits in this patient cohort make it an appealing therapeutic modality in TBI. Unfortunately, the literature has not shown benefit when hypothermia is applied to the severe TBI population, either as a therapy (in an attempt to reduce elevated intracranial pressure) or as a prophylactic measure (in attempts to maintain normal intracranial pressure) [27,35,36]. In addition, some studies have suggested there may be a harm associated with cooling patients with TBI below normothermia and its use is currently not recommended. The landmark studies by Clifton in the NABISH studies ultimately did not support therapeutic hypothermia in the first 6 h of injury while suggesting some benefit in the EDH group [37]. Significant controversy still exists as to timing and duration of hypothermia. Targeted temperature management, as opposed to prophylactic hypothermia, is currently the prevailing concept but lacks evidence as to the degree of hypothermia or normothermia, duration of hypothermia, as well as when to initiate and stop.

9.7 Seizure prophylaxis

Seizure activity, either generalized or focal, is relatively common with an incidence as high as 12% occurrence after severe TBI, and antiepileptic drugs routinely are employed in the management of patients with brain injury. Seizures are typically categorized as early posttraumatic seizures (PTS) (less than 7 days from initial injury) and late PTS (greater than 7 days postinjury). Early PTS are at risk of increasing metabolic demand and ICP during a vulnerable phase of TBI recovery. While late PTS have less impact on the acute physiology of brain injury, they are known to result in a higher recurrence rate long-term. The acute phase of brain injury may benefit from seizure prophylaxis with varying degrees of benefit per the type of injury to prevent secondary neurologic injury. These may include injury patterns such as intraparenchymal contusions, intracranial hemorrhage, or penetrating injuries [2]. There is no evidence to suggest that the long-term use of antiepileptic medications is effective for seizure prophylaxis in patients sustaining TBI beyond the initial week following injury. Clinical trials of antiepileptic drugs for prophylaxis in TBI have focused on the use of two particular agents, valproate and phenytoin [38]. While phenytoin appears to be the most studied AED in TBI, according to some consensus guidelines [38] evidence exists that a third agent, levitiracetam, has become a commonly utilized antiepileptic in TBI owing to its lack of frequent side effects and broad therapeutic window [39]. Current guidelines [2] do not recommend one agent over the other but acknowledge the well-established safety of phenytoin, and the less supported safety and effectiveness of levitiracetam.

Steroids: One of the few class 1 BTF guidelines is the recommendation against administration of steroids after TBI based on the results of the CRASH trial. As a result, we do not discuss this option beyond not recommending this therapy.

Beyond therapies and interventions aimed at directly reducing ICP and associated edema, there are several intensive care measures routinely employed in the care of TBI patients that are supported by the evidence. We discuss one such measure here that is well supported as a standard of care practice: the use of prophylaxis against venous thromboembolism (VTE). VTE is a feared, posttraumatic, complication in the ICU given its significant incidence, as high as 58% in an untreated population [40]. Within all-comers in the cohort of traumatically injured patients, specific risk factors for VTE include injury to the spinal cord, fractures of the pelvis or long bones of the leg, a recent surgery, the need for blood transfusion, and elderly age [41]. With regards to TBI, there is some evidence that major head injury is also a risk factor in the general population subgroups [42]. Both venous compression devices (graduated compression devices and pneumatically powered sequential devices) as well as prophylactic-dose subcutaneous heparin are effective in reducing the risk of VTE. In one study performed by Dennis et al. [43], the authors described a reduction in the incidence of VTE from 8.98% to 2.9% with the aforementioned prophylaxis. Both low-dose heparin and sequential venous compression prophylaxis were shown by this study to be equally efficacious. In clinical practice, sequential compression devices are often preferred due to the relative contraindication of anticoagulant use in patients with TBI associated with hemorrhage [44], though some guidelines recommend prophylactic dose low-molecular-weight heparin as soon as deemed clinically safe to do so. It must be noted, however, that there is a paucity of data to suggest when the initiation of pharmacoprophylaxis for VTE is considered "safe," particularly in patients with TBI associated with intracranial hemorrhage. In patients with known associated intracranial hemorrhage, the use of scheduled CT scans separated by between 12 and 24 hours has been employed to assess for stability of a given hemorrhage and as a marker of when low-molecular-weight heparin might be safely started [44]. The use of a prophylactic occlusive filter device in the inferior vena cava amongst those patients not suitable for low-molecular-weight heparin prophylaxis is a controversial topic and most authorities do not recommend this as a routine means of prophylaxis for VTE due to a lack of evidence regarding efficacy.

The therapeutic options for severe TBI are still limited and constrained by the lack of successful clinical trials to provide level I evidence. However, although not discussed here, the number of monitoring techniques and the evolution of multimodal monitoring are increasing. The effectiveness of multimodal monitoring has yet to be fully demonstrated but may allow for the development of different therapeutics and surrogate markers to aid in the therapy and management of severe TBI patients.

References

[1] Majdan M, Brazinova A, Rusnak M, Leitgeb J. Outcome prediction after traumatic brain injury: comparison of the performance of routinely used severity scores and multivariable prognostic models. J Neurosci Rural Pract 2017;8:20—9.

[2] Carney N, Totten AM, O'Reilly C, et al. Guidelines for the management of severe traumatic brain injury, fourth edition. Neurosurgery 2017;80:6—15.

[3] Bickell WH, Wall Jr. MJ, Pepe PE, et al. Immediate versus delayed fluid resuscitation for hypotensive patients with penetrating torso injuries. N Engl J Med 1994;331:1105—9.

[4] Pietropaoli JA, Rogers FB, Shackford SR, Wald SL, Schmoker JD, Zhuang J. The deleterious effects of intraoperative hypotension on outcome in patients with severe head injuries. J Trauma 1992;33:403—7.

[5] Dash HH, Chavali S. Management of traumatic brain injury patients. Korean J Anesthesiol 2018;71:12—21.

[6] Bouma GJ, Muizelaar JP. Cerebral blood flow, cerebral blood volume, and cerebrovascular reactivity after severe head injury. J Neurotrauma 1992;9(Suppl. 1):S333—48.

[7] Carrera E, Schmidt JM, Fernandez L, et al. Spontaneous hyperventilation and brain tissue hypoxia in patients with severe brain injury. J Neurol Neurosurg Psychiatry 2010;81:793—7.

[8] Muizelaar JP, Marmarou A, Ward JD, et al. Adverse effects of prolonged hyperventilation in patients with severe head injury: a randomized clinical trial. J Neurosurg 1991;75:731—9.

[9] Albanese J, Viviand X, Potie F, Rey M, Alliez B, Martin C. Sufentanil, fentanyl, and alfentanil in head trauma patients: a study on cerebral hemodynamics. Crit Care Med 1999;27:407—11.

[10] Pinaud M, Lelausque JN, Chetanneau A, Fauchoux N, Menegalli D, Souron R. [Effects of Diprivan on cerebral blood flow, intracranial pressure and cerebral metabolism in head injured patients]. Ann Fr Anesth Reanim 1991;10:2—9.

[11] Roberts I, Sydenham E. Barbiturates for acute traumatic brain injury. Cochrane Database Syst Rev 2012;12: CD000033.

[12] Trapani G, Altomare C, Liso G, Sanna E, Biggio G. Propofol in anesthesia. Mechanism of action, structure-activity relationships, and drug delivery. Curr Med Chem 2000;7:249—71.

[13] Kang TM. Propofol infusion syndrome in critically ill patients. Ann Pharmacother 2002;36:1453—6.

[14] Jooste EH, Muhly WT, Ibinson JW, et al. Acute hemodynamic changes after rapid intravenous bolus dosing of dexmedetomidine in pediatric heart transplant patients undergoing routine cardiac catheterization. Anesth Analg 2010;111:1490—6.

[15] Aryan HE, Box KW, Ibrahim D, Desiraju U, Ames CP. Safety and efficacy of dexmedetomidine in neurosurgical patients. Brain Inj 2006;20:791—8.

[16] Zorumski CF, Izumi Y, Mennerick S. Ketamine: NMDA receptors and beyond. J Neurosci 2016;36:11158—64.

[17] Gardner AE, Dannemiller FJ, Dean D. Intracranial cerebrospinal fluid pressure in man during ketamine anesthesia. Anesth Analg 1972;51:741—5.

[18] Grathwohl KW, Black IH, Spinella PC, et al. Total intravenous anesthesia including ketamine versus volatile gas anesthesia for combat-related operative traumatic brain injury. Anesthesiology 2008;109:44—53.

[19] Kolenda H, Gremmelt A, Rading S, Braun U, Markakis E. Ketamine for analgosedative therapy in intensive care treatment of head-injured patients. Acta Neurochir (Wien) 1996;138:1193—9.

[20] Cromartie III. RS. Rapid anesthesia induction in combat casualties with full stomachs. Anesthesia Analgesia 1976;55:74—6.

[21] Sibley A, Mackenzie M, Bawden J, Anstett D, Villa-Roel C, Rowe BH. A prospective review of the use of ketamine to facilitate endotracheal intubation in the helicopter emergency medical services (HEMS) setting. Emerg Med J 2011;28:521—5.

[22] Vespa P, Prins M, Ronne-Engstrom E, et al. Increase in extracellular glutamate caused by reduced cerebral perfusion pressure and seizures after human traumatic brain injury: a microdialysis study. J Neurosurg 1998;89:971—82.

[23] Bhutta AT, Schmitz ML, Swearingen C, et al. Ketamine as a neuroprotective and anti-inflammatory agent in children undergoing surgery on cardiopulmonary bypass: a pilot randomized, double-blind, placebo-controlled trial. Pediatr Crit Care Med 2012;13:328—37.

[24] Chang Y, Lee JJ, Hsieh CY, Hsiao G, Chou DS, Sheu JR. Inhibitory effects of ketamine on lipopolysaccharide-induced microglial activation. Mediators Inflamm 2009;2009:705379.

[25] Knapp JM. Hyperosmolar therapy in the treatment of severe head injury in children: mannitol and hypertonic saline. AACN Clin Issues 2005;16:199−211.

[26] Boone MD, Oren-Grinberg A, Robinson TM, Chen CC, Kasper EM. Mannitol or hypertonic saline in the setting of traumatic brain injury: what have we learned? Surg Neurol Int 2015;6:177.

[27] Marion DW, Penrod LE, Kelsey SF, et al. Treatment of traumatic brain injury with moderate hypothermia. N Engl J Med 1997;336:540−6.

[28] Sakellaridis N, Pavlou E, Karatzas S, et al. Comparison of mannitol and hypertonic saline in the treatment of severe brain injuries. J Neurosurg 2011;114:545−8.

[29] Prabhakar H, Singh GP, Anand V, Kalaivani M. Mannitol versus hypertonic saline for brain relaxation in patients undergoing craniotomy. Cochrane Database Syst Rev 2014;CD010026.

[30] Muralidharan R. External ventricular drains: management and complications. Surg Neurol Int 2015;6: S271−4.

[31] Phan K, Moore JM, Griessenauer C, et al. Craniotomy versus decompressive craniectomy for acute subdural hematoma: systematic review and meta-analysis. World Neurosurg 2017;101:677−85 e2.

[32] Timofeev I, Santarius T, Kolias AG, Hutchinson PJ. Decompressive craniectomy—operative technique and perioperative care. Adv Tech Stand Neurosurg 2012;38:115−36.

[33] Sahuquillo J, Arikan F. Decompressive craniectomy for the treatment of refractory high intracranial pressure in traumatic brain injury. Cochrane Database Syst Rev 2006;CD003983.

[34] Hutchinson PJ, Kolias AG, Timofeev IS, et al. Trial of decompressive craniectomy for traumatic intracranial hypertension. N Engl J Med 2016;375:1119−30.

[35] Aibiki M, Maekawa S, Yokono S. Moderate hypothermia improves imbalances of thromboxane A2 and prostaglandin I2 production after traumatic brain injury in humans. Crit Care Med 2000;28:3902−6.

[36] Jiang J, Yu M, Zhu C. Effect of long-term mild hypothermia therapy in patients with severe traumatic brain injury: 1-year follow-up review of 87 cases. J Neurosurg 2000;93:546−9.

[37] Clifton GL, Allen S, Barrodale P, et al. A phase II study of moderate hypothermia in severe brain injury. J Neurotrauma 1993;10:263−71 discussion 73.

[38] Yerram S, Katyal N, Premkumar K, Nattanmai P, Newey CR. Seizure prophylaxis in the neuroscience intensive care unit. J Intensive Care 2018;6:17.

[39] Jones KE, Puccio AM, Harshman KJ, et al. Levetiracetam versus phenytoin for seizure prophylaxis in severe traumatic brain injury. Neurosurg Focus 2008;25:E3.

[40] Hammond FM, Meighen MJ. Venous thromboembolism in the patient with acute traumatic brain injury: screening, diagnosis, prophylaxis, and treatment issues. J Head Trauma Rehabil 1998;13:36−50.

[41] Geerts WH, Code KI, Jay RM, Chen E, Szalai JP. A prospective study of venous thromboembolism after major trauma. N Engl J Med 1994;331:1601−6.

[42] Knudson MM, Ikossi DG. Venous thromboembolism after trauma. Curr Opin Crit Care 2004;10:539−48.

[43] Dennis JW, Menawat S, Von Thron J, et al. Efficacy of deep venous thrombosis prophylaxis in trauma patients and identification of high-risk groups. J Trauma 1993;35:132−8 discussion 8−9.

[44] Cothren CC, Smith WR, Moore EE, Morgan SJ. Utility of once-daily dose of low-molecular-weight heparin to prevent venous thromboembolism in multisystem trauma patients. World J Surg 2007;31:98−104.

Classical TBI biomarkers

S100 biomarkers in patients with traumatic brain injury

Henriette Beyer[1], Peter Biberthaler[2] and Viktoria Bogner-Flatz[3]

[1]Trauma Surgery Klinikum rechts der Isar, Munich, Germany [2]Department of Trauma Surgery, Klinikum rechts der Isar, School of Medicine, Technical University of Munich, Munich, Germany [3]Department of General, Trauma and Reconstructive Surgery, Emergency Medicine Ludwig Maximilians University, Munich, Germany

10.1 Introduction

The wide spectrum of symptoms associated with trauma-induced craniocerebral injury traumatic brain injury (TBI) is challenging medical personnel tasked with treating trauma patients in emergency rooms worldwide. In particular, the diagnosis of mild TBI is difficult to secure as a fraction of affected patients can still exhibit intracranial damage without manifesting severe symptoms. In recent research the use of several protein biomarkers is discussed as an additional means of diagnosis in addition to established imaging methods. These markers are accessible via immunoassay of sampled blood and believed to permit inference regarding the severity of TBI and patient outcome [1]. One such marker, S100B, is already used clinically to facilitate better assessment of patients exhibiting less severe symptoms of craniocerebral injury in some countries [2]. The family of S100 proteins was first described by Moore et al. in 1965 [3]. S100B was characterized as a marker for neural damage during the 1980s [4]. In 1995 the interrelation of S100B and craniocerebral injury was investigated by Ingebrigtsen et al. [5].

10.2 Biomarker family S100

Altered enzyme activities, metabolites or proteins are regarded as biomarkers if they express a physiological or pathological condition [6]. The S100 proteins were studied with regards to their function as biomarkers in several studies.

10.4.1 General characteristics

The name is derived from the protein's complete solubility in ammonium sulfate of neutral pH value [3]. S100 is a comparably small homodimer protein with a molecular weight of nine to fourteen ku [7]. There are 20 members of the S100 protein family that have been identified and their biological effects have been investigated (cf. Table 10.1). To confirm family membership, amino acid sequences and structural features must be examined [8].

S100 comprises two monomers, alpha and beta, which define the naming scheme used to denominate the different isoforms [9]. Mostly, S100B is used as a collective term for dimers containing at least one monomer of the "B-variant" [10]. To discuss different applications of proteins of this family the nomenclature used throughout the literature is sometimes unclear. For example, S100A1B (heterodimer composed of S100A1 and S100B subunits) and S100BB (homodimer composed of two S100B subunits) are both referred to as S100B in the literature, as they both contain a beta-subunit [10,11].

S100 can be characterized as a calcium binding protein [8]. In human cells, calcium holds an essential role in signal transduction. A special "motif" is needed to bind calcium and transfer signals. The best-known motif is the "EF-hand," which is built of a helix−loop−helix structure [12,13], and of which S100 contains two forming a dimer [12].

10.4.2 Biological functions

Proteins of the S100 family participate in physiological processes but can also indicate pathological states. Physiologically, S100 family proteins perform intra- as well as extracellular functions. S100 functions within the cells span a range of diverse processes, including but not limited to cell-to-cell communication, proliferation, differentiation, apoptosis, metabolic functions, and calcium-homeostasis [13]. Extracellular S100 proteins mostly participate in immune responses, tissue development and repair, as well as tumor cell invasion [13].

Clinically the indicative utility is discussed in the context of several varying illnesses. For example, high levels of S100 A8, 9, and 12 can be found in acute or chronic inflammatory disorders like rheumatic arthritis [14]. But the diagnostic informative value in general is limited, because if there is a second disease, the biomarkers would not discriminate, e.g., while S100A12 is found in general lung disorders, it is likely to indicate early stage lung injury in septic patients [13,15].

10.4.3 Family member S100B

The most researched isoform of the S100 family is S100B. Its characteristic as a biomarker for TBI is already used clinically [2]. The utilization of S100B is similar to that of Troponin I and the CK-MB enzyme as indicators for myocardial infarctions, as its concentration is measured in blood samples.

TABLE 10.1 S100 family.

	Tumor associated		Biological and pathological functions (mainly other than tumor)			
Name	Downregulated ↓ Upregulated ↑ Tissue	Consequence	Expressed in/interaction with	Intracellular function	Extracellular function	Maybe involved in...
S100-A1			Skeletal muscle fibers Cardiomyocytes Certain neuronal populations	Muscle	Ca^{2+}-Transport	calcification of bones and cartilage
S100-A2	↓ + ↑	↓ means poor prognosis			Immune System	
S100-A3			Hair root cells, some astrocytomas	Epithelial cell differentiation, hair cuticular barrier formation	-	Hair protection from oxidative damage
S100-A4	↑	Stimulates cell survival, motility, and invasion	Cytoskeletal proteins		Immune System and allergic response	Metastatic/ tumor progression, T-cell-infiltration in primary tumors, cardioprotective
S100-A5	↑ (in bladder cancers and recurrent meningiomas)					
S100-A6	Many tumors	Implicated in tumorigenesis, survival of neuroblastoma cells	Many cells	Cell proliferation, cytoskeletal dynamics, inhibits actions between Hsp → favors/ inhibits apoptosis	Stimulates lactogen II secretion from trophoblasts and insulin release	Secretory processes, allergic responses
S100-A7	↑ Breast cancer	Restricted to estrogen receptor alpha-negative			Overexpressed in inflammatory skin disease, antimicrobial responses (reduces E.coli), Immune system	Prevent generation of amyloidogenic peptides (Alzheimer's Disease)
S100-A8			Keratinocytes (a.o.)	Immune System; Myeloid cell differentiation	upregulated by corticosteroids (Immune System)	

(Continued)

TABLE 10.1 (Continued)

| Name | Tumor associated | | Biological and pathological functions (mainly other than tumor) | | | |
	Downregulated ↓ Upregulated ↑ Tissue	Consequence	Expressed in/interaction with	Intracellular function	Extracellular function	Maybe involved in…
S100-A9			Interaction with S-100A8	Inhibits myeloid differentiation	Protective in Asthma, Immune System	RAGE-ligand →autoimmune diseases
S100-A10		Essential for migration of tumor-promoting macrophages into tumor sites		Tethering Plasma membrane proteins, Downregulated in depressive-like states (interaction with serotonin-receptors)	Leukemia, Fibrinolysis, Angiogenesis, Immune System, Bluetongue-virus	
S100-A11				Inhibits and stimulates cell growth (dependent on ligand), DNA-repair	Collagen, chondrocytes, osteoarthritis progression	
S100-A12			Constitutively in neutrophils, inducible in macrophages and smooth muscle cells; epithelial cells	Vascular remodeling (aortic aneurysms), vessel calcification, chemokine secretion in human airway (allergic inflammation)	Immune system	Modulation of interactions between cytoskeleton and membranes, (anti-)chaperone-like functions
S100-A13				Stress-induced release of fibroblast growth factor and IL-1alpha		Angiogenesis
S100-A14		Cancer suppressor (p53 pathway)				
S100-A15				—	In keratinocytes in inflamed skin, antimicrobial activity	
S100-A16 ↑				Adipogenesis-promoting, negative impact on insulin sensitivity	—	

S100-B		Astrocytes, certain neuronal populations, Schwann cells, melanocytes, chrondrocytes, adipocytes, skeletal myofibers and associated satellite cells, certain dendritic cell and lymphocyte populations (usw)	Stimulator of cell proliferation and migration, inhibitor of apoptosis and differentiation → neurodegenerative diseases, cardiac remodeling after infarction, melanomagenesis and gliomagenesis; elevation in serum correlates with mood disorders, schizophrenia; outcome predictor in traumatic brain injury	Intraventricular infusion induces neurogenesis within the hippocampus (enhanced cognitive function), myoblast proliferation, Schwann cell migration, T-cell interaction	Accumulation contributes to neuroinflammation
S100-G		Many tissues	Cytosolic Ca buffer, transport of S100 proteins through membranes	–	
S100-P	Mediates tumor growth, drug resistance and metastasis (RAGE dependent)				
S100-Z	↓ (several tumors)	–	–		

In humans, some "functions" may have influence on tumors as well (most tumor-related "functions" are intracellular).

" – " Means no function reported; if empty -> function appears in tumor respectively biological/pathological.

Sometimes no attribution to certain cells -> empty box.

All subunits described as homodimers; may have some other functions as heterodimers (like S100A1B).

From Donato R, Cannon BR, Sorci G, Riuzzi F, Hsu K, Weber DJ, Geczy CL. Functions of S100 proteins. Curr Mol Med 2013.

10.4.1.1 Special characteristics of S100B

S100B is secreted mainly from astrocytes and cannot traverse the blood—brain barrier under normal physiologic conditions [6]. Therefore concentration in CSF is expected to be higher than in serum [6,16]. The physiological level of S100B in CSF is believed to be between 0.8—3.1 µg/L (mean 1.5 µg/L in women, 1.9 µg/L in men) [17], in serum between 0.02—0.15 µg/L [17]. There is evidence that age and sex influences the level of S100B in CSF [17,18].

Depending on the concentration, it has different effects on neurons, astrocytes, and microglia [13]: low levels of S100B are thought to stimulate astrocyte proliferation [17], whereas high levels encourage inflammation [19]. The amount of S100B released is regulated by several factors, including catecholamines [18] or glutamate [20] as stimulating neurotransmitters, and high glucose as a possible decreasing condition [21].

While S100B is often described as a brain-specific biomarker, it is also synthesized in other tissues such as adipocytes, chondrocytes, melanocytes, Langerhans cells, cardiomyocytes, and skeletal muscle fibers [22]. This additional synthesis, as well as the patient's ethnicity, needs to be considered when assessing the concentration of S100B in serum samples. Abdesselam et al. showed that the physiologic concentration correlates with ethnicities. Black people for example have a median S100B concentration twice as high as Caucasians [17].

10.4.1.2 Mechanism of pathologic increase of S100B

The mechanism of the pathologic increase in serum levels of S100B is still the subject of current research. There are two main options discussed. First, the influence of pathologies on expression, release, and metabolism of S100B are considered [22]. Holdenrieder et al. examined various benign pulmonary, gynecological, urological, autoimmune, and gastrointestinal diseases to detect the influence of the level of S100B. They evaluated malign diseases like breast, ovarian, gastric, liver, or bladder cancer as well, and none of them showed increased levels of S100B [23].

Second, the opening of the blood—brain barrier, and therefore increased release of S100B, is a possible mechanism [23]. This would include apoplexy [24], neurodegenerative diseases such as multiple sclerosis [25], premorbid Alzheimer's [26], subarachnoidal hemorrhage [27], or vasospasms [28] as a possible influencer of pathologic increased serum level.

10.4.1.3 Half-life and elimination of S100B

Another important factor during the assessment of S100B levels in samples is half-life, which is considered to be below 60 minutes [6]. The half-life of S100B is also affected by diseases or events such as skin cancer (half-life of up to 90 minutes) or TBI (half-life of up to 120 minutes) [29]. S100B's main elimination mechanism is by kidney filtration, but disturbed liver function is believed to also cause increased concentrations [30].

10.3 Clinical applications of S100B

A wide range of possible applications for the S100 protein family is currently being discussed with possible therapeutic as well as diagnostic purposes. S100B is already actively used for applications in dermatology and neurosurgery. Further applications in the experimental phase are schizophrenia [31], depression, and suicidality, as well as lung and ovarian cancer [32].

10.4.4 Applications in dermatology

Usage of S100B as a tumor marker is currently limited to melanoma, with its first usage reported by Gaynor et al. [33]. The occurrence of S100 protein in these tumor cells is deducted from their shared neuroectodermal origin. In the following two decades, melanoma-related research of S100 applications continued. In 2002 Molina et al. investigated the sensitivity and specificity of serum concentrations of S100, regarding benign as well as severe illnesses [30]. In their research, they found S100 to be an expedient biomarker for melanoma, while also highlighting the possibility of false positives due to liver or kidney illness [34]. They speculate that heightened S100 concentrations hint at liver metastases [30] and suggest it may serve as an indication of measuring S100B for monitoring therapy. Unfortunately, detection and diagnosis are not reasonable clinical strategies, due to low sensitivity [35].

The heterodimer S100A1B is found in melanocytes [36], and Bolander et al. further showed that for the adoption of S100B as a tumor marker the differentiation of isoforms during concentration measurement is important. S100BB concentrations show higher correlation with a relapse risk of melanoma compared to S100A1 concentrations or S100B concentrations at large [36].

10.4.5 Applications in neurosurgery

Even without a clearly identified pathological mechanism, the correlation of several neurological and neurosurgical clinical pictures with increased S100B concentration are evident. These include subarachnoid hemorrhage, TBI, and cerebral infarcts [24]. Depending on the medical condition, different benefits can be gained by employing the biomarker. In the case of subarachnoid hemorrhage, the marker is utilized best to forecast complications and general prognosis, as cerebral damage develops over a time span of minutes to hours after the trigger [37]. Wiesman et al. showed a positive correlation between S100B and an early onset neurological deficit [27]. They found the protein to be an indicator of equal sensitivity compared to the clinically used Hunt-und-Hess Score [27,38,39].

In the case of TBI, the immediate cerebral damage means that the biomarker function of S100B should instead be utilized as early as possible due to the short half-time mentioned. As of now the S100B serum concentration is used as a criterion for exclusion of cerebral lesions clinically [2]. If a patient shows minor or no symptoms of TBI, and an additional negative S100 test with serum concentration below 0.01 µg/L, the treating physician can forego the classical imaging methods. This decreases radiation exposure for patients and cost for the institution [40]. Usage of the S100 test to predict the ultimate patient outcome is nevertheless controversial.

This differentiation of isoforms regarding their function as biomarkers seems to be critical for neurosurgical patients too. A study by Nylén shows that the isoform S100BB concentration better correlates with patient outcome and is therefore better suited to support predictions [40].

10.4 Current state of research regarding neurosurgical implications of S100B

Several aspects of S100 biomarker utilization in the context of TBI are subject to current research efforts. This is closely related to the question of which extracerebral sources and other influences (like intoxicants) have an impact on S100B level. Another controversial point is the ideal timing for concentration determination and its half-life in serum.

Finally, the clinically important question is regarding the effectiveness of S100B concentration as a predictor of the severity of injury and patient outcomes. Which conclusions can be drawn at what level of certainty from an increased concentration? This is crucial to the question of whether S100B diagnostics can meaningfully impact TBI diagnosis.

10.4.6 Studies regarding diagnostic application of S100B

Many of the current studies directly investigating S100B support its assistance in TBI diagnosis. Their results show that utilization of S100B can be the exclusion of tomographic imaging, and scans can be reduced by a third for mild TBI [41]. Research regarding appropriate threshold values for exclusion has been performed, with a goal to maximize sensitivity. Depending on the cohort observed, the sensitivity for a cutoff level of $0.1\,\mu g/L$ S100B in serum is 0.95 [41] to 0.99 [42]. Biberthaler et al. employed a multicenter study of 1309 mild TBI patients, defined by GCS of 13 to 15 and at least one additional symptom. Müller et al. surveyed a smaller collective of 226 patients selected according to the same criteria.

Symptoms exhibited by patients with mild TBI are often highly subjective and variable. While some symptoms and parameters like anticoagulation treatment or patient age are objectively quantifiable, their relations to patient outcome are variable. Other factors, such as retrograde amnesia, headache, and dizziness, depend on subjective patients rating in the first place. Therefore objective parameters to assess severity are welcome to increase the quality of diagnosis. Unden et al. came to the same evaluation of S100B: in combination with other clinical parameters it is a valuable instrument of diagnosis [43].

10.4.1.4 Influence of alcohol intoxication on diagnostic outcome

Another characteristic of the patient collective is the coincidence of mild TBI and alcohol intoxication. This further complicates diagnostic testing based on patient valuation. For up to 45% of patients, it is not obvious to the treating physician whether the observed symptoms are triggered by alcohol ingestion or trauma [42]. S100B biomarker concentration in serum is independent of blood alcohol concentration and thus constitutes at least one objective factor in assessing these patients [23,44].

10.4.1.5 β-error in diagnostics

Since the sensitivity does not reach 100%, patients with symptoms of mild TBI and S100B concentrations below the cutoff threshold of 0.1 µg/L might still develop cerebral lesions. Müller et al. calculated the number of patients affected to be 1.5%. They analyzed the lesions in these missed incidents to be minor and without therapeutic consequences [41]. This benign failure mode of the biomarker screening is due to the concentration of S100B scaling well with the severity of trauma.

10.4.7 Studies regarding half-life and elimination of S100B

The half-life and elimination of the S100 protein are critical if the results are to be used to diagnose TBI status. Following cardiac surgery, the half-life of S100B is 25 minutes [45]. In contrast, Townend et al. measured the half-life to be 97 minutes in a study with TBI patients [46]. Another study examined posttraumatic enzyme kinetics and elimination in 65 rodents in order to find the optimal time for measurement of S100B. In rats, serum concentration of S100B is stable up to 24 hours after TBI [47]. Ultimately, rodent results do not seem to be transferrable to human patients since studies in humans show rapid elimination of S100 proteins from serum [46]. Still, elimination times in humans do depend on kidney function [30] and ethnicity [48].

10.4.8 Studies regarding extracerebral sources of S100B

The influence of extracerebral sources, such as S100 synthesis in bone and muscle tissues, have been investigated and confirmed by Pelinka et al. From a clinical perspective this means that fractures, body fat, and muscular mass need to be included into the evaluation of S100 levels. Pelinka et al. found that hemorrhagic shock was associated with a rise in S100 concentration during a clinical study to quantify the influence of major fractures on S100B response to TBI. A bone fracture study, without cranial involvement in rats, suggested a compensation factor to be calculated [49]. These results and those of Pelinka et al. clearly show S100B to be elevated by extracerebral release mechanisms in polytraumatic patients [50]. Pham et al. on the other hand did not find S100B concentrations to be influenced by extracerebral sources or BMI [50].

10.4.9 Prognostic value of S100B

Outside of direct diagnostic applications, S100B could also indicate mortality. In combination with other potential biomarkers, such as GFAP, a correlation between serum concentrations and survival rate after TBI were found by Pelinka et al. in a time series study [1]. A decrease of S100B concentration within a time span of no longer than 36 hours after the traumatic incident indicated a higher chance of survival when compared to persistently increased values.

10.5 Conclusion

S100B is an expedient parameter complementing the diagnostic tool set for mild TBI. Measurements of the protein currently provide valuable information during patient admission in the emergency department. Under certain circumstances the S100B measurement can replace a traditional CT imaging scan, although imaging methods are still faster compared to determination of S100B serum levels [51]. During longer hospitalization, S100B levels can also provide insights regarding patient progression and outcome. A declining S100B concentration within 48 hours of admission indicates a positive progression [52]. Constant or increasing concentrations indicate complications followed by negative patient progression [53]. Therefore to track the development of S100B levels at least one subsequent measurement is advised after the initial test. Regardless, for the successful clinical application of S100B biomarker tests a definitive threshold value is needed. Threshold values between 0.1 µg/L and 0.2 µg/L are advised by the ACEP [54]. With high sensitivity and low specificity, S100B biomarker tests are best applied as criteria for exclusion. Increased S100B concentration does not conclusively prove cerebral damage but a physiological concentration in adult patients admitted with TBI does rule out cerebral damage with sufficient certainty. Due to the multiple potential sources of S100 proteins both ACEP and the Scandinavian Guidelines recommend S100b diagnostics only in cases of isolated TBI. Polytraumatic patients are explicitly excluded from the list of applications for these biomarkers [38,54].

Following Scandinavian Guidelines (2013) and recommendations of ACEP (2008), this subsequent advice arises for the management of acute TBI:

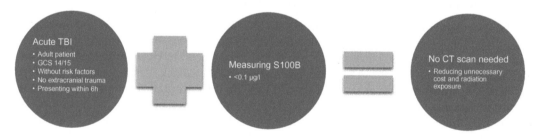

References

[1] Pelinka LE, Kroepfl A, Leixnering M, Buchinger W, Raabe A, Redl H. GFAP versus S100B in Serum after Traumatic Brain Injury: Relationship to Brain Damage and Outcome. Journal of Neurotrauma 2004;21 (11):1553−61 2004 Nov.

[2] Unden J, Ingebrigtsen T, Romner B. Scandinavian Neurotrauma Committee (SNC). Scandinavian guidelines for initial management of minimal, mild and moderate head injuries in adults: an evidence and consensus-based update. BMC Medicine 2013 Feb 25;11:50.

[3] Moore BW. A soluble protein characteristic of the nervous system. Biochemical and biophysical research communications 1965 Jun 9;19(6):739−44.

[4] Sindic CJ, Chalon MP, Cambiaso CL, Laterre EC, Masson PL. Assessment of damage to the central nervous system by determination of S-100 protein in the cerebrospinal fluid. Journal of Neurology, Neurosurgery, and Psychiatry 1982 Dec;45(12):1130−5.

[5] Ingebrigtsen T, Romner B, Kongstad P, Langbakk B. Increased serum concentrations of protein s-100 after minor head injury: a biochemical serum marker with prognostic value? Journal of Neurology, Neurosurgery, and Psychiatry 1995 Jul;59(1):103−4.

[6] Dash PK, Zhao J, Hergenroeder G, Moore AN. Biomarkers for the Diagnosis, Prognosis, and Evaluation of Treatment Efficacy for Traumatic Brain Injury. Neurotherapeutics: The Journal of the American Society for Experimental NeuroTherapeutics 2010 Jan;7(1):100−14.

[7] Donato R. S100: a multigenic family of calcium-modulated proteins of the EF-hand type with intracellular and extracellular functional roles. The International Journal of Biochemistry & Cell Biology 2001 Jul;33(7):637−68.

[8] Zimmer DB, Cornwall EH, Landar A, Song W. The S100 Protein Family: History, Function, and Expression. Brain Research Bulletin 1995;37(4):417−29.

[9] Isobe T, Ishioka N, Okuyama T. Structural relation of two S-100 proteins in bovine brain: subunit composition of S-100a protein. European Journal of Biochemistry 1981 Apr;115(3):469−74.

[10] Nylen K, Öst M, Csajbok LZ, Nilsson I, Hall C, Blennow K, Nellgard B, Rosengren L. Serum levels of S100B, S100A1B and S100BB are all related to outcome after severe traumatic brain injury. Acta Neurochirurgia 2008 Mar;150(3):221−7.

[11] Kligman D, Hilt DC. The S100 Protein Family. Trends in Biochemical Sciences 1988 Nov;13(11):437−43.

[12] Chazin WJ. Relating Form and Function of EF-hand Calcium Binding Proteins. Accounts of Chemical Research 2011 Mar 15;44(3):171−9.

[13] Strynadka NCJ, James MNG. Crystal structures of the helix-loop-helix calcium-binding proteins. Annual Review of Biochemistry 1989;58:951−98.

[14] Donato R, Cannon BR, Sorci G, Riuzzi F, Hsu K, Weber DJ, Geczy CL. Functions of S100 Proteins. Current Molecular Medicine 2013 Jan;13(1):24−57.

[15] Baillet A, Trocme C, Berthier S, Arlotto M, Grange L, Chenau J, Quétant S, Sève M, Berger F, Juvin R, Morel F, Gaudin P. Synovial fluid proteomic fingerprint: S100A8, S100A9 and S100A12 proteins discriminate rheumatoid arthritis from other inflammatory joint diseases. Rheumatology 2010 Apr;49(4):671−82.

[16] Kikkawa T, Sato N, Kojika M, Takahashi G, Aoki K, Hoshikawa K, Akitomi S, Shozushima T, Suzuki K, Wakabayashi G, Endo S. Significance of measuring S100A12 and sRAGE in the serum of sepsis patients with postoperative acute lung injury. Digestive Surgery 2010;27(4):307−12.

[17] Petzold A, Keir G, Lim D, Smith M, Thompson EJ. Cerebrospinal fluid (CSF) and serum S100B: release and wash-out pattern. Brain Research Bulletin 2003 Aug 15;61(3):281−5.

[18] Abdesselam OB, Vally J, Adem C, Foglietti M-J, Beaudeux J-L. Reference Values for Serum S-100B Protein depend on the race of individuals. Clinical Chemistry 2003 May;49(5):836−7.

[19] Nygaard O, Langbakk B, Romner B. Age- and sex-related changes of S-100 protein concentrations in cerebrospinal fluid and serum in patients with no previous history of neurological disorder. Clinical Chemistry 1997 Mar;43(3):541−3.

[20] van Engelen B, Lamers K, Gabreels F, Wevers R, van Geel WJA, Borm G. Age-related changes of neuron-specific enolase, S-100 protein, and myelin basic protein concentrations in cerebrospinal fluid. Clinical chemistry 1992 Jun;38(6):813−16.

[21] Selinfreund R, Barger S, Pledger W, Van Eldik L. Neurotrophic protein S100beta stimulates glial cell proliferation,. Proceedings of the National Academy of Sciences 1991 May 1;88(9):3554−8.

[22] Suzuki F, Kato K, Nakajima T. Hormonal regulation of adipose S-100 protein release. Journal of Neurochemistry 1984 Nov;43(5):1336−41.

[23] Ciccarelli R, Di Iorio P, Bruno V, Battaglia G, Alimonte ID, Onofrio MD, Nicoletti F, Caciagli F. Activation of A1 adenosine or mGlu3 metabotropic glutamate receptors enhances the release of Nerve Growth Factor and S100beta protein from cultured astrocytes. Glia 1999 Sep;27(3):275−81.

[24] Morbini P, Villa C, Campo I, Zorzetto M, Inghilleri S, Luisetti M. The receptor for advanced glycation end products and its ligands: a new inflammatory pathway in lung disease?,. Modern Pathology 2006 Nov;19(11):1437−45.

[25] Thelin EP, Nelson DW, Bellander B-M. A review of the clinical utility of serum S100B protein levels in the assessment of traumatic brain injury,. Acta Neurochirugia 2017 Feb;159(2):209−25.

[26] Holdenrieder S, Spelsberg F, Hatz R, Waidelich R, Untch M, Hofmann K, Wehnl B, Heinemann V, Stieber P. Pattern of S100-release in benign and malignant diseases beside malignant melanoma,. J Lab Med 2013;37 (1):21−8.

[27] Calcagnile O, Holmen A, Chew M, Unden J. S100B levels are affected by older age but not by alcohol intoxication following mild traumatic brain injury. Scandinavian Journal of Trauma, Resuscitation and Emergency Medicine 2013 Jul 6;21:52.

[28] Büttner T, Weyers S, Postert T, Sprengelmeyer R, Kuhn W. S-100 protein: serum marker of focal brain damage after ischemic territorial MCA infarction. Stroke 1997 Oct;28(10):1961−5.

[29] Wiesmann M, Missler U, Hagenström H, Gottmann D. S-100 Protein Plasma Levels after Aneurysmal subarachnoid haemorrhage. Acta Neurochirurgia 1997;139(12):1155−60.

[30] De Vries J, Snels S, Menovsky T, Lemmens WA, De Reus H, Lamers K, Grotenhuis J. Peri-operative levels of S-100 protein in serum: marker for surgical manipulation and postoperative complications,. Minimal Invasive Neurosurgery 2003 Feb;46(1):33−6.

[31] Jackson RG, Samra GS, Radcliffe J, Clark GH, Price CP. The early fall in levels of S-100 beta in traumatic brain injury,. Clinical Chemistry and Laboratory Medicine 2000 Nov;38(11):1165−7.

[32] Molina R, Navarro J, Filella X, Castel T, Ballesta AM. S-100 Protein Serum Levels in Patients with benign and malignant diseases: false-positive results related to liver and renal function,. Tumorbiology 2002 Jan-Feb;23 (1):39−44.

[33] Hong W, Zhao M, Li H, Peng F, Wang F, Li N, Xiang H, Su Y, Huang Y, Zhang S, Zhao G, Rubai Z, Mao L, Lin Z, Fang Y, Zhang Q, Xie B. Higher Plasma S100B Concentrations in Schizophrenia Patients, and Dependently associated with inflammatory markers,. Scientific Reports 2016 Jun 9;6:27584.

[34] Yen M-C, Huang Y-C, Kan J-Y, Kuo P-L, Hou M-F, Hsu Y-L. S100B Expression in breast cancer as a predictive marker for cancer metastasis. Int J Oncol 2018 Feb;52(2):433−40.

[35] Usui A, Kato K, Abe T, Murase M, Tanaka M, Takeuchi E. S-100ao protein in blood and urine during open heart surgery. Clinical Chemistry 1989 Sep;35(9):1942−4.

[36] Alber B, Hein R, Garbe C, Caroli U, Luppa PB. Multicenter evaluation of the analytical and clinical performance of the Elecsys S100 immunoassay in patients with malignant melanoma. Clinical Chemistry and Laboratory Medicine 2005;43(5):557−63.

[37] Bolander A, Agnarsdottir M, Wagenius G, Strömberg S, Ponten F, Ekman S, Brattström D, Larsson A, Einarsson R, Ullenhag G, Hesselius P, Bergqvist M. Serological and immunohistochemical analysis of S100 and new derivates as markers for prognosis in patients with malignant melanoma. Melanoma Research 2008 Dec;18(6):412−19.

[38] Unden J, Astrand R, Waterloo K, Ingebrigtsen T, Bellner J, Reinstrup P, Andsberg G, Romner B. Clinical significance of serum S100B levels in neurointensive care. Journal of Neurocritical Care 2007;6(2):94−9.

[39] Vos PE, van Gils M, Beems T, Zimmerman C, Verbeek MM. Increased GFAP and S100beta but not NSE serum levels after subarachnoid haemorrhage are associated with clinical severity. European Journal of Neurology 2006 Jun;13(6):632−8.

[40] Weiss N, Sanchez-Pena P, Roche S, Beaudeaux JL, Colonne C, Coriat P, Puybasset L. Prognosis value of Plasma S100B Protein Levels after subarachnoid aneurysmal hemorrhage. Anesthesiology 2006 Apr;104 (4):658−66.

[41] Biberthaler P, Linsenmeier U, Pfeifer K-J, Kroetz M, Mussack T, Kanz K-G, Hoecherl EF, Jonas F, Marzi I, Leucht P, Jochum M, Mutschler W. Serum S-100B concentration provides additional information for the indication of computed tomography in patients after minor head injury. Shock 2006 May;25(5):446−53.

[42] Müller K, Townend W, Biasca N, Unden J, Waterloo K, Romner B, Ingebrigtsen T. S100B Serum Level predicts Computed Tomography Findings after Minor Head Injury. The Journal of Trauma Injury, Infection, and Critical Care 2007 Jun;62(6):1452−6.

[43] Unden J, Romner B. Can Low Serum Levels of S100B Predict Normal CT Findings After Minor Head Injury in Adults?: An Evidence-Based Review and Meta-Analysis. Journal of Head Trauma and Rehabilitation 2010 Jul-Aug;25(4):228−40.

[44] Biberthaler P, Mussack T, Wiedemann E, Gilg T, Soyka M, Koller G, Pfeifer KJ, Linsenmaier U, Mutschler W, Gippner-Steppert C, Jochum M. Elevated Serum Levels of S-100B reflect the extent of Brain Injury in alcohol intoxicated patients after mild head trauma,. Shock 2001 Aug;16(2):97−101.

[45] Jönsson H, Johnsson P, Höglund P, Alling C, Blomquist S. The elimination of S100B and renal function after cardiac surgery,. Journal of Cardiothoracic and Vascular Anesthesia 2000 Dec;14(6):698−701.

[46] Townend W, Dibble C, Abid K, Vail A, Sherwood R, Lecky F. Rapid elimination of protein S-100B from serum after minor head trauma. Journal of Neurotrauma 2006 Feb;23(2):149−55.

[47] Rothoerl RD, Brawanski A, Woertgen C. S-100B Protein Serum Levels After Controlled Cortical Impact Injury in the Rat. Acta Neurochirurgia 2000;142(2):199−203.

[48] Van Eldik L, Wainwright M. The Janus face of glial-derived S100B: beneficial and detrimental functions in the brain,. Restorative Neurology and Neuroscience 2003;21(3-4):97−108.

[49] Pelinka LE, Szalay L, Jafarmadar M, Schmidhammer R, Redl H, Bahrami S. Circulating S100B is increased after bilateral femur fracture without brain injury in the rat. British Journal of Anaesthesia 2003 Oct;91 (4):595−7.

[50] Pham N, Fazio V, Cucullo L, Teng Q, Biberthaler P, Bazarian JJ, Janigro D. Extracranial Sources of S100B do not affect Serum levels. PLoS ONE 2010 Sep 10;5(9).

[51] Yang Z, Yan W, Cai H. S100A12 provokes mast cell activation: a potential amplification pathway in asthma and innate immunity. Journal of Allergy and Clinical Immunology 2007 Jan;119(1):106−14.

[52] Kapural M, Krizanac-Bengez L, Barnett G, Perl J, Masaryk T, Apollo D, Rasmussen P, Mayberg M, Janigro D. Serum S-100beta as a possible marker of blood-brain barrier disruption. Brain Research 2002 Jun 14;940(1-2):102−4.

[53] Kanner AA, Marchi N, Fazio V, Mayberg MR, Koltz MT, Siomin V, Stevens GHJ, Masaryk T, Ayumar B, Vogelbaum MA, Barnett GH, Janigro D. Serum S100beta: A Noninvasive Marker of Blood-Brain Barrier Function and Brain Lesions. Cancer 2003 Jun 1;97(11):2806−13.

[54] Marchi N, Rasmussen P, Kapural M, Fazio V, Kight K, Mayberg M, Kanner A, Ayumar B, Albensi B, Cavaglia M, Janigro D. Peripheral markers of brain damage and blood-brain barrier dysfunction. Restorative Neurology and Neuroscience 2003;21(3-4):109−21.

Pathophysiology and clinical implementation of traumatic brain injury biomarkers: neuron-specific enolase

S. Bezek[1], Peter Biberthaler[2], I. Martinez-Espina[1] and Viktoria Bogner-Flatz[3]

[1]Emergency Medicine Baylor College of Medicine, Houston, TX, United States [2]Department of Trauma Surgery, Klinikum rechts der Isar, School of Medicine, Technical University of Munich, Munich, Germany [3]Department of General, Trauma and Reconstructive Surgery, Emergency Medicine, Ludwig Maximilians University, Munich, Germany

11.1 Introduction

Enolase is a catalytic enzyme found mainly in cellular cytosol that is essential to fermentation as well as glucose catabolism and production. Its enzymatic properties were discovered in 1934 by Lohman and Meyerhof. Enolase, also known as phosphopyruvate hydratase, converts 2-phosphoglycerate (2-PG) into phosphoenolpyruvate (PEP) and water in the second to last step of glycolysis [1]. Enolase can also function in the reverse direction during gluconeogenesis. Enolase is enzymatically activated in a two-step process by metal ions, most effectively by magnesium, thus forming a metal ion−activated enzyme complex [2,3].

Enolase is present in various human cells as specific isoforms consisting of a combination of two α, β, or γ subunits called dimeric isozymes. Enolase homodimers, $\alpha\alpha$, $\beta\beta$, and $\gamma\gamma$ predominate in human tissue; however, the heterodimers $\alpha\beta$ and $\alpha\gamma$ are present as well [4,5]. Enolase 1 is encoded by the ENO1 gene and consists of isoenzymes containing the α subunit. It is known as nonneuronal enolase (NNE) and is present in a variety of tissues including adipose, brain (supportive cells), liver, spleen, and kidney. Enolase 2, also known as neuron-

TABLE 11.1 Description of three enolase isoforms.

Type of enolase	Recognized name	Subunit	Distribution	Subunit dimers
Enolase 1	Nonneuronal enolase	ENO1 gene encodes α subunit	Adipose, brain (support cells), liver, spleen, and kidney*	$\alpha\alpha$, $\alpha\gamma$, $\alpha\beta$
Enolase 2	Neuron-specific enolase	ENO2 gene encodes γ subunit	Neurons and neuroendocrine tissue, neuronal support cells*	$\gamma\gamma$, $\alpha\gamma$
Enolase 3	Muscle-specific enolase	ENO3 gene encodes β subunit	Muscle cells	$\beta\beta$, $\alpha\beta$

*$\alpha\gamma$ found in small amounts in erythrocytes and platelets.

specific enolase (NSE), is encoded by the ENO2 gene and consists of isoenzymes containing the γ subunit. It is present in high concentrations in the neuronal and neuroendocrine tissues. Enolase 3 is a muscle specific enolase (MSE) encoded by the ENO3 gene and consists of isoenzymes containing the β subunit that is found in the muscle cells [6–9] (Table 11.1). Each enolase isoform can be differentiated via immunological means while the five isozymes can be distinguished via DEAE-cellulose chromatography [10].

11.2 Neuron-specific enolase basics—physiology and pathophysiology

Neuron-specific enolase exists as two dimeric isozymes: $\gamma\gamma$ or $\alpha\gamma$. The homodimeric isozyme, $\gamma\gamma$, is found in neurons and neuroendocrine cells. The heterodimeric isozyme, $\alpha\gamma$, is found in the neuronal cellular support system which consists of cells such as astrocytes, microglia, oligodendrocytes, and meningeal fibroblasts. Additionally, both erythrocytes and platelets contain a small amount of NSE in the $\alpha\gamma$ isozyme form [11,12]. Like other enolases, NSE exhibits not only important intracellular enzymatic properties but is also critical to the regulatory functions in growth, cell differentiation, regeneration, repair, inflammation, apoptosis, and cell death.

Zheng et al. showed that NSE enhances the PI3K/Akt and MAPK/ERK signaling pathways and thereby seems to influence survival and regeneration of neuronal cells [13]. Conversely, this enhancement of the PI3K/Akt and MAPK/ERK signaling pathways is also connected to the RhoA/Rho kinase pathway which can trigger inflammation with resultant neuronal death and subsequent regeneration [14,15]. Haque et al. concluded in their systematic review on the role of NSE in cerebral spinal cord injury: NSE activates proinflammatory pathways that trigger neurodegeneration and early NSE blocking may have potential as a new pharmacological target to prevent secondary neuronal damage [16,17].

Normally, NSE is not secreted into the extracellular space. However, under various conditions of neuronal damage and death, the homodimer γ isoform of NSE is released into the extracellular space and can be measured in CSF or serum [18]. NSE release is partly due to leakage and partly due to upregulation of NSE, in order to initiate repair mechanisms and maintain homeostasis [19]. Because of this, NSE has been utilized as a biomarker to assess neuronal injury. In healthy individuals, NSE has a very low serum baseline (10 ng/mL) and half-life of 24–30 hours [20].

11.3 Neuron-specific enolase as a biomarker in pathological conditions

NSE increase in the human body has been described under various pathological conditions such as neoplasms. The use of NSE as a biomarker was first described by Prinz and Marangos as a marker of neuroendocrine tumor [21]. To date, NSE is considered to be the most useful tumor marker for diagnosis, prognosis, and subsequent surveillance of small cell lung cancer [22,23].

Additionally, in nonsmall cell lung cancer and in neuroendocrine tumors, NSE upregulation is noted in the blood. NSE can also be used as a marker for diagnosis and therapy surveillance of neuroblastoma, in which levels above 100 ng/mL are associated with poor outcome [24,25]. In metastatic melanoma and seminoma of different stages, elevated NSE levels could be detected in the blood and correlated to progression and prognosis [26,27].

Aside from malignancies, NSE upregulation has been linked to neurological conditions in neurodegenerative diseases such as Huntington's disease (HD), Friedreich's ataxia, hereditary spastic paraplegia, Parkinson's disease (PD), Alzheimer's disease (AD), and amyotrophic lateral sclerosis (ALS) [15,28—34]. Other pathological conditions that demonstrate elevated NSE include retinal detachment, hereditary optic neuropathy [35—37], as well as diabetic neuropathy [38,39].

Neuronal damage due to infectious diseases such as bacterial meningitis or encephalitis, in the central nervous system, also involves NSE elevations [40—42]. In addition, some research groups have reported that NSE levels in critically ill septic patients may have utility as a marker of neuronal injury in sepsis [43—45].

11.4 Neuron-specific enolase after ischemic brain damage

NSE is one of the most studied biomarkers to assess the prognosis of neurological outcome after cardiac arrest. Despite this, appropriate cutoff levels remain challenging [46]. In cardiogenic shock states or cardiac arrest-associated hypoperfusion, NSE is released into the blood and CSF as a result of hypoxic brain cell damage [47], with peak serum concentrations at 72 hours after cardiac arrest [48]. Multiple studies strengthen the use of NSE for prognosis after cardiac arrest as a proxy for severity of neuronal damage due to anoxia [20]. Daubin et al. found that in postarrest, comatose patients, high NSE levels (>97 ng/dL) had 100% positive predictive value of having a poor outcome within 3 months, such as death or persistent vegetative state [49]. Choosing the appropriate time for NSE measurement after cardiac arrest seems to be challenging and highly variable. Some authors measured NSE at 72 hours, while others recommended measuring at different times during the first 48 hours [50]. Einav et al. reported that low NSE levels on days 1 and 3 are predictors for good neurological outcome [51]. In contrast, the American Academy of Neurology states NSE levels of greater than 33 μg/L at days 1 to 3 to be a reliable prediction marker of unfavorable neurological outcomes [52]. Streitberger et al. recently found in a multicenter trial including 1053 patients that values of less than or equal to 17 μg/L argue against hypoxic-ischemic encephalopathy, and that high neuron-specific enolase serum concentrations reliably predicted poor outcome at ICU discharge (no false positives at a 90 μg/L) [53]. These differences show there are still controversies about appropriate cutoff values and standardized time points for prognosing neurological outcome using NSE serum biomarkers. Importantly, other sources of NSE and confounders like left ventricular assist devices, intraaortic balloon pump, or therapeutic hypothermia (TH) should be considered [54]. Since the advent of TH, studies show that NSE levels can be reduced in cardiac arrest patients who have undergone TH. Additionally, NSE cutoffs that prognosticate poor outcomes are higher than in patients who have not undergone TH [55,56]. These interesting findings are likely the result of a reduction in ischemic neuronal damage by TH and indicate an important topic for further study utilizing NSE as a biomarker in postcardiac arrest patients. In pediatric postcardiac arrest resuscitation, NSE has turned out to be a reliable biomarker for unfavorable neurologic outcome; however, like adults, standardized NSE cutoffs in children also remain unclear and need to be prospectively evaluated [57,58].

Ischemic stroke is another etiology of brain hypoxia that induces increased NSE levels in the blood. The implications for using NSE and other biomarkers in ischemic stroke are encouraging. The respective levels of biomarkers could potentially help in assessing the size of affected stroke region (infarct volume), severity of stroke, or in predicting stroke outcomes [22]. In a systematic review by Ahmad et al., several studies revealed a strong correlation between NSE levels, infarct volume, clinical course, and long-term outcome [59–62]. Maximum NSE levels within 72 hours of admission depend on the degree of disability on admission and can be used to predict both resultant disability and short-term outcome after acute ischemic stroke [63]. Zaheer et al. studied 75 patients after ischemic stroke and reported strong correlation between NSE serum levels, infarct volume, and 30-day functional neurological outcome [64]. Alternatively, there are a few studies that could find significant correlations in NSE levels with clinical stroke characteristics. Specifically, Brouns et al. studied NSE, along with other biomarkers, in the cerebrospinal fluid (CSF) of patients who suffered an acute ischemic stroke and found that NSE levels did not correlate to stroke characteristics, whereas other CSF biomarkers did correlate to stroke parameters, such as stroke severity and outcome [65,66].

An interesting investigation by Kim et al. showed that performing serial NSE analysis over multiple days following an ischemic stroke might be useful to risk stratify patients at risk for complications such as hemorrhagic conversion. Some patients experience a second peak in NSE levels and those patients, as well as those who had a large initial lesion, were at an increased risk for transformation from ischemic to hemorrhagic stroke [67].

11.5 Neuron-specific enolase in brain trauma

11.5.1 Mild traumatic brain injury

Biomarkers in mild TBI (mTBI) have clinical applications for risk management, decision-making, predicting neurocognitive complications such as postconcussion syndrome and overall, long-term outcomes. NSE elevation in mTBI indicates neuronal damage and has been studied by numerous investigators [68]. De Krujik et al. compared NSE levels in mTBI patients with those of healthy controls and found NSE only slightly higher in patients with mTBI, which questions the reliability of NSE assessment in mTBI [69]. On the other hand, Topolovec-Vranic et al. investigated the use of biomarkers for outcome prognostication after mTBI and found elevated NSE levels in 65% of patients. They concluded that early biomarker assessment, such as NSE, combined with the use of other common determinants such as performing a thorough clinical history and examination may add value to the early prognostication of mTBI outcome such as PCS [70]. Buonora et al. suggested the use of a multivariate biomarker assessment strategy, one that utilizes six biomarkers, including NSE to assess mTBI and provide early detection of patients at risk for development of neuropathological sequelae [71].

One of the worrisome consequences in a small subset of patients who suffer an mTBI is the development of PCS. PCS has been found to impact the health-related quality of life of affected individuals and can be physically, emotionally, and financially taxing. Patients who develop PCS may suffer from a variety of physical manifestations which may include chronic headaches, dizziness, nausea and vomiting, and postural stability. They may also suffer from neurocognitive symptoms such as difficulty concentrating which may derail academic study or work duties. Some may even suffer from neuropsychiatric symptoms which include depression, anxiety, and suicidality [72]. Unfortunately, initial clinical findings alone may not be sufficient in prognosticating whether a patient with mTBI will develop PCS. Mercier et al. analyzed and discussed the prognostic value of NSE for prediction of PCS after mTBI in a systematic review evaluating 10 studies. They concluded that there is no evidence of an association between independent NSE serum levels and early or persistent postconcussion symptoms after mTBI [73]. Some studies revealed a significant connection between NSE levels and headache and diminished neuropsychological performance [69] or physical examination in mid-term outcome [70]. Additionally, authors noted that in mTBI, NSE levels had no association with important functional neurological outcome parameters like Glasgow Outcome Scale (GOS) assessment or return to work at 6 and 15 months.

One area currently of interest to researchers, clinicians, and the general public is chronic traumatic encephalopathy (CTE) that is caused by multiple mTBI over time. This is most commonly seen in particular athletes (boxers, football players) and other high-risk individuals such as military personal who are exposed to repetitive traumatic brain injuries [74]. A review by Pan et al. suggests that serum NSE measurements may be less optimal than CSF measurements in predicting CTE due to concern of contamination from NSE in hemolyzed erythrocytes, in addition to being less useful in the setting of mTBI [75].

There is a single observational-cross control study that measured long-term NSE serum levels in boxers after a 2-month resting period. They found that NSE levels were nearly doubled in the boxers versus the control population. The authors hypothesized that NSE might be a suitable biomarker to indicated chronic neuronal decay as a consequence of frequent repetitive mTBI [76]. Overall, expect this to be a highly researched topic in the next decade.

Other studies have looked at the implication of biomarker assessment in evaluating and managing a concussion in athletes and considered if there is a distinction between biomarkers in injured and noninjured athletes. O'Connell et al. performed a systematic review regarding the use of biomarkers in sports-related concussions; however, they found that NSE would not be an optimal biomarker in this setting. Overall S100B holds the most promise and studies reviewed indicated that serial S100B measurements can distinguish injured from noninjured patients; however, the clinical significance remains uncertain [77].

Overall, NSE seems to have rather poor utility in functioning as a biomarker for risk stratification, management, and outcome prediction of mTBI.

11.6 Moderate and severe traumatic brain injury

Although the use of NSE biomarkers for mTBI is limited, studies evaluating the application of NSE as a biomarker in moderate and severe TBI seem to be more encouraging. One of the first studies looking at NSE as a biomarker in severe TBI was performed by Dauberschmit and colleagues. This small study divided patients with TBI into two groups based on survival to hospitalization. The study showed a statistically significant difference in NSE plasma and CSF levels between the survivor and deceased groups who initially presented with TBI, with levels higher in the deceased group [78]. Another group demonstrated the predictive potential of elevated NSE biomarkers in CSF within the first 3 days to predict brain death in severe TBI patients [79]. A systemic review and meta-analysis by Cheng et al. examined 14 studies to determine the prognostic value of NSE biomarkers in moderate and severe TBI. They concluded that higher NSE concentrations are associated with adverse outcomes (GOS ≤ 3) and higher mortality. They found a positive association with mortality and the NSE serum threshold needed to attain 100% sensitivity for mortality was 20 µg/L. Nevertheless, the authors explained that, overall, there remains a lack of standardization in NSE assays, the use of cutoff values, and the optimal sampling time points [80].

It should be recognized that TBI diagnosis, prognostication, and management decisions are not determined solely on one piece of information, such as a particular biomarker. Instead, clinicians will analyze multiple data points to facilitate the medical decision-making process—these include historical features, physical examination, determination of Glasgow Coma Score, laboratory tests, and radiological imaging such as a computed tomography scan (CT) or magnetic resonance imaging (MRI). An interesting study by Gradisek et al. examined the prognostic ability of the biomarkers SB100, glial fibrillary acid protein (GFAP), and NSE in relation to clinical and radiological parameters to determine long-term mortality (1-year) after severe TBI upon admission. It was determined, similar to prior studies, that elevated NSE levels were higher in nonsurvivors. When the prognostic model utilizing the three parameters of clinical, radiological, and biochemical data were analyzed, it was found that unlike GFAP and SB100, NSE was not significant enough to predict 1-year mortality [81].

A study by Herrmann et al. looked at the relationship between NSE levels and CT scan findings in patients with TBI. They found higher, more persistent NSE levels in those with moderate to severe TBI as compared to mTBI. They also found a correlation between elevated NSE levels and volume of cerebral contusions seen on CT scan. There were varied biochemical release patterns elucidated from the serial NSE blood samples analyzed. These patterns differed based on radiological findings discovered on head CT primary such as cortical contusions, diffuse axonal injury (DAI) and signs of cerebral edema without focal mass lesions [82]. An additional study by Chabok et al., reveals pertinent data related to radiographical findings of TBI and NSE biomarkers in patients with DAI. They were trying to determine predictive values of NSE, especially those who had only mild findings of DAI on CT scan. This is particularly valuable as DAI is a devastating cause of TBI—often leaving patients in a persistent vegetative state. It is caused by shearing forces that injure or disrupt the axons of neuronal cells [83]. This study found that elevated serum NSE levels in patients with DAI within the first 3 days were associated with poor outcomes despite initially mild CT findings. In fact, at 72 hours NSE levels of about 51.8 μg/L could predict death with 100% sensitivity and specificity in patients with DAI [84].

Clinical management of those who have moderate to severe TBI can be challenging and special care is taken to prevent secondary insults to the brain that may be caused by brain swelling and hypoperfusion. There are several studies on the correlation of NSE blood levels with intracranial pressure (ICP), cranial perfusion, and mortality prediction after TBI. Stein et al. found an interesting, albeit weak correlation of elevated NSE in CSF (cerebrospinal fluid) with intracranial hypertension and cerebral hypotension in severe TBI [85].

Another research group, Olivecrona et al., demonstrated a correlation between elevated NSE and maximal ICP and minimal cerebral perfusion pressure. They also showed concordance with numerous studies that elevated NSE (at 72 hours) had the highest predictive power regarding survival. Interestingly, they comment on the fact that therapies designed to prevent secondary insults and the effects these therapies have on biomarker release are relatively unknown to date [86]. An earlier study on severe TBI patients treated with standardized therapy to reduce ICP also considered whether these therapies impact biomarker release. The authors could not correlate any prognostic value from NSE assessment after 3 and 12 months regarding outcome, and thereby hypothesized that treatment strategies might influence biomarker release patterns as well [87]. There are, to our knowledge, no studies looking at the use of NSE in monitoring treatment success in severe TBI.

In the largest retrospective TBI outcome study to date, Thilen et al. support prior findings regarding NSE as a biomarker in TBI. This study considered patients presenting with TBI over a 9-year study period and included independent analysis of NSE both alone and in combination with SB100 in predicting outcomes. NSE levels can be used to determine survivability after TBI, but do not seem to correlate with favorable or unfavorable outcomes such as GOS. Notably, NSE in combination with S100B did not provide added information to aid in prognostication of outcomes over S100B, independently [88]. Thilen and colleagues followed up their retrospective analysis with a systemic review regarding the serial sampling of various serum protein biomarkers, including NSE in TBI. This review elucidates typical patient characteristics, assays used to measure NSE, the sampling frequency, the half-life of NSE, and the trend of NSE over time. The typical patient includes mild–severe TBI. Various assays exist, and like S100B, they are readily available in clinical practice. The sampling frequency most often varies from 6, 12, to 24 hours. Extracranial contribution of NSE from hemolysis plays a contribution in total serum levels over time. Half-life varies, likely based on the severity from 12–72 hours or longer. Trends show that usually NSE peaks and then declines over time; however, it should be noted that a slower decline or a second peak are correlated with more severe injuries/unfavorable outcome and progressing injuries, respectively [89].

Blood CNS biomarkers may also be useful post mortem as a supplement to the standard autopsy [90]. There are several studies that report elevated NSE concentrations post mortem after fatal TBI, which leads to the consideration of using a simple blood test in the deceased as an option for a focused, fast, and cost-effective cause of death [91].

11.7 Neuron-specific enolase in children

The use of biomarkers may be another modality for clinicians to utilize when risk stratifying pediatric patients presenting with a TBI. TBI is common in children and although clinical guidelines exist to standardize and guide management, diagnostic imaging using a head CT may be necessary [92]. In children, performing a CT scan of the head carries increased lifetime risk of cancers due to the radiation exposure, which is both age and dose dependent. Additionally, children may require sedation in order to acquire quality images, which carries a risk of clinical decompensation and is resource intensive.

Geyer et al. focused on S100B and NSE in mild pediatric TBI and thereby compared two different clinical groups in children, mTBI (GCS 13−15 with clinical symptoms) and a head contusion group (GCS of 15 without clinical symptoms). Neither biomarker could distinguish between the two groups, which suggests relevant limitations of those biomarkers in the diagnostic use of mTBI in children [93]. When considering moderate and severe TBI, there are some studies that reveal a potential use of NSE in predicting short-term neurological disability [19]. Shore et al. reported similar findings with respect to NSE levels in CSF having an inverse relationship to GCS/GOS overall. However, upon subgroup analysis, they noted significant limitations in the ability to assess neurological injury severity (GCS/GOS) in children below 4 years old and those who were victims of inflicted trauma as opposed to accidental trauma [94]. A systematic literature review of biomarkers as outcome predictors in pediatric patients with severe TBI was performed by Daoud et al. They showed that blood NSE levels in pediatric patients did not correlate to outcomes such as mortality or functional status after discharge (GOS); however, CSF NSE levels that were elevated did correlate with poor outcomes [95].

A subsequent meta-analysis was performed by Nakhjavan-Shahraki et al., that specifically assessed NSE in predicting brain injury outcomes. Analysis showed a significant heterogeneity between the studies. Mean serum NSE level was higher in children with TBI and predicted unfavorable outcome when compared than normal children. Subgroup analysis showed that NSE has different values in predicting TBI, depending on the outcome under assessment [96]. Mean CSF NSE level was significantly higher in children with TBI and predicted unfavorable outcomes when compared to normal children. Because of the limited studies, subgroup analysis was unable to be performed. Overall, these results, given the significant heterogeneity and small sample size suggest a rather restricted usefulness of NSE in diagnosis and outcome prognosis for pediatric TBI beyond what is already known.

11.8 Limitations of neuron-specific enolase as a traumatic brain injury biomarker

There are several serious drawbacks and limitations of NSE that should be kept in mind if utilizing it as a biomarker. As discussed previously, the brain is not the only source of NSE. It is also present in erythrocytes and hemolysis can significantly influence the use of serum NSE as a biomarker. Because of this potential confounder, it is recommended to consider hemolysis in parallel with serum NSE testing [97]. Studies recommend using either a hemolysis correction factor or performing a hemolysis index prior to utilizing serum NSE [98]. Planche et al. suggest measuring serum NSE only in samples with a hemolytic index ≤ 10 [99]. Secondly, consideration of NSE as a biomarker in poly-trauma has yet to be elucidated. Pelinka et al. reported NSE upregulation in rats after kidney and liver ischemia and in major, multiple trauma in the absence of any head injury [100]. In another animal study, elevated NSE was also found in rats after bilateral femur fractures and hemorrhagic shock without CNS involvement [47]. This needs further study in human subjects, but indicates a relevant overassessment of head injury severity in the presence of polytrauma. Another critical issue is the biomarker release pattern, which makes the optimal sampling time point of NSE challenging. Additionally, NSE biomarker kinetics have a broad range and may or may not be affected by therapeutic modalities to reduce secondary brain injury. For example, serum NSE has a relatively long half-life and thus a slower decline than other markers such as S100B [88], which makes NSE measurement over a short time period to monitor progress or guide therapy challenging [101]. Finally, as discussed earlier, differing NSE assays and varying cutoff points for NSE measurements also pose limits to standardization across studies.

11.9 Conclusion

In summary, NSE has been shown to be an effective biomarker in some pathological conditions, such as neuroendocrine cancers and hypoxic brain injury. However, they have shown less utility in traumatic brain injury. Overall, both CSF and serum NSE biomarkers are most useful in predicting mortality in moderate to severe traumatic brain injuries in adults. There is little utility to using NSE biomarkers to diagnose or prognosticate in mild traumatic brain injury. There is limited evidence that in adults, higher or prolonged levels of NSE predict worse outcome, maximum ICP, and severity of traumatic brain damage, both clinically and on CT radiography. In pediatric patients, there is moderate evidence that an inverse relationship between NSE and predicted neurological outcome and mortality exists in children with nonaccidental trauma and >4 years old. There is a significant propensity towards CSF level providing a stronger correlation to predicting outcomes. NSE has multiple limitations and overall, it consistently performs worse in outcome analysis than other biomarkers, such as S100B in the same patient population.

References

[1] Lohman K, Meyerhof O. Enzymatic transformation of phosphoglyceric acid into pyruvic and phosphoric acid. Biochem Z 1934;273:60−72.
[2] Valle BL. Zinc and metalloenzymes. Adv Prot Chem 1955;10:317−84.
[3] Faller LD, Baroudy BM, Johnson AM, Ewall RX. Magnesium ion requirements for yeast enolase reactivity. Biochemistry 1977;16:3864−9.
[4] Marangos PJ, Zis AP, Clark RL, Goodwin FK. Neuronal, non-neuronal and hybrid forms of enolase in brain: structural, immunological and functional comparisons. Brain Res 1978;150:117−33.
[5] Kato K, Asai R, Shimizu A, Suzuki F, Ariyoshi Y. Immunoassay of three enolase isozymes in human serum and in blood cells. Clin Chim Acta 1983;127:353−63.
[6] Pancholi V. Multifunctional alpha-enolase: its role in diseases. Cell Mol Life Sci 2001;58(7):902−20.
[7] Merkulova T, Dehaupas M, Nevers MC, Creminon C, Alameddine H, Keller A. Differential modulation of alpha, beta and gamma enolase isoforms in regenerating mouse skeletal muscle. Eur J Biochem 2000;267 (12):3735−43.

[8] Shimizu A, Suzuki F, Kato K. Characterization of alpha alpha, beta beta, gamma gamma and alpha gamma human enolase isozymes, and preparation of hybrid enolases (alpha gamma, beta gamma and alpha beta) from homodimeric forms. Biochim Biophys Acta 1983;748(2):278–84.

[9] Piast M, Kustrzeba-Wojcicka I, Matusiewicz M, Banas T. Molecular evolution of enolase. Acta Biochim Pol 2005;52(2):507–13.

[10] Suzuki F, Umeda Y, Kato K. Rat brain enolase isozymes: purification of three forms of enolase. J Biochem 1980;87:1587–94.

[11] Deloulme JC, Helies A, Ledig M, Lucas M, Sensenbrenner M. A comparative study of the distribution of alpha- and gamma-enolase subunits in cultured rat neural cells and fibroblasts. Int J Dev Neurosci 1997;15 (2):183–94.

[12] Marangos PJ, Campbell IC, Schmechel DE, Murphy DL, Goodwin FK. Blood platelets contain a neuron-specific enolase subunit. J Neurochem 1980;34:1254–8.

[13] Zheng J, Liang J, Deng X, Chen X, Wu F, Zhao X, et al. Mitogen activated protein kinase signaling pathways participate in the active principle region of Buyang Huanwu decoction-induced differentiation of bone marrow mesenchymal stem cells. Neural Regen Res 2012;7(18):1370–7.

[14] Hafner A, Obermajer N, Kos J. Gamma-enolase C-terminal peptide promotes cell survival and neurite outgrowth by activation of the PI3K/Akt and MAPK/ERK signalling pathways. Biochem J 2012;443(2):439–50.

[15] Haque A, Polcyn R, Matzelle D, Banik NL. New insights into the role of neuron-specific enolase in neuroinflammation, neurodegeneration, and neuroprotection. Brain Sci 2018;8(2):33.

[16] Haque A, Capone M, Matzelle D, Cox A, Banik NL. Targeting enolase in reducing secondary damage in acute spinal cord injury in rats. Neurochem Res 2017;42(10):2777–87.

[17] Polcyn R, Capone M, Hossain A, Matzelle D, Banik NL, Haque A. Neuron specific enolase is a potential target for regulating neuronal cell survival and death: implications in neurodegeneration and regeneration. Neuroimmunol Neuroinflamm 2017;4:254–7.

[18] Wu HM, Huang SC, Hattori N, Glenn TC, Vespa PM, Yu CL, et al. Selective metabolic reduction in gray matter acutely following human traumatic brain injury. J Neurotrauma 2004;21(2):149–61.

[19] Bandyopadhyay S, Hennes H, Gorelick MH, Wells RG, Walsh-Kelly CM. Serum neuron-specific enolase as a predictor of short-term outcome in children with closed traumatic brain injury. Acad Emerg Med 2005;12 (8):732–8.

[20] Gul SS, Huesgen KW, Wang KK, Mark K, Tyndall JA. Prognostic utility of neuroinjury biomarkers in post out-of-hospital cardiac arrest (OHCA) patient management. Med Hypotheses 2017;105:34–47.

[21] Prinz RA, Marangos PJ. Serum neuron-specific enolase: a serum marker for nonfunctioning pancreatic islet cell carcinoma. Am J Surg 1983;145(1):77–81.

[22] Isgro MA, Bottoni P, Scatena R. Neuron-specific enolase as a biomarker: biochemical and clinical aspects. Adv Exp Med Biol 2015;867:125–43.

[23] Quoix E, Purohit A, Faller-Beau M, Moreau L, Oster JP, Pauli G. Comparative prognostic value of lactate dehydrogenase and neuron-specific enolase in small-cell lung cancer patients treated with platinum-based chemotherapy. Lung Cancer 2000;30(2):127–34.

[24] Zeltzer PM, Marangos PJ, Evans AE, Schneider SL. Serum neuron-specific enolase in children with neuroblastoma. Relationship to stage and disease course. Cancer 1986;57(6):1230–4.

[25] Zeltzer PM, Marangos PJ, Sather H, Evans A, Siegel S, Wong KY, et al. Prognostic importance of serum neuron specific enolase in local and widespread neuroblastoma. Prog Clin Biol Res 1985;175:319–29.

[26] Fossa SD, Klepp O, Paus E. Neuron-specific enolase—a serum tumour marker in seminoma? Br J Cancer 1992;65(2):297–9.

[27] Wibe E, Hannisdal E, Paus E, Aamdal S. Neuron-specific enolase as a prognostic factor in metastatic malignant melanoma. Eur J Cancer 1992;28A(10):1692–5.

[28] Chaves ML, Camozzato AL, Ferreira ED, Piazenski I, Kochhann R, Dall'Igna O, et al. Serum levels of S100B and NSE proteins in Alzheimer's disease patients. J Neuroinflammation 2010;7:6.

[29] Ciancarelli I, De Amicis D, Di Massimo C, Sandrini G, Pistarini C, Carolei A, et al. Influence of intensive multifunctional neurorehabilitation on neuronal oxidative damage in patients with Huntington's disease. Funct Neurol 2015;30(1):47–52.

[30] Dincel GC, Atmaca HT. Role of oxidative stress in the pathophysiology of toxoplasma gondii infection. Int J Immunopathol Pharmacol 2016;29(2):226–40.

[31] Schaf DV, Tort AB, Fricke D, Schestatsky P, Portela LV, Souza DO, et al. S100B and NSE serum levels in patients with Parkinson's disease. Parkinsonism Relat Disord 2005;11(1) 39–4.

[32] Schmidt FM, Mergl R, Stach B, Jahn I, Schonknecht P. Elevated levels of cerebrospinal fluid neuron-specific enolase (NSE), but not S100B in major depressive disorder. World J Biol Psychiatry 2015;16(2):106–13.

[33] Schon EA, Manfredi G. Neuronal degeneration and mitochondrial dysfunction. J Clin Invest 2003;111 (3):303–12.

[34] Vasiljevic B, Maglajlic-Djukic S, Gojnic M, Stankovic S. The role of oxidative stress in perinatal hypoxic-ischemic brain injury. Srp Arh Celok Lek 2012;140(1–2):35–41.

[35] Dunker S, Sadun AA, Sebag J. Neuron specific enolase in retinal detachment. Curr Eye Res 2001;23(5):382–5.

[36] Quintyn JC, Pereira F, Hellot MF, Brasseur G, Coquerel A. Concentration of neuron-specific enolase and S100 protein in the subretinal fluid of rhegmatogenous retinal detachment. Graefes Arch Clin Exp Ophthalmol 2005;243(11):1167–74.

[37] Yee KM, Ross-Cisneros FN, Lee JG, Da Rosa AB, Salomao SR, Berezovsky A, et al. Neuron-specific enolase is elevated in asymptomatic carriers of Leber's hereditary optic neuropathy. Invest Ophthalmol Vis Sci 2012;53 (10):6389–92.

[38] Li J, Yan M, Zhang Y, Xie M, Yan L, Chen J. Serum neuron-specific enolase is elevated as a novel indicator of diabetic retinopathy including macular oedema. Diabet Med 2015;32(1):102–7.

[39] Sandhu HS, Butt AN, Powrie J, Swaminathan R. Measurement of circulating neuron-specific enolase mRNA in diabetes mellitus. Ann N Y Acad Sci 2008;1137:258–63.

[40] Bartek Jr. J, Thelin EP, Ghatan PH, Glimaker M, Bellander BM. Neuron-specific enolase is correlated to compromised cerebral metabolism in patients suffering from acute bacterial meningitis; an observational cohort study. PLoS One 2016;11(3):e0152268.

[41] Song TJ, Choi YC, Lee KY, Kim WJ. Serum and cerebrospinal fluid neuron-specific enolase for diagnosis of tuberculous meningitis. Yonsei Med J 2012;53(6):1068–72.

[42] Pratamastuti D, Indra Gunawan P, Saharso D. Serum neuron specific enolase is increased in pediatric acute encephalitis syndrome. Korean J Pediatr 2017;60(9):302–6.

[43] Anderson BJ, Reilly JP, Shashaty MGS, Palakshappa JA, Wysoczanski A, Dunn TG, et al. Admission plasma levels of the neuronal injury marker neuron-specific enolase are associated with mortality and delirium in sepsis. J Crit Care 2016;36:18–23.

[44] El Shimy MS, El-Raggal NM, El-Farrash RA, Shaaban HA, Mohamed HE, Barakat NM, et al. Cerebral blood flow and serum neuron-specific enolase in early-onset neonatal sepsis. Pediatr Res 2018;84(2):261–6.

[45] Yao B, Zhang LN, Ai YH, Liu ZY, Huang L. Serum S100beta is a better biomarker than neuron-specific enolase for sepsis-associated encephalopathy and determining its prognosis: a prospective and observational study. Neurochem Res 2014;39(7):1263–9.

[46] Stammet P, Collignon O, Hassager C, Wise MP, Hovdenes J, Aneman A, et al. Neuron-specific enolase as a predictor of death or poor neurological outcome after out-of-hospital cardiac arrest and targeted temperature management at 33 degrees C and 36 degrees C. J Am Coll Cardiol 2015;65(19):2104–14.

[47] Pelinka LE, Jafarmadar M, Redl H, Bahrami S. Neuron-specific-enolase is increased in plasma after hemorrhagic shock and after bilateral femur fracture without traumatic brain injury in the rat. Shock 2004;22 (1):88–91.

[48] Rosen H, Sunnerhagen KS, Herlitz J, Blomstrand C, Rosengren L. Serum levels of the brain-derived proteins S-100 and NSE predict long-term outcome after cardiac arrest. Resuscitation 2001;49(2):183–91.

[49] Daubin C, Quentin C, Allouche S, Etard O, Gaillard C, Seguin A, et al. Serum neuron-specific enolase as predictor of outcome in comatose cardiac-arrest survivors: a prospective cohort study. BMC Cardiovasc Disord 2011;11:48.

[50] Storm C, Nee J, Sunde K, Holzer M, Hubner P, Taccone FS, et al. A survey on general and temperature management of post cardiac arrest patients in large teaching and university hospitals in 14 European countries-The SPAME trial results. Resuscitation 2017;116:84–90.

[51] Einav S, Kaufman N, Algur N, Kark JD. Modeling serum biomarkers S100 beta and neuron-specific enolase as predictors of outcome after out-of-hospital cardiac arrest: an aid to clinical decision making. J Am Coll Cardiol 2012;60(4):304–11.

[52] Wijdicks EF, Hijdra A, Young GB, Bassetti CL, Wiebe S. Quality standards subcommittee of the American Academy of N. Practice parameter: prediction of outcome in comatose survivors after cardiopulmonary

resuscitation (an evidence-based review): report of the Quality Standards Subcommittee of the American Academy of Neurology. Neurology 2006;67(2):203–10.

[53] Streitberger KJ, Leithner C, Wattenberg M, Tonner PH, Hasslacher J, Joannidis M, et al. Neuron-specific enolase predicts poor outcome after cardiac arrest and targeted temperature management: a multicenter study on 1,053 patients. Crit Care Med 2017;45(7):1145–51.

[54] Taccone F, Cronberg T, Friberg H, Greer D, Horn J, Oddo M, et al. How to assess prognosis after cardiac arrest and therapeutic hypothermia. Crit Care 2014;18(1):202.

[55] Tiainen M, Roine RO, Pettila V, Takkunen O. Serum neuron-specific enolase and S-100B protein in cardiac arrest patients treated with hypothermia. Stroke 2003;34:2881–6.

[56] Steffen IG, Hasper D, Ploner CJ, Schefold JC, Dietz E, Martens F, et al. Mild therapeutic hypothermia alters neuron specific enolase as an outcome predictor after resuscitation: 97 prospective hypothermia patients compared to 133 historical non- hypothermia patients. Crit Care 2010;14:R69.

[57] Fink EL, Berger RP, Clark RS, Watson RS, Angus DC, Richichi R, et al. Serum biomarkers of brain injury to classify outcome after pediatric cardiac arrest. Crit Care Med 2014;42(3):664–74.

[58] Kramer P, Miera O, Berger F, Schmitt K. Prognostic value of serum biomarkers of cerebral injury in classifying neurological outcome after paediatric resuscitation. Resuscitation 2018;122:113–20.

[59] Ahmad O, Wardlaw J, Whiteley WN. Correlation of levels of neuronal and glial markers with radiological measures of infarct volume in ischaemic stroke: a systematic review. Cerebrovasc Dis 2012;33 (1):47–54.

[60] Oh SH, Lee JG, Na SJ, Park JH, Choi YC, Kim WJ. Prediction of early clinical severity and extent of neuronal damage in anterior-circulation infarction using the initial serum neuron-specific enolase level. Arch Neurol 2003;60(1):37–41.

[61] Oh SH, Lee JG, Na SJ, Park JH, Kim WJ. The effect of initial serum neuron-specific enolase level on clinical outcome in acute carotid artery territory infarction. Yonsei Med J 2002;43(3):357–62.

[62] Wunderlich MT, Lins H, Skalej M, Wallesch CW, Goertler M. Neuron-specific enolase and tau protein as neurobiochemical markers of neuronal damage are related to early clinical course and long-term outcome in acute ischemic stroke. Clin Neurol Neurosurg 2006;108(6):558–63.

[63] Pandey A, Shrivastava AK, Saxena K. Neuron specific enolase and c-reactive protein levels in stroke and its subtypes: correlation with degree of disability. Neurochem Res 2014;39(8):1426–32.

[64] Zaheer S, Beg M, Rizvi I, Islam N, Ullah E, Akhtar N. Correlation between serum neuron specific enolase and functional neurological outcome in patients of acute ischemic stroke. Ann Indian Acad Neurol 2013;16 (4):504–8.

[65] Brouns R, De Vil B, Cras P, De Surgeloose D, Marien P, De Deyn PP. Neurobiochemical markers of brain damage in cerebrospinal fluid of acute ischemic stroke patients. Clin Chem 2010;56(3):451–8.

[66] Gonzalez-Garcia S, Gonzalez-Quevedo A, Fernandez-Concepcion O, Pena-Sanchez M, Menendez-Sainz C, Hernandez-Diaz Z, et al. Short-term prognostic value of serum neuron specific enolase and S100B in acute stroke patients. Clin Biochem 2012;45(16–17):1302–7.

[67] Kim BJ, Kim YJ, Ahn SH, Kim NY, Kang DW, Kim JS, et al. The second elevation of neuron-specific enolase peak after ischemic stroke is associated with hemorrhagic transformation. J Stroke Cerebrovasc Dis 2014;23 (9):2437–43.

[68] Wang KK, Yang Z, Zhu T, Shi Y, Rubenstein R, Tyndall JA, et al. An update on diagnostic and prognostic biomarkers for traumatic brain injury. Expert Rev Mol Diagn 2018;18(2):165–80.

[69] De Kruijk JR, Leffers P, Menheere PP, Meerhoff S, Rutten J, Twijnstra A. Prediction of post-traumatic complaints after mild traumatic brain injury: early symptoms and biochemical markers. J Neurol Neurosurg Psychiatry 2002;73(6):727–32.

[70] Topolovec-Vranic J, Pollmann-Mudryj MA, Ouchterlony D, Klein D, Spence J, Romaschin A, et al. The value of serum biomarkers in prediction models of outcome after mild traumatic brain injury. J Trauma 2011;71(5 Suppl 1):S478–86.

[71] Buonora JE, Yarnell AM, Lazarus RC, Mousseau M, Latour LL, Rizoli SB, et al. Multivariate analysis of traumatic brain injury: development of an assessment score. Front Neurol 2015;6:68.

[72] Scholten AC, Haagsma JA, Andriessen TM, Vos PE, Steyerberg EW, van Beeck EF, et al. Health-related quality of life after mild, moderate and severe traumatic brain injury: patterns and predictors of suboptimal functioning during the first year after injury. Injury 2015;46(4):616–24.

[73] Mercier E, Tardif PA, Cameron PA, Emond M, Moore L, Mitra B, et al. Prognostic value of neuron-specific enolase (NSE) for prediction of post-concussion symptoms following a mild traumatic brain injury: a systematic review. Brain Inj 2018;32(1):29–40.

[74] Stern PhD RA, Riley BS DO, Daneshvar MA DH, Nowinski BA CJ, Cantu MD RC, McKee MD AC. Long-term consequences of repetitive brain trauma: chronic traumatic encephalopathy. PM&R 2011;3:S460–7.

[75] Pan J, Connolly ID, Dangelmajer S, Kintzing J, Ho AL, Grant G. Sports-related brain injuries: connecting pathology to diagnosis. Neurosurgical Focus FOC 2016;40(4):E14.

[76] Zetterberg H, Tanriverdi F, Unluhizarci K, Selcuklu A, Kelestimur F, Blennow K. Sustained release of neuron-specific enolase to serum in amateur boxers. Brain Inj 2009;23(9):723–6.

[77] O'Connell B, Kelly AM, Mockler D, Oresic M, Denvir K, Farrell G, et al. Use of blood biomarkers in the assessment of sports-related concussion-a systematic review in the context of their biological significance. Clin J Sport Med 2017.

[78] Dauberschmidt R, Marangos PJ, Zinsmeyer J, Bender V, Klages G, Gross J. Severe head trauma and the changes of concentration of neuron-specific enolase in plasma and in cerebrospinal fluid. Clin Chim Acta 1983;131(3):165–70.

[79] Bohmer AE, Oses JP, Schmidt AP, Peron CS, Krebs CL, Oppitz PP, et al. Neuron-specific enolase, S100B, and glial fibrillary acidic protein levels as outcome predictors in patients with severe traumatic brain injury. Neurosurgery 2011;68(6):1624–30 discussion 30-1.

[80] Cheng F, Yuan Q, Yang J, Wang W, Liu H. The prognostic value of serum neuron-specific enolase in traumatic brain injury: systematic review and meta-analysis. PLoS One 2014;9(9):e106680.

[81] Gradisek P, Osredkar J, Korsic M, Kremzar B. Multiple indicators model of long-term mortality in traumatic brain injury. Brain Inj 2012;26(12):1472–81.

[82] Herrmann M, Jost S, Kutz S, Ebert AD, Kratz T, Wunderlich MT, et al. Temporal profile of release of neuro-biochemical markers of brain damage after traumatic brain injury is associated with intracranial pathology as demonstrated in cranial computerized tomography. J Neurotrauma 2000;17(2):113–22.

[83] Povlishock JT, Becker DP, Cheng CL, Vaughan GW. Axonal change in minor head injury. J Neuropathol Exp Neurol 1983;42(3):225–42.

[84] Chabok SY, Moghadam AD, Saneei Z, Amlashi FG, Leili EK, Amiri ZM. Neuron-specific enolase and S100BB as outcome predictors in severe diffuse axonal injury. J Trauma Acute Care Surg 2012;72(6):1654–7.

[85] Stein DM, Kufera JA, Lindell A, Murdock KR, Menaker J, Bochicchio GV, et al. Association of CSF biomarkers and secondary insults following severe traumatic brain injury. Neurocrit Care 2011;14(2):200–7.

[86] Olivecrona Z, Bobinski L, Koskinen LO. Association of ICP, CPP, CT findings and S-100B and NSE in severe traumatic head injury. Prognostic value of the biomarkers. Brain Inj 2015;29(4):446–54.

[87] Olivecrona M, Rodling-Wahlstrom M, Naredi S, Koskinen LO. S-100B and neuron specific enolase are poor outcome predictors in severe traumatic brain injury treated by an intracranial pressure targeted therapy. J Neurol Neurosurg Psychiatry 2009;80(11):1241–7.

[88] Thelin EP, Jeppsson E, Frostell A, et al. Utility of neuron-specific enolase in traumatic brain injury; relations to S100B levels, outcome, and extracranial injury severity. Crit Care 2016;20:285.

[89] Thelin EP, Zeiler FA, Ercole A, et al. Serial sampling of serum protein biomarkers for monitoring human traumatic brain injury. Dynamics: A Syst Rev Front Neurol 2017;8:300.

[90] Sieber M, Dressler J, Franke H, Pohlers D, Ondruschka B. Post-mortem biochemistry of NSE and S100B: A supplemental tool for detecting a lethal traumatic brain injury? J Forensic Leg Med 2018;55:65–73.

[91] Ondruschka B, Pohlers D, Sommer G, Schober K, Teupser D, Franke H, et al. S100B and NSE as useful post-mortem biochemical markers of traumatic brain injury in autopsy cases. J Neurotrauma 2013;30(22):1862–71.

[92] Kuppermann Prof N, Holmes Prof JF, Dayan MD PS, et al. Identification of children at very low risk of clinically-important brain injuries after head trauma: a prospective cohort study. Lancet 2009;374:1160–70.

[93] Geyer C, Ulrich A, Grafe G, Stach B, Till H. Diagnostic value of S100B and neuron-specific enolase in mild pediatric traumatic brain injury. J Neurosurg Pediatr 2009;4(4):339–44.

[94] Shore PM, Berger RP, Varma S, Janesko KL, Wisniewski SR, Clark RS, et al. Cerebrospinal fluid biomarkers versus glasgow coma scale and glasgow outcome scale in pediatric traumatic brain injury: the role of young age and inflicted injury. J Neurotrauma 2007;24(1):75–86.

[95] Daoud H, Alharfi I, Alhelali I, Charyk Stewart T, Qasem H, Fraser DD. Brain injury biomarkers as outcome predictors in pediatric severe traumatic brain injury. Neurocrit Care 2014;20(3):427–35.

[96] Nakhjavan-Shahraki B, Yousefifard M, Oraii A, Sarveazad A, Hosseini M. Meta-analysis of neuron specific enolase in predicting pediatric brain injury outcomes. EXCLI J 2017;16:995−1008.

[97] Ramont L, Thoannes H, Volondat A, Chastang F, Millet MC, Maquart FX. Effects of hemolysis and storage condition on neuron-specific enolase (NSE) in cerebrospinal fluid and serum: implications in clinical practice. Clin Chem Lab Med 2005;43(11):1215−17.

[98] Verfaillie CJ, Delanghe JR. Hemolysis correction factor in the measurement of serum neuron-specific enolase. Clin Chem Lab Med 2010;48(6):891−2.

[99] Planche V, Brochet C, Bakkouch A, Bernard M. [Importance of hemolysis on neuron-specific enolase measurement]. Ann Biol Clin (Paris) 2010;68(2):239−42.

[100] Pelinka LE, Hertz H, Mauritz W, Harada N, Jafarmadar M, Albrecht M, et al. Nonspecific increase of systemic neuron-specific enolase after trauma: clinical and experimental findings. Shock 2005;24(2):119−23.

[101] Ingebrigtsen T, Romner B. Biochemical serum markers of traumatic brain injury. J Trauma 2002;52 (4):798−808.

Traumatic brain injury biomarkers glial fibrillary acidic protein/ubiquitin C-terminal hydrolase L1

Gary James Mitchell

Emergency Trauma Centre, Royal Brisbane and Womens Hospital, Brisbane, QL, Australia

The need to perform a computed tomography (CT) scan in a patient potentially suffering a traumatic brain injury (TBI) involves accurate risk stratification with the aim of predicting if the patient has suffered an intracranial hemorrhage which may require operative management.

Concussion and minor TBI (m-TBI) are often used interchangeably. m-TBI is diagnosed if the initial Glasgow Scoring System (GCS) is 13–15 after an injury. Patients with an m-TBI will have a normal CT scan in 90% of cases, with less than 1% requiring neurosurgical intervention [1]. Concussion is on the spectrum of m-TBI as there is a functional rather than an anatomical disturbance and, by definition, the patient should have no anatomical changes on CT imaging. For the purpose of this chapter we will use both terms interchangeably.

Clinician objectivity of symptoms in m-TBI and the ongoing treatment, including therapeutic interventions and best practice for physical and cognitive rest, are still debated. Biomarkers specific for TBI could be a massive step toward more clearly answering the questions about ongoing care.

In more severe forms of TBI, where management is currently based on neurosurgical interventions after the acute injury, biomarkers have the potential to help predict severity and outcome as well as playing an important role in tailoring appropriate treatment.

Two such biomarkers, which have shown promising results in both risk stratifying patients to perform a CT scan and diagnosing m-TBI, are ubiquitin C-terminal hydrolase L1 (UCHL-1) and glial fibrillary acidic protein (GFAP).

12.1 Computed tomography imaging

The obvious indication to perform a CT imaging scan of the brain is to rule out an intracranial hemorrhage that may require neurosurgical intervention, such as subdural, epidural, intraventricular, parenchymal, subarachnoid, and petechial hemorrhage. It could be further hypothesized that all degrees of TBI from mild to severe will have some form of nerve pathway injury within the brain which will not be obvious on conventional neuro-imaging and a novel biomarker could potentially provide an added benefit to diagnosing an injury.

Currently, for patients with a suspected TBI emergency physicians utilize clinical decision rules (CDRs) such as the Canadian, New Orleans, or Nexus CT rules in adults, and the PEACRN and CATCH in pediatric patients to determine the pretest probability for intracranial traumatic injury. In the context of head injury, these CDRs have been shown to significantly reduce the number of CT scans physicians ordered for patients who have suffered an m-TBI [2–4] thus reducing the inadvertent potential risk to patients of performing a CT (radiation-induced carcinogenesis), as well as departmental issues associated with costs and patient flow.

However, despite using these CDRs, CT scans are often ordered unnecessarily, often due to fear of litigation, patient and family requests, lack of experience in applying the rules, and departmental flow issues. A highly sensitive and specific biomarker could potentially reduce an inadvertent CT scan being ordered in the event of a suspected TBI.

The ALERT-TBI study published in the *Lancet Neurology* investigated two blood-based biomarkers to predict traumatic intracranial injuries on head CT acutely after TBI [5]. Subsequently, the US Food and Drug Administration (FDA) approved assays for these biomarkers (UCHL-1 and GFAP) for commercialization—the first TBI biomarker assays in the United States.

The study reported on 1977 patients from 22 recruited sites and included patients who presented within 12 hours of their head injury, and who were investigated with a CT scan and venepuncture performed in the emergency department (ED). Patients presenting with a TBI and a GCS level of 9–15 were selected to then undergo both a CT and biomarker analysis. The authors of the ALERT-TBI study hypothesized that GFAP and UCH-L1 would reduce unnecessary head CT scanning, which was described as "overused and resource intensive."

12.2 Ubiquitin C-terminal hydrolase L1 and glial fibrillary acidic protein

Ubiquitin is found in nearly all cells of the body and is a regulatory protein.

UCH-L1, a specific isoform of ubiquitin, is primarily found in central neurons and in the neuroendocrine system but has also been found in the testis, ovaries, and kidneys [6].

GFAP is a member of the intermediate filament family of cytoskeletal proteins which provide a structural support to the neuroglia. Neuroglia assist in maintaining homeostasis, form myelin, and protect neurons in both the peripheral and central nervous systems. GFAP has also been detected in other cells throughout the body outside of the central nervous system—such as Schwann cells, myoepithelial cells, chondrocytes, fibroblasts, and lymphocytes [7].

GFAP and UCH-L1 have been used together in m-TBI biomarker analysis measuring the different types of cells potentially injured in TBI. UCH-L1 has been found in more diffuse brain injuries compared to GFAP, which is suggested to be raised in more focal injuries [1,8].

The assay performed for the ALERT-TBI study combined both biomarkers and was an in vitro enzyme-linked immunosorbent assay (ELISA) providing a semiquantitative measurement of both UCH-L1 and GFAP [9].

The UCH-L1 and GFAP proteins are measured and reported separately. Both biomarker results are needed to obtain a final brain traumatic indicator (BTI) result. BTI will be reported as a "positive result" if either or both UCH-L1 and GFAP are above the predetermined cutoff [9].

12.3 Predetermined cutoff and validation

The reference ranges for both biomarkers in the ALERT-TBI study were determined from an independent group of 334 adults who had suffered an m-TBI described as GCS13−15. There were no significant differences for race or gender but there was a trend of higher levels for both biomarkers in association with increasing age, especially over the age of 60 years [9].

Two other studies have attempted to validate the biomarkers in patients with a TBI. Papa et al. [1] studied the time course and diagnostic accuracy of both biomarkers with mild to moderate TBI (MMTBI), along with testing the biomarkers to identify traumatic intracranial lesions on CT scan and the prediction of needing a neurosurgical intervention. The study had two groups of trauma patients recruited. The first group included patients with MMTBI and the second group was composed of patients without MMTBI (Table 12.1)

In the second study, Posti et al. [7] studied the levels of GFAP and UCH-L1 in patients with acute orthopedic injuries. One group had m-TBI with a normal CT scan and the other group had no evidence of an m-TBI (Table 12.1).

The reference ranges used to identify a positive result as used in the ALERT-TBI study were inconsistent for both biomarkers in the studies by Papa et al. [1] and Posti et al. [7] (Table 12.1) due to the different assays used between companies.

12.4 Biomarker performance

The ALERT-TBI study combined both proteins to determine reportable status for TBI (Table 12.1) with the combined biomarkers having a sensitivity of 0.973 for prediction of acute intracranial injury on CT for all with patients suffering an m-TBI (GCS13−15). However, GFAP alone had a sensitivity of 0.963 (95% CI 0.91−0.99), with a negative predictive value of 0.995 (0.998−0.99) for TBI [10]. The authors acknowledge that the diagnostic improvement of both biomarkers over GFAP alone was not statistically significant.

TABLE 12.1 Comparing studies.

		Bazarian et al.: ALERT-TBI	Papa et al.: Time course and diagnostic accuracy of glial and neuronal blood biomarkers GFAP UCH-L1 in a large cohort of trauma patients with and without m-TBI	Posti et al.: GFAP and UCH-L1 are not specific biomarkers for mild CT—Negative TBI
Study inclusion		GCS 9–15 with nonpenetrating TBI + head CT and blood collected within 12 h	2 cohorts: • All trauma patients without MMTBI • All trauma patients + MMTBI	2 cohorts: • Orthopedic injury without TBI • m-TBI (normal CT scan) + / − Orthopedic trauma
Objectives		Sensitivity and negative predictive value of the biomarkers for the detection of traumatic intracranial injury on CT		
Study numbers		1977	584 • Trauma + without MMTBI—259 (44.3%) • Trauma + with MMTBI—325 (55.7%)	166 • Isolated orthopedic injury—73 (44%) • m-TBI + / − orthopedic injury—93 (56%)
Threshold for abnormal result	GFAP	0.08 ng/mL	0.03 ng/mL	0.3 ng/mL
	UCHL1	0.01 ng/mL	0.1 ng/mL	0.16 ng/mL

CT, computed tomography; *GCS*, Glasgow scoring system; *GFAP*, glial fibrillary acidic protein; *m-TBI*, minor TBI; *MMTBI*, mild to moderate TBI; *UCHL1*, ubiquitin C-terminal hydrolase L1.

Papa et al. reported a similar finding while investigating the time course of detection of both biomarkers after a mild or moderate TBI. They found the combination of GFAP and UCH-L1 marginally outperformed GFAP alone at enrollment and at 8, 36, 60, and 168 hours; however, the differences were not significant.

For TBI biomarkers to be useful in determining the safe discharge of patients with a head injury, the negative predictive value of 1.00 ($n = 8$) in the ALERT-TBI study (0.995–1.00) would support this.

In ALERT-TBI the overall positive predictive value (PPV) of the biomarkers in patients with minor-TBI and a GCS 14–15 was 0.088 (0.073–0.105) but for neurosurgically manageable lesions ($n = 8$) the PPV was 0.006 (0.003–0.012)

This supports the biomarkers as a useful "rule out" test but less so of a "rule in" test.

12.4.1 Vignette

Military personnel are very prone to concussive episodes and more severe TBIs from blast injuries. In potentially injured soldiers, the implications of a suspected TBI are not only the extraction of the soldier from combat but also access and transportation for a CT scan. This can be logistically difficult and dangerous. The potential to screen military personnel with possible TBI using biomarkers could reduce the number of retrievals for CT imaging. From the ALERT-TBI study the sensitivity of the combined biomarkers for detecting intracranial lesions on CT was 0.976 (0.931−0.995) in patients with GCS 9−15 and 0.973 (0.924−0.994) in patients with an initial GCS of 14−15. Significantly the sensitivity was 1.00 (0.631−1.00) for the identification of patients with neurosurgical manageable lesions ($n = 8$). Therefore the potential use of screening military personnel using the GFAP/UCH-L1 proteins, where CT scanning is immediately unobtainable, would appear to be useful.

However, with the overall specificity at 0.34 (0.32−0.37) there is still the potential of retrieving patients for a CT scan inappropriately and therefore use needs to be limited to patients for whom there is a persisting concern for a neurosurgical lesion.

12.5 Specificity of glial fibrillary acidic protein/ubiquitin C-terminal hydrolase L1

For biomarkers to be useful clinically, specificity for TBI is crucial. GFAP and UCHL1 were initially thought to be brain-specific biomarkers, but they exist in tissues outside the CNS. Elevated levels of both biomarkers have been detected in patients following seizures and strokes [7]. Additionally, there are concerns there is a statistically significant elevation of both biomarkers after orthopedic injuries. This is of relevance in multitrauma patients who often have multisystem involvement and thus the biomarkers could be raised by a cause other than a TBI.

The pathological process for elevated protein levels after an orthopedic injury is thought to be due to GFAP and UCH-L1 expression in chondrocytes and fibroblasts in peripheral bone marrow and joint cartilage. Therefore after orthopedic injury there may be detectable levels of the biomarkers in circulating blood, but to date, conflicting results have been reported [11,12].

Posti et al. found levels of GFAP were higher in patients with orthopedic injuries without central nervous system involvement than CT negative patients with an m-TBI and/or orthopedic injuries on arrival day, but did find that levels trended equal over time. Levels of UCH-L1 in this study were not significantly different between patients with orthopedic injuries and patients with an m-TBI and negative CT scan.

This contrasts with the study by Papa et al. when looking at time course and diagnostic accuracy of both biomarkers for TBI. Here the authors found higher concentrations of both biomarkers in patients with MMTBI compared to controls with orthopedic injuries without a mild or moderate TBI.

Potential causes for the contradicting results include patients possibly having suffered a concomitant m-TBI but not meeting the definitions each study had produced for these inclusion criteria. Posti et al. measured biomarkers within 24 hours but Papa et al. measured biomarkers within 4 hours of injury and subsequently every 4 hours in the first 24-hour period. Finally, as mentioned earlier, there was no standardization in the level deemed a positive result between the assays used in each study. This discrepancy is particularly important in the evaluation of the clinical relevance of TBI biomarkers in both diagnosing m-TBI and for performing a CT scan in multitrauma patients.

12.5.1 Vignette

One potential scenario for utilization of TBI biomarkers is in decision-making about expedited operative care for multitrauma patients with unstable vital signs and potentially uncontrolled hemorrhage in addition to a possible TBI.

The decision to perform a CT scan prior to theater to diagnose a concurrent intracranial hemorrhage and have neurosurgical involvement could potentially delay operating when hemorrhage control would be a priority. However, if TBI biomarkers suggested TBI this could help risk stratify if there has been an intracranial bleed and expedite neurosurgical involvement. A rapid, sensitive, and specific biomarker could potentially play a role in this decision-making process.

12.6 Glial fibrillary acidic protein and ubiquitin C-terminal hydrolase L1 trends over time

Papa et al. looked at the individual and combined accuracy of the GFAP and UCH-L1 biomarkers over time in trauma patients with and without TBI. One thousand eight hundred and thirty-one blood samples were taken from 584 recruited patients over a 7-day period. The aim was to detect the presence of mild or moderate TBI from those trauma patients without TBI, identify traumatic intracranial lesions on CT scan, and identify patients requiring neurosurgical intervention.

Both biomarkers had a detectable serum level within 1 hour after injury in 318 of 325 multitrauma patients presenting with a MMTBI with a GCS 13–15.

The control group of trauma patients who had not suffered a TBI was defined as not having suffered a loss of consciousness, amnesia, or altered sensorium after injury. However, these limited inclusion factors are not exhaustive, as patients with an m-TBI may have subtle neurocognitive abnormalities or delayed symptoms which may not have been identified.

GFAP was detectable in all trauma patients with or without MMTBI within 1 hour but peaked at 20 hours and was still detectable at 7 days. In patients with mild or moderate TBI, GFAP was significantly higher (median 0.112 ng/mL) compared to trauma controls (median 0.008 ng/mL) and remained higher than the control group at nearly all other time points.

UCH-L1 was shown to rapidly rise to peak levels at 8 hours in all trauma patients and decreased over a 48-hour period with some baseline fluctuations. Compared to the trauma control group, UCH-L1 was significantly higher in the mild and moderate TBI group (0.258 ng/mL vs. 0.171 ng/mL $P < .001$). Papa et al. reported similar findings, with UCH-L1 shown to peak on arrival compared to values at day 1.

These findings suggest UCH-L1 may be useful as an acute marker to identify TBI and therefore rule out the need for transferring patients from the sporting arena, military theater, or rural hospitals for CT imaging. GFAP, having a later peak and shorter half-life, may be more useful in patients with persisting symptoms of an m-TBI or delayed presentations within a 48-hour period.

12.7 Use in m-traumatic brain injury

A key finding in the ALERT-TBI study was that the biomarkers yielded 10 times more positive test results than positive CT scans for TBI. This suggests that the biomarkers may detect more subtle TBI degrees of injury. This requires validation using higher neuroimaging modalities such as functional MRI (f-MRI), which has shown promise in diagnosing m-TBI or concussion but is expensive and logistically difficult to use in the majority of patients in the clinical setting.

After patients have suffered an m-TBI there is a variation in management strategies including the optimum time frames for both physical and cognitive rest and the potential role of rehabilitation. The GFAP and UCH-L1 biomarkers may help answer these questions and add a level of objectivity if used alongside current cognitive and subjective symptom reporting after interventions are implemented.

For medical practitioners and patients, confidence of diagnosis is required in both the acute and ongoing periods after an m-TBI, as symptoms reported may be due to concussion or other conditions such as middle ear imbalance, dehydration, or whiplash. In the first 48 hours post injury setting of TBI, the biomarkers may be useful if a clinical diagnosis of concussion is unclear. However, they would be less useful in postconcussion syndrome (PCS) as this is diagnosed if symptoms are persisting for up to 2 weeks after the initial injury.

In one study [13], somatization was reported in 55% of patients suffering alleged PCS. Therefore the diagnosis and management can often be difficult in this group of patients with persisting symptoms. The potential of the UCH-L1 and GFAP proteins to quantify ongoing neuronal injury along with current conventional neuropsychological testing may add a level of objectivity in the management of patients with PCS.

12.7.1 Vignette

In the professional sporting arena, athletes who have suffered a concussion during competition or training may underreport symptoms in order to return to the competitive environment. This may place the athlete at significant risk of further injury, underperformance, and potentially significant long-term cognitive issues. The optimum time to rehabilitate and return to intensive training is still much debated and currently relies on both subjective patient reporting of symptoms and objective neurocognitive testing. However, despite clinical recovery and symptom improvement, there is still concern that the functional disturbance associated with a concussion may still persist. GFAP and UCH-L1 proteins may identify the subtle functional disturbance of brain functioning during a concussive episode, and may be used not only as an aid to diagnosis but also in conjunction with current best practice to return athletes to the sporting environment.

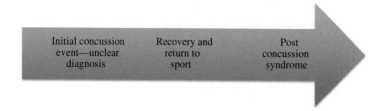

FIGURE 12.1 Potential points in patient presentation to measure biomarkers in patients suffering m-TBI.

This is particularly important in the professional sporting environments where athletes often need to partake in an accelerated return to sport with both potential adverse health outcomes and careers being constantly balanced with medical staff. This role requires investigation and validation (Fig. 12.1).

12.8 Future directions

The GFAP and UCHL1 TBI biomarkers have an emerging role and significant potential to transform aspects of contemporary clinical care. However, there are a number of aspects that require rigorous investigation. Specifically, the correlation of the GFAP and UCHL1 biomarkers to patient outcomes must be considered to clarify if they will add new information to patient care and management decisions.

The potential to use the GFAP and UCH-L1 biomarkers to triage those patients who may not benefit from CT imaging to rule out an intracranial hemorrhage could allow for the reassurance of patients and physicians, especially when CT scanning is not easily available, such as in rural and remote healthcare settings. Significant economic benefits for health services are also possible if the assays provide accurate high-throughput and rapid turnaround. The comparative benefit of TBI biomarkers to current CDRs in settings with accessible CT availability needs further study as the impact and safety of reducing CT investigation in this cohort is unknown.

The value of assessing biomarkers on every m-TBI patient and potentially using serial measurements to define recovery is unknown as it is estimated that 90% of concussions will recover within 14 days. As with all TBI biomarkers, GFAP and UCH-L1 are unlikely to be beneficial unless their role, e.g., for the subgroup of patients who show both red flags for postconcussion syndrome (mental health patients, chronic migraine sufferers, multiple previous concussions) or need a tailored return to sport, academia, or work activities can be well-defined. In the subset of patients where concussion is suspected but not clear and no CT scan is warranted, further validation and clinical context needs to be applied before biomarker testing will be a standard of care in their assessment and management.

A cutoff value to determine a positive result needs to be obtained in future research and standardized in future clinical studies and assays. This standard is required to enable comparative validation studies to reliably identify how GFAP and UCH-L1 could impact current clinical practice. The specificity of both biomarkers is unclear and further research needs to be taken into other potential causes for raised GFAP and UCH-L1. Patients may have suffered an associated secondary injury with their concussion and elevated biomarkers may predispose them to an unwarranted CT brain or even ongoing neuroimaging. This seems to be particularly relevant to the group of patients suffering concurrent orthopedic injuries.

As with all potential biomarkers being researched for m-TBI, GFAP and UCH-L1 have the potential to add or strengthen evidence for interventions, which may modify disease outcome. The trends in biomarkers after therapeutic or nontherapeutic interventions could be particularly prominent in helping define the optimum time for rest or to return patents to cognitive and physical activities such as work or the sporting environment.

With all this in mind, it is extremely important to consider the impact of any new enhancements and pathological tests on health service costs and patient volume and outcome. A logical and evidence-based strategy would need to be developed in order to select the patient population who would benefit from biomarker testing within the constraints of the healthcare system.

References

[1] Papa L, Lewis L, et al. Serum levels of ubiquitin C-terminal hydrolase distinguish mild traumatic brain injury from trauma controls and are elevated in mild and moderate traumatic brain injury patients with intracranial lesions and neurosurgical intervention. J Trauma Acute Care Surg 2012;72(5):1335−44.

[2] Stiell IG, Wells G, et al. The Canadian CT head rule for patients with minor head injury. Lancet 2001;357:1391−6.

[3] Haydel MJ, Preston CA, et al. Indications for computed tomography in patients with minor head injury. N Engl J Med 2000;343:100−5.

[4] Smits M, Dippel DWJ, et al. Predicting intracranial traumatic findings on computed tomography in patients with minor head injury: the CHIP prediction rule. Ann Intern Med 2007;146:397−405.

[5] Bazarian J, Biberthaler P, et al. Serum GFAP and UCH-L1 for prediction of absence of intracranial injuries on head CT (ALERT-TBI): a multicenter observational study. Lancet Neurol 2018; S1474−4422(18)30275-8.

[6] Zetterberg M, Sjolander A, et al. Ubiquitin carboxy-terminal hydrolase L1 *(UCHL1)* S18Y polymorphism in Alzheimer's disease. Molecular Neurodegeneration. 2010; 5: 11.

[7] Posti J, Hossain I, et al. Glial fibrillary acidic protein and ubiquitin C-terminal hydrolase-L1 are not specific biomarkers for mild CT-negative traumatic brain injury. J Neurotrauma 2017. Available from: https://doi.org/10.1089/neu.2016.4442.

[8] Mondello S, Papa L, et al. Neuronal and glial markers are differently associated with computed tomography findings and outcome in patients with severe traumatic brain injury: a case control study. Crit Care 2011;15: R156.

[9] Banyan BTI Catalog. https://banyanbio.com/assets/files/000175_vA-IFU-Banyan-BTI.pdf.

[10] Maas A, Lingsma H. ALERT-TBI study on biomarkers for TBI: has science suffered? Lancet Neurol 2018; (18):30275−8.

[11] Fellenberg J, Lehner B, et al. Silencing of the UCHL1 gene in giant cell tumors of bone. Int J Cancer 2010;127:1804−12.

[12] Hsu S, Lai M, et al. Ubiquitin carboxyl-terminal hydrolase L1 (UCHL1) regulates the level of SMN expression through ubiquitination in primary spinal muscular atrophy fibroblasts. Clin Chim Acta 2010;411:1920−8.

[13] Perrine K, Gibalsi J. Somatization in post-concussion syndrome: a retrospective study. Cureus 2016;8(8):e743.

Neurofilaments light chain/ Neurofilaments heavy chain

Shoji Yokobori, Ryuta Nakae and Hiroyuki Yokota

Department of Emergency and Critical Care Medicine, Nippon Medical School, Tokyo, Japan

13.1 Introduction

Typically, neuronal biomarkers are proteins that can be repeatedly and safely measured from biofluids, providing clinicians with specific information regarding the brain and spinal cord. The ideal biomarker is uniquely present in the central nervous system and accurately reflects the extent of neuronal damage (specificity), is highly abundant and easily detectable (sensitivity), and is useful for measuring therapeutic efficacy. With these concepts in mind, the present chapter focuses on the role of cerebrospinal fluid (CSF) neurofilament (NF) levels as biomarkers of axonal structure.

NFs are a major cytoskeletal component in axons. The NF heteropolymer consists of light chain (NFL, 68 kDa), medium chain (NFM, 150 kDa), heavy chain (NFH, 190−210 kDa), and α-internexin polypeptides [1,2]. NF subunits are localized in the neuronal soma [3], following which they are transported to and accumulate in disconnected axons after injury [4]. The phosphorylated form of the heavy subunit (pNFH) is thus specific to axons and can be detected in the blood via an immunoassay after various neuronal injuries in rats [5,6]. Following axonal injury, an influx of calcium activates calcineurin, altering the phosphorylation state and the repelling forces of the NF sidearms and forming areas of NF compaction accompanied by marked local loss of cytoskeletal integrity [7,8]. Subsequently, activated calpain and caspase-3 mediate the dephosphorylation and proteolysis of phosphorylated NFs (pNFs), causing them to collapse into tightly packed bundles in the centers of axons [9]. These modifications reduce the stability of pNFs and thus the caliber of injured axons. Subsequently, this process promotes pNF degradation, which results in the formation of axonal retraction balls and disconnection. Experiments involving rat models have revealed that NFM (150 kDa) levels are upregulated between 6 and 24 hours after injury [10]. Significant serum levels of pNFH fragments can be observed as early as 6 hours after neuronal injury in rats, with levels peaking between 12 and 48 hours and decreasing to baseline by day 7 [5]. In this previous study, the two peaks in serum levels of NFH fragments

Biomarkers for Traumatic Brain Injury
DOI: https://doi.org/10.1016/B978-0-12-816346-7.00013-0

corresponded to primary and secondary axotomy, respectively. However, because secondary axotomy was more severe than primary axotomy, the second peak was sharper than the first [5]. Because blood is quicker, safer, and more convenient to obtain than CSF, assays of serum pNFH may represent a more convenient method for the specific assessment of axonal damage in patients with diffuse axonal TBI. In this chapter, we review the feasibility of this protein biomarker for diagnostic and prognostic purposes (see Table 13.1).

13.2 Neurofilament for traumatic brain injury diagnosis

Rapid triage and decision-making in the treatment of TBI present a challenge for those working in resource-poor environments such as battlefield and prehospital settings. Thus additional tools for guiding TBI treatment are required. For example, glial fibrillary acidic protein (GFAP) and ubiquitin carboxy-terminal hydrolase L1 (UCH-L1) were recently approved by the US FDA for the detection of brain trauma associated with mild TBI and concussion. Recent evidence also suggests that NFs can be used as diagnostic biomarkers for distinguishing axonal and focal injury.

In 2005 Shaw et al. demonstrated that serum pNFH expression increases following experimental spinal cord injury (SCI) and TBI in rats. In this previous study, higher levels of serum pNFH were detected in rat models, peaking at 2 days postinjury [5]. Zurek et al. first reported the efficacy of serum NFH measurement for predicting the injury type and outcome in children with TBI [11]. In this study, levels of NFH were significantly higher in patients with diffuse axonal injury (DAI) on initial CT scans [11]. In another study, Vajtr et al. compared serum NFH concentrations between DAI ($n = 10$) and focal injury ($n = 28$), revealing that median serum NFH levels were higher in patients with DAI than in those with focal TBI up to 10 days after admission [12]. In this study, the median serum S100B concentration was higher in patients with focal mass lesions (1.72 vs 0.37 μg/L, $P < .05$) than in patients with DAI throughout the 10-day hospitalization period. In contrast, median serum pNFH levels were higher in patients with DAI than in those with focal TBI (0.625 vs 0.139 ng/L, $P < .05$) during the same period. Time-dependent profiles revealed that serum pNFH levels increased between days 4 and 10 in both groups, with values ranging from 0.263 to 1.325 ng/L in patients with DAI, and from 0.103 to 1.108 ng/L in patients with focal injuries [12].

More recently, Gaston et al. reported that serum levels of pNFH were significantly higher on day 1 in patients with mild TBI (GCS:13−15) who exhibited positive CT findings (CT +) ($P < .008$) than in those who exhibited negative CT findings (CT-). The area under the curve (82.5%) for the CT + group versus the CT-group was significant ($P = .021$), with a sensitivity of 87.5% and a specificity of 70%, using a cutoff of 1071 pg/mL for serum pNFH. Gaston et al. concluded that pNFH levels may be useful in determining which individuals require CT imaging to assess the severity of their injury [13].

A 2017 case series by Ljungqvist et al. demonstrated the efficacy of NFL as a marker for DAI [14]. In this study, the authors measured acute serum concentrations of NFL in nine patients with severe TBI and DAI using a novel ultrasensitive single molecule array (SIMOA) assay. Ljungqvist et al. analyzed the relationships between NFL concentrations and MRI findings in the acute stage, as well as those between clinical outcomes and

TABLE 13.1 Previous studies of neurofilament proteins in human patients with TBI.

Authors (Year)	Biofluid (Serum/CSF)	Type of neurofilament (NFL, NFH)	Number of patients, Cohort	Design	Timing of sampling	Primary outcome/purpose	Details	Reference journal
Zurek et al. (2011)	Serum	pNFH	49 children with TBI	Prospective	After admission and every 24 h for a maximum of 6 consecutive days	Diagnostic/prognostic biomarker of DAI	Levels of pNFH on days 2–4 were significantly higher in patients with poor outcomes at 6 months (GOS = 1) than in other patients ($P = .027$; $P = .019$; $P = .01$). Levels of pNF-H were significantly higher in patients with diffuse axonal injury on initial CT scans ($P = .004$).	Brain Inj 2011;25:221–226.
Vajtr et al. (2012)	Serum	pNFH	Patients with DAI ($n = 10$) and focal ($n = 28$) injuries	Retrospective	After admission and every 24 h for a maximum of 10 consecutive days	Comparison of biomarker concentration between patients with DAI and focal TBI.	Median serum pNFH levels were higher in patients with DAI than in those with focal TBI (0.625 vs 0.139 ng/L, $P < .05$) throughout the 10-day hospitalization period.	Soud Lek 2012;57:7–12.
Ljungqvist et al. (2017)	Serum	NFL	Nine patients with severe TBI and DAI	Case series	Acute phase	The authors examined the relationships between NFL concentrations and MRI findings in the acute stage, as well as those between clinical outcomes and magnetic resonance diffusion tensor imaging (MR-DTI) parameters at 12 months.	Mean NFL levels were 30 times higher among patients than controls. NFL levels completely discriminated between patients and controls. Serum NFL levels were well-correlated with MR-DTI parameters, with higher NFL concentrations in patients with higher trace (R(2) = 0.79) and lower fractional anisotropy (FA) (R (2) = 0.83) values.	J Neurotrauma 2017;34:1124–1127.

(Continued)

TABLE 13.1 (Continued)

Authors (Year)	Biofluid (Serum/ CSF)	Type of neurofilament (NFL, NFH)	Number of patients, Cohort	Design	Timing of sampling	Primary outcome/ purpose	Details	Reference journal
Martinez-Morillo et al. (2015)	Serum	NFM	106 serum samples from 12 patients with TBI and 68 serum samples from 68 patients with mild TBI	Prospective	Not mentioned	To evaluate the NFM concentration in the serum of healthy individuals and patients with brain damage	A total of 44% of patients with mild TBI exhibited increased NFM concentration, with significantly higher levels ($P = .01$) in patients with polytrauma.	Clin Chem Lab Med 2015;53:1575–1584.
Gaston et al. (2014)	Serum	pNFH	Mild TBI ($n = 34$)	Prospective	Days 1 and 3 after injury	To characterize NFH levels as a predictor of injury severity in patients with mild TBI (mTBI).	A significant inverse correlation was observed between serum pNFH levels and GCS scores. Serum pNFH levels were significantly higher in patients with mTBI in the CT-positive group ($P < .008$) than in those in the CT-negative group. The area under the curve (82.5) for the CT-positive group versus the CT-negative group was significant ($P = .021$), with a sensitivity of 87.5% and a specificity of 70%, using a cutoff of 1071 pg/mL for serum pNFH.	J Neurosurg 2014;121:1232–1238.
Zurek et al. (2012)	Serum	pNFH	63 children with TBI	Prospective	Every 24 h for a maximum of six consecutive days.	To predict long-term outcomes in children with TBI	Levels of pNFH increased significantly faster in patients with worse GOS scores and those who had died ($P < .001$; $P = .001$)	Acta Neurochir 2012;154:93–103.

Study	Source	Biomarker	Patients	Design	Timing	Objective	Findings	Reference
Shibahashi et al. (2016)	Serum	pNFH	32 Patients with TBI (GCS score of 13 or less on admission).	Prospective	24 and 72 h after TBI	To elucidate the usefulness of serum pNFH as a prognostic indicator for patients with TBI.	Serum pNFH levels at 24 h after injury were a good predictive marker of death at 6 months ($P < .001$, optimal cutoff value: 240 pg/mL, AUC: 0.93). The serum pNFH value at 72 h after injury was correlated with an unfavorable outcome (vegetative state or death) at 6 months ($P < .01$), with a cutoff value of 80 pg/mL.	J Neurotrauma 2016;33:1826–1833.
Shahim et al. (2016)	Serum	NFL	Patients with severe TBI (sTBI) ($n = 72$) versus controls ($n = 35$).	Prospective	On admission	To compare the diagnostic and prognostic utility of NFL with the established blood biomarker S100B.	Serum NFL levels were markedly higher in patients with sTBI than in controls. NFL levels at admission yielded an AUC of 0.99 for the detection of TBI versus controls (AUC of 0.96 for S100B), and this AUC increased to 1.00 at day 12 (cf. 0.65 for S100B). Initial NFL levels predicted poor clinical outcomes at 12 months. In contrast, S100B was not related to outcomes.	Sci Rep 2016;6:36791.

Abbreviations: *AUC*, Area under the curve; *CSF*, cerebrospinal fluid; *DAI*, diffuse axonal injury; *GCS*, Glasgow Come Scale; *GOS*, Glasgow Outcome Scale; *NFL*, neurofilament light chain; *NFM*, neurofilament medium chain; *pNFH*, phosphorylated neurofilament heavy chain; *TBI*, traumatic brain injury.

magnetic resonance diffusion tensor imaging (MR-DTI) parameters at 12 months. Mean NFL concentrations were 30 times higher in patients than in controls. Furthermore, NFL levels completely discriminated between patients and controls. The authors also noted a relationship between serum NFL levels and MR-DTI parameters, with higher NFL concentrations in patients with higher trace ($R^2 = 0.79$) and lower fractional anisotropy (FA) ($R^2 = 0.83$) values. These results suggest that serum NFL levels reflect the severity of DAI [14].

Although these previous studies clarify the potential role of NFH as a biomarker for distinguishing DAI from focal injury, comparatively less evidence has been obtained regarding NFM as a biomarker for TBI. In 2015 Martinez-Morillo et al. evaluated NFM in the CSF and serum of healthy individuals and patients with mild-to-severe TBI. NFM levels were increased in patients with stroke and TBI, and 44% of patients with mild TBI exhibited increased NFL and NFM concentrations, which was significantly higher in patients with polytrauma [15]. However, further studies are required to verify these findings, and to compare sensitivity among NFL, NFM, and NFH levels.

13.3 Neurofilament levels for detecting secondary brain injury

The major prognostic factor after TBI is the severity of the primary brain injury. Following impact, a delayed secondary brain injury cascade is set in motion. While primary brain injury itself is unavoidable, the focus of medical treatment for TBI is the prevention of secondary brain injury. Therefore an adequate understanding of the pathology of this secondary injury is required in the treatment of patients with TBI.

DAI is now recognized to typically involve a more progressive, slower response characterized by transient, traumatically induced, neurochemically magnified disruptions of the axonal membrane and its associated ion channels over the course of 24 hours, thereby leading to uncontrollable calcium influx [16]. These mechanisms induce subsequent failure of axoplasmic transportation, pooling of intraaxonal contents, and separation of the axon from its distal part, thus creating a retraction ball of axoplasm. This process, termed delayed or secondary axotomy, occurs over the course of 24—72 hours from the traumatic impact. As one cannot observe these histological changes in living humans, biomarkers are essential for tracking the progression of secondary brain injury.

In the field of neurocritical care, advanced continuous cerebral monitoring has been applied for the detection of secondary brain injury. To date, the measurement of intracranial pressure (ICP) is widely accepted as the standard method of cerebral monitoring. Indeed, ICP monitoring is strongly suggested by the recent TBI treatment guidelines [17].

Previous studies have indicated that cleaved-Tau (C-tau) [18], neuron-specific enolase (NSE) [19], S100B [20,21], GFAP [22,23], and α-II spectrin breakdown products (SBDPs) [24] represent potential biomarkers for ICP [25]. However, no studies have investigated the efficacy of NF measurement for continuous clinical monitoring, possible due to differences in effective half-life among TBI biomarkers [26]. The kinetic profile of pNFH in the serum differs somewhat from that of many other biomarkers. Although several biomarkers peak and then decline within a few days after injury, the concentration of pNFH continues to increase. This continuous increase occurred over 6 consecutive days in one pediatric population [27], and between 4 and 10 days after injury in another study [12].

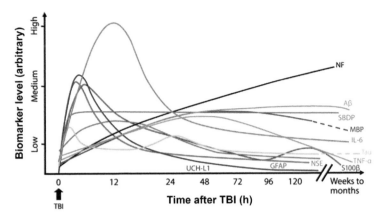

FIGURE 13.1 **Kinetics of TBI biomarkers.** Schematic representation depicting the rise and fall of serum or plasma biomarkers of TBI for which representative kinetic data were available. Separate long-term values (months to weeks) are included when possible. *Aβ*, amyloid beta; *GFAP*, glial fibrillary acidic protein; *IL-6*, interleukin 6; *MBP*, myelin basic protein; *NF*, neurofilament; *NSE*, neuron-specific enolase; *SBDP*, spectrin breakdown product; *TBI*, traumatic brain injury; *TNF-α*, tumor necrosis factor alpha; *UCH-L1*, Ubiquitin carboxyl-terminal hydrolase L1. Source: *Adapted from Adrian H, Marten K, Salla N, Lasse V. Biomarkers of traumatic brain injury: temporal changes in body fluids. eNeuro. 2016;3.*

Proteins with shorter serum availability, such as S100B, may be superior to proteins such as NFL for the purpose of detecting secondary brain injury [26]. In terms of biological characteristics, NFs exhibit decreased temporal resolution relative to other biomarkers, as well as a longer half-life (see Fig. 13.1) [28].

In contrast, the longer bioavailability of NF may be advantageous for detecting chronic posttraumatic disorder [29]. Bagnato et al. measured CSF levels of NFL in 10 patients who developed a severe disorder of consciousness following TBI (time since brain injury: 309 ± 169 days). NFL concentrations were very high in all 10 patients, ranging from 2.4 to 60.5 times the upper normal limit (median value: 4458 pg/mL; range: 695–23,000 pg/mL). Such findings may also aid in outcome prediction among patients with severe TBI.

13.4 Neurofilament levels for outcome prediction in patients with traumatic brain injury

Outcome prediction following TBI is essential for determining the direction of future treatment. Zurek et al. examined the prognostic properties of NFs in pediatric patients with TBI. In this study, outcomes were evaluated at 6 months using the Glasgow Outcome Scale (GOS) in all patients, and NFH levels increased significantly faster in patients who exhibited worse GOS scores or died [27]. More recently, Shibahashi et al. demonstrated that pNFH may represent an outcome biomarker in adult patients with TBI: [30] Serum pNFH levels at 24 hours after injury were effective in predictive death at 6 months after injury, with an optimal cutoff value of 240 pg/mL and an area under the curve of 0.930 [30]. An additional study suggested that serum NFL levels may be useful for assessing the severity of neuronal injury and predicting outcomes following severe TBI [31].

Shahim et al. reported higher levels of serum NFL in patients with lower GOS scores at 12 months after injury (R = −0.34, $P = 0.010$). In contrast, there was no significant difference in the levels of S100B based on GOS category [31].

Taken together, these findings indicate that serum NF levels may be more appropriate than conventional biomarkers (e.g., S100B) for predicting prognosis in patients with TBI.

13.5 Serum biomarkers of cardiac arrest/ultimate ischemic brain damage

Cardiac arrest (CA) results in global ischemic brain injury in humans. Moreover, the return of spontaneous circulation (ROSC) is strongly influenced by the severity of CA and neuronal damage. In our preliminary pilot study, we measured and compared several serum biomarkers for brain damage (NSE, S100B, pNFH) and inflammatory cytokine levels (interleukin-6; L-6) in patients discharged from the hospital following CA. This 1-year prospective observational study was performed at an urban tertiary emergency medical center.

Our study included patients with cardiogenic or suspected cardiogenic out-of-hospital CA (OHCA) who had been transferred to the emergency room at our institution. Blood samples obtained at admission were centrifuged at 2500 rpm for 10 min, and the sera were stored at −80ₒC until batch biomarker analyses. Commercial sandwich enzyme-linked immunosorbent assay kits were used to detect S100B (EMD Millipore Corporation, Billerica, MA) and pNFL levels (BioVendor, Brno, Czech Republic) based on previously described protocols [32]. NSE detection was performed using an electrochemiluminescence immunoassay (Roche Diagnostics, Mannheim, Germany). Levels of the inflammatory cytokine IL-6 were detected using the Human IL-6 RAYFAST system (RAYFAST, Toray, Tokyo), which provides rapid serum IL-6 measurements [33].

Our results indicated that patients without ROSC exhibited significantly higher serum concentrations of NSE, S100B, and IL-6 than patients with ROSC, although there was no significant difference in pNFH levels (see Table 13.2).

TABLE 13.2   Differences in neurological and inflammatory biomarkers between ROSC and non-ROSC groups.

	ROSC group ($n = 26$)	Non-ROSC group ($n = 26$)	P-value
Brain biomarkers			
Neuron-specific enolase, ng/mL	24.2 (19.1−44.4)	61.4 (39.4−91.7)	<0.001
S100-β, pg/mL	1562.6 (884.1−2286.6)	2515.7 (1946.9−2999.9)	<0.001
pNFH, pg/mL	40.7 (0.0−184.4)	35.6 (0.0−118.5)	0.78
Inflammatory cytokine levels			
IL-6, pg/mL	42.0 (23.5−144.0)	116.0 (35.0−972.0)	0.04

Data are shown as number (%) or median (interquartile range).
IL-6: interleukin 6; *pNFH*, phosphorylated neurofilament heavy chain; *ROSC*, return of spontaneous circulation.

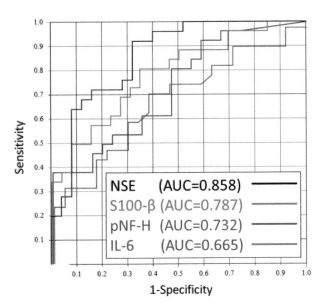

FIGURE 13.2 **The receiver operating characteristic curve for discriminating between patients who did and did not experience ROSC.** The receiver operating characteristic curve analysis was performed using serum brain and inflammatory biomarkers. The strongest predictor of ROSC in the ED was NSE, which provided an AUC of 0.858. *AUC,* area under the curve; *ED,* emergency department; *IL-6,* interleukin-6; *NSE,* neuron-specific enolase; *pNFH,* phosphorylated neurofilament heavy chain; *ROSC,* return of spontaneous circulation.

We also compared the area under the curve (AUC) for each biomarker (Fig. 13.2). Among all neurological and inflammatory biomarkers, the receiver operating characteristic curve analysis revealed that an NSE cutoff value of 40.6 ng/mL provided the greatest AUC for discriminating between ROSC and non-ROSC cases (AUC = 0.858). This finding clearly demonstrates that pNF is not sensitive for detecting ischemic brain damage caused by CA, relative to NSE or S100B. As previously discussed, the biokinetic properties of each biomarker are quite different: That is, NSE and S100B concentrations peak more quickly than those of pNF (see Fig. 13.1). Therefore pNF levels may not be advantageous for the diagnosis of acute ischemia in patients with CA.

13.6 Conclusion

In this chapter, we reviewed recent studies and described our preliminary clinical experience regarding NFs as biomarkers of global ischemic brain injury. Overall, the accumulated evidence suggests that NFs, which exhibit unique biokinetic properties relative to conventional neurological biomarkers, can be used as a diagnostic biomarker of DAI. However, the duration of bioavailability is longer for NFs, resulting in decreased temporal resolution when compared with other biomarkers. Due to delays in peak concentrations of pNF after TBI, pNF levels do not appear suitable for detecting immediate TBI or ischemic brain injury, or for monitoring secondary brain injury in intensive care settings. However, because they reflect the destruction of axonal structures, NFs may be appropriate for predicting TBI prognosis.

References

[1] Petzold A. Neurofilament phosphoforms: surrogate markers for axonal injury, degeneration and loss. J Neurol Sci 2005;233:183–98.

[2] Julien JP, Mushynski WE. Neurofilaments in health and disease. Prog Nucleic Acid Res Mol Biol 1998;61:1–23.

[3] Hamberger A, Huang YL, Zhu H, Bao F, Ding M, Blennow K, et al. Redistribution of neurofilaments and accumulation of beta-amyloid protein after brain injury by rotational acceleration of the head. J Neurotrauma 2003;20:169–78.

[4] Chen XH, Meaney DF, Xu BN, Nonaka M, McIntosh TK, Wolf JA, et al. Evolution of neurofilament subtype accumulation in axons following diffuse brain injury in the pig. J Neuropathol Exp Neurol 1999;58:588–96.

[5] Shaw G, Yang C, Ellis R, Anderson K, Parker Mickle J, Scheff S, et al. Hyperphosphorylated neurofilament NF-H is a serum biomarker of axonal injury. Biochem Biophys Res Commun 2005;336:1268–77.

[6] Anderson KJ, Scheff SW, Miller KM, Roberts KN, Gilmer LK, Yang C, et al. The phosphorylated axonal form of the neurofilament subunit NF-H (pNF-H) as a blood biomarker of traumatic brain injury. J Neurotrauma 2008;25:1079–85.

[7] Jafari SS, Maxwell WL, Neilson M, Graham DI. Axonal cytoskeletal changes after non-disruptive axonal injury. J Neurocytol 1997;26:207–21.

[8] Buki A, Povlishock JT. All roads lead to disconnection?—traumatic axonal injury revisited. Acta Neurochir (Wien) 2006;148:181–93 discussion 93-94.

[9] Park E, Liu E, Shek M, Park A, Baker AJ. Heavy neurofilament accumulation and alpha-spectrin degradation accompany cerebellar white matter functional deficits following forebrain fluid percussion injury. Exp Neurol 2007;204:49–57.

[10] Kang SK, So HH, Moon YS, Kim CH. Proteomic analysis of injured spinal cord tissue proteins using 2-DE and MALDI-TOF MS. Proteomics 2006;6:2797–812.

[11] Zurek J, Bartlova L, Fedora M. Hyperphosphorylated neurofilament NF-H as a predictor of mortality after brain injury in children. Brain Inj 2011;25:221–6.

[12] Vajtr D, Benada O, Linzer P, Samal F, Springer D, Strejc P, et al. Immunohistochemistry and serum values of S-100B, glial fibrillary acidic protein, and hyperphosphorylated neurofilaments in brain injuries. Soud Lek 2012;57:7–12.

[13] Gatson JW, Barillas J, Hynan LS, Diaz-Arrastia R, Wolf SE, Minei JP. Detection of neurofilament-H in serum as a diagnostic tool to predict injury severity in patients who have suffered mild traumatic brain injury. J Neurosurg 2014;121:1232–8.

[14] Ljungqvist J, Zetterberg H, Mitsis M, Blennow K, Skoglund T. Serum neurofilament light protein as a marker for diffuse axonal injury: results from a case series study. J Neurotrauma 2017;34:1124–7.

[15] Martinez-Morillo E, Childs C, Garcia BP, Alvarez Menendez FV, Romaschin AD, Cervellin G, et al. Neurofilament medium polypeptide (NFM) protein concentration is increased in CSF and serum samples from patients with brain injury. Clin Chem Lab Med 2015;53:1575–84.

[16] Pettus EH, Christman CW, Giebel ML, Povlishock JT. Traumatically induced altered membrane permeability: its relationship to traumatically induced reactive axonal change. J Neurotrauma 1994;11:507–22.

[17] Carney N, Totten AM, O'Reilly C, Ullman JS, Hawryluk GW, Bell MJ, et al. Guidelines for the management of severe traumatic brain injury Fourth Edition Neurosurgery 2017;80:6–15.

[18] Zemlan FP, Jauch EC, Mulchahey JJ, Gabbita SP, Rosenberg WS, Speciale SG, et al. C-tau biomarker of neuronal damage in severe brain injured patients: association with elevated intracranial pressure and clinical outcome. Brain Res 2002;947:131–9.

[19] Stein DM, Kufera JA, Lindell A, Murdock KR, Menaker J, Bochicchio GV, et al. Association of CSF biomarkers and secondary insults following severe traumatic brain injury. Neurocrit Care 2011;14:200–7.

[20] Olivecrona Z, Bobinski L, Koskinen LO. Association of ICP, CPP, CT findings and S-100B and NSE in severe traumatic head injury. Prognostic value of the biomarkers. Brain Inj 2015;29:446–54.

[21] Raabe A, Grolms C, Sorge O, Zimmermann M, Seifert V. Serum S-100B protein in severe head injury. Neurosurgery 1999;45:477–83.

[22] Pelinka LE, Kroepfl A, Leixnering M, Buchinger W, Raabe A, Redl H. GFAP versus S100B in serum after traumatic brain injury: relationship to brain damage and outcome. J Neurotrauma 2004;21:1553–61.

[23] Pelinka LE, Kroepfl A, Schmidhammer R, Krenn M, Buchinger W, Redl H, et al. Glial fibrillary acidic protein in serum after traumatic brain injury and multiple trauma. J Trauma 2004;57:1006—12.

[24] Brophy GM, Pineda JA, Papa L, Lewis SB, Valadka AB, Hannay HJ, et al. AlphaII-Spectrin breakdown product cerebrospinal fluid exposure metrics suggest differences in cellular injury mechanisms after severe traumatic brain injury. J Neurotrauma 2009;26:471—9.

[25] Yokobori S, Hosein K, Burks S, Sharma I, Gajavelli S, Bullock R. Biomarkers for the clinical differential diagnosis in traumatic brain injury—a systematic review. CNS Neurosci Ther 2013;19:556—65.

[26] Thelin EP, Zeiler FA, Ercole A, Mondello S, Buki A, Bellander BM, et al. Serial sampling of serum protein biomarkers for monitoring human traumatic brain injury dynamics: a systematic review. Front Neurol 2017;8:300.

[27] Zurek J, Fedora M. The usefulness of S100B, NSE, GFAP, NF-H, secretagogin and Hsp70 as a predictive biomarker of outcome in children with traumatic brain injury. Acta Neurochir 2012;154:93—103 discussion.

[28] Adrian H, Marten K, Salla N, Lasse V. Biomarkers of traumatic brain injury: temporal changes in body fluids. eNeuro 2016;3.

[29] Bagnato S, Grimaldi LME, Di Raimondo G, Sant'Angelo A, Boccagni C, Virgilio V, et al. Prolonged cerebrospinal fluid neurofilament light chain increase in patients with post-traumatic disorders of consciousness. J Neurotrauma 2017;34:2475—9.

[30] Shibahashi K, Doi T, Tanaka S, Hoda H, Chikuda H, Sawada Y, et al. The Serum phosphorylated neurofilament heavy subunit as a predictive marker for outcome in adult patients after traumatic brain injury. J Neurotrauma 2016;33:1826—33.

[31] Shahim P, Gren M, Liman V, Andreasson U, Norgren N, Tegner Y, et al. Serum neurofilament light protein predicts clinical outcome in traumatic brain injury. Sci Rep 2016;6:36791.

[32] Yang Z, Bramlett HM, Moghieb A, Yu D, Wang P, Lin F, et al. Temporal profile and severity correlation of a panel of rat spinal cord injury protein biomarkers. Mol Neurobiol 2018;55:2174—84.

[33] Koyama K, Ohba T, Ishii K, Jung G, Haro H, Matsuda K. Development of a quick serum IL-6 measuring system in rheumatoid arthritis. Cytokine 2017;95:22—6.

Tau protein, biomarker for traumatic brain injury

Pablo Tovar

Emergency Medicine, Baylor College of Medicine, Houston, TX, United States

14.1 Introduction

The effects of traumatic brain injury can vary from subtle to life altering with possible negative long-term impact on quality of life. Traumatic brain injury results in functional as well as structural changes in the brain. These structural changes are a result of axonal injury and can manifest as neurologic, cognitive, and behavior abnormalities [1]. Repetitive traumatic brain injury can result in chronic traumatic encephalopathy, a disease characterized by hyperphosphorylated tau and fibrillary tangles [2,3]. Tau protein can be cleaved and can make their way into cerebral spinal fluid (CSF) and serum [4]. There is a growing need to supplement and enhance the clinical diagnosis of traumatic brain injury with objective diagnostic biomarkers. Using tau protein as a biomarker for traumatic brain injury may aid in the diagnosis of traumatic brain injury and potentially help us better characterize and measure the degree of brain injury and dysfunction as well as assist in determining prognosis and outcomes.

14.2 Pathophysiology

Tau protein was first isolated in 1975 and described as a microtubule-associated protein involved in microtubule formation and stability [5]. Tau proteins are predominately intracellular soluble proteins that are found in the brain and central nervous system but are also found in the extracellular space. Six isoforms of tau proteins have been identified in human brain tissue and exist mostly in an unfolded form with little tendency to aggregate. The longest tau isoform contains as many as 85 potential phosphorylation sites. The phosphorylation of these sites results in physiological changes in tau function which may alter its binding to microtubules and ultimately affect the stabilization and assembly of microtubules [5]. Studies have indicated that the phosphorylation, in particular hyperphosphorylation of tau, is thought to result in increased tau aggregation as has been noted in Alzheimer's and other tauopathies such as traumatic brain injury [6]. The aggregation of hyperphosphorylated, misfolded tau results in the accumulation of insoluble tau protein tangles. These aggregates of tau tangles impair cellular function and have been associated with cellular death [7]. Following traumatic brain injury tau proteins are released into the CSF and serum [8]. It is this extracellular tau protein that is the focus of many studies evaluating traumatic brain injury.

14.3 Tau as a biomarker in cerebral spinal fluid

Tau proteins measured in the CSF of individuals with traumatic brain injury have been found to be higher than those in healthy individuals and patients with other tauopathies [9]. Neselius et al. investigated the impact of acute traumatic brain injury in 30 Olympic boxers. CSF tau protein levels were measured 1–6 days after a boxing match and also after resting for 14 days. The levels of tau protein in the CSF were found to be elevated when compared to the control group, thus suggesting the association between traumatic brain injury and elevated tau protein levels [10]. Studies have also shown an association between tau protein levels in the CSF and poor prognosis and recovery after traumatic brain injury [9,11]. Zemlan et al. compared initial tau levels in the CSF, initial Glasgow Coma Scale (GCS) and elevated intracranial pressure as predictors of clinical outcomes. They found that patients with traumatic brain injury had tau protein levels 40,000 times higher than the levels normally found in the CSF of healthy individuals. The study also found that individuals with poorer outcomes based on the Glasgow Outcome Scale (GOS) at discharge had tau protein levels 10 times higher than individuals with good outcomes [9]. One of the limitations of this study was that the latency period between the initial traumatic brain injury and collection of tau protein was not studied. Variability in arrival time to the hospital and collection time may affect the degree of tau elevation. Similar results were noted in a study by Ost et al., researchers in this study found that patients with severe traumatic brain injury (GCS 3–8) had tau protein levels in the CSF greater than 702 pg/mL. CSF tau protein levels greater than 702 pg/mL were associated with poor outcomes as defined by an Extended Glasgow Outcome Score (GOS-E) of 1–4 [12].

14.4 Tau as a biomarker in the blood

Tau protein as a biomarker in blood would be advantageous over the need to identify tau proteins in CSF as it would be more cost-effective and can be collected much quicker and less invasively than CSF fluid. Studies in military personnel with a history of traumatic brain injury have found increased serum levels of tau proteins in their serum suggesting that tau protein may be a useful biomarker in the evaluation of traumatic brain injury [13]. Liliang et al. collected serum tau levels on patients who arrived to the hospital within 6 hours of suffering severe traumatic brain injury as defined by a GCS equal to or less than 8. Patients with good outcome, as defined by GOS, were found to have average serum tau protein levels of 51.6 pg/mL, while patients with poor outcomes were found to have an average serum tau protein level of 436.2 pg/mL. The receiver operating characteristic curve demonstrated that a tau protein level greater than or equal to 114 pg/mL had a 88% sensitivity and 94% specificity for predicting poor outcomes [14]. This study also suggests that there is an association between elevated tau protein levels in the serum, severity of brain injury, and poor prognosis. A study by Wang et al. also examined serum tau protein levels in patients with traumatic brain injury. Their serum tau protein levels were compared to their initial GCS and GOS-E at 1 year. Serum tau protein levels in all degrees of traumatic brain injury peaked around 2 days after brain injury. It was also noted that tau protein levels were significantly higher in patients with severe traumatic brain injury compared to those with mild or moderate traumatic brain injury. Tau protein levels >116.04 mg/mL on day 2 resulted in a 93.75% sensitivity and 92.5% specificity for predicting a poor outcome. Patients with a tau protein level >372.1 pg/mL on day 2 had a 100% sensitivity and 83.33% specificity for 1-year mortality in the severe traumatic brain injury group [3]. Like the Liliang study, this highlights the association between elevated serum tau proteins levels, severity of injury, and future prognosis.

On the other hand, some studies have found serum tau proteins to be unreliable as early biomarkers for the detection of traumatic brain injury, in particular patients with mild traumatic brain injury [15]. Wuthisuthimethawee et al. studied 44 patients with mild traumatic brain injury defined by GCS 13–15 on arrival. The average blood collection time was less than 1 hour from injury. Tau protein levels above .1 pg/dL were not detected in any of the study participants [15]. It is suspected that tau protein levels in this study were not detected in the serum as there is likely a latency period from the time of axonal injury and the transportation of tau proteins into the serum. In another study, Bulut et al. investigated the diagnostic value of serum tau proteins in individuals with mild traumatic brain injury. Although the study found serum tau protein levels were mildly higher in individuals with mild traumatic brain injury, the study did not demonstrate a statistical difference between serum tau proteins levels after mild traumatic brain injury and those of the healthy patients in the control group [16]. Kavalci et al. evaluated the correlation between serum tau protein concentrations and abnormal cranial CT after traumatic brain injury and also concluded that tau protein levels, although elevated, were not statistically significant in their study when compared to the control group [17]. Although some studies have shown that any detectable level of tau protein in the serum is associated with a greater likelihood of intracranial injury and poorer outcome, others have noted limitations of tau as a serum biomarker [18]. More studies are needed to further evaluate the possibility of the use of tau protein as a serum biomarker.

14.5 Conclusion

Since tau proteins were first described in 1975, tau proteins have been studied as potential biomarkers for use in clinical medicine. Researchers have been hard at work to identify a biomarker with high enough specificity and sensitivity to be used as a tool to facilitate diagnoses, risk stratification, and prognosis of patients after traumatic brain injury. Although further studies will be needed to better assess the quantitative and temporal variations of tau protein levels in the CSF and serum after traumatic brain injury, studies have shown an association between elevations of tau proteins and severity of injury and future outcomes. Evidence thus far suggests that tau proteins may prove useful as a biomarker for traumatic brain injury.

References

[1] Guskiewicz KM. Association between recurrent concussion and late-life cognitive impairment in retired professional football players. Neurosurgery 2005;57(4):719−26; discussion 719-26.
[2] Goedert M. Propagation of tau aggregates. Mol Brain 2017;10(1):18.
[3] McKee AC, Stein TD, Nowinski CJ, et al. The spectrum of disease in chronic traumatic encephalopathy. Brain 2013;136(1):43−64.
[4] Wang J. Serum τ protein as a potential biomarker in the assessment of traumatic brain injury. Exp Ther Med 2016;11(3):1147−51.
[5] Weingarten MD. A protein factor essential for microtubule assembly. Proc Natl Acad Sci USA 05/1975;72 (5):1858−62.
[6] Grundke-Iqbal I. Abnormal phosphorylation of the microtubule-associated protein tau (tau) in Alzheimer cytoskeletal pathology. Proc Natl Acad Sci USA 07/1986;83(13):4913−17.
[7] Agoston DV. Biofluid biomarkers of traumatic brain injury. Brain Inj. 2017;31(9):1195−203.
[8] Takahashi K. Serum tau protein level serves as a predictive factor for neurological prognosis in neonatal asphyxia. Brain Dev 2014;36(8):670−5.
[9] Zemlan FP. C-tau biomarker of neuronal damage in severe brain injured patients: association with elevated intracranial pressure and clinical outcome. Brain Res 2002;947(1):131−9.
[10] Neselius S. CSF-biomarkers in olympic boxing: diagnosis and effects of repetitive head trauma. PLoS One 2012;7(4):e33606.
[11] Magnoni S. Tau elevations in the brain extracellular space correlate with reduced amyloid-β levels and predict adverse clinical outcomes after severe traumatic brain injury. Brain 2012;135:1268−80.
[12] Ost M. Initial CSF total tau correlates with 1-year outcome in patients with traumatic brain injury. Neurology 2006;67(9):1600−4.
[13] Olivera A. Peripheral total tau in military personnel who sustain traumatic brain injuries during deployment. JAMA Neurol 2015;72(10):1109−16.
[14] Liliang P. Tau proteins in serum predict outcome after severe traumatic brain injury. J Surg Res 2010;160 (2):302−7.
[15] Wuthisuthimethawee P. Serum cleaved tau protein and traumatic mild head injury: a preliminary study in the Thai population. Eur J Trauma Emerg Surg 2013;39(3):293−6.
[16] Bulut M. Tau protein as a serum marker of brain damage in mild traumatic brain injury: preliminary results. Adv Ther 2006;23(1):12−22.
[17] Kavalci C. The value of serum tau protein for the diagnosis of intracranial injury in minor head trauma. Am J Emerg Med 2007;25(4):391−5.
[18] Shaw GJ. Serum cleaved tau protein levels and clinical outcome in adult patients with closed head injury. Ann Emerg Med 2002;39(3):254−7.

Novel TBI biomarkers

Neurogranin

Julian Pohlan[1], Bernd A. Leidel[2] and Tobias Lindner[3]

[1]Department of Radiology, Campus Mitte, Charité—Universitätsmedizin Berlin, Berlin,
Germany [2]Department of Emergency Medicine, Campus Benjamin Franklin, Charité—
Universitätsmedizin Berlin, Berlin, Germany [3]Department of Acute & Emergency Medicine,
Campus Virchow-Klinikum, Charité—Universitätsmedizin Berlin, Berlin, Germany

The protein neurogranin (Ng) is currently discussed as a future biomarker in traumatic brain injury (TBI). Ng levels in blood plasma and cerebrospinal fluid seem to reflect organ-specific damage to the brain. This chapter will explain the function of Ng in health and disease in the historical context. We will also provide an overview of the disease entities where the biomarker neurogranin might play a role in future.

15.1 Historical background

Neurogranin, abbreviated as Ng, was first mentioned in 1990 by Alfonso Represa and his colleagues. Electron microscopy localized Ng in granule-like structures of hippocampal and cortical pyramidal cells of the central nervous system (CNS) [1]. One year earlier, the researchers had already purified p17, later referred to as Ng, from the bovine brain [2]. Further ultrastructural analyses of neuronal tissue yielded a postsynaptic localization of Ng (see Fig. 15.1) [3]. It took another 8 years from its discovery to understand the underlying genetics in more detail [4]. The discovery of aberrant behavior in mice who lack Ng gave birth to analyses in pathological states of the brain [5,6]. Since then scientific interest in Ng has been growing steadily, with respect to preclinical as well as clinical research (see Fig. 15.2).

15.2 Physiologic function

Ng, or P17, is a relatively small 78-amino-acid protein of mainly intracellular localization. It is known to be a protein kinase C substrate [2].

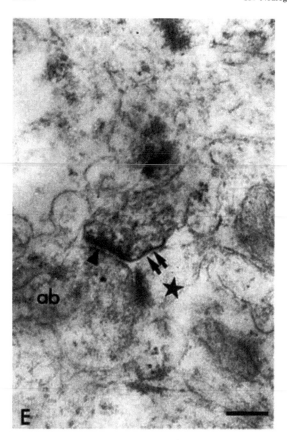

FIGURE 15.1 Ultrastructure with granular neurogranin immune reactivity in a dendritic spine head in cytoplasm, at the postsynaptic density (arrow head) and subsynaptic membrane (double arrows) [3].

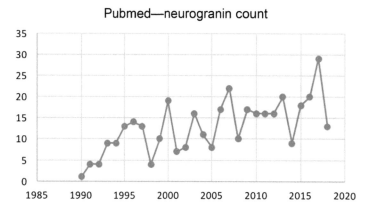

FIGURE 15.2 Count of neurogranin hits on PubMed over time.

Protein kinase C itself belongs to a multiisoform family of serine/threonine kinases involved in many physiological and pathological cellular processes. Principally, its translocation to cellular endomembranes, and thereby activation, depends on the presence of second messengers, such as calcium, diacylglycerol, and phosphatidylinositol 4,5-bisposphonate [7].

First, experimental induction of long-term potentiation (LTP) depends on the activation of PKC and subsequent Ng phosphorylation [8]. It has been shown that Ng phosphorylation by the PKC pathway lessens its binding probability with calmodulin (CaM), as depicted below. Ng phosphorylation also correlates with LTP magnitude, possibly reflecting Ng effects on memory [9].

Second, nonphosphorylated Ng binds to CaM in the presence of low intracellular calcium [10]. The Ca^{2+}/CaM complex can activate Ca^{2+}/CaM-dependent protein kinase II (CaMKII). As a downstream effect, LTP is fostered with enhanced synaptic transmission. Phosphorylation of Ng by PKC will lower the probability of binding CaM, thus modulating LTP [5,11]. Further, Ng binds both the N- and C-domains of CaM modulating calcium-binding kinetics. Both the availability and calcium saturation of CaM can be controlled by Ng. This provides interesting insights into calcium—CaM signaling in neurons [12]. Live-cell confocal microscopy shows that CaM in dendritic spines is mainly mobile. The diffusion rate of CaM seems to be regulated by Ng. Correspondingly, the effect of Ng on synaptic strength can partly be explained by targeting CaM within dendritic spines [13]. It is known that in the resting state there are low levels of free CaM, most of it bound to Ng or GAP-43. As predicted by simulations, LTP is strongly diminished in knockout of Ng. Upon induction of LTP, CaM seems to be provided mainly by rapidly dissociating CaM—Ng complexes [14].

Third, Ng can associate with cellular endomembranes upon binding to phosphatidic acid (PA). Phosphorylation by PKC will prevent Ng binding to PA [15]. In low-calcium states CaM binding to Ng will inhibit its binding to PA. It has been proposed that PA allows the recruitment of Ng to intracellular areas of demand [16,17].

Ng also seems to be critical for activation of α-amino-3-hydroxy-5-methyl-4-isoxazole-propionic acid (AMPA) receptors. Loss of Ng will consequently lead to sensitized long-term synaptic depression (LTD) as seen in the mouse visual cortex [18].

As a conclusion, Ng plays an important role in linking PKC and Ca/CaM messaging with relevance for synaptic plasticity. The complex interplay between Ng and memory-relevant neuronal structures remains partly to be elucidated [16]. (Fig. 15.3)

Ng gene (NRGN) encodes the aforementioned brain-specific protein. It is a 12-kb gene with four exons and three introns lying at Chromosome 11 (11q24). Mature mRNA spans 1.3 kb. Comparison with rat and goat protein yielded minimal changes in amino acids with no change in binding capacity to CaM or PKC [4]. Importantly, thyroid hormones were found to control NRGN expression [19].

The physiologic function of Ng is also implied by knockout experiments. Ng null mutant ($Ng^{-/-}$) mice were found to be viable animals with impaired memory function as well as altered emotional processing [5].

Morris water maze test and Barnes maze revealed deficits in spatial navigation of $Ng^{-/-}$ mice. Heterozygote $Ng^{+/-}$ were not significantly different from wild-type controls. The authors concluded that one allele of the NRGN might yield sufficient protein concentrations in the CNS. Besides the memory impairment, the authors noted anxiety-related behaviors in Ng-deficient mice. Confirmed by the light—dark transition test, the authors hypothesized an altered stress response in $Ng^{-/-}$ mice. Knockout of Ng might therefore produce an anxiety-like phenotype with consequences for learning and memory [6]. Accordingly, Ng enrichment leads to the reversal of neurocognitive defects in Ng null mutant mice [20].

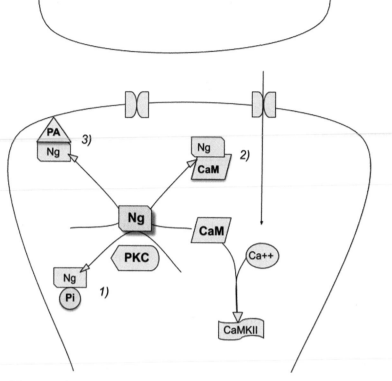

FIGURE 15.3   Schematic of neurogranin function and states in cellular processes, that is, the postsynaptic cell in the central nervous system.
1. PKC-mediated phosphorylation of Ng.
2. CaM associates with Ng in the absence of Calcium.
3. Ng is associated with membranes upon binding with PA.
PA, phosphatidic acid; *Ng*, neurogranin; *CaM*, calmodulin; *PKC*, protein kinase C; *Ca*$^{2+}$, calcium; *CaMKII*, Ca^{2+}/CaM-dependent protein kinase II. The membranous pores are representative of different channels such as N-methyl-D-aspartate receptor (*NMDA-R*) and α-amino-3-hydroxy-5-methyl-4-isoxazolepropionic acid (*AMPA-R*). *Source: Adapted from Diez-Guerra FJ. Neurogranin, a link between calcium/calmodulin and protein kinase C signaling in synaptic plasticity. IUBMB Life 2010;62(8):597–606.*

15.3 Pathophysiology of brain disorders

Ng expression and localization seem to be altered in pathological states of neuronal tissue. The following part of this chapter will guide the reader through different brain-specific disease entities. In disease, Ng has been found to be displaced from its intracellular location into the extracellular space and thus in blood and cerebrospinal fluid. Using those two biofluids, Ng quantification will mirror neuronal disintegration.

15.3.1 Neurodegeneration

Research on rodent models of Alzheimer's disease (AD) suggests that Ng can restore amyloid β—mediated impairment of synaptic transmission, thereby underlining its role in the pathogenesis [11]. As synaptic degeneration progresses in AD, Ng will be released from postsynaptic structures into adjacent tissue [21]. It has been found that especially CSF Ng concentrations seem to mirror the disease activity in humans [22]. One study found specific elevations of Ng in AD, compared with vascular dementia and other types of dementia. Apparently, different epitopes can be used for targeting Ng as three CSF tests were evaluated as equivalent [23]. Others confirmed the specifically elevated CSF Ng in AD compared with healthy subjects and frontotemporal dementia in a cross-sectional study. The authors also found significant correlation of CSF Ng with total tau and hyper-phosphorylated tau in CSF, that is, current standard biomarkers of AD [22].

More recently, Ng has been evaluated in mild cognitive impairment (MCI) which is considered an early stage of AD. With CSF Ng levels being high, patients also had poor baseline memory scores. Also, CSF Ng predicted memory as well as executive function decline over time. In fact, the highest levels of Ng in CSF were associated with a rapid decline of memory and executive function in patients. The authors claimed a prognostic relevance of Ng in MCI and AD given their results [24].

Similarly, a potential role of Ng has recently been described in Parkinson's disease (PD). The authors found that overexpressed α-synuclein can bind Ng in mice. They correlated this with altered interaction of Ng and α-synuclein in human brains of patients with PD. Besides, phosphorylated Ng levels were decreased in the superior temporal cortex of human brains in PD [25].

15.3.2 Neuroinflammation

One study found that Ng reflects disease activity in relapsing remitting multiple sclerosis with response to treatment. This further highlights a potential role of Ng in the evaluation of new therapies in chronic diseases of the brain [26].

15.3.3 Neuropsychiatric conditions

Ng variants were found to be related to schizophrenia [27,28]. A meta-analysis of genome-wide association studies confirmed rs12807809 variation in the Ng gene to be significantly associated with schizophrenia [29].

Another group used functional magnetic resonance tomography to evaluate healthy subjects' performances in cognitive tests after genotyping for NRGN rs12807809. Interestingly, the NRGN variants was associated with differential neural functioning in the anterior and posterior cingulum, that is, areas of episodic memory processing known to be dysfunctional in schizophrenia [30].

Surprisingly, evaluation in Huntington's disease yielded that CSF Ng does not reflect disease processes [31].

Interestingly, Ng in the nucleus accumbens interfered with tolerance induction via ethanol exposure in a preclinical model. Concluding, dysfunctional or absent Ng might increase susceptibility to addiction [32]. Along this line, chronic cocaine abuse decreased the expression of Ng in mice. Given the role of thyroid hormones in the expression of Ng the authors also evaluated thyroid receptor signaling. This revealed interference of cocaine with the required heterodimerization of thyroid hormone receptor and retinoid X receptor in Ng transcriptional activation [33].

15.3.4 Neurovascular

Ng has been evaluated in acute ischemic stroke with measurement of plasma and CSF Ng in 50 patients. The correlation of CSF Ng with stroke volume yielded a cutoff of 5 mL stroke volume as assessed with magnetic resonance imaging (MRI). Thus minor and major

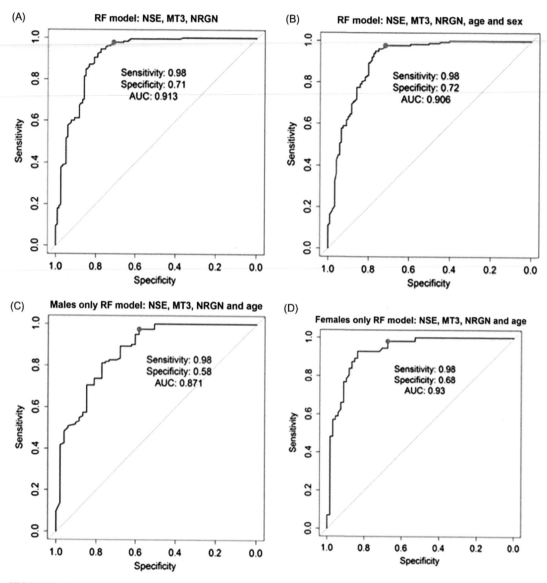

FIGURE 15.4 Receiver operator characteristics (ROC) curves for random forest models including Ng, MT3, and NSE with respect to age and gender [38].

strokes might be differentiated using Ng. Correspondingly, plasma Ng and stroke volume were positively correlated in this retrospective analysis [34].

15.4 Neurogranin and traumatic brain injury

With Ng being a brain-specific protein, a benefit in diagnosing TBI was hypothesized. One of the major advantages of Ng is clearly that it can be measured in whole blood samples. Research now partly aims at evaluating a potential role of Ng in avoiding CT overuse in mild TBI (mTBI).

Yang et al. assessed Serum neurogranin ELISA in TBI and healthy controls with 76 TBI in total. The authors found significantly elevated Ng values in TBI compared with healthy controls, although the control group differed significantly from TBI cases—age, gender, and race were all significantly different in both groups. One other limitation to this study is the asymmetric group size with possible overestimation of the effect size [35].

Unexpectedly, Shahim et al. did not find significant Ng elevations in CSF samples from 16 patients with postconcussion syndrome as compared with neurologically healthy controls. However, the sample size was comparatively small. In addition, the study assessed Ng in chronic trauma and not acutely elevated Ng values after a defined hit [36].

The investigators of the HeadSMART study enrolled patients with TBI for longitudinal assessment. Biomarkers including Ng were evaluated in addition to standard clinical, neuropsychological, and CT examinations [37]. A recent analysis from the HeadSMART trial assessed a three-biomarker panel of Ng, neuron-specific enolase, and metallothionein 3 (MT3) in patients with mild traumatic brain injury (mTBI). The study included a total of 179 mTBI patients compared with healthy controls. The results suggest a benefit of combined biomarker testing for an accurate diagnosis of mTBI with accuracy rates varying from 72%–100% (see Fig. 15.4). In particular, early samples taken less than 2 hours from the incident seemed to be predictive with 100% accuracy. However, the study had a limited number of probes in this subgroup (10/10) [38].

Further high-quality studies are needed to confirm these results and confirm the role of Ng in establishing a diagnosis of TBI or mTBI.

15.5 Conclusions

- Ng might serve as a biomarker for traumatic brain injury in future.
- Ng can be measured both in cerebrospinal fluid and serum.
- Mentioned first in 1990, after its discovery in bovine brain isolates, interest in the brain-specific protein has strongly increased.
- In concert with other biomarkers, the use of Ng measurement could help avoid cranial computed tomography (cCT) overuse and thereby reduce radiation exposure in patients with TBI.
- Literature suggests that Ng might add to the diagnostic repertoire in other brain-related disorders such as Alzheimer's or stroke.

- Replication of data as well as more high-quality, prospective studies are needed in order to establish Ng as a biomarker.

References

[1] Represa A, Deloulme JC, Sensenbrenner M, Ben-Ari Y, Baudier J. Neurogranin: immunocytochemical localization of a brain-specific protein kinase C substrate. J Neurosci 1990;10(12):3782–92.

[2] Baudier J, Bronner C, Kligman D, Cole RD. Protein kinase C substrates from bovine brain. Purification and characterization of neuromodulin, a neuron-specific calmodulin-binding protein. J Biol Chem 1989;264 (3):1824–8.

[3] Neuner-Jehle M, Denizot J-P, Mallet J. Neurogranin is locally concentrated in rat cortical and hippocampal neurons. Brain Res 1996;733(1):149–54.

[4] Martinez de Arrieta C, Perez Jurado L, Bernal J, Coloma A. Structure, organization, and chromosomal mapping of the human neurogranin gene (NRGN). Genomics 1997;41(2):243–9.

[5] Pak JH, Huang FL, Li J, et al. Involvement of neurogranin in the modulation of calcium/calmodulin-dependent protein kinase II, synaptic plasticity, and spatial learning: a study with knockout mice. Proc Natl Acad Sci USA 2000;97(21):11232–7.

[6] Miyakawa T, Yared E, Pak JH, Huang FL, Huang KP, Crawley JN. Neurogranin null mutant mice display performance deficits on spatial learning tasks with anxiety related components. Hippocampus 2001;11 (6):763–75.

[7] Igumenova TI. Dynamics and membrane interactions of protein kinase C. Biochemistry 2015;54(32):4953–68.

[8] Chen S-J, Sweatt JD, Klann E. Enhanced phosphorylation of the postsynaptic protein kinase C substrate RC3/neurogranin during long-term potentiation. Brain Res 1997;749(2):181–7.

[9] Zhong L, Kaleka KS, Gerges NZ. Neurogranin phosphorylation fine-tunes long-term potentiation. Eur J Neurosci 2011;33(2):244–50.

[10] Gerendasy DD, Sutcliffe JG. RC3/neurogranin, a postsynaptic calpacitin for setting the response threshold to calcium influxes. Mol Neurobiol 1997;15(2):131–63.

[11] Kaleka KS, Gerges NZ. Neurogranin restores amyloid beta-mediated synaptic transmission and long-term potentiation deficits. Exp Neurol 2016;277:115–23.

[12] Hoffman L, Chandrasekar A, Wang X, Putkey JA, Waxham MN. Neurogranin alters the structure and calcium binding properties of calmodulin. J Biol Chem 2014;289(21):14644–55.

[13] Petersen A, Gerges NZ. Neurogranin regulates CaM dynamics at dendritic spines. Sci Rep 2015;5:11135.

[14] Zhabotinsky AM, Camp RN, Epstein IR, Lisman JE. Role of the neurogranin concentrated in spines in the induction of long-term potentiation. J Neurosci 2006;26(28):7337–47.

[15] Domínguez-González I, Vázquez-Cuesta Silvia N, Algaba A, Díez-Guerra FJ. Neurogranin binds to phosphatidic acid and associates to cellular membranes. Biochemical J 2007;404(1):31–43.

[16] Diez-Guerra FJ. Neurogranin, a link between calcium/calmodulin and protein kinase C signaling in synaptic plasticity. IUBMB Life 2010;62(8):597–606.

[17] Zhong L, Cherry T, Bies CE, Florence MA, Gerges NZ. Neurogranin enhances synaptic strength through its interaction with calmodulin. EMBO J 2009;28(19):3027–39.

[18] Han KS, Cooke SF, Xu W. Experience-dependent equilibration of AMPAR-mediated synaptic transmission during the critical period. Cell Rep 2017;18(4):892–904.

[19] de Arrieta CM, Morte B, Coloma A, Bernal J. The human RC3 gene homolog, NRGN contains a thyroid hormone-responsive element located in the first intron. Endocrinology 1999;140(1):335–43.

[20] Huang FL, Huang K-P, Boucheron C. Long-term enrichment enhances the cognitive behavior of the aging neurogranin null mice without affecting their hippocampal LTP. Learn Mem 2007;14(8):512–19.

[21] Lista S, Hampel H. Synaptic degeneration and neurogranin in the pathophysiology of Alzheimer's disease. Expert Rev Neurother 2017;17(1):47–57.

[22] Lista S, Toschi N, Baldacci F, et al. Cerebrospinal fluid neurogranin as a biomarker of neurodegenerative diseases: a cross-sectional study. J Alzheimers Dis 2017;59(4):1327–34.

[23] Willemse EAJ, De Vos A, Herries EM, et al. Neurogranin as cerebrospinal fluid biomarker for Alzheimer disease: an assay comparison study. Clin Chem 2018.

[24] Headley A, De Leon-Benedetti A, Dong C, et al. Neurogranin as a predictor of memory and executive function decline in MCI patients. Neurology 2018;90(10):e887–95.

[25] Koob AO, Shaked GM, Bender A, Bisquertt A, Rockenstein E, Masliah E. Neurogranin binds alpha-synuclein in the human superior temporal cortex and interaction is decreased in Parkinson's disease. Brain Res 2014;1591:102–10.

[26] Novakova L, Axelsson M, Khademi M, et al. Cerebrospinal fluid biomarkers as a measure of disease activity and treatment efficacy in relapsing-remitting multiple sclerosis. J Neurochemistry 2017;141(2):296–304.

[27] Stefansson H, Ophoff RA, Steinberg S, et al. Common variants conferring risk of schizophrenia. Nature 2009;460(7256):744–7.

[28] Shen YC, Tsai HM, Cheng MC, Hsu SH, Chen SF, Chen CH. Genetic and functional analysis of the gene encoding neurogranin in schizophrenia. Schizophr Res 2012;137(1–3):7–13.

[29] Donohoe G, Walters J, Morris DW, et al. A neuropsychological investigation of the genome wide associated schizophrenia risk variant NRGN rs12807809. Schizophr Res 2011;125(2):304–6.

[30] Krug A, Krach S, Jansen A, et al. The effect of neurogranin on neural correlates of episodic memory encoding and retrieval. Schizophr Bull 2013;39(1):141–50.

[31] Byrne LM, Rodrigues FB, Johnson EB, et al. Cerebrospinal fluid neurogranin and TREM2 in Huntington's disease. Sci Rep 2018;8(1):4260.

[32] Reker AN, Oliveros A, Sullivan 3rd JM, et al. Neurogranin in the nucleus accumbens regulates NMDA receptor tolerance and motivation for ethanol seeking. Neuropharmacology 2018;131:58–67.

[33] Kovalevich J, Corley G, Yen W, Kim J, Rawls SM, Langford D. Cocaine decreases expression of neurogranin via alterations in thyroid receptor/retinoid X receptor signaling. J Neurochemistry 2012;121(2):302–13.

[34] De Vos A, Bjerke M, Brouns R, et al. Neurogranin and tau in cerebrospinal fluid and plasma of patients with acute ischemic stroke. BMC Neurol 2017;17(1):170.

[35] Yang J, Korley FK, Dai M, Everett AD. Serum neurogranin measurement as a biomarker of acute traumatic brain injury. Clin Biochem 2015;48(13–14):843–8.

[36] Shahim P, Tegner Y, Gustafsson B, et al. Neurochemical aftermath of repetitive mild traumatic brain injury. JAMA Neurol 2016;73(11):1308–15.

[37] Peters ME, Rao V, Bechtold KT, et al. Head injury serum markers for assessing response to trauma: design of the HeadSMART study. Brain Inj 2017;31(3):370–8.

[38] Peacock WF, Van Meter TE, Mirshahi N, et al. Derivation of a three biomarker panel to improve diagnosis in patients with mild traumatic brain injury. Front Neurol 2017;8:641.

Myelin basic protein in traumatic brain injury

Stanley L. Wu

Baylor College of Medicine, Houston, TX, United States

16.1 Myelin basic protein

Myelin in the central nervous system (CNS) is derived from the plasma membrane of the oligodendrocyte and in the peripheral nervous system formed from Schwann cells. In 1962 it was described as consisting of two major proteins: a proteolipid and a basic protein, also referred to as the A1 protein [1]. When injected at low levels in Freund's adjuvant, the A1 protein induces experimental allergic encephalomyelitis, which is a demyelinating paralytic disease. This had been reproduced in many animal and human studies [2−4]. Today, the structure of Myelin basic protein (MBP) is much more well described. It is a protein involved in the myelination of axons in the CNS and functions to maintain the structure of the nerves, but more importantly it provides insulation to impulse conduction and more precisely increase the transmission of action potentials across the myelinated axons [5].

In CNS myelin is approximately 30%−40% water, 70%−80% lipid, and 15%−25% protein [5−7]. The protein component includes myelin basic protein, myelin oligodendrocyte glycoprotein and proteolipid protein. The lipid components include, galactocerebroside which is the most abundant, sphingomyelin which strengthens the myelin sheath, and cholesterol, which is essential to myelin formation [5].

In this chapter we will begin with our current knowledge of myelin in the scientific literature. Because MPB is the major component of myelin we will make the assumption that studies that are measuring myelin and those which study MPB are nearly equivalent. To date, there is very little exploration of the use of MPB as a marker for traumatic brain injury, but we can make some basic theories based on the current literature about what we can expect to expand in the near future when measuring MBP in these clinical situations.

221

16.1.1 Myelin and multiple sclerosis

Myelin's association with demyelination is much better known in the pathophysiology of MS, which is a chronic autoimmune, inflammatory neurologic disease of the CNS. Antibodies destroy the myelin and cause varying degrees of axonal damage [8]. Often cerebral spinal fluid (CSF) is sampled to look for MBP. In some studies, varying levels of MBP seem to indicate disease severity. Levels greater than 9 ng/mL are suggestive of active demyelinating disease. Levels between 4 and 8 ng/mL suggest slowly progressive, chronic disease or recovery from an acute episode of myelin breakdown. Levels less than 4 ng/mL indicate remission or no myelin breakdown [9,10]. However, other studies have shed light on the wide variation in MBP's specificity for MS [11]. Greene published a retrospective cross-sectional study of 16,690 CSF samples comparing the performance of MBP and two other CSF markers for diagnosis of MS: oligoclonal bands (OCB) and immunoglobulin G (IgG) index. Greene found that MBP did not increase diagnostic sensitivity or specificity when used in combination with OCB and/or IgG index and concluded that MBP is unnecessary and overused. Other non-MS-related causes of MBP found in CSF at elevated levels include bleeding of the CNS, CNS trauma, certain encephalopathies, infections of the CNS, and stroke [12].

While MBP may be too nonspecific for the differentiation of MS from other types of central demyelinating diseases, we explore the possibility of its use in traumatic brain injury (TBI). Because the myelin sheath insulates axons, we know that axonal damage will therefore cause myelin damage in traumatic brain injury. In a study of 25 TBI cases with 57 controls, MBP concentrations for the test group after 5 days was markedly greater than the controls (10.49 +/− 6.97 vs. 0.11 +/− 0.01 ng/mL, $P < .01$). This small study lends support for the use of MBP as a marker in TBI [13].

The level of CSF MBP in TBI may be relevant, but perhaps calcium should be looked at more closely as the causative agent to nerve damage, as suggested by a 2013 study published in *Brain Sciences*. A group of researchers studied 66 guinea pig optic nerves and applied a 2-hour stretch to them and measured their outcomes. Using electron microscopy, the authors found that central myelin injury contributes to axonal degeneration following traumatic brain injury and they hypothesized that elevated levels of calcium disrupt MBP and potentiate areas of myelin delamination secondary to increased waves of calcium depolarization [14].

Perhaps measuring serum or CSF myelin is not the optimal approach, and instead advanced neuroimaging as a surrogate of the brain chemistry is more effective. Spader and Dean studied collegiate football and rugby sports players brains in an attempt to identify early minor TBI using MRI. The researchers measured myelin water fraction as a surrogate to measure myelin content in 12 male players with a minor TBI and compared them with 10 nonplayers brains. The study was then repeated after 3 months. While the impact is small with such a small sample, the study found that myelin water fraction was higher in the brains of the players versus the nonplayers. The authors concede that it is uncertain if the increased myelin was a reflection of axon neuropathology or disorderly remyelination causing hypermyelination [15].

A similar study of 11 hockey players after one mild TBI showed transiently reduced myelin water fraction at 2 weeks post injury and recovered by 2 months post injury [16]. Again, larger cohorts need to be studied.

A systematic review of published literature on advanced neuroimaging, fluid biomarkers, and genetic testing in the assessment of sport-related concussions was published in 2017. This was a comprehensive search of Medline, PubMed, CINAHL, PsycInfo, Scopus, and Cochrane Library from January 2000 to December 2016 in which 98 studies were included, 76 of which were on neuroimaging, 16 on biomarkers, and six on genetic testing. All studies were graded on the quality of the data and the level of evidence obtained. Their conclusion was that there is some importance for these types of tests, however, the level of which is still undetermined and requires further validation [17]. The result of this study was then used in part in the 2017 published consensus article by the Concussion in Sport Group on concussion in children and adolescents which concluded that the use of biomarkers in the assessment or management of sports-related concussions has "limited application" and that there is "a need for more objective means to assess the presence/severity of sports related concussions in athletes" [18].

16.1.2 Summary and future study

The paucity of current research and sound data on myelin basic protein in cases of TBI is highlighted by the "limited" endorsement by the Concussion in Sport Group. With the current knowledge, MBP is at best a nonspecific marker of past TBI. We could extrapolate current data on MS research and myelin to extend to traumatic brain injury patients, however, there are no studies regarding the temporal relationship between levels of MPB and a traumatic brain injury, or the differentiation between acute versus chronic brain injury, specifically. Future studies should focus on narrowing down its level of sensitivity and specificity. Perhaps the marker could be used as a negative predicative marker for the lack of traumatic brain injury. Currently no such studies exist.

References

[1] Bunge MB, Bunge RP, Pappas GD. Electron microscopic demonstration of connections between glia and myelin sheaths in the developing mammalian central nervous system. J Cell Biol 1962;12:448–53. Available from: https://doi.org/10.1083/jcb.12.2.448.

[2] Einstein ER, Robertson DM, Dicaprio JM, Moore W. The isolation from bovine spinal cord of a homogeneous protein with encephalitogenic activity. J Neurochem 1962;9:353–61.

[3] Eylar EH, Salk J, Beveridge GC, Brown LV. Experimental allergic encephalomyelitis. An encephalitogenic basic protein from bovine myelin. Arch Biochem Biophys 1969;132(1):34–48.

[4] Kies MW, Thompson EB, Alvord EC. The relationship of myelin proteins to experimental allergic encephalomyelitis. Ann NY Acad Sci 1965;122:148–60.

[5] Salzer JL, Zalc B. Myelination. Curr Biol 2016;26(20):R971–5. Available from: https://doi.org/10.1016/j.cub.2016.07.074.

[6] Chrast R, Saher G, Nave KA, Verheijen MH. Lipid metabolism in myelinating glial cells: lessons from human inherited disorders and mouse models. J Lipid Res 2011;52(3):419–34. Available from: https://doi.org/10.1194/jlr.R009761.

[7] Stoffel W, Bosio A. Myelin glycolipids and their functions. Curr Opin Neurobiol 1997;7(5):654–61. Available from: https://doi.org/10.1016/s0959-4388(97)80085-2.

[8] Goldenberg MM. Multiple sclerosis review. P T 2012;37(3):175–84.

[9] Ohta M, Ohta K. Detection of myelin basic protein in cerebrospinal fluid. Expert Rev Mol Diagn 2002;2(6):627–33. Available from: https://doi.org/10.1586/14737159.2.6.627.

[10] Cohen SR, Herndon RM, McKhann GM. Radioimmunoassay of myelin basic protein in spinal fluid. An index of active demyelination. N Engl J Med 1976;295(26):1455−7. Available from: https://doi.org/10.1056/NEJM197612232952604.

[11] Greene DN, Schmidt RL, Wilson AR, Freedman MS, Grenache DG. Cerebrospinal fluid myelin basic protein is frequently ordered but has little value: a test utilization study. Am J Clin Pathol 2012;138(2):262−72. Available from: https://doi.org/10.1309/AJCPCYCH96QYPHJM.

[12] Mukherjee A, Vogt RF, Linthicum DS. Measurement of myelin basic protein by radioimmunoassay in closed head trauma, multiple sclerosis and other neurological diseases. Clin Biochem 1985;18(5):304−7.

[13] Su E, et al. Increased CSF concentrations of myelin basic protein after TBI in infants and children: absence of significant effect of therapeutic hypothermia. Neurocrit Care 2012;17(3):401−7. Available from: https://doi.org/10.1007/s12028-012-9767-0.

[14] Maxwell WL. Damage to myelin and oligodendrocytes: a role in chronic outcomes following traumatic brain injury? Brain Sci 2013;3(3):1374−94. Available from: https://doi.org/10.3390/brainsci3031374.

[15] Spader HS, et al. Prospective study of myelin water fraction changes after mild traumatic brain injury in collegiate contact sports. J Neurosurg 2018;1−9. Available from: https://doi.org/10.3171/2017.12.JNS171597.

[16] Wright AD, et al. Myelin water fraction is transiently reduced after a single mild traumatic brain injury—a prospective Cohort study in collegiate hockey players. PLoS One 2016;11(2):e0150215. Available from: https://doi.org/10.1371/journal.pone.0150215.

[17] McCrea M, et al. Role of advanced neuroimaging, fluid biomarkers and genetic testing in the assessment of sport-related concussion: a systematic review. Br J Sports Med 2017;51(12):919−29. Available from: https://doi.org/10.1136/bjsports-2016-097447.

[18] McCrory P, et al. Consensus statement on concussion in sport-the 5. Br J Sports Med 2017;51(11):838−47. Available from: https://doi.org/10.1136/bjsports-2017-097699.

Analytical testing consideration

Antibody selection, evaluation, and validation for analysis of traumatic brain injury biomarkers

Robert J. Webber[1], Richard M. Sweet[2] and Douglas S. Webber[1]

[1]Research & Diagnostic Antibodies, Las Vegas, NV, United States [2]School of Medicine, University of California San Francisco and Renal Department, Zuckerberg San Francisco General Hospital, San Francisco, CA, United States

17.1 Introduction

Man's quest for new knowledge, including new clinical diagnostic tests, innovative medical devices, and novel drug therapies for numerous medical conditions, has involved the development of better and more sophisticated tools, instruments, and analytical equipment to assist in the collection and analysis of data to answer ever increasingly complex questions. The tools used for biomedical investigation range from electron microscopes to interplanetary space stations and include biological molecules such as enzymes, proteins that function as a biological catalyst, and antibodies, immunoglobulins secreted by activated B lymphocytes as part of the adaptive immune response. The binding of an antibody to its epitope on the antigen is a prime example of exquisite three-dimensional molecular shape recognition and specificity at the antibody's binding site, and therein lays the immense utility of immunological methods and procedures. Antigen binding to an antibody has often been compared to a key fitting precisely into a lock. While this visual analogy is a good first approximation, it doesn't account for conformational epitopes nor for cross-reactions by structurally related molecules with weaker binding affinity/avidity due to an imperfect molecular fit into the antibody's binding site.

Three main types of antibodies are in current biomedical research use: polyclonal antisera, monoclonal antibodies, and recombinant antibodies. Each of these has their strengths and weaknesses compared to the other types. Recombinant chimeric antibodies are created by inserting the V_L and V_H domains with the desired antigen binding specificity onto the constant domains of another species' IgG immunoglobulin, for example the variable domains of a mouse monoclonal antibody onto a human IgG_1 backbone scaffold. The resulting mouse/human chimeric antibody retains only approximately 30% of the original mouse antibody amino acid sequence. Humanized antibodies are genetically engineered by grafting each of the complementarity determining regions (CDRs) from an antibody with the desired antigen binding specificity into the corresponding CDRs of another antibody, for example, grafting the CDRs from a mouse monoclonal antibody into a human IgG_1 antibody. The resulting humanized antibody only retains approximately 9% of the original mouse antibody amino acid sequence. By eliminating much or almost all of the mouse protein from the recombinant antibody, some types of interference in immunological procedures are abolished, such as interference from human antimouse antibodies (HAMA).

Antibodies of known antigen specificity are widely used in biomedical research for procedures such as Western immunoblots, immunohistochemistry, immunocytochemistry, flow cytometry, enzyme immunoassays (EIAs), affinity purification, and immunoprecipitation, and they are the cornerstones on which much basic research, drug development, and clinical in vitro diagnostic (IVD) tests are based. Brain-specific biomarkers for traumatic brain injury (TBI) in blood, serum, or plasma can be detected and quantitated using well-established and widely accepted immunoprocedures that are currently applied to the analysis of a variety of other types of biomarkers for various conditions. These same methods can also be applied to cerebral spinal fluid (CSF) samples, in addition to blood, serum, and plasma specimens. However, since biomarkers for TBI may only be present in extremely low concentrations, a highly sensitive analytical procedure will be necessary to accurately detect and measure any brain-specific analyte that can serve as a biomarker for TBI.

Locating an existing source of a desired antibody for a specific application or procedure is however often a daunting task, and sometimes isn't possible since an antibody may not have yet been developed for the specific antigen of interest or that is suitable for a particular immunotechnique [1,2]. Two initial concerns regarding any antibody used in an immunological procedure should be kept in mind while trying to find an appropriate antibody. One major concern is the quality of the antibody—it should be a high-quality antibody. Ideally, the antibody should be high titer, have a high affinity/avidity for its antigen, and have minimal nonspecific binding. The second major concern is recognizing that not every antibody is suitable for all types of immunological procedures. For example, an antibody might perform well in a Western blot but fail completely when used in an immunohistochemical staining procedure [3]. It should always be kept in mind that not all antibodies are suitable for all types of immunotechniques.

17.2 Finding the right antibody for a specific research application

A step-by-step guide of how to find a suitable antibody for a specific application is illustrated (Fig. 17.1) and described below, including how to evaluate the possible candidate antibodies [3–7], and how to validate the immunoprocedure using the selected antibody with points to consider as one progresses through the process [1–14]. Finding/locating an existing antibody that will serve a specific research purpose is often the most difficult and time-consuming part of the entire process [1,2]. There are hundreds of

Antibody Selection, Evaluation, and Validation Guide

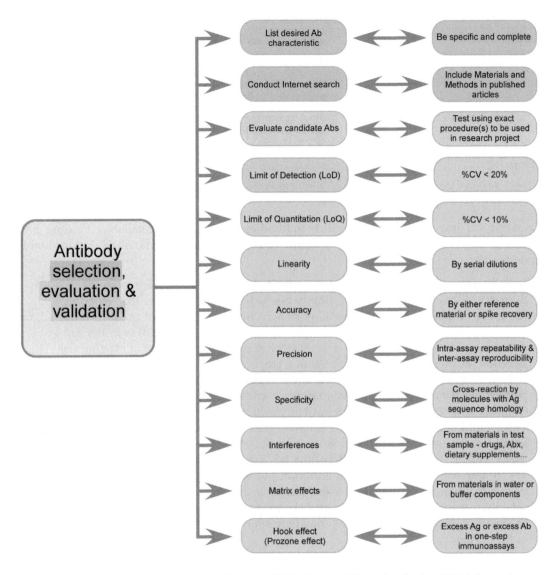

FIGURE 17.1   A step-by-step guide for antibody selection (highlighted in green), evaluation (highlighted in purple), and validation (highlighted in orange) for biomarkers of traumatic brain injury. *Ab*, antibody; *Abx*, antibiotics; *Ag*, antigen; %CV, percent coefficient of variation.

TABLE 17.1   Resource providers for guidelines to antibody selection, evaluation, and characterization and for immunoassay validation.

Resource provider	Website URL
PubMed	https://www.ncbi.nlm.nih.gov/pubmed/
Clinical and Laboratory Standards Institute	https://clsi.org/
FDA Office of In Vitro Diagnostics	https://www.fda.gov/medicaldevices/ productsandmedicalprocedures/invitrodiagnostics/default.htm
EU In Vitro Diagnostic Medical Devices	http://ec.europa.eu/growth/single-market/european-standards/ harmonised-standards/iv-diagnostic-medical-devices_en
National Biomarker Development Alliance [10]	http://nbdabiomarkers.org/
Research Resource Identifiers (RRIDs) [11]	https://scicrunch.org/resources/about/guidelines

thousands, if not millions, of research antibodies commercially available. Finding and selecting the best antibody for a specific research application is often a formidable undertaking.

1. Initially, try to list all the characteristics desired in the antibody. For example, is a fluorescent- or enzyme-labeled antibody needed, or is an antibody that will only recognize and bind to a single member of a multiprotein family of proteins required, or is an antibody that will immunoprecipitate its antigen necessary? It is important to define as many of the desired characteristics as possible *in advance* of starting the selection, evaluation, and assay validation steps.

   Note: It is also important to define the acceptance criteria in advance of actually performing the evaluation and validation procedures.
2. Conduct an internet search for an antibody with the desired characteristics (Table 17.1). This should also include searching the Materials and Methods sections of published literature, for example on the PubMed web site of the National Center for Biotechnology Information (NCBI) at the US National Library of Medicine.
3. Try to find at least three different antibodies to test and evaluate initially [10,11]. Also, be mindful that many distributors sell the same antibody under a different name and catalog number. If possible, try to find the primary producer of the antibody because they will probably be much more knowledgeable about the performance characteristics of the antibody.

17.3 Antibody evaluation and initial characterization

1. Test each of the antibodies to be evaluated for suitability in the immunological procedure under the *exact* conditions it will be used during the research project. Start with the three best candidates identified, and then if none of those meet the predefined acceptance criteria, test some additional antibodies. If none of the available antibodies

meet the acceptance criteria, consider other approaches, such as conducting another internet search using slightly different search parameters, or collaborating with someone who already has published using an antibody they developed, or revising the acceptance criteria. Alternatively, be prepared to develop the necessary antibody either in-house or under contract by a commercial supplier of custom antibodies.

2. Depending upon what information is already known about the antibody, it may be wise/prudent to conduct additional characterization studies. For example, it might be useful to check the antibody's affinity/avidity; or to epitope map the antibody's binding site on its antigen; or if the epitope is known, to use synthetic peptide analogs of the epitope to establish a competitive binding procedure or for peptide blocking experiments.

3. For an antibody that didn't perform well during the initial evaluation procedure, don't give up on it because it might be useful in some other procedure: for example, to affinity purify its antigen from a cell culture lysate. Just because an antibody didn't perform well in one procedure, doesn't necessarily mean it won't work well in a different type of immunoprocedure.

17.4 Immunological test method characteristics and validation

Once an antibody has been evaluated and met the evaluation acceptance criteria, the immunological test method to be used during the research project should be validated (Fig. 17.1). Validation procedures are conducted to ensure that the test method is accurate, specific, and reproducible over the concentration range that the analyte will be detected or measured [12−14]. All analytic immunological test procedures are indirect measurements of the antibody's analyte based upon the binding of the antibody to its epitope on the analyte. Standardization of each analytical test method depends upon measuring known quantities of either a reference standard or the purified analyte to generate a standard curve. The test result for an individual sample is calculated from the standard curve. However, since an international reference standard only exists for a very few clinically important immunoassays, analyte standardization remains an issue for the vast majority of analytic immunoassay tests. Calibrating immunoassays based upon different preparations of the analyte as standard material is very difficult to achieve. When developing an immunoassay for a biomarker for TBI, it would be prudent to build a large quantity of a primary in-house reference gold standard early during the validation process that can be stored stably and used periodically to calibrate secondary in-house assay standards. If an interlaboratory discrepancy develops, it can potentially be resolved and reconciled by comparing each laboratory's in-house gold standard.

Immunoassay validation provides an assurance of test method dependability during routine use. The specific types of procedures used to validate a test method vary for different types of immunoprocedures. Generally, validation studies include limit of detection (LoD); limit of quantitation (LoQ); linearity (by serial dilutions); accuracy (by spike recovery); precision (by intraassay repeatability and interassay reproducibility); specificity; interferences; and possibly also matrix effects and hook effect (prozone effect). Below are examples of performance characteristics often determined during validation studies on an immunological test method. This list is not meant to be all inclusive, nor should it be interpreted that all of these analytical/test methods are necessary applicable to all types of immunological test procedures.

1. The LoD is defined as the lowest amount of an analyte that can be detected in a sample with a (stated) probability [15,16]. Operationally, LoD is the lowest amount of an analyte that can be consistently differentiated from the absence of that substance in a sample with a stated level of confidence using a specific test procedure. The results of the tests can be evaluated by signal-to-noise ratio (S:N ratio) or by the percent coefficient of variation (%CV). Typically, the LoD is the amount of an analyte where the %CV declines to less than 20%.

2. The LoQ is defined as the lowest amount of an analyte that can be quantitatively determined in a sample with stated acceptance accuracy and precision, under stated experimental conditions [15,16]. Operationally, LoQ is the lowest amount of an analyte that can be accurately and reproducibly measured in a sample, and typically is the amount of an analyte where the %CV declines to less than 10%.

3. Linearity is tested by measuring serial dilutions of multiple samples spiked with high quantities of the analyte to determine the concentration vs. assay measurement relationship across a range of concentrations using a specific analytical procedure [17]. If a linear relationship is not found, a nonlinear mathematical model can be used. The aim is to develop a mathematical model, either linear or nonlinear, that approximates the concentration vs. measurement relationship as closely as possible.

4. Accuracy of a test method is defined as how close the test results are for a specific analyte as compared to the true amount of the analyte contained in the sample tested [18−22]. If available, accuracy can be determined using certified reference material. Alternatively, accuracy can be established through spike recovery experiments: it is calculated as the difference between the average value determined and the true value and is reported with confidence intervals.

5. Precision is usually assessed by determining the intraassay repeatability and interassay reproducibility of an immunological test method [19−22]. Intraassay %CVs less than 10% and interassay %CVs less than 15% are generally acceptable for most types of analytical immunoprocedures. These values primarily reflect and are closely related to the technical performance of an immunological test method by the person performing the test.

6. Specificity is the ability to unmistakably detect or measure the analyte of interest by an immunological test method in the presence of other sample components [23]. An antibody's epitope is typically only six to eight amino acids long, and therefore usually just a small part of the whole analyte. Thus molecules similar to the analyte that contain the same sequence will also bind to the antibody during analytical test procedures, and depending upon the type of immunoassay being performed, their binding can lead to incorrectly high test results (a false positive) or incorrectly low test results (a false negative). The types of molecules that can cause interference in immunoassays include pre- and proforms of the analyte; degradation fragments of the analyte that retain the epitope, such as lower molecular weight bands in Western immunoblots; and structurally related molecules that contain a region with sequence homology to the

analyte's epitope, such as other members of a multiprotein family of proteins. For example, neuronal nitric oxide synthase (nNOS) is involved in neural transmission and is a member of the nitric oxide synthase family of isozymes (EC 1.14.13.39). This family of three structurally related isozymes also includes the inducible (iNOS) and the endothelial (eNOS) forms of the enzyme, and each form has very different physiological functions. All three enzymes produce NO, and they share approximately 60%−70% homology in their respective DNA and amino acid sequences. However, if investigating nNOS as a possible biomarker for TBI using an antibody that binds to a region where the amino acids are the same, the immunoassay will not differentiate between these three isozymes. Only an immunoassay based upon an antibody whose epitope is located in a region of nNOS where its amino acid sequence is different from its two other family members will be able to correctly determine the level of nNOS in a sample that might also contain either iNOS or eNOS. Specificity can be determined by testing if any interference occurs in the measurement of known amounts of the analyte in the presence of a potential interfering (cross-reacting) material. Interference in an immunological test procedure can also be caused by components in the test sample [23]: for example, whole blood, serum, and plasma samples can contain drugs, antibiotics, dietary supplements, and/or components of food recently digested. These can have a variety of detrimental effects on the immunoprocedure including inhibiting antibody binding, increasing the assay background, and lowering the signal-to-noise ratio (S:N ratio). Drugs that might be used to treat a person with a specific disease or condition can be tested at $1\times$, $3\times$, and $10\times$ the expected serum/plasma level in the test procedure to determine if it might have an effect on the test results. The dietary supplement biotin (vitamin B_7) has been shown to interfere with certain immunoassays that use a biotin-labeled component as part of the assay system (Fig. 17.2), and resulted in the US FDA issuing a warning letter for certain types of clinical IVD tests [24]. Depending upon the assay format, free biotin can either increase or decrease the measured amount of a biomarker/analyte when the assay method uses a biotin and avidin/streptavidin/neutravidin binding step. It would probably be wise to avoid designing and developing any new immunological test methods to be used as clinical diagnostics in the future that involve a biotin and avidin/streptavidin/neutravidin binding procedure.

7. Matrix effects in an immunological test procedure can be caused by contaminants in the water used to dilute buffers and wash solutions or by other components added to a buffer or wash solution used in a test method [25]. For example, the water used to dilute a $10\times$ concentrated assay buffer will constitute 90% of the liquid in the assay buffer when actually used in the test procedure. Low quality water has often been the root cause for many immunological test procedure failures. Similarly, the quality of materials used to make a buffer or wash solution can have major detrimental effects on a test method. For example, bovine serum albumin (BSA) is routinely used in many assay buffers, and not all grades/preparations of BSA are suitable. It is often necessary to screen multiple lots/batches of BSA to identify one that will work well in a specific test procedure. After finding a "good" batch, many labs will order a large quantity, that is, enough for 18−24 months, to avoid having to rescreen a new batch every few months. This same process is also applicable to all other components, such as NaCl,

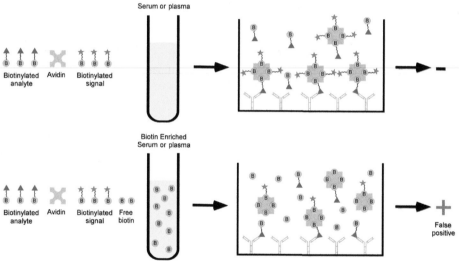

FIGURE 17.2   Two examples of how large doses of the dietary supplement biotin (vitamin B₇) ingested shortly before a blood sample is drawn for analysis can interfere with the test results of immunoassays. (A) Interference in a sandwich immunoassay in which biotin in the sample interferes with the binding of labeled-avidin to the biotin-labeled detection antibody and results in a decreased assay measurement. In this example the biotin in the sample results in a false-negative test result. (B) Interference in a competitive binding immunoassay in which the biotin in the sample interferes with the avidin binding to the biotinylated signal and results in decreased assay measurement. In this example the biotin in the sample results in a false-positive test result.

dibasic sodium phosphate, monobasic sodium phosphate, Tris-salts, detergent(s), and any other component added to either a buffer or wash solution. For this reason, decades ago the legacy commercial clinical IVD test companies adopted closed assay systems, in part, to eliminate anything being added to any reagent used in their clinical tests, and thereby, they could maintain very tight control over the quality and performance of all reagents and components needed for a clinical immunoassay.

8. Hook effect (or prozone effect) is an immunoassay problem that results in false negatives or inaccurately low test results. The effect can be caused by either analyte/antigen excess or antibody excess, and occurs almost exclusively in one-step sandwich immunoassays in which a washing step is *not* included between the capture and detection antibody incubations.

17.5 Diagnostic sensitivity and specificity, positive predictive value, negative predictive value, positive and negative likelihood ratios, and diagnostic odds ratio

The results of immunological test procedures are often expressed in 2×2 contingency tables (Table 17.2) [26–29]. The data contained in the contingency table is used to calculate a number of important test procedure characteristics including diagnostic sensitivity and specificity (Table 17.3). Also calculated from the data in the contingency table are the test procedure's positive predictive value (PPV), negative predictive value (NPV), positive likelihood ratio (LR +), negative likelihood ratio (LR−), and diagnostic odds ratio (DOR) (Table 17.3).

Diagnostic sensitivity (Table 17.3) is defined as the ability of a test procedure to correctly identify individuals who have a specific condition or disease [8,26], and is calculated as Sensitivity = (TP/TP + FN). For example, an immunoassay may have been demonstrated to have a 90% sensitivity which means that if 100 individuals known to have a specific condition or disease are tested, the results will correctly identify 90 of the 100 cases as positive. The other 10 individuals who were tested also have the condition or disease, but the incorrect test result will be negative: this is called a false-negative test result (Table 17.2). A test method's diagnostic sensitivity becomes very important when attempting to rule out a dangerous condition or disease. Thus the more sensitive a test method is, the fewer false-negative test results are reported which failed to identify the existence of a specific condition or disease even though it was present.

TABLE 17.2 2×2 Contingency table example.

	Individuals have the condition or disease	Individuals do not have the condition or disease
Positive test result	True positive (TP)	False positive (FP)
Negative test result	False negative (FN)	True negative (TN)

See Simundic AM. Measures of diagnostic accuracy: basic definitions. J Int Fed Clin Chem Lab Med 2009;19:26–9.

TABLE 17.3   Immunological test procedure characteristics derived from 2×2 contingency tables.

Characteristic	Calculation	Comment
Sensitivity	TP/(TP + FN)	Not dependent upon disease prevalence in population
Specificity	TN/(TN + FP)	Not dependent upon disease prevalence in population
Positive predictive value	PPV = TP/(TP + FP)	Is dependent upon disease prevalence in population
Negative predictive value	NPV = TN/(TN + FN)	Is dependent upon disease prevalence in population
Positive likelihood ratio	LR + = Sensitivity/(1 − Specificity)	Not dependent upon disease prevalence in population
Negative likelihood ratio	LR − = (1 − Sensitivity)/Specificity	Not dependent upon disease prevalence in population
Diagnostic odds ratio	DOR = (TP/FN)/(FP/TN)	Not dependent upon disease prevalence in population

DOR, Diagnostic odds ratio; *FN*, false negative; *FP*, false positive; *LR +* , positive likelihood ratio; *LR −* , negative likelihood ratio; *NPV*, negative predictive value; *PPV*, positive predictive value; *TN*, true negative; *TP*, true positive.
See Simundic AM. Measures of diagnostic accuracy: basic definitions. J Int Fed Clin Chem Lab Med 2009;19:26−9.

Diagnostic specificity (Table 17.3) is defined as the ability of a test to correctly exclude people who do not have a specific condition or disease [8,26], and is calculated as Specificity = (TN/TN + FP). For example, a specific immunoassay may have been demonstrated to have a 95% specificity. If 100 healthy people are tested using that immunoassay, only 95 of those 100 healthy individuals will yield a negative test result, and therefore be found not to have that specific condition or disease. The other five individuals tested also do not have that specific condition or disease, but their incorrect test result will be positive: this is called a false positive (Table 17.2). The higher a test's specificity is, the fewer "false-positive" test results it yields. A false-positive test result may lead to a misdiagnosis.

Neither sensitivity nor specificity are affected by the prevalence of the condition or disease in the population (Table 17.3). Although few, if any, immunological test procedures are correct 100% of the time, most that have been cleared for marketing by a governmental regulatory agency yield only a small percentage of false-positive or false-negative test results.

PPV is defined as the proportion of individuals with a condition or disease who yield a positive test result in the total number of positive test results [8,27]; it is calculated from the 2×2 contingency table as PPV = (TP/TP + FP); and it is affected by the prevalence of the condition or disease in the patient population examined.

NPV is defined as the proportion of individuals without a condition or disease who yield a negative test result in the total number of negative test results [8,27]; it is calculated from the 2×2 contingency table as NPV = (TN/TN + FN); and it is also affected by the prevalence of the condition or disease in the patient population examined.

Because both PPV and NPV are strongly influenced by the prevalence of a condition or disease in the patient population examined (Table 17.3), these predictive values should only be used with the specific patient population for which they were derived, and they should not be applied to other patient populations where the disease prevalence may be different.

Positive likelihood ratio (LR +) is the ratio of the expected test result in individuals with a condition or disease to the individuals without the condition or disease [8,28]. LR + is a very useful indication of the accuracy of a test, and is calculated as LR + = Sensitivity/(1-Specificity). Operationally, the LR + value indicates how many more times likely a positive test result is to be obtained for an individual with a condition or disease than in someone who does not have the condition or disease. The LR + value is one of the best measures of a rule-in diagnostic test result: the higher the LR + value, the better indicator the test is for having a specific condition or disease. Most good clinical IVD tests have a LR + value >10.

Negative likelihood ratio LR − is the ratio of the probability that a negative test result will be obtained for an individual who actually has a specific condition or disease to the probability that a negative test result will be obtained from someone who does not have the condition or disease [8,28], and is calculated as LR − = (1−Sensitivity)/Specificity. Operationally, the LR − value indicates how many times less likely a negative test result will be obtained in an individual with a condition or disease than in someone who does not have the condition or disease. The LR − value is one of the best measures of a rule-out diagnostic test result: the lower the LR − value, the better indicator the test is for *not* having a specific condition or disease. Most good clinical IVD tests have a LR − value <0.1.

Since both the LR + value and the LR − value are calculated from the sensitivity and specificity of a diagnostic test, and since neither sensitivity nor specificity are affected by disease prevalence in a population (Table 17.3), neither the LR + value nor the LR − value are influenced by disease prevalence in a population. Thus the likelihood ratios for an immunological test procedure derived for one patient population are also applicable to other patient populations provided the definition of the condition or disease remains unchanged.

DOR is the ratio of the odds of a positive test result in people with the condition or disease relative to the odds of a positive test result in people without the condition or disease [29]. The DOR is calculated as DOR = (TP/FN)/(FP/TN). Operationally, the DOR can be viewed as the ratio of the odds of disease in people who test positive relative to the odds of disease in people who test negative. The DOR value can range from zero to infinity where higher values indicate better test method differentiation. The DOR is also not affected by the prevalence of the condition or disease in different patient populations as long as the definition of the condition or disease is not changed (Table 17.3).

17.6 Antibodies for traumatic brain injury

Other chapters in this book have presented detailed information about brain-specific proteins used as blood/serum/plasma biomarkers or as CSF biomarkers of TBI including ubiquitin C-terminal hydrolase L1 (UCHL-1), S100 calcium-binding protein B (S100B), glial fibrillary acidic protein (GFAP), neuron-specific enolase (NSE), neurofilaments L and H (NFL/NFH), Tau, brain-derived neurotrophic factor (BDNF), neurogranin, myelin basic protein (MBP), and inflammatory interleukin (IL) markers. Much of the research performed on these potential biomarkers of TBI has been conducted using specific antibodies and immunological test methods [30–33]. In a recent systematic review and meta-analysis of clinical studies conducted on S100B, GFAP, NSE, UCHL-1, Tau, and neurofilament proteins to evaluate these as blood biomarkers for diagnosing intracranial lesions on CT scan after mild TBI, Mondello and associates found that there were serious problems with the design, analysis, and reporting of many of the existing clinical study reports [33]. Further, based on their findings, Mondello and colleagues emphasized the need for methodologically rigorous studies focused on the biomarker's intended use, which included defining standardized, validated, and reproducible analytical procedures [33]. This study highlights the difficulty in assimilating together and analyzing clinical data gathered by different investigators using different procedures even though they are studying and researching the same clinical condition, mild TBI.

Future studies can be envisioned in which other proteins may be investigated as potential biomarkers of mild TBI. This includes [1] the two types of acetylcholine receptors (AChR)—the muscarinic AChRs and nicotinic AChRs; the serotonin (5-hydroxy-tryptamine) receptors; the opioid receptors; and the dopamine receptors. Since these cell receptors are tightly associated membrane proteins, they may be released during cell injury as components of microvesicles, such as microparticles, exosomes, or apoptotic bodies. Concurrent disruption of the blood–brain barrier could result in the release of the microvesicles into the peripheral circulation where they could be captured and analyzed. Commercial antibodies are available for these and many more potential brain-specific proteins that might serve as a blood biomarkers for mild TBI in specific cell types and possibly also specific regions of the brain.

17.7 What to report in a research publication

Numerous groups of investigators have published articles regarding the information that should be reported for the antibodies when reporting results of experimental biomedical research including immunological procedures [3–14]. However, a consensus does not currently appear to exist and a thorough review of this controversial topic is outside the scope of this chapter. While a consensus doesn't exist, most agree on a number of basic pieces of information that should be included in the Materials and Methods section of all publications using an antibody for any immunological procedure.

If a commercially available antibody has been used in prior published articles for the same immunoprocedure, the pieces of information that should be reported are the vendor's name and address; the name of the antibody; the type of antibody; its catalog number; and the lot number used. If any additional antibody characterization or test method validation studies were conducted, those results should also be included.

If the antibody has not been used in a previous publication, then additional characterization and assay validation data should be reported. The recommended amount of additional information and the type of data varies greatly in different recommended guidelines [3–14]. For example, Bordeaux and associates [7] proposed that for an antibody to be validated, it must be shown to be specific, selective, and reproducible in the test procedure for which it is to be used. Uhlen et al. [4] recommended five conceptual pillars should be utilized for antibody validation in an application specific manner. The five pillars were developed during an ad hoc working group on antibody validation and were suggested to be used as guidelines to assure antibody reproducibility. Weller [5] has proposed 10 basic rules that must be met for an antibody to be validated, and therefore understood and repeatable by other investigators. Weller also developed a checklist to be completed as each rule is finished (5—see Supplemental data). Further, Andresson and colleagues [12] produced a list of 10 validation parameters by which they recommend all immunological test procedures should be validated. They suggest specific procedures to be used to accomplish each of the 10 validation parameters, and developed template spreadsheets for data collection and analysis and to facilitate standardize presentation of validation reports (12—see Supplemental data). While a considerable amount of overlap exists among these guidelines [3–14], significant differences also exist between them. Thus until a widely accepted consensus is reached within the biomedical research community, it remains the responsibility of each individual research team to decide how detailed their antibody evaluation and immunological test method validation should be to adequately validate their procedures. The steps proposed herein are a balanced approach which is flexible depending upon the antibody being evaluated and the type of immunological procedure being validated while still providing sufficient experimental data to assure the antibody detects/measures the appropriate analyte and the test method is adequately characterized to allow other researchers to successfully reproduce the test procedure in their laboratory.

17.8 Concluding remarks

The Glasgow Coma Score (GCS) is the procedure most often used to determine the severity of a possible brain injury. Future studies on immunological test procedures for mild TBI should be focused on developing a biomarker-based test for TBI that correlates closely with the GCS as an initial screening tool for emergency room patient evaluation. Also, since current biomarkers can detect an injury to certain types of neuronal tissue, a future goal should be to develop immunoassays which will correlate the location of an injury to damage in a specific area of the brain as seen on imaging studies. Ideally, one or more biomarker-based immunological test procedure will be developed that correlates closely to the results obtained by imaging studies and the GCS during initial patient evaluation for individuals with possible TBI. A panel of biomarker-based immunoassays for mild TBI should be developed and validated to monitor a patient's condition until it stabilizes or resolves. Additionally, a validated biomarker or panel of tests-based test for TBI might accelerate the discovery and testing of a candidate therapy to effectively treat mild TBI.

References

[1] Acharya P, Quinlan A, Neumeister V. The ABCs of finding a good antibody: how to find a good antibody, validate it, and publish meaningful data. F1000Res 2017;6:851.

[2] Pauly D, Hanack K. How to avoid pitfalls in antibody use. F1000Res 2015;4:691.

[3] Lee JW, Devanarayan V, Barrett YC, et al. Fit-for-purpose method development and validation for successful biomarker measurement. Pharm Res 2006;23:312–28.

[4] Uhlen M, Bandrowski A, Carr S, et al. A proposal for validation of antibodies. Nat Methods 2016;13:823–6.

[5] Weller MG. Ten basic rules of antibody validation. Anal Chem Insights 2018;13:1–5.

[6] Reiss PD, Min D, Leung MY. Working towards a consensus for antibody validation. F1000Res 2014;3:266.

[7] Bordeaux J, Welsh AW, Agarwal S, et al. Antibody validation. Biotechniques 2010;48:197–209.

[8] Simundic AM. Measures of diagnostic accuracy: basic definitions. J Int Fed Clin Chem Lab Med 2009;19:203–11.

[9] Guidance for Industry. Bioanalytical method validation. Fed Regist 2001;66:28526–7.

[10] Poste G, Compton CC, Barker AD. The national biomarker development alliance: confronting the poor productivity of biomarker research and development. Expert Rev Mol Diagn 2015;15:211–18.

[11] Bandrowski A, Brush M, Grethe JS, et al. The resource identification initiative: a cultural shift in publishing. F1000Res 2015;4:134.

[12] Andreasson U, Perret-Liaudet A, van Waalwijk van Doorn LJ, et al. A practical guide to immunoassay method validation. Front Neurol 2015;6:179.

[13] Fosang AJ, Colbran RJ. Transparency is the key to quality. J Biol Chem 2015;290:29692–4.

[14] Rosenblatt M. An incentive-based approach for improving data reproducibility. Sci Transl Med 2016;8 (336):336ed5.

[15] Clinical and Laboratory Standards Institute. Protocols for determination of limits of detection and limits of quantitation, approved guideline. CLSI Document EP17. Wayne, PA: CLSI; 2004, 19087-1846, USA.

[16] Clinical and Laboratory Standards Institute. Evaluation of detection capability for clinical laboratory measurement procedures. 2nd ed. Wayne, PA: CLSI Document EP17A2E. CLSI; 2012, 19087-1846, USA.

[17] Clinical and Laboratory Standards Institute. Evaluation of the linearity of quantitative measurement procedures: a statistical approach; approved guideline. Wayne, PA: CLSI Document EP6-A. CLSI; 2003, 19087-1846, USA.

[18] Clinical and Laboratory Standards Institute. User protocol for evaluation of qualitative test performance; approved guideline. Wayne, PA: CLSI Document EP12-A2. CLSI; 2008, 19087-1846, USA.

[19] Clinical and Laboratory Standards Institute. Evaluation of precision performance of quantitative measurement methods; approved guideline. 2nd ed. Wayne, PA: CLSI Document EP05-A2. CLSI; 2004, 19087-1846, USA.

[20] Clinical and Laboratory Standards Institute. Evaluation of precision of quantitative measurement procedures; approved guideline. 3rd ed. Wayne, PA: CLSI document EP05A3. CLSI; 2014, 19087-1846, USA.

[21] ISO 5725-1. Accuracy (trueness and precision) of measurement methods and results—part 1: general principles and definitions; 1994.

[22] ISO 5725-2. Accuracy (trueness and precision) of measurement methods and results—part 2: basic method for the determination of repeatability and reproducibility of a standard measurement method; 1994.

[23] Clinical and Laboratory Standards Institute. Interference testing in clinical chemistry; approved guideline. 2nd ed. Wayne, PA: CLSI document EP07-A2. CLSI; 2005, 19087-1846, USA.

[24] FDA Safety Communication. The FDA warns that biotin may interfere with lab tests. November 2017, <https://www.fda.gov/medicaldevices/safety/alertsandnotices/ucm586505.htm> [accessed 5.11.18].

[25] Clinical and Laboratory Standards Institute. Evaluation of matrix effects; approved guideline. 2nd ed. Wayne, PA: CLSI document EP14-A2. CLSI; 2005, 19087-1846, USA.

[26] Altman DG, Bland JM. Diagnostic tests 1: sensitivity and specificity. BMJ 1994;308:1552.

[27] Altman DG, Bland JM. Diagnostic tests 2: predictive values. BMJ 1994;309:102.

[28] Deeks JJ, Altman DG. Diagnostic tests 4: likelihood ratios. BMJ 2004;329:168–9.

[29] Glas AS, Lijmer JG, Prins MH, et al. The diagnostic odds ratio: a single indicator of test performance. J Clin Epidemiol 2003;56:1129–35.

[30] Papa L, Edwards D, Ramia M. Exploring serum biomarkers for mild traumatic brain injury Chapter 22 In: Kobeissy FH, editor. Brain neurotrauma: molecular, neuropsychological, and rehabilitation aspects. Boca Raton, FL: CRC Press/Taylor & Francis; 2015.

[31] Zerrerberg H. Blennow. Fluid biomarkers for mild traumatic brain injury and related conditions. Nat Rev Neurol 2016;12:563−74.

[32] Kim HJ, Tsao JW, Stanfill AG. The current state of biomarkers of mild traumatic brain injury. J Clin Invest Insight 2018;3(1):e97105.

[33] Mondello S, Sorinol A, Czeiter E, et al. Blood-based protein biomarkers for the management of traumatic brain injuries in adults presenting to emergency departments with mild brain injury: a living systematic review and meta-analysis. J Neurotrauma 2017;34:1−21.

Sensitive immunoassay testing platforms

Maximo J. Marin[1] and Xander M.R. van Wijk[2]

[1]Department of Pathology, Keck School of Medicine, University of Southern California, Los Angeles, CA, United States [2]Department of Pathology, Pritzker School of Medicine, The University of Chicago, Chicago, IL, United States

18.1 Brief introduction to traumatic brain injury and current state of testing

Currently, as discussed throughout other chapters, the diagnosis of traumatic brain injury (TBI) is made through a combination of a neuroevaluation, for example by means of the Glasgow Coma Scale (GCS), and radiologic imaging, mostly consisting of computed tomography (CT). CT has the ability to detect focal structural lesions [1] and, in general, GCS scores, especially in the more severe cases, correlate well with CT pathological findings [2,3]. However, CT imaging lacks the sensitivity to detect axonal injury, also called diffuse axonal injury or traumatic axonal injury (TAI) [1,4]. A significant portion, approximately 80%, of the reported TBI cases are classified as concussions or mild/moderate TBI (mTBI) [5,6]. mTBI can often have a significant amount of TAI that is not detected or is underestimated by CT [4]. Further, TAI is a major predictor of neurologic outcome [7]. Thus in cases where TAI is the primary injury, head CT scans are poor predictors of outcome. Many cases of TBI may go unnoticed without using magnetic resonance imaging (MRI) [8]. However, MRI use has been limited as it is less cost-effective, has limited on-site availability, and requires longer imaging time than CT. Yet, even in cases where both CT and MRI are used, findings still do not predict neurocognitive function at any stage of mTBI, or outcome after 1-year of initial injury [8].

TBI patients are at risk for long-term neuropsychiatric and psychological symptoms [9,10]. Symptoms of mTBI are synonymous with postconcussive syndrome [11,12]. These symptoms include headaches, nausea, sleep disturbance, fatigue, irritability, depression, impatience, forgetfulness, poor concentration, cognitive impairment, and blurred vision. Currently, no existing test identifies subclinical TBI/mTBI, or patients who will suffer long-term TBI sequelae. The prognostic and diagnostic clinical tools for risk stratification of TBI patients are still limited. These challenges have created a need for the development of biomarkers that target the pathophysiological processes at the cellular and molecular level, which ultimately could be used to supplement or improve prognostic information and diagnosis.

18.2 Brief overview of neural tissue and cell types

The brain, like many other organs, is composed of different types of cells that are necessary to provide the proper structure and function needed for everyday performance. The principle unit of the brain is the neuron. Neurons have a unique ability to receive, store, and transmit information through electrical and chemical signals. A neuron consists of a cell body (soma), dendrites, and an axon. In general, input and output signals are conveyed by dendrites and axons, respectively. Supporting cell types within the neural tissue are generally called glial cells. Glial cells are divided into subtypes which are astrocytes, oligodendrocytes, and microglial cells. In general, glial cells are considered cells that provide support for neurons in numerous biological processes (such as metabolism, tissue repair, and regeneration), provide support for the blood–brain barrier (BBB), provide myelin for neuronal axons, and play a role during inflammation. It is from these cells, that is, neurons and glial cells, that most, if not all, TBI biomarkers will originate (Fig. 18.1).

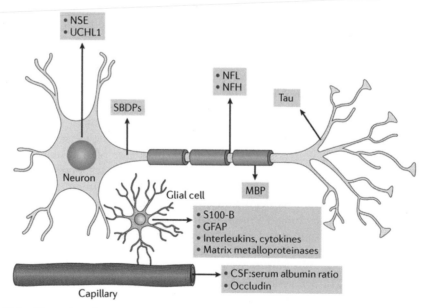

FIGURE 18.1　Illustration of common neural tissue cells and the cellular location of potential TBI biomarkers. *Reprinted from Zetterberg H, Blennow K. Fluid biomarkers for mild traumatic brain injury and related conditions. Nat Rev Neurol 2016;12:563–74. With permission from Macmillan Publishers Ltd.*

18.3 Discussion of biomarkers and their limitations in testing for mild/moderate traumatic brain injury

18.3.1 Fluid type

Although there is precedence for using cerebral spinal fluid (CSF) for testing central nervous system (CNS) biomarkers, this section will primarily focus on the use of biomarkers in the setting of the peripheral blood. The main advantages of using CSF is that it communicates readily with neural interstitial fluid that bathes the neurons and so detection of biomarkers in CSF should reflect neural tissue injury [13]. However, the disadvantage is that the required lumbar puncture is much more invasive than venipuncture. Furthermore, most automated, clinical laboratory assays are approved for use with blood samples rather than other bodily fluid samples. We believe that blood testing is the future for TBI testing. However, it should be noted that using blood sampling for TBI biomarkers is not without difficulty and this will be addressed further in this chapter.

18.3.2 Food and Drug Administration—approved laboratory test and limitations

In general, many of the current (potential) TBI biomarkers, which include S100B, glial fibrillary acidic protein (GFAP), neuron-specific enolase (NSE), ubiquitin carboxy terminal hydrolase L1 (UCH-L1), neurofilaments (NF), myelin basic protein (MBP), spectrin breakdown products (SBDP), tau, microtubule-associated protein-2 (MAP2), and amyloid β, correlate with head injury [14]. Of those biomarkers, GFAP has excelled as it correlates with findings of TAI, GCS, CT, and TBI severity [15,16]. GFAP is a structural protein located in astrocytes and released upon injury [14,17,18]. Another marker that has done well in studies is UCH-L1. UCH-L1 is an enzyme located in the cytoplasm of neurons [13,14,18,19]. One study showed that it outperformed GFAP when the goal was to reduce CT scans in patients with mTBI [20]. In accordance with these and other studies, the FDA recently approved the first blood test to aid in the evaluation of mTBI/concussion [21].

This test, the Banyan Biomarkers Brain Trauma Indicator (BTI), is used to rule out those suspected mTBI cases which do not need to undergo imaging. Essentially, low levels of GFAP and UCH-L1 predict the absence of intracranial injury seen on CT, with the goal to decrease the use of CT. In a landmark study the sensitivity and negative predictive value of the combined UCH-L1 and GFAP test for the detection of intracranial injury were 97.6% and 99.6%, respectively [22]. The positive predictive value, however, was only 9.5%. Furthermore, as mentioned above, head CT has poor sensitivity for detection of axonal injury and many TBI cases ($\sim$80%) are classified as mTBI, in which axonal injury seems to be an important component of the pathology [23]. Additionally, one study showed that GFAP and UCH-L1 lack the ability to rule out concussion/mTBI reliably [24]. Further, other studies have shown that up to 25% of mTBI cases have levels of UCH-L1 and GFAP below limits of quantification with current assays [17]. Thus the Banyan TBI test has a limited scope of use and does not adequately address the CT-negative mTBI cases.

18.3.3 Biomarkers more specific to axonal injury/mild or moderate traumatic brain injury

As discussed in the previous section, although UCH-L1 and GFAP are markers that have shown promise, there is a serious concern as to whether these two biomarkers have the ability to identify patients that have mTBI without any CT identifiable injury. Biomarkers that have shown potential in detecting mTBI are proteins involved in neuronal axon injury [14,18,19]. For example, intermediate filaments are essential components of the axonal cytoskeleton of the neurons. One major intermediate filament of the neuron is called NF and is specific to axonal injury [14,18,19,25]. NFs are assembled from NF triplet proteins [14,17,19]. Specifically, NF light (NF-L) has demonstrated the ability to identify patients with mTBI/concussion [13,14,17,26]. However, most of the studies used CSF samples. In one study that analyzed serum samples from moderate to severe TBI cases, NF-L concentration, measured by a standard immunoassay, correlated to TBI outcome but did not show correlation with TAI or intracranial injury by CT [27]. Furthermore, when comparing levels of NF-L in the CSF and serum with a standard immunoassay, that is, enzyme-linked immunosorbent assay (ELISA), there is only weak correlation [27,28]. It is noted that this immunoassay is not recommended for blood measurements by the manufacturer. The correlation is better with a slightly more sensitive electrochemiluminescence (ECL) assay and best with the ultrasensitive Simoa assay (see below for a description of the Simoa technology) [28].

Another potential biomarker for neuronal axonal injury is tau protein. Tau microtubule-associated protein is located in the neuron and is abundant in the axons [13,14,18,19,25,29]. Studies have consistently shown that tau levels are elevated in CSF after mild and severe head injury and correlate well with outcomes [13,18,30−33]. In serum, distinctly elevated tau levels are associated with a poor outcome and poor GCS [34]. Serum tau levels are significantly higher in high-risk compared to low-risk mTBI patients, however, the level in low-risk mTBI patients is comparable to healthy volunteers [35]. Further evidence shows serum tau is a poor predictor of mTBI, CT lesions, and has weak prognostic value [36−40]. It is important to note that these studies used conventional immunoassay testing. Meaning, these assays, typically used for CSF, may not be adequate to accurately detect low levels of tau in blood.

18.4 The need for multiplexed and sensitive assays

18.4.1 Why do we need multiplexed assays?

The pathology of TBI is a complex process. Biomarker detection depends on the mechanism, site(s), extent of head injury, chronicity, primary cell origin of injury, biomarker peak levels, baseline and peak concentrations, and half-life [14,29,41,42]. The pathophysiological complexity is reflected by the patterns that emerge when evaluating the biomarkers of TBI (see Table 18.1).

One possible solution to evaluating TBI with biomarkers could be through the use of multiplexed assays. For example, before the discovery and prominent clinical use of

TABLE 18.1 Representative TBI biomarkers cell origin and time dependent changes in blood.

Protein	Cell origin	Time to peak	Time return to baseline	Concentration baseline (ng/mL)	Concentration peak (ng/mL)	Serum half-life
S100B	Astrocyte	12–27 h	96 h	<0.05	>1.13	1.5 h
GFAP	Astrocyte	3–20 h	>24 h	<0.03	0.48	
NSE	Neuron	15 h	25–48 h	<15	21	24 h
UCH-L1	Neuron	8 h	24 h	<0.09	0.23	
NF-L	Neuron		>15 d[a]	<0.01[b]		
MBP	Oligo	1.5–8 h	>83 d	0.15	0.17	
SBDP	Several	1 h to 6 d				
Tau	Neuron	1 h		<0.04	1.68–8.69	
MAP2	Neuron	6 months				
Amyloid Beta	Neuron	24 h to 6 d				

[a]*From Al Nimer F, Thelin E, Nystrom H, et al. Comparative assessment of the prognostic value of biomarkers in traumatic brain injury reveals an independent role for serum levels of neurofilament light. PLoS One 2015;10(7):e0132177.*
[b]*From Shahim P., Zetterberg H., Tegner Y., Blennow K. Serum neurofilament light as a biomarker for mild traumatic brain injury in contact sports. Neurology. 2017;88(19):1788–94.*
GFAP, glial fibrillary acidic protein; MAP2, microtubule-associated protein-2; MBP, myelin basic protein; NF-L, neurofilaments light; NSE, neuron-specific enolase; SBDP, spectrin breakdown products; UCH-L1, ubiquitin carboxy terminal hydrolase L1.
Adapted from Kornguth S, Rutledge N. Integration of biomarkers into a signature profile of persistent traumatic brain injury involving autoimmune processes following water hammer injury from repetitive head impacts. Biomarkers Insights 2018;13. With permission from SAGE Publishing.

cardiac troponin (cTn), biomarker testing for an acute myocardial infarction included a "cardiac panel." This panel included LDH (and possibly its isoforms), myoglobin, and CK-MB. Although each of these markers had their limitations, the panel's advantage was to provide complementary and comprehensive data for the characterization of a possible evolving infarction. However, these cardiac biomarkers were not multiplexed in the technical sense, but the information that was produced would be used by clinicians similarly to multiplexed assays in the clinical setting. Thus a panel of biomarkers that are multiplexed could be used to inform clinicians of a potential TBI case.

18.4.2 The barriers of traumatic brain injury biomarker testing in blood: the need for ultrasensitive assays

Detection of CNS-specific biomarkers in blood has two large barriers to overcome. First, once the neural tissue has been injured, the biomarkers have to make their way effectively through a biophysical barrier, the BBB, and then into the bloodstream. Detection of CNS biomarkers in the peripheral blood may be limited by a number of factors such as clearance from the blood (via liver and or kidney), proteolytic degradation, binding to carrier proteins, and variable permeability of biomarker proteins crossing the BBB due to the proteins' inherent properties, like molecular size and charge [17]. Due to differences in these properties, some biomarkers may be more suited to cross the BBB than others. This is a major problem in that many biomarkers that have excellent specificity for TBI may not be used in a clinical setting if the current assays cannot detect the molecule at sufficiently low enough concentrations.

The second barrier to consider is the dilutional effect of the blood volume once the biomarker reaches the peripheral bloodstream [44]. When comparing CSF volume versus blood volume, the average adult CSF volume is approximately 0.15 L, while the average adult blood volume is approximately 5.5 L. The blood to CSF volume ratio is approximately 30−40. The low-level concentration of TBI biomarkers in the peripheral blood leads to a technical limitation with the use of most conventional immunoassays.

Both of these barriers can be ameliorated by having assays that can detect these biomarkers at very low concentrations. Thus developing high-sensitive assays can be a solution [25]. To develop an intuition for high-sensitive testing and the potential it has with mTBI cases, we will integrate our discussion with the hallmark analyte for high-sensitive testing, cTn.

cTn is a protein highly specific for myocardium [45] and when found in the bloodstream generally indicates myocardial injury. However, before cTn testing was available, traditional testing for suspected acute myocardial infarction (AMI) included clinical exam/presentation and blood testing for nonspecific cardiac markers such as total CK, CK-MB, LDH, and electrocardiogram (ECG) [45]. When cTn became available, the clinical landscape changed dramatically. When a patient with suspected AMI had a negative ECG, cTn set a precedence with its specificity and sensitivity for myocardial injury despite a negative or nonspecific ECG. Further, as cTn assays became more sensitive and cTn was detected at earlier time points, cTn began to assume a larger role as the predominant biomarker over other biomarkers such as CK-MB [46]. Guidelines shifted to include cTn not only as a screening tool but also as a diagnostic gold standard along with ECG and clinical presentation. Essentially, cTn became important for risk stratification, rule-out purposes in an emergency setting, diagnosis, and prognosis. With the introduction of highly sensitive cTn assays, the diagnosis of an AMI (or rule-out) can be made even earlier [47,48], leading to early triage and treatment. Similar to the evolution of cTn testing in AMI, assays for CNS-specific biomarkers that are highly/ultrasensitive may lead to early evaluation of TBI and better detection of mTBI.

Thus to be able to detect the low concentrations of CNS-derived proteins in blood early after injury, highly/ultrasensitive (immuno)assays are needed [25]. Although multiple sensitive immunoassay platforms exist, such as Milliplex, V-plex, high sensitivity ELISAs, Imperacer, proximity extension, and proximity ligation assays (PEA and PLA), the single-molecule array (Simoa) and single-molecule counting (SMC) technologies have the highest sensitivity. The remainder of this chapter will focus on these two ultrasensitive immunoassays.

18.5 Digital enzyme-linked immunosorbent assay using single-molecule arrays

18.5.1 Measurement principles

Unlike the conventional ELISA, which operates in an analog manner, the so-called digital ELISA developed by Quanterix Corporation isolates single beads in an array of

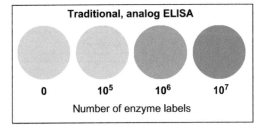
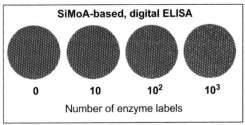

- Reaction volume = 100×10^{-6} L
- Diffusion of product = dilution = limited sensitivity
- Millions of molecules needed to overcome background and reach detection limit

- Reaction volume = 50×10^{-15} L
- Diffusion of product defeated by sealing = no dilution = single molecule sensitivity
- One molecule needed to overcome background and reach detection limit

FIGURE 18.2   Comparison between a traditional, analog ELISA and the Simoa-based, digital ELISA. *Reprinted from Rissin DM et al. Measurement of single protein molecules using digital ELISA. In: Wild D, editor. The immunoassay handbook theory and applications of ligand binding, ELISA and related techniques. 4th ed.; 2013. p. 223–42. Copyright (2013) Elsevier. With permission from Elsevier.*

femtoliter (fL; 10^{-15} L)-sized wells and counts wells that are "on" (a bead containing labeled target molecule) or "off" (a bead without labeled target molecule). Fig. 18.2 shows a comparison between the traditional, analog ELISA and the digital ELISA, which is based on the single-molecule array, or Simoa for short. The foundation of the digital ELISA lies in the Walt Lab at Tufts University (now at Harvard Medical School), where they used Simoa for the study of kinetics and inhibition of *single* enzymes [50–53]. They showed that the production of fluorescent molecules, that is, resorufin, by a single enzyme (ß-galactosidase) in the setting of the ultralow (~ 50 fL) volume of a Simoa well was sufficient to allow detection by a standard fluorescence microscope. It is this ultralow volume that allows rapid accumulation of fluorescence and circumvents the issue of dilution into a large reaction volume as in the traditional ELISA or other conventional immunoassays. Two patents that are the foundation of this technology are assigned to Tufts University and are exclusively licensed to Quanterix, which was established in 2007 in Massachusetts, USA.

Fig. 18.3 shows a schematic overview of the digital ELISA. The technology has been well described in the peer-reviewed literature and works as follows [49,54–59]. First, microscopic paramagnetic beads ($\sim 2.7 \mu$m in diameter) that are conjugated with capture antibody using standard carbodiimide chemistry are incubated with a sample containing the target molecule of interest, a brain-derived protein, for example (Step A). After sequential incubations with a detection antibody (biotinylated using standard modification of primary amines, typically resulting in 5–9 biotins per antibody) and a streptavidin-ß-galactosidase (SßG) enzyme conjugate that binds to biotin (Step B), the fluorogenic enzyme substrate resorufin-ß-D-galactopyranoside (RPG) is added and beads are transferred via a microfluidic system to the Simoa (Step C). The Simoa used in the fully automated HD-1 analyzer is 3×4 mm in size and contains 216,000 wells, each with a 40-fL volume (Fig. 18.4). The HD-1 analyzer uses a DVD-sized disc containing 24 arrays together with

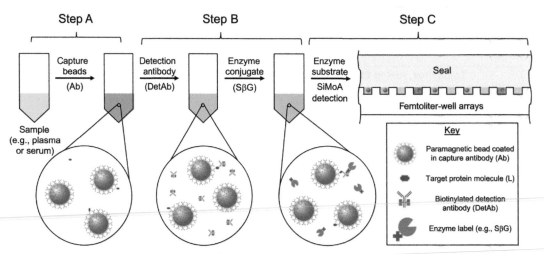

FIGURE 18.3 Schematic overview of the Simoa-based, digital ELISA. See text for details on the different steps. *Reprinted from Chang L, et al. Single molecule enzyme-linked immunosorbent assays: theoretical considerations. J Immunol Met 2012;378(1−2):102−15. Copyright (2012) Elsevier. With permission from Elsevier.*

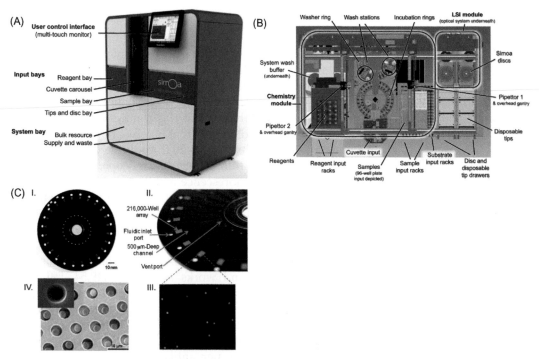

FIGURE 18.4 (A) External view of the fully automated Simoa HD-1 analyzer. (B) Schematic overview of the internal components. (C) Simoa disc. (I) Bottom view. (II) Close-up view. (III) Fluorescent microscopy image of an array showing several active beads ("on" wells). (IV) Scanning electron microscopy image of an array showing wells with single beads. *Adapted from Wilson DH, et al. The simoa HD-1 analyzer: a novel fully automated digital immunoassay analyzer with single-molecule sensitivity and multiplexing. J Lab Autom. 2016;21(4):533−47. Copyright (2016) SAGE Publishing. With permission from SAGE Publishing.*

the accompanying 24 microfluidic systems. The arrays are aligned radially to allow manufacturing using cyclic olefin polymer by an injection molding technique based on DVD manufacturing methods. The size of the wells (4.25 μm diameter, 3.25 μm depth, and 8 μm center-to-center spacing) was purposely designed so that only one bead can fit per well. Finally, addition of fluorocarbon oil washes away beads that did not settle into a well and the organic oil seals off the aqueous solution inside the wells. Wells with beads that contain the labeled target molecule will rapidly build up resorufin, a fluorescent molecule that is maximally excited at ~572 nm.

The array is imaged by a standard charge-coupled device (CCD) camera. Note that the high local concentration of fluorescence, that is, high signal-to-background, via enzymatic amplification within a well makes it possible to use low-cost cameras and excitation sources. Two fluorescent images are taken at 574/615 nm 30 seconds apart to capture the resorufin signal. A fluorescent signal that increases from the first to the second image is considered to be from an "on" well (labeled target molecule present). An increase in fluorescence is required to exclude fluorescent debris such as dust particles. Furthermore, an image is taken at 490/530 nm, which identifies the wells that contain a bead through polymer autofluorescence. Wells that contain a bead, but show no fluorescent signal, are considered "off" wells, that is, there is no labeled target molecule. Typically, 500,000 beads are used per sample of which 25,000−50,000 settle into wells in 90 seconds and are imaged.

Images are analyzed by customized software and the number of "on" and "off" wells are quantified. Although the fraction of "on" wells (f_{on}) could be used to construct a calibration curve, the use of a different output measure, that is, the average number of enzyme-labeled target molecules per bead (AEB), allows for a linear response over a wider range and a wide analytical measurement range by combining digital and analog modes, as explained below. As an excess of capture antibody-conjugated beads (500,000 beads, with ~80,000 antibodies each) is used, this drives the equilibrium towards target−antibody complexes. Importantly, the probability of beads containing 0, 1, 2, etc. labeled target molecules follows the Poisson distribution (Eq. (18.1)). If the average number of events (μ) is known (in this case μ is AEB), the probability of exactly v events (in this case v is the number of enzyme-labeled target molecules per bead) is given by:

$$P_{\mu}(v) = e^{-\mu}\left(\frac{\mu^{v}}{v!}\right) \tag{18.1}$$

From the Poisson distribution it follows that at a high bead-to-target ratio (low AEB), the vast majority of beads contain either 0 or 1 labeled target molecules (and thus enzymes). For example, a 25 μL sample of a 4 fM target protein solution contains ~60,000 molecules. Assuming every target protein is captured and labeled, the AEB is 60,000/ 500,000 = 0.12. The Poisson distribution predicts that of these 500,000 beads, 88.7% will not carry an enzyme, 10.7% carry one, and 0.6% carry two. With higher target molecule concentrations (higher AEB), more beads will carry two or more enzymes. As more beads carry more than one enzyme, f_{on} does not increase proportionally to the target molecule concentration. In contrast, AEB does increase linearly up to ~50%−70% of active beads (Fig. 18.5A). However, a bead with two enzymes, in terms of fluorescent signal, is

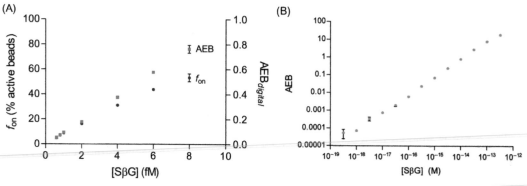

FIGURE 18.5   (A) The average enzyme-linked target molecules per bead (AEB; *red squares*) has a wider linear range than the fraction of active beads (*f*on; *blue circles*). (B) Example of a calibration curve using the AEB determined by both digital (Eq. 18.3 in text), up to 10 fM, and analog (Eq. 18.4 in text), from 31.6 fM, modes, spanning a 6-log dynamic range. (C) The switch from digital (*blue line*) to analog (*red line*) mode is based on the coefficient of variation (CV) of both modes. Below ∼0.7 *f*on the digital mode is used, above the analog mode is used. *Adapted from* [56]: *Rissin DM, et al. Simultaneous detection of single molecules and singulated ensembles of molecules enables immunoassays with broad dynamic range. Anal Chem. 2011;83(6):2279−85. Copyright (2011) American Chemical Society. With permission from the American Chemical Society.*

practically indistinguishable from a bead with one or three enzymes. This poses a problem in the measurement of AEB, as beads can only be counted as "on" or "off." Rearrangement of the Poisson distribution equation (Eqs. (18.2) and (18.3)) when v is 0 ("off" fraction) offers a solution: it allows f_{on} to be converted into an AEB value.

$$\mu = -\ln\left[P_\mu(0)\right] \tag{18.2}$$

$$\mu = -\ln\left[1 - f_{on}\right] = AEB_{digital} \tag{18.3}$$

However, once every bead contains at least one enzyme, this approach fails. Therefore at higher target molecule concentrations, the AEB is determined using an analog measurement approach.

In the analog mode, the average fluorescent intensity is determined from the "on" wells ($\bar{I}_{bead}$) and converted to AEB using the average single enzyme fluorescent intensity ($\bar{I}_{single}$)

taken from a sample that contains less than 10% active beads (usually a low calibrator), by the following equation:

$$AEB_{analog} = \frac{f_{on} \times \bar{I}_{bead}}{\bar{I}_{single}} \tag{18.4}$$

Using this approach, the digital and analog modes are seemingly meshed into one calibration curve, allowing for a wide dynamic range, typically >4 logs (Fig. 18.5B). The actual switch from digital to analog is made based on the imprecision profile of the two different modes, as quantified by the coefficient of variation (CV). The CV of the digital mode increases with the fraction of active beads, as the number of active beads does not increase proportionally with the increase in analyte concentration (due to more beads with two or more enzymes). At ~70% active beads, the CV of the analog mode is lower than that of the digital mode, and this is where the switch from digital to analog mode is made (Fig. 18.5C).

Finally, the Simoa technology also has the option of multiplexing, that is, the measurement of multiple target molecules of interest within one reaction. Beads with different capture antibodies are encoded with different fluorescent dyes and different intensities of dyes, not unlike the xMAP technology by Luminex Corporation. Multiplexing does introduce optical scatter into neighboring wells when measuring both high abundance (AEB >1) and low abundance (AEB ~0.01) target molecules simultaneously. This is computationally corrected for during image processing. The maximum number of analytes that can be simultaneously measured is 10, as there are restrictions on the encoding of the beads and on antibody compatibility.

18.5.2 Performance

The Simoa-based, digital ELISA technology is on average ~1000-fold more sensitive than conventional commercial assays [49]. The limit of detection (LOD) for some representative assays is given in Table 18.2. For example, in the era of highly sensitive troponin testing, the Simoa digital ELISA test for cTn I (cTnI) v2.0 is the most sensitive with an LOD of 13 fg/mL (0.013 ng/L; using 50 μL sample) [60], more sensitive even than the Erenna immunoassay by Singulex Inc. based on SMC (LOD of 200 fg/mL with 50 μL sample), as described below [61]. The Simoa assay was able to detect cTnI in 34 samples that previously had an undetectable cTnI (<0.006 ng/mL) using a contemporary cTnI assay (Siemens Ultra cTnI) [62]. Using Simoa, cTnI is detectable in 93% of healthy individuals ($n = 400$) [63]. The imprecision (CV) of Simoa assays is generally less than 10%, except at concentrations that approach the LOD and limit of quantitation (LOQ), the latter calculated as the concentration at which the CV is 20% [59,64]. The upper limit of calibration range of the cTnI assay is 300 ng/L, spanning ~4.4 logs. The upper limit of the dynamic range is 1200 ng/L, which includes a 4× autodilution.

The Simoa HD-1 analyzer is a fully automated analyzer that can handle 5 mL, 7 mL, and 10 mL primary tubes as well as 1 mL pediatric sample cups. It was designed for both research and clinical laboratories and has random/continuous access operation with stat capability (priority sample processing). Time to first result is generally 1 hour (45–77 min), with new results every 45 seconds and an overall instrument throughput of

TABLE 18.2 Limit of detection (LOD) of some representative Simoa-based, digital ELISA assays and comparison with commercial analog tests.

Protein	Simoa LOD (fg/mL)	Fold increase in sensitivity over best commercial analog test
IL-1ß	1	57
TNF-α	3	35
GM-CSF	3	87
P24	5	3000
IL-6	5	8
PSA	6	1667
Aß42	20	2500
Tau	20	3000
IL-1α	24	42
GLP-1	33	333
Troponin I	50[a]	60
p-Tau-231	50	ND
p-Tau-181	100	600

[a]The LOD of the newest version of the troponin I assay (v2.0) is 13 fg/mL on the HD-1 analyzer.
Adapted from Rissin DM et al. Measurement of single protein molecules using digital ELISA. In: Wild D, editor. The immunoassay handbook theory and applications of ligand binding, ELISA and related techniques. 4th ed.; 2013. p. 223–42. Copyright (2013) Elsevier. With permission from Elsevier.

66 samples per hour. "Walk-away time," that is, time interval without operator intervention, is 4.5 hours. A typical sample volume is 20–50 μL. More details are provided in [59]. The Simoa HD-1 analyzer is not (yet) approved by the FDA, however, private laboratories are offering laboratory-developed tests (LDTs) using the technology. Assays can also be performed in an "off-line" format in which a technician performs assay incubation and wash steps similar to a standard ELISA protocol with resuspension of beads and automated washing with magnetic separation of beads using a separate plate shaker and washer. The assay plate is then loaded onto the SR-X benchtop reader for single-molecule detection on Simoa discs. This instrument has a smaller footprint and allows for a more flexible workflow. Quanterix also aims to develop an ultrasensitive point-of-care device.

In summary, the Simoa technology provides opportunities for both research and clinical laboratories to precisely measure low concentrations of brain-derived proteins in blood. As the Simoa technology depends on the interaction of a biotinylated detection antibody with a streptavidin-enzyme conjugate, it may be subject to interference by biotin in blood after taking high-dose biotin supplements. This is not specific to the Simoa technology and biotin interference has been shown for conventional immunoassays that use the biotin–streptavidin linkage methodology [65–67]. Importantly, a recent application note showed that plasma biotin did not interfere with Simoa assays.

18.5.3 Applications in neurology/traumatic brain injury

Quanterix offers Simoa assays for multiple biomarkers involved in neurology (Table 18.3). For example, the assays for GFAP and UCH-L1 are an order of magnitude more sensitive than the Banyan Biomarkers assays based on chemiluminescent ELISA that have reportable ranges of 10–320 pg/mL and 80–2560 pg/mL, respectively. Quanterix also offers neurology multiplex assays. Using 46 μL of sample, the Neurology 4-Plex assay measures four biomarkers that have been associated with TBI, that is, NF-light, Tau, GFAP, and UCH-L1 (NF-light is a registered trademark of Uman Diagnostics, and GFAP and UCH-L1 are registered trademarks of Banyan Biomarkers, with which Quanterix reached licensing agreements) [82]. There is also the option to develop customized assays on the Simoa platform using the "home-brew" kit. In addition, Quanterix has a CLIA-certified service laboratory where samples can be sent for analysis and custom assays can be developed for the customer.

The Simoa neurology assays have been used in both experimental and clinical research on TBI; example references are given in Table 18.3. These ultrasensitive assays are able to measure brain-derived proteins in serum/plasma in healthy individuals and allow for

TABLE 18.3 Simoa neurology assays.

Protein	LOD (pg/ mL)	LOQ (pg/ mL)	Upper limit of dynamic range (pg/mL)	Median endogenous [plasma] (pg/mL)	Sample volume (μL)	Sample type[b]	Example references in TBI research
Aß40	0.522	1.23	800	65.97	32.5	C, E	[69]
Aß42	0.044	0.137	400	4.70	32.5	C, E	[69–72]
α-Synuclein	0.955	4.12	10,000	4145	19	C, E, S	
BDNF	0.011	0.034	64,000	11,306	33	C, E, S	
GFAP	0.211	0.686	4000	88.0	46	C, E, S	[71,73–75]
NF-light	0.038	0.174	2000	5.33	46	C, E, S	[73–79]
NSE	1.296	9.88	120	7845	2	C, E, S	
pNF-heavy	0.663	2.88	8400	30.82	55	C, E, S	
p-Tau-181[a]	0.23	5.16	1080	36.8	46	C, E, S	
p-Tau-231	0.293	1.03	2000	22.0	46	C, E	[69]
Tau	0.019	0.061	360	1.65	46	C, E, S	[69–71,73,77,78,80,81]
TDP43	0.20	0.41	4800	2.29	45	C, E, S	
UCH-L1	1.05	3.43	20,000	9.51	46	C, E, S	[73]

[a]p-Tau-181 is not yet released, preliminary data based on CSF measuring.
[b]C = CSF, E = EDTA plasma, S = serum.
LOD, limit of detection; LOQ, limit of quantitation; TBI, traumatic brain injury; GFAP, glial fibrillary acidic protein; NF-L, neurofilaments light; NSE, neuron-specific enolase; ubiquitin carboxy terminal hydrolase L1 (UCH-L1)
Data from Simoa Neurology Assay Flyer. <https://www.quanterix.com/resources/product-brochures/simoa-neurology-assay-flyer>; July 2017 [accessed 5.1.2019]. Example references using these assays in TBI research are given in the last column.

detection of changes in concentrations after injury and may be able to detect concentration differences in relation to time after injury or severity of injury. This is especially true for tau protein, which has very low concentrations in the blood. For example, using the Simoa assay, concussed ice hockey players had increased concentrations of (total) tau in plasma (median 10.0 pg/mL), compared to preseason values (median 4.5 pg/mL), and the tau concentration was highest immediately after concussion and decreased during rehabilitation [80].

Using the Neurology 4-Plex Simoa assay, plasma GFAP had the highest discriminative ability to distinguish between normal and abnormal CT head scans with an area under the curve (AUC) of 0.88, compared to UCH-L1 (AUC 0.86), tau (AUC 0.77), and NF-L (AUC 0.84); the AUC of the combination of these four biomarkers was 0.90 [82]. Similarly, the combination of plasma tau, NF-L, and GFAP (proteins associated with different pathophysiologic mechanisms) showed a good discriminatory power (AUC 0.80, 95% CI 0.69−0.90) for detection of MRI abnormalities [73]. Lastly, measurement of inflammatory biomarkers and analysis of exosomes using ultrasensitive assays may also have a role in TBI research and diagnosis [69,70,83].

18.6 Single-molecule counting

18.6.1 Measurement principles

The Erenna immunoassay, previously referred to as Zeptyx, is based on SMC technology and has been developed by Singulex Inc (California, USA) [61,84]. Similar to Simoa, the basis of this assay is a standard sandwich type ELISA on microscopic paramagnetic beads (1 μm diameter) (Fig. 18.6). Beads are coated with capture antibody via a biotin−streptavidin interaction and after incubation with sample, fluorophore-labeled detection antibody is added. In addition to the bead-based assay, a plate-based assay can also be used, where the capture antibodies are directly coated to the ELISA plate. Where in a regular ELISA the whole ensemble is then measured using a plate reader, in digital ELISA and SMC singular events are counted. After standard sandwich ELISA incubations and washing steps, in the digital ELISA the sample is transferred into the Simoa; however, in SMC the detection antibodies are eluted from the complex using a 4 M urea or low-pH glycine solution that disrupts antibody−antigen interactions. A small elution volume (20 μL) is used to concentrate signal and enhance the SMC process. The elution solution is transferred into a 384-well plate with a 0.2-μm filter and centrifuged to separate the beads from the detection antibodies. The 384-well plate is placed in the Erenna system, and a few μL solution is transferred into a 100-μm diameter capillary flow cell. As the solution passes a small interrogation space (5 μm), fluorophore-labeled detection antibodies that were eluted from the target protein are excited using a laser. The emitted light is detected using a confocal system with a photon detector. The flow rate and small interrogation space are set that only one molecule is counted at a time. Emitted photons with a signal intensity 5−6 SD over background are counted in short increments (bins, 10 μs−1 ms dependent on the instrument) over a 1-minute interval or until 1000 events are detected. Similar to digital ELISA, a wide

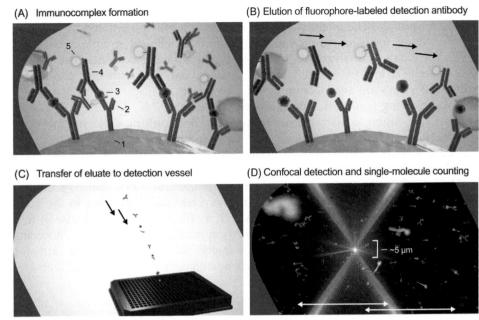

FIGURE 18.6 Overview of single-molecule counting technology. (A) Formation of immunocomplexes similar to standard immunoassays such as ELISA; 1: magnetic bead; 2: capture antibody; 3: target analyte; 4: detection antibody; 5: fluorophore. (B) The antibody—antigen interactions are disrupted using a high-molar urea or low-pH glycine solution, freeing the labeled detection antibodies. (C) The eluate containing the labeled antibodies is transferred to a 384-well detection plate. (D) Labeled detection antibodies are detected using a confocal laser microscope directly scanning the plate as depicted (Clarity and SMCxPRO systems), or are detected using a flow system (Erenna system). *Adapted with permission from MilliporeSigma. Learn how Single Molecule Counting (SMC™) technology works using the SMCxPRO™ Instrument. 2019; http://www.emdmillipore.com/US/en/20190412_170026. Accessed August 20th, 2019.*

dynamic range (~4.5 logs) is obtained by combining different (digital and analog) output measurements. At low concentrations, the number of detected, single-molecule, events (DE) is counted. At intermediate to high concentrations, when there is a significant chance of having twomolecules in the same counting event, the sum of photons in all the DEs is counted (corrected for estimated background photons), termed events photons (EP). At the highest analyte concentrations when EPs start to saturate, total light (total photons; TP) is measured by the sum of all photons. This TP measurement is comparable to total light intensity measured on a whole ensemble analog plate reader [61,85].

MilliporeSigma has acquired exclusive rights on Singulex's SMC technology for research applications. They offer the first-generation Erenna system and the newer, second-generation instrument SMCxPRO [86]. The main difference between the two systems is that in the Erenna system the eluted sample is transferred from the 384-well plate and read in a capillary flow system, whereas in the SMCxPRO instrument the eluted sample is directly read through the bottom of the 384-well plate using a confocal laser system. The 642-nm laser scans 275 μm above the surface of a 384-well flat bottom plate. While maintaining the high sensitivity of the Erenna system, this system has a smaller footprint and is more affordable. The Singulex Clarity system is a fully automated in vitro diagnostics system with a focus on improved throughput for clinical samples. Similar to the SMCxPRO, the eluate is analyzed using a well-based scanning confocal laser system. The Clarity uses both DE and EP, but not TP, for data analysis. Currently only the cTnI and C. diff toxins A/B assays are available on the Clarity system.

While multiplexing is not offered on any of the current SMC devices, it is theoretically possible by using multiple distinct fluorophores. In fact, multiplex determination of IL-4, IL-6, and IL-10 using three fluorophores and three accompanying laser and detection systems has been shown by Singulex's R&D department [85]. Photon detection is also based on microplate scanning (and not the flow system). In addition to Alexa 647 used in the Erenna, SMCxPRO, and Clarity systems, the fluorophores ATTO532 and BV421 were used together with lasers with 405, 520, and 635 nm wavelengths. According to the authors, a fourth near-infrared laser could be added, as well as fluorophores that excite at the same but emit at different wavelengths, possibly allowing multiplexing of four or more analytes. Considering the need for multiplexing and Quanterix Simoa's multiplexing capabilities, it is probable that multiplexing will be offered on next-generation SMC instruments.

18.6.2 Performance

Similar to Simoa, SMC is an ultrasensitive platform with assay LODs in the pg/mL to fg/mL range (Table 18.4). The technology has a good precision with CVs generally less than 10%, except for concentrations approaching the LOQ/LOD. The LOD depends on the sample volume that is used; for example for cTnI the LOD is 0.11 ng/L (fg/mL) using 100 μL sample, 0.2 ng/L using 50 μL, and 1.2 ng/L using 10 μL [61]. The LOD of the cTnI assay on the automated Singulex Clarity is 0.12 ng/L using 100 μL sample and the upper

TABLE 18.4   Limit of detection (LOD) of some representative SMC (Erenna) assays depending on sample volume.

Protein	Sample volume (μL)	SMC LOD (pg/mL)	Sample volume (μL)	SMC LOD (pg/mL)
MCP-1	200	0.03	20	0.25
RANTES	100	0.05	20	0.3
VEGF	100	0.12	20	0.55
IL-8	50	0.12	20	0.3
IL-1α	200	0.01	20	0.1
IL-7	200	0.02	10	0.3
IL-6	100	0.01	10	0.13
TNF-α	200	0.02	10	0.4
IL-1ß	150	0.02	10	0.3
cTnI	100	0.11	10	1.2

Adapted from Todd J, et al. Ultrasensitive flow-based immunoassays using single-molecule counting. Clin Chem. 2007;53(11):1990−5. With permission from the American Association for Clinical Chemistry.

limit of the dynamic range is 25,000 ng/L, spanning >5 logs [87]. Similar to Simoa, cTnI could be detected in a high percentage of large cohorts (n >500) of healthy volunteers, that is, 96.8%−100% [87,88]. Many investigational studies have taken advantage of the sensitivity of Singulex cTnI assay, for example in exercise-induced myocardial ischemia and in ruling out functionally relevant coronary artery disease [89,90]. The Singulex Clarity cTnI assay has received the CE mark in Europe and Singulex has filed a 510(k) premarket notification submission with the US Food and Drug Administration (FDA) for approval in the United States. The Singulex Clarity platform is a fully automated analyzer that can process batches of up to 48 samples at a time and has an average throughput of 24 samples per hour. The time to first result is 32 minutes (for the *C. diff* toxins A/B assay). Twelve different assays can be loaded at one time and the walk-away time is 90 minutes [91]. Singulex is also focusing on developing a point-of-care instrument that will have the same sensitivity as the Clarity. The SMCxPRO, which requires off-line sample preparation can analyze a full 384-well plate in 2.75 hours. With 4−30 seconds read time per sample it is significantly faster than the Erenna system (typical read time of 8 hours for a full 384-well plate) [86]. Similar to Simoa and conventional immunoassays, with the use of a biotin−streptavidin linker SMC may be sensitive to biotin interference.

18.6.3 Applications in neurology/traumatic brain injury

To our knowledge, the SMC platforms have not (yet) been used for research or clinical applications in TBI. The neurology assay kits commercially available are for amyloid beta 1−40 (Aβ40) and amyloid beta 1−42 (Aβ42) on the SMCxPRO and Erenna platforms. The LOQs of these assays are 5.86 and 0.98 pg/mL, respectively, which is a factor of five to sevenfold less sensitive than the corresponding Simoa assays, but adequately sensitive to detect these peptides in plasma of (most) healthy individuals. Aβ40 and Aβ42 are part of the amyloid beta plaque which is a hallmark of Alzheimer's disease (AD), but these peptides have also been studied in relation to TBI [69−72]. Similar to Quanterix, Singulex has a CLIA-licensed, CAP-accredited laboratory that provides testing using SMC technology. There is also the option to develop your own SMC assays and several groups have developed assays that are highly specific for Aβ oligomers (over Aβ monomers) and studied CSF samples, with LOQs of 0.15−6.25 pg/mL [92−94]. Visinin-like protein-1 (VILIP-1) has also been studied as a marker of neuronal injury in AD using the Erenna platform in plasma and CSF [95]. Furthermore, SMC technology has been used to quantify mutant Huntington protein, which is present in CSF at very low levels, for the first time in Huntington's disease patients [96]. A large number of cytokine assay kits are commercially available for the Erenna and SMCxPRO platforms and interleukin 17F (IL-17F) has been studied using SMC in patients with multiple sclerosis [97].

18.7 Concluding remarks

To be able to use blood as a fluid for measurement of TBI biomarkers, ultrasensitive immunoassays are needed to measure the low concentrations of CNS-derived proteins in blood. Both Simoa (Quanterix) and SMC (Singulex) technologies are ultrasensitive technologies that are available on fully automated analyzers aimed toward implementation in the clinical laboratory. The Singulex Clarity has gained the CE mark in Europe and is pending FDA approval for the United States. However, after writing of this chapter, in June 2019, Singulex unexpectedly stopped operations without providing an official explanation for the abrupt closing. The SMC technology is still available through MilliporeSigma. Quanterix Simoa HD-1 has not (yet) been approved for clinical use in either Europe or the USA as of writing of this chapter. Although a lot of TBI research has been performed using Simoa technology, similar results should be achievable using SMC. Given the complex pathology of TBI, any laboratory test that helps in its evaluation will most likely benefit from a multiplexed approach in which multiple biomarkers are measured that represent different aspects of the pathology and differential timing after injury. Multiplexing is available using Simoa, but not (yet) with SMC technology. Theoretically, SMC technology is amenable to multiplexing. Although seemingly challenging today, Quanterix aims to develop a point-of-care device, which may aid the evaluation of TBI "in the field," for example, for application by the military or the National Football League.

References

[1] Teasdale G, Maas A, Lecky F, Manley G, Stocchetti N, Murray G. The Glasgow Coma Scale at 40 years: standing the test of time. Lancet Neurol 2014;13(8):844–54.
[2] Bruns Jr J, Hauser WA. The epidemiology of traumatic brain injury: a review. Epilepsia 2003;44(s10):2–10.
[3] Lee TT, Aldana PR, Kirton OC, Green BA. Follow-up computerized tomography (CT) scans in moderate and severe head injuries: correlation with Glasgow Coma Scores (GCS), and complication rate. Acta Neurochir (Wien) 1997;139(11):1042–7 discussion 1047–1048.
[4] Mittl RL, Grossman RI, Hiehle JF, et al. Prevalence of MR evidence of diffuse axonal injury in patients with mild head injury and normal head CT findings. AJNR Am J Neuroradiol 1994;15(8):1583–9.
[5] Bazarian JJ, McClung J, Shah MN, Cheng YT, Flesher W, Kraus J. Mild traumatic brain injury in the United States, 1998–2000. Brain Inj 2005;19(2):85–91.
[6] Bigler ED. Neuropsychology and clinical neuroscience of persistent post-concussive syndrome. J Int Neuropsychol Soc 2008;14(1):1–22.
[7] Medana IM, Esiri MM. Axonal damage: a key predictor of outcome in human CNS diseases. Brain 2003;126 (Pt 3):515–30.
[8] Lee H, Wintermark M, Gean AD, Ghajar J, Manley GT, Mukherjee P. Focal lesions in acute mild traumatic brain injury and neurocognitive outcome: CT versus 3 T MRI. J Neurotrauma 2008;25(9):1049–56.
[9] Schwarzbold M, Diaz A, Martins ET, et al. Psychiatric disorders and traumatic brain injury. Neuropsychiatr Dis Treat 2008;4(4):797–816.
[10] Vanderploeg RD, Curtiss G, Belanger HG. Long-term neuropsychological outcomes following mild traumatic brain injury. J Int Neuropsychol Soc 2005;11(3):228–36.
[11] Carroll LJ, Cassidy JD, Peloso PM, et al. Prognosis for mild traumatic brain injury: results of the WHO collaborating centre task force on mild traumatic brain injury. J Rehabil Med 2004;(43 Suppl):84–105.
[12] Schneiderman AI, Braver ER, Kang HK. Understanding sequelae of injury mechanisms and mild traumatic brain injury incurred during the conflicts in Iraq and Afghanistan: persistent postconcussive symptoms and posttraumatic stress disorder. Am J Epidemiol 2008;167(12):1446–52.
[13] Zetterberg H, Blennow K. Fluid biomarkers for mild traumatic brain injury and related conditions. Nat Rev Neurol 2016;12(10):563–74.
[14] Adrian H, Marten K, Salla N, Lasse V. Biomarkers of traumatic brain injury: temporal changes in body fluids. eNeuro 2016;3(6).
[15] Papa L, Lewis LM, Falk JL, et al. Elevated levels of serum glial fibrillary acidic protein breakdown products in mild and moderate traumatic brain injury are associated with intracranial lesions and neurosurgical intervention. Ann Emerg Med 2012;59(6):471–83.

[16] Okonkwo DO, Yue JK, Puccio AM, et al. GFAP-BDP as an acute diagnostic marker in traumatic brain injury: results from the prospective transforming research and clinical knowledge in traumatic brain injury study. J Neurotrauma 2013;30(17):1490−7.

[17] Bogoslovsky T, Gill J, Jeromin A, Davis C, Diaz-Arrastia R. Fluid biomarkers of traumatic brain injury and intended context of use. Diagnostics (Basel) 2016;6(4).

[18] Jones A, Jarvis P. Review of the potential use of blood neuro-biomarkers in the diagnosis of mild traumatic brain injury. Clin Exp Emerg Med 2017;4(3):121−7.

[19] Kim HJ, Tsao JW, Stanfill AG. The current state of biomarkers of mild traumatic brain injury. JCI Insight 2018;3(1).

[20] Welch RD, Ayaz SI, Lewis LM, et al. Ability of serum glial fibrillary acidic protein, ubiquitin C-terminal hydrolase-L1, and S100B to differentiate normal and abnormal head computed tomography findings in patients with suspected mild or moderate traumatic brain injury. J Neurotrauma 2016;33(2):203−14.

[21] FDA authorizes marketing of first blood test to aid in the evaluation of concussion in adults, <https://www.fda.gov/newsevents/newsroom/pressannouncements/ucm596531.htm>; 2018 [accessed 25.1.19].

[22] Bazarian JJ, Biberthaler P, Welch RD, et al. Serum GFAP and UCH-L1 for prediction of absence of intracranial injuries on head CT (ALERT-TBI): a multicentre observational study. Lancet Neurol 2018;17 (9):782−9.

[23] Kirov II, Tal A, Babb JS, et al. Proton MR spectroscopy correlates diffuse axonal abnormalities with post-concussive symptoms in mild traumatic brain injury. J Neurotrauma 2013;30(13):1200−4.

[24] Lewis LM, Schloemann DT, Papa L, et al. Utility of serum biomarkers in the diagnosis and stratification of mild traumatic brain injury. Acad Emerg Med 2017;24(6):710−20.

[25] Zetterberg H, Blennow K. Fluid markers of traumatic brain injury. Mol Cell Neurosci 2015;66(Pt B):99−102.

[26] Blennow K, Brody DL, Kochanek PM, et al. Traumatic brain injuries. Nat Rev Dis Prim 2016;2:16084.

[27] Al Nimer F, Thelin E, Nystrom H, et al. Comparative assessment of the prognostic value of biomarkers in traumatic brain injury reveals an independent role for serum levels of neurofilament light. PLoS One 2015;10 (7):e0132177.

[28] Kuhle J, Barro C, Andreasson U, et al. Comparison of three analytical platforms for quantification of the neurofilament light chain in blood samples: ELISA, electrochemiluminescence immunoassay and Simoa. Clin Chem Lab Med 2016;54(10):1655−61.

[29] Agoston DV, Shutes-David A, Peskind ER. Biofluid biomarkers of traumatic brain injury. Brain Inj 2017;31 (9):1195−203.

[30] Neselius S, Brisby H, Theodorsson A, Blennow K, Zetterberg H, Marcusson J. CSF-biomarkers in Olympic boxing: diagnosis and effects of repetitive head trauma. PLoS One 2012;7(4):e33606.

[31] Ost M, Nylen K, Csajbok L, et al. Initial CSF total tau correlates with 1-year outcome in patients with traumatic brain injury. Neurology 2006;67(9):1600−4.

[32] Franz G, Beer R, Kampfl A, et al. Amyloid beta 1−42 and tau in cerebrospinal fluid after severe traumatic brain injury. Neurol 2003;60(9):1457−61.

[33] Zemlan FP, Jauch EC, Mulchahey JJ, et al. C-tau biomarker of neuronal damage in severe brain injured patients: association with elevated intracranial pressure and clinical outcome. Brain Res 2002;947 (1):131−9.

[34] Liliang PC, Liang CL, Weng HC, et al. Tau proteins in serum predict outcome after severe traumatic brain injury. J Surg Res 2010;160(2):302−7.

[35] Bulut M, Koksal O, Dogan S, et al. Tau protein as a serum marker of brain damage in mild traumatic brain injury: preliminary results. Adv Ther 2006;23(1):12−22.

[36] Guzel A, Karasalihoglu S, Aylanc H, Temizoz O, Hicdonmez T. Validity of serum tau protein levels in pediatric patients with minor head trauma. Am J Emerg Med 2010;28(4):399−403.

[37] Kavalci C, Pekdemir M, Durukan P, et al. The value of serum tau protein for the diagnosis of intracranial injury in minor head trauma. Am J Emerg Med 2007;25(4):391−5.

[38] Bazarian JJ, Zemlan FP, Mookerjee S, Stigbrand T. Serum S-100B and cleaved-tau are poor predictors of long-term outcome after mild traumatic brain injury. Brain Inj 2006;20(7):759−65.

[39] Ma M, Lindsell CJ, Rosenberry CM, Shaw GJ, Zemlan FP. Serum cleaved tau does not predict postconcussion syndrome after mild traumatic brain injury. Am J Emerg Med 2008;26(7):763−8.

[40] Morris M, Maeda S, Vossel K, Mucke L. The many faces of tau. Neuron 2011;70(3):410–26.

[41] Kornguth S, Rutledge N. Integration of biomarkers into a signature profile of persistent traumatic brain injury involving autoimmune processes following water hammer injury from repetitive head impacts. Biomark Insights 2018;13 1177271918808216.

[42] Nortje J, Menon DK. Traumatic brain injury: physiology, mechanisms, and outcome. Curr Opin Neurol 2004;17(6):711–18.

[43] Shahim P, Zetterberg H, Tegner Y, Blennow K. Serum neurofilament light as a biomarker for mild traumatic brain injury in contact sports. Neurology 2017;88(19):1788–94.

[44] Zetterberg H, Smith DH, Blennow K. Biomarkers of mild traumatic brain injury in cerebrospinal fluid and blood. Nat Rev Neurol 2013;9(4):201–10.

[45] McPherson RA, Pincus MR Henry's clinical diagnosis and management by laboratory methods; 2017.

[46] Saenger AK, Jaffe AS. Requiem for a heavyweight: the demise of creatine kinase-MB. Circulation 2008;118 (21):2200–6.

[47] Keller T, Zeller T, Peetz D, et al. Sensitive troponin I assay in early diagnosis of acute myocardial infarction. N Engl J Med 2009;361(9):868–77.

[48] Reichlin T, Hochholzer W, Bassetti S, et al. Early diagnosis of myocardial infarction with sensitive cardiac troponin assays. N Engl J Med 2009;361(9):858–67.

[49] Rissin DM, Wilson DH, Duffy DC. Measurement of single protein molecules using digital ELISA. In: Wild D, editor. The immunoassay handbook. theory and applications of ligand binding, ELISA and related techniques. 4th ed 2013. p. 223–42.

[50] Rissin DM, Walt DR. Digital readout of target binding with attomole detection limits via enzyme amplification in femtoliter arrays. J Am Chem Soc 2006;128(19):6286–7.

[51] Rissin DM, Walt DR. Digital concentration readout of single enzyme molecules using femtoliter arrays and Poisson statistics. Nano Lett 2006;6(3):520–3.

[52] Gorris HH, Rissin DM, Walt DR. Stochastic inhibitor release and binding from single-enzyme molecules. Proc Natl Acad Sci U S A 2007;104(45):17680–5.

[53] Rissin DM, Gorris HH, Walt DR. Distinct and long-lived activity states of single enzyme molecules. J Am Chem Soc 2008;130(15):5349–53.

[54] Chang L, Rissin DM, Fournier DR, et al. Single molecule enzyme-linked immunosorbent assays: theoretical considerations. J Immunol Methods 2012;378(1–2).

[55] Rissin DM, Kan CW, Campbell TG, et al. Single-molecule enzyme-linked immunosorbent assay detects serum proteins at subfemtomolar concentrations. Nat Biotechnol 2010;28(6):595–9.

[56] Rissin DM, Fournier DR, Piech T, et al. Simultaneous detection of single molecules and singulated ensembles of molecules enables immunoassays with broad dynamic range. Anal Chem 2011;83(6):2279–85.

[57] Kan CW, Rivnak AJ, Campbell TG, et al. Isolation and detection of single molecules on paramagnetic beads using sequential fluid flows in microfabricated polymer array assemblies. Lab Chip 2012;12(5):977–85.

[58] Rissin DM, Kan CW, Song L, et al. Multiplexed single molecule immunoassays. Lab Chip 2013;13 (15):2902–11.

[59] Wilson DH, Rissin DM, Kan CW, et al. The simoa HD-1 analyzer: a novel fully automated digital immunoassay analyzer with single-molecule sensitivity and multiplexing. J Lab Autom 2016;21(4):533–47.

[60] Troponin I HD-1 Data Sheet. <https://www.quanterix.com/sites/default/files/assays/Simoa_Troponin-I_Data_Sheet_HD-1.pdf>; 2018 [accessed 24.1.19].

[61] Todd J, Freese B, Lu A, et al. Ultrasensitive flow-based immunoassays using single-molecule counting. Clin Chem 2007;53(11):1990–5.

[62] Wu AH, van Wijk XM. A new ultra-high sensitivity troponin I assay for chest pain patients with no evidence of troponin I using a conventional assay. Clin Biochem 2015;48(4–5):358–9.

[63] Mastali M, Fu Q, Sobhani K, Merz NB, Van Eyk J. Ultra-high sensitive cardiac troponin I baseline levels are affected by age and sex. Circulation 2018;136:A19167.

[64] Wilson DH, Hanlon DW, Provuncher GK, et al. Fifth-generation digital immunoassay for prostate-specific antigen by single molecule array technology. Clin Chem 2011;57(12):1712–21.

[65] The FDA warns that biotin may interfere with lab tests: FDA safety communication, <https://www.fda.gov/medicaldevices/safety/alertsandnotices/ucm586505.htm>; 2017 [accessed 31.12.18].

[66] Colon PJ, Greene DN. Biotin interference in clinical immunoassays. JALM 2018;2(6):941–51.

[67] Li J, Wagar EA, Meng QH. Comprehensive assessment of biotin interference in immunoassays. Clin Chim Acta 2018;487:293—8.

[68] Simoa Neurology Assay Flyer. <https://www.quanterix.com/resources/product-brochures/simoa-neurology-assay-flyer>; July 2017 [accessed 5.1.19].

[69] Kenney K, Qu BX, Lai C, et al. Higher exosomal phosphorylated tau and total tau among veterans with combat-related repetitive chronic mild traumatic brain injury. Brain Inj 2018;32(10):1276—84.

[70] Gill J, Mustapic M, Diaz-Arrastia R, et al. Higher exosomal tau, amyloid-beta 42 and IL-10 are associated with mild TBIs and chronic symptoms in military personnel. Brain Inj 2018;32(10):1277—84.

[71] Bogoslovsky T, Wilson D, Chen Y, et al. Increases of plasma levels of glial fibrillary acidic protein, tau, and amyloid beta up to 90 days after traumatic brain injury. J Neurotrauma 2017;34(1):66—73.

[72] Mondello S, Buki A, Barzo P, et al. CSF and plasma amyloid-beta temporal profiles and relationships with neurological status and mortality after severe traumatic brain injury. Sci Rep 2014;4:6446.

[73] Gill J, Latour L, Diaz-Arrastia R, et al. Glial fibrillary acidic protein elevations relate to neuroimaging abnormalities after mild TBI. Neurology 2018;91(15):e1385—9.

[74] Korley FK, Nikolian VC, Williams AM, Dennahy IS, Weykamp M, Alam HB. Valproic acid treatment decreases serum glial fibrillary acidic protein and neurofilament light chain levels in swine subjected to traumatic brain injury. J Neurotrauma 2018;35(10):1185—91.

[75] Hossain I, Mohammadian M, Takala RS, et al. Early levels of GFAP and NF-L in predicting the outcome of mild TBI. J Neurotrauma 2018.

[76] Cheng WH, Stukas S, Martens KM, et al. Age at injury and genotype modify acute inflammatory and neurofilament-light responses to mild CHIMERA traumatic brain injury in wild-type and APP/PS1 mice. Exp Neurol 2018;301(Pt A):26—38.

[77] Joseph JR, Swallow JS, Willsey K, et al. Elevated markers of brain injury as a result of clinically asymptomatic high-acceleration head impacts in high-school football athletes. J Neurosurg 2018;1—7.

[78] Wallace C, Zetterberg H, Blennow K, van Donkelaar P. No change in plasma tau and serum neurofilament light concentrations in adolescent athletes following sport-related concussion. PLoS One 2018;13(10): e0206466.

[79] Shahim P, Gren M, Liman V, et al. Serum neurofilament light protein predicts clinical outcome in traumatic brain injury. Sci Rep 2016;6:36791.

[80] Shahim P, Tegner Y, Wilson DH, et al. Blood biomarkers for brain injury in concussed professional ice hockey players. JAMA Neurol 2014;71(6):684—92.

[81] Olivera A, Lejbman N, Jeromin A, et al. Peripheral total tau in military personnel who sustain traumatic brain injuries during deployment. JAMA Neurol 2015;72(10):1109—16.

[82] Korley FK, Yue JK, Wilson DH, et al. Performance evaluation of a multiplex assay for simultaneous detection of four clinically relevant traumatic brain injury biomarkers. J Neurotrauma 2018.

[83] Devoto C, Arcurio L, Fetta J, et al. Inflammation relates to chronic behavioral and neurological symptoms in military personnel with traumatic brain injuries. Cell Transpl 2017;26(7):1169—77.

[84] Wu AH, Fukushima N, Puskas R, Todd J, Goix P. Development and preliminary clinical validation of a high sensitivity assay for cardiac troponin using a capillary flow (single molecule) fluorescence detector. Clin Chem 2006;52(11):2157—9.

[85] Gilbert M, Livingston R, Felberg J, Bishop JJ. Multiplex single molecule counting technology used to generate interleukin 4, interleukin 6, and interleukin 10 reference limits. Anal Biochem 2016;503:11—20.

[86] Hwang J, Banerjee M, Venable AS, et al. Quantitation of low abundant soluble biomarkers using high sensitivity single molecule counting technology. Methods 2018.

[87] Garcia-Osuna A, Gaze D, Grau-Agramunt M, et al. Ultrasensitive quantification of cardiac troponin I by a Single Molecule Counting method: analytical validation and biological features. Clin Chim Acta 2018;486:224—31.

[88] Apple FS, Ler R, Murakami MM. Determination of 19 cardiac troponin I and T assay 99th percentile values from a common presumably healthy population. Clin Chem 2012;58(11):1574—81.

[89] Lee G, Twerenbold R, Tanglay Y, et al. Clinical benefit of high-sensitivity cardiac troponin I in the detection of exercise-induced myocardial ischemia. Am Heart J 2016;173:8—17.

[90] Walter JE, Honegger U, Puelacher C, et al. Prospective validation of a biomarker-based rule out strategy for functionally relevant coronary artery disease. Clin Chem 2018;64(2):386—95.

VI. Analytical testing consideration

[91] Singulex. Singulex Clarity System. <https://www.singulex.com/singulex-clarity-system/> [accessed 27.2.19].

[92] Esparza TJ, Zhao H, Cirrito JR, et al. Amyloid-beta oligomerization in Alzheimer dementia versus high-pathology controls. Ann Neurol 2013;73(1):104−19.

[93] Savage MJ, Kalinina J, Wolfe A, et al. A sensitive abeta oligomer assay discriminates Alzheimer's and aged control cerebrospinal fluid. J Neurosci 2014;34(8):2884−97.

[94] Yang T, O'Malley TT, Kanmert D, et al. A highly sensitive novel immunoassay specifically detects low levels of soluble Abeta oligomers in human cerebrospinal fluid. Alzheimers Res Ther 2015;7(1):14.

[95] Tarawneh R, D'Angelo G, Macy E, et al. Visinin-like protein-1: diagnostic and prognostic biomarker in Alzheimer disease. Ann Neurol 2011;70(2):274−85.

[96] Wild EJ, Boggio R, Langbehn D, et al. Quantification of mutant huntingtin protein in cerebrospinal fluid from Huntington's disease patients. J Clin Invest 2015;125(5):1979−86.

[97] Hartung HP, Steinman L, Goodin DS, et al. Interleukin 17 F level and interferon beta response in patients with multiple sclerosis. JAMA Neurol 2013;70.

Clinical mass spectrometry and its applications in traumatic brain injuries

Y. Victoria Zhang and Putuma P. Gqamana

Pathology and Laboratory Medicine University of Rochester Medical Center, Rochester, NY, United States

19.1 Introduction of mass spectrometry platform

The mass spectrometer (MS) is a modern analytical instrument that is used to determine the mass and structural connectivity of charged chemical species in a high vacuum. Any chemical species that can be volatilized and charged can be analyzed by a MS. MS has a long history in medical research with the initial major milestones traced back to 1910, based on a compendium of recent review articles published online by *Nature* at https://www.nature.com/milestones/milemassspec/timeline/index.html. MS technology has evolved over time owing to a few significant innovations in chemistry and physics, which were duly recognized universally and accordingly awarded the Nobel Prize. With all the exciting developments, the basic schematic design of the MS instrument remained unchanged. Shown in Fig. 19.1 are the three central and enduring components, namely the ionization source, the mass analyzer, and the detecting device.

Each of the three components plays a unique and complementary function. The ionization source is used to vaporize and charge analytes into gas phase ions, which are then focused and transmitted via ion optics onto the mass analyzer. The mass analyzer is the core of the MS which is used to determine the mass over charge ratio (m/z). The analyzer's sensitivity, specificity, and duty cycle determine its overall performance and the utility of different models on the bench. Finally, the detector captures and amplifies the transient signals for quantitative analysis.

Many innovations in physics and engineering have transformed the components of the MS, thereby allowing the instrument to grow from being initially a major technology in

Biomarkers for Traumatic Brain Injury
DOI: https://doi.org/10.1016/B978-0-12-816346-7.00019-1

265

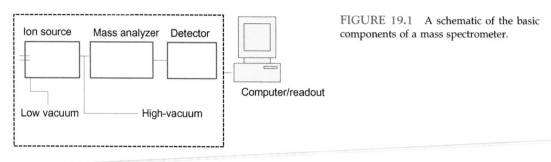

FIGURE 19.1   A schematic of the basic components of a mass spectrometer.

the analysis of atoms and isotopes to the analysis of the more complex and larger chemical particles [1,2]. These innovations included the development of powerful mass analyzers such as the quadrupole, the time-of-flight (TOF), and the orbitrap analyzers, as well as the discovery of soft ionization methods.

In particular, the flexibility in the modular design in MS which allows for the mixing of different sources and analyzers opened up opportunities for diversified applications and the powerful utility of MS technology. For example, the ability to access more than one ionization source in one instrument allows for versatility in the analysis of both polar and nonpolar analytes, whereas the combination of the same or different mass analyzers (e.g., triple quadrupole [QqQ], TOF-TOF, and quadrupole–TOF) allows for higher MS resolution, analytical specificity, powerful structural interrogation, as well as sophisticated quantitative analysis of complex mixtures [3].

In recent decades, gas (GC) and liquid (LC) chromatography have been incorporated into the workflow for mass spectrometry to further broaden the applications of this platform. In total, these culminated in the modern analytical instrumentation and hybrid techniques of GC and LC with mass spectrometry; that is, GC-MS and LC-MS or GC-MS/MS and LC-MS/MS respectively. These have since become the foundation of analytical platforms for industry, pharma, and the health sciences. We will discuss the evolvement and functions of the ion source and mass analyzers in more detail in the following session.

19.2 Fundamentals of clinical mass spectrometry

All analytes have to be ionized to be detected by MS instruments. Different types of ionization methods exist for different types of analytes. In general the polar analytes are more readily ionizable and nonpolar analytes are difficult to ionize. Traditional ionization methods include electron ionization (EI) [4], chemical ionization (CI) [5], and many other flavors, such as field desorption (FD), field ionization (FI), plasma desorption (PD), secondary ion MS (SIMS), and fast atom bombardment (FAB) [6–9]. However, two landmark soft-ionization approaches—electrospray ionization (ESI) [10,11] and laser desorption ionization (LDI) [12]—have transformed modern mass spectrometry from being a niche application in industrial and synthetic chemistry to more transformative biological and clinical applications.

John B. Fenn and Koichi Tanaka were subsequently honored with the Nobel Prize in Chemistry in 2002 for the discovery of ESI and LDI and their use in the MS analysis of high-molecular-weight biomolecular species [12,13]. Due to the unmatched utility of these new soft ionization methods in the analysis of thermally labile biomolecules, such as proteins and oligonucleotides, ESI and MALDI [14], a variant of LDI, drove much of what has become state-of-the-art in biological mass spectrometry of the modern era. ESI in particular lent itself very well to the coupling of LC and MS due to the compatibility of LC elution with ESI sources.

19.2.1 Types of ionization methods

19.2.1.1 Electrospray ionization

A simple schematic of the ESI source can be shown Fig. 19.2. In ESI the analyte ions are extracted from the solution spray under high voltage (<5 kV) into the MS inlet. The ESI mechanisms are not quite clear yet, but nonetheless the most common and accepted theory attributes ESI to the stretching of charged and liquid droplets in the sample spray into what is called the Taylor cone, whereby the devolution into gas phase ions can occur via coulombic explosion and/or ion evaporation; the latter which can be assisted by a hot gas envelope. Typically the solution spray is doped with weak organic acids such as formic acid, which function as proton donors to provide the charges for the analytes in solution. Hence, one of the main advantages of ESI is the ability to produce multiply charged analytes in very basic biomolecules, such as polypeptides and large proteins. Multiple charging produces low m/z ions from high MW species, thereby allowing such analytes to be detected inside the typical upper mass limit of 3500 m/z units. Therefore, ESI enabled the analysis of large and small molecules and has played an essential role for "-omics" research such as proteomics and metabolomics research. It is also one of the most commonly used ionization methods for clinical applications in diagnostic laboratories.

19.2.1.2 Atmospheric pressure chemical ionization

In addition to ESI, other ionization sources that can be coupled to LC include the atmospheric pressure CI (APCI) and atmospheric pressure photoionization (APPI) sources [15,16]. Some vendors supply MSs which are readily fitted with dual ESI and APCI sources, or adaptable atmospheric pressure ionization (API) source compartments, whereby ionization modes can be used interchangeably, without a significant cost in instrument downtime. Nonetheless, APCI and ESI are different and occur by different

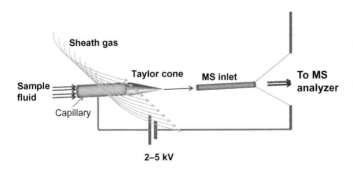

FIGURE 19.2 A schematic representation of the ESI process is shown with analyte ions extracted from the sample fluid into the MS inlet under high voltage (2–5 kV). This complex ionization process involves the formation of the Taylor cone from charged droplets, which then devolves into gas phase ions via coulombic explosion and/or ion evaporation, the latter of which can be assisted by a gas envelope.

charging mechanisms, despite producing mostly the protonated species, $M(H^+)$ from molecule M with $M + 1$ in m/z, given a charge, $z = 1$.

Unlike ESI, APCI benefits not from ions preformed in solution but rather from the CI cascade which is triggered by charging from a corona discharge needle at ~ 3 kV to a counter electrode, which is placed between the analyte aerosol spray (eluting from the thin capillary) and the high-vacuum inlet. Hence, the APCI source offers a much needed complementarity to ESI by being more universal and compatible to less ionizable, less polarizable analytes. In addition, since APCI derives most charging from a post spray event, it is less affected by matrix effects than ESI which derives most charging from the condensed phase.

19.2.1.3 Atmospheric pressure photoionization

Another atmospheric ionization source which is similar to the APCI in configuration is the APPI source, whereby charging is derived from a discharge lamp, usually a Kr lamp (10 eV), instead of the corona discharge. It can also be fitted in the same multiple source housing as both ESI and APCI. In direct APPI, photoionization occurs by the removal of valence electrons from the analyte, consistent with first ionization potentials (IP), whereas in dopant APPI mode, a molecule with a low enough IP (<11 eV) is used to trigger a cascade of ion–molecule reactions, such as secondary ionizations, charge exchange, etc., at atmospheric pressure, much like in APCI. This source is also very useful in the ionization of analytes with IP <11 eV, but which are less polarizable and less ionizable by ESI. Most LC mobile phases, such as water, methanol, and acetonitrile, have IP > 11 eV and are inert to ionization by this source.

19.2.1.4 Matrix-assisted laser desorption ionization

Together with ESI, matrix-assisted LDI (MALDI), is the major breakthrough invention for mass spectrometry. It offers one of the most important ionization methods for biological MS in general. Unlike ESI and other API sources discussed above, MALDI is predominantly a high-vacuum ionization source, much like most MS ionization methods which preceded the API sources. Nonetheless, many vendors do supply MS instruments that are fitted with adaptable sources that can house the atmospheric pressure (AP) MALDI configuration.

In the MALDI process, the analyte sample—which may be a biofluid droplet, a few micron thin tissue section, or a biopsy—is uniformly coated with matrix crystals on the sample plate, by direct droplet deposition or using a nanospray coating device. The matrix is usually a photon-absorbing Lewis acid such as alpha-cyano-4-hydroxy-cinnaminic acid (CHCA). The dried sample plate, which can host as many as 384 sample spots or more, or as many as 12 matrix-coated fresh tissue sections, or formalin fixed paraffin embedded tissues, is then placed on the source inside the MS instrument and allowed to pump down to high vacuum. Laser pulses are then bombarded on the sample spots under high vacuum to evaporate the solid sample and to eject analyte ions, which are produced from gas phase proton transfer reactions between the sample and the matrix. The gas phase ions are voltage accelerated through a field-free time of flight (TOF) tube to a detector (See Fig. 19.3).

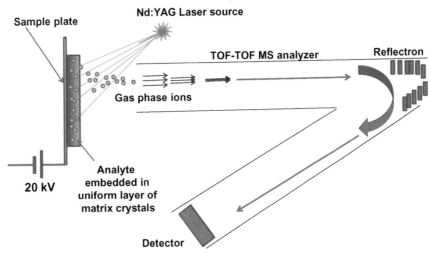

FIGURE 19.3   A schematic representation of the MALDI process is shown above. The analyte sample is embedded inside matrix crystals and uniformly deposited on a spot on the sample plate. The matrix is usually a photon-absorbing Lewis acid like CHCA. The dried sample plate, which can host as many as 384 sample spots or more, is then placed on the source inside the MS instrument. Laser pulses are then bombarded on the sample spots under high vacuum to evaporate the solid sample and to eject analyte ions, which are produced from gas phase proton transfer reactions between the sample and the matrix. The gas phase ions are voltage accelerated through a field-free time of flight (TOF) tube to a detector.

MALDI, coupled with a TOF mass analyzer (MALDI-TOF MS), has been used for large molecules (e.g., proteins, peptides, and lipids) analysis to offer mass "fingerprinting" for various disease conditions in biological samples for biomarker discovery research. Recently, MALDI-TOF stepped into the clinical diagnostic field as the main innovation for microorganism identification in the clinical microbiology labs to offer faster turnaround time for general microbiology testing and infectious disease control [17–25]. Active studies have also taken place for tissue imaging and histopathological analysis of surgical slides to offer opportunities to support anatomic pathology services in the future [26–29].

19.2.2 Mass analyzers

19.2.2.1 Overview

Whereas the performance of ionization sources is considered to be the bottleneck for a mass spectrometry analysis, mass analyzers represent the nexus of signal quality control. This core MS component, its integrity, engineering, and geometry determine the fundamental quantitative relationship between a controlled property of the electromagnetic field and m/z of the ions under study. A brief summary of different mass analyzers, their most popular utility, and figures of merit are summarized in Tables 19.1 and 19.2. In Table 19.1 the mass analyzers are represented in terms of their field energy range, their analysis function and utility, whereas in Table 19.2 they are briefly evaluated in terms of their performance features. For example, the orbitrap mass analyzers are high-resolution mass

TABLE 19.1   Various types of mass analyzers are represented in terms of their field energy range, analysis function, and utility.

Type of analyzer	Field energy range	Measured quantity	m/z Resolution	Scanning/ Trapping	Utility
Magnetic sector (B)	keV	mv/z	High res	Scanning	Research
Electrostatic sector (E)	keV	mv^2/z	High res	Scanning	Research
Time of flight (TOF)	keV	flight time (t)	High res	Scanning	All
Quadrupole (Q)	eV	m/z	Low res	Scanning	Commercial, research
Quadrupole ion trap (QIT)	eV	m/z	Low res	Trapping	Research
Linear ion trap (LIT)	eV	m/z	Low res	Trapping	Research
Ion cyclotron resonance (ICR)	eV	m/z	High res	Trapping	Research
Orbitrap	eV	m/z	High res	Trapping	Research

analyzers and have been used in an increasing number of applications in the clinical setting, yet the QqQ mass analyzers, which are low-resolution mass analyzers, are more commonly preferred in clinical diagnostics because of the speed advantage and higher cost-effectiveness. Hence, QqQ mass analyzers, as well as quadrupole-TOF (Q-TOF) instruments are the most commonly used analyzers in clinical diagnostics, with the latter employing the TOF analyzer to compensate for the speed and m/z resolution.

19.2.2.2 Time of flight mass analyzers

The TOF mass analyzer is based on the measurement of flight times of ions of a certain kinetic energy moving translationally in a field-free tube. Typically 20 kV accelerated ions of 1000 m/z units, flying along a 2-meter-long and linear drift tube, will reach the detector within flight times of the order of tens of microseconds (μs). TOF analyzers are typically coupled to a MALDI source because of the pulsed nature of these sources, which complements the timing devices. In addition, TOF analyzers can be assembled as a Q-TOF in tandem to a quadrupole mass analyzer, or as a TOF-TOF reflectron in order to increase the flight path and enhance the resolution with respect to a single linear TOF mass analyzer. Q-TOF mass analyzers are most often of the Q-TOF-TOF reflectron configuration. Hence, tandem MS utility which is analogous to a QqQ can be obtained, albeit with higher m/z resolution.

19.2.2.3 Triple-quadrupole mass analyzers

The QqQ is the most popular mass analyzer used in tandem MS instruments. It is assembled from three quadrupole ion guides (Q1, q2, and Q3), two of which serve as mass analyzers (Q1 and Q3), and one of which is used as a collision cell or transmitting device (q2). The combination of the different functions of the three parts provides the diverse functions of the QqQ instrument and enables it to be the most popular analyzer for clinical

TABLE 19.2 Various types of mass analyzers are represented in terms of their performance as evaluated from figures of merit such as mass range, resolution, and speed amongst others.

Figures of merit	TOF	Q	QIT	B/E sectors	ICR	Orbi
Mass range (m/z)	>250,000	1000–2500	1000–2500	25,000	Depends on magnetic strength (B)	100–2500
Resolution	$>10^3$	0.7, 0.4 FWHM	0.7, 0.4 FWHM	$>10^3$	$>10^4$	$>10^4$
Exact m/z	At low m/z	n/a	n/a	At low m/z	Best	Best
Sensitivity	Low-mid	Highest	High	Low-mid	Low-mid	Low-mid
All ion detection	n/a	n/a	n/a	n/a	Best	Best
Ion storage	n/a	n/a	Good	n/a	Better	Better
Speed	Fast	Fastest	Mid	Fast	Slow	Slow
Dynamic range	Mid-high	Highest	High	Mid-high	Mid-high	Mid-high
Quantification	Good in Q-TOF	Best	Good	n/a	n/a	n/a
MS/MS modes	MS2	MS2	MS2	MS^n $(n>2)$	MS^n $(n>2)$	MS^n $(n>2)$
Sampling	LC-based/MALDI pulsed	LC-based	LC-based	Variable	Variable	LC-based
Simplicity	Medium	Simple	Simple	Good	Complex	Complex
Cost/performance	High	Best	Good	High	Highest	Higher
Disadvantage	Pulsed source, cost, size	Low res	Low res	Pulsed source, cost, size	Magnet, cost, size	Cost

functions. Its popularity is due to its flexibility and diversity of functions from different scan modes, which we will describe in detail and are represented by the general schematic shown in Fig. 19.4.

These transitions/scan modes are shown in terms of filled circles, to denote fixed m/z selection (filtering MS event), as well as empty circles to denote scanning, according to a representation popularized by Kondrat and Cooks [3]. The QqQ can function as a single quad analyzer when the collision cell stays idle and does not have any additional functions. In this case, the Q1 mass analyzer can be used as a mass filter, allowing only ions of selected m/z values to pass, which is referred to as selected ion monitoring (SIM) or single scan. It can also allow the scanning and collection of a full spectrum, that is, the transmission of all ions of allowable m/z values, which is referred as full scan. However, in addition to the generic full MS scans and SIM used for preliminary surveys at either Q1 or Q3, many linked scans and mass filters can be performed with both quadrupoles used in tandem.

Examples of linked-scan modes shown in Fig. 19.4 include the precursor-ion scan, product-ion scan, and neutral-loss scan, all of which involve permutations of MS filtering and linked scanning, following or preceding CID accordingly. For example, in the precursor-ion scan, MS1 scanning is linked to fixed selection at MS2, whereas in the product-ion scan, MS2 scanning is linked to fixed selection at MS1. On the other hand, a neutral loss scan involves both MS1 and MS2 scanning for a given MS1/MS2 relationship

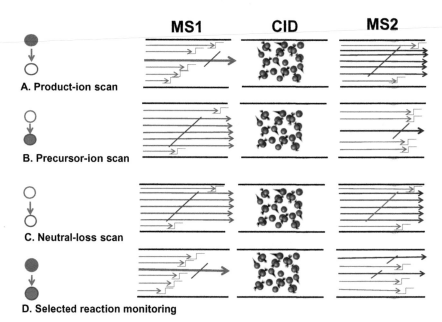

FIGURE 19.4   A general schematic for tandem MS linked scans depicting the ion transitions from precursor ions at MS1 to product ions at MS2. These transitions can also be shown in terms of filled circles, to denote fixed m/z selection (filtering MS event), as well as empty circles to denote scanning, according to a representation popularized by Kondrat and Cooks [3].

of M_i/M_i-N, whereby M_i and M_i-N pertain to the m/z values of the precursor and product ions, respectively, with N denoting the molecular weight (MW) of neutral fragment loss in the decomposition.

The last example shown in Fig. 19.4 is of a particular interest to the modern applications in quantitative analysis, especially in clinical mass spectrometry. This pertains to single-reaction monitoring (SRM), which is essentially a double-stage SIM to measure the precursor ion in Q1, break down the analyte of interest in q2, and measure the signature product ion in Q3. It is typical to measure more than one product ion for one analyte of interest to increase the specificity of the identification and confidence in quantitation. In the meantime, many SRMs can be performed for many analytes during one MS run, which is referred to as multiple-reaction monitoring (MRM). This is presented to the instrument as a list of many precursor-ion/product-ion pairs; to be filtered and monitored during the same analysis. The SRM and MRM modes provide the possibility for the most selective, efficient, and sensitive tandem MS modes that are used in routine and quantitative analysis.

The MRM technology is feasible in many MS/MS configurations from a wide assortment of mass analyzers (see Tables 19.1 and 19.2). However, mass analyzers based on radio frequency (rf) ion guides and multipoles are particularly effective at the implementation of this technology, because of fast-switching rates, the robustness in the acquisition and processing of complex and noisy transients. This feature has allowed for the high-throughput LC-tandem MS analysis of complex mixtures to be realized—in mass analyzers such as the QqQ, quadrupole-ion traps (Q-IT, LTQ-Orbitrap, LTQ-FTICR, etc.), and Q-TOF MSs [30,31].

Typically, for MRM applications in quantitative clinical analysis and elsewhere, at least two transitions per analyte are recommended for the reliable quantification with one SRM being for quantification and the other for additional confirmation and additional levels of specificity for each analyte. Modern instruments are capable of analyzing a large number of MRMs in one experiment while maintain high confidence and specificity in each compound's identification and quantification. For instance, in one study for the LC-MS/MS analysis of drugs of abuse in urine, as many as 1000 transitions (MRM) were processed in a 10-minute run, allowing the highly accurate and reliable quantitative analysis of more than 100 analytes [32]. In addition, two state-of-the-art mass analyzers were compared, namely the QqQ and quadrupole-orbitrap instruments (QExactive, Thermo Fisher Scientific), whereby the performance of the QqQ instrument was slightly better in terms of sensitivity and speed of processing [32].

Despite not having the highest mass accuracy amongst mass analyzer (see Table 19.2), the QqQ MS, produces the best performance in terms of dynamic range, sensitivity, cost, and speed. The LC-QqQ-MS instrument remains the flagship of LC-MS/MS instruments virtually amongst all vendors of modern analytical instruments. Its use is growing considerably in the clinical environment and prototypes of these instruments, such as the classical and self-contained clinical chemistry analyzer instrument, already exist (https://sciex.com/about-us/press-releases/vitamin-d-clearance). It has become the most reliable workhorse and the most robust of the many mass analyzers employed in LC-MS/MS technology with a multitude of clinical applications of LC-MS/MS in clinical diagnostics.

19.3 Clinical applications of mass spectrometry

19.3.1 Overview

Clinical mass spectrometry has generated a lot of interest since the 1950s and the advancements in the technology have enabled even faster growth in clinical applications in the 21st century. New clinical tests continue to be developed, new applications are being explored, and the instruments themselves continue to push boundaries in sensitivity and selectivity for more and broader clinical applications. Some early publications (1950–1978) on clinical mass spectrometry applications included the GC-MS studies of urine β-mercaptolactate-cystines, neutral fecal steroids, dansyl derivatized biogenic amines, urinary acids, etc. [33–38]. The MS analysis of amino acids and urine organic acids would form the core of the earliest MS applications in newborn metabolic screening for inborn errors of metabolism (IEM), such as phenylketonuria (PKU) and various inherited disorders of organic acid metabolism. The MS analysis of inherited disorders of fatty acid metabolism, especially for small, medium, and long-chain acylcarnitines would soon dominate MS applications in IEM [39–42]. In addition, derivatization and GC-MS analysis was the dominant platform in the analysis of metabolites and mixtures for decades, until the arrival of LC-MS/MS and particularly with QqQ MS which became more prominent toward the beginning of the 21st century.

Some major clinical applications of modern LC-MS/MS include newborn screening/IEM, clinical toxicology, drug of abuse testing and pain management, endocrinology and hormone testing, and therapeutic drug monitoring. Recent applications include microorganism identification and clinical proteomics testing for proteins and peptides. Some active research and emerging areas include tissue imaging and real-time surgical testing using mass spectrometry [43–52]. We will use some of the examples to illustrate the functions of mass spectrometry in clinical labs.

19.3.2 Clinical toxicology: drugs of abuse and pain management

Drugs of abuse and pain management are two areas that have played an important role in broadening applications of mass spectrometry. This application fully utilized the specificity and multiplexing capabilities of the mass spectrometry platform and is used to confirm positive identifications of individual drugs after presumptive results from immunoassays for a drug class. The differences between the immunoassay and MS will be discussed in more depth in a later section of this chapter highlighting the unique capabilities of the mass spectrometry platform that give it an advantage. The common categories for drugs of abuse include, but are not limited to, amphetamines and methamphetamines, benzodiazepines, buprenorphine, barbiturates, cocaine, methadone, marijuana, and opiates. They are typically developed in individual panels for qualitative conformation or quantitative results. A more detailed discussion of the sensitivity of LC-MS for drug analysis is shown in Section 19.4.2.

19.3.3 Endocrinology/steroid hormones

The quantification of steroid hormones plays an important role in the diagnosis and treatment of endocrine disorders. There are hundreds of steroids found in humans and all have similar chemical structures. Despite tremendous advances in the analysis of steroids by automated immunoassay, problems still remain, particularly reflected in lack of specificity, sensitivity, and associated matrix effects, as well as limited dynamic range for many analytes. LC-MS/MS has played an important role in providing accurate results for analysis of many of the steroid hormones such as testosterone, estrogen, and free forms of steroid hormones (e.g., free thyroid hormones). The unique advantages of LC-MS/MS with regards to sensitivity will also be discussed in detail in a later section of the chapter.

19.3.4 Therapeutic drug monitoring

The development of the immunosuppressive medication sirolimus (rapamycin) led to the necessity of monitoring its concentration in transplant patients, due, in part, to its narrow therapeutic window. As additional immunosuppressants were developed, methods have been easily modified to quantify a number of these drugs, with tacrolimus, sirolimus, everolimus, and cyclosporine often analyzed in one analytical run [53–56]. These assays are typically performed by LC-MS/MS due to the unavailability or lack of specificity of immunoassay-based tests. At the beginning, the development of the antibodies targeted to those compounds was challenging. LC-MS/MS stepped in as a powerful platform to analyze those compounds without the need for generating specific antibodies. The inactive metabolites of these substances have been shown to interfere with immunoassays and LC-MS/MS provided a great level of specificity to identify and quantify the compounds of interest that immunoassays are not able to achieve. As other classes of immunosuppressants have been in clinical use, additional methods have been developed to measure their concentrations. Other TDM examples also include antidepressants (e.g., amitriptyline), antiepileptics (e.g., lamotrigine and leveritacetam), antifungals (e.g., posaconazole), and pain management (e.g., buprenorphine). These methods are essential to support clinical decision and dose adjustment to serve personalized treatment for patients.

19.3.5 Targeted mass spectrometer assay for clinical proteomics

LC-MS/MS assays for clinical proteomics to analyze peptides and proteins are areas of great interest and growth, although only a few clinical laboratories are running them on a routine basis. The one that remains prominent is the thyroglobulin assay in serum or plasma, which combines the power of immunoenrichment to LC-MS/MS [57]. This assay has played an essential role in establishing the framework and pathways in developing and validating protein assays on LC-MS/MS. It paved the road for clinical proteomics assays to serve the patient needs that are not served by current immunoassays. It also stimulated discussions on the complexity of transferring protein markers into routine clinical diagnostic practices which require rigorous validations and a robust process for targeted clinical LC-MS/MS analysis. These challenges include discordance between laboratories with the enrichment protocols, as well as the uncertainties in the variable digestion protocols that are used to generate the tryptic peptides. Nonetheless efforts are afoot to standardize validation protocols for quantitative clinical proteomics, especially with regard to interlaboratory concordance and harmonization. Studies have shown consistent results among different labs which were using different calibrators and sample preparation steps [57]. This showed great promise for broader applications of targeted mass spectrometry assays for peptides and proteins in a routine clinical lab. This chapter will later discuss further the future prospects of such protein/peptide-based LC-MS/MS assays, especially for diagnostics in traumatic brain injuries (TBI), where proteins/peptides primarily serve as candidate biomarkers.

Overall, mass spectrometry, particularly QqQ mass spectrometry has played an unprecedented role in clinical applications. It has been used in multiple disciplines in laboratory medicine. Drug of abuse, pain management, endocrine, and clinical proteomics are examples of applications illustrating the value of mass spectrometry in serving patients' needs in day-to-day clinical practices. All of these functions are due to the unique advantages of this powerful technology over the traditional methods, such as immunoassay, in providing a complementary platform for clinical diagnostics.

19.4 Comparing immunoassays to clinical mass spectrometer

To date, the above clinical applications constitute the bulk of what is considered clinical mass spectrometry for clinical diagnosis to directly serve the patients' needs on a day-to-day basis. The usage of LC-MS/MS continues to increase rapidly and the growth is due to several significant advantages over the traditional immunoassay methods.

19.4.1 Specificity

First and foremost, LC-MS/MS provides a higher level of specificity for compound identification. Therefore it has been one of the major technologies complementary to immunoassays as a confirmatory platform for drugs of abuse, pain management, and forensic toxicology. LC-MS/MS in this area is promising to resolve the false positive or false negative concerns due to cross-reactivity and poor specificity that plague immunoassays.

The lack of specificity is considered widely to be the major weakness of immunoassays, since antibodies can be cross-reactive with many protein isoforms and other structurally similar molecules, instead of uniquely responding to one designated analyte. In addition, interactions between antigen probes and autoantibodies in human biofluids can further complicate the analytical performance and accuracy of immunoassays. On the other hand, LC-MS/MS is a lot more specific to designated analytes, be they small isomeric molecules or protein isoforms. The advantages in specificity in LC-MS/MS assays accrue from multiple levels of analytical verification within the experiment; that is, LC verification as well as tandem MS verification. First, the unique LC retention times (RT) of analytes distinguish them from other components in the mixture. Second, the molecular weight information confirmed by an MS experiment confers an additional level of specificity. Eventually, the MRM transitions will further distinguish isobaric analytes that may be coeluting. Additionally, even in cases where only precursor scans are performed, high-resolution mass spectrometry can be used to differentiate similar nominal m/z of precursor ions up to the fourth decimal, as is done in the case of quadrupole-orbitrap instruments. As such, clinical mass spectrometry in various eclectic configurations can be used to distinguish protein isoforms and structurally similar small molecules which otherwise would cross-react with the antibody probe in an IA.

19.4.2 Sensitivity

LC-MS/MS typically have higher sensitivity and therefore are able to detect lower concentrations of compounds. The cutoffs for immunoassay-based screening methods and LC-MS/MS-based confirmation assays for commonly available drug of abuse compounds/classes are shown in Table 19.3. Although the cutoffs can vary from lab to lab for LC-MS/MS assays, they are overall much lower than the immunoassays. The high sensitivity provides a great advantage for LC-MS/MS to detect compounds at lower concentration and be the confirmatory testing complementary to the screening tests for drug of abuse.

Furthermore, the high sensitivity can provide additional medical benefits for assays such as testosterone when immunoassay has very limited sensitivity at the low-level end. In this particular case, testosterone measurement is important for both males and females with the circulating levels varying from <7 to more than 1200 ng/dL, depending on age and gender. However, immunoassays have struggled to accurately measure typical low-level concentrations. A comprehensive study of 10 different immunoassays indicated that at lower concentrations (300 ng/dL or 10.4 nmol/L) immunoassays could contribute to two- to even fivefolds of difference (200%−500%) in measuring testosterone in women and children and men with hypogonadism [58]. This can create serious concerns in the diagnosis of endocrine and reproductive diseases. LC-MS/MS assays for testosterone show significantly improved accuracy at the low concentration and overall dynamic range, with

TABLE 19.3 The sensitivity of a LC-MS/MS assay from our reference laboratory is compared to that of the Thermo Fisher DRI (IA). The data shows that LC-MS/MS assay has cutoffs more than one order of magnitude lower than the IA.

Cut-offs for common drug of abuse assays: immunoassay vs. LC-MS/MS (ng/mL)		
Assay	Immunoassay	LC-MS/MS
Amphetamines	1000	20
Barbiturates	200	50
Benzodiazepines	200	20
Cocaine	300	5
Methadone	100	10
Opiates	300	20
Oxycodone	100	20
THC	50	5

improved lower limits of quantification compared to immunoassays. It is recommended to use LC-MS/MS for testosterone testing in pediatric patients, women, and low-testosterone men for accurate measurement and clinical diagnosis [58].

19.4.3 Multiplexing capability

Multiplexing is another unique feature for LC-MS/MS which has resulted in it gaining in popularity. As mentioned above, since LC-MS/MS can detect each analyte uniquely independent of other structurally similar molecules, it is possible in principle that many analytes can be detected simultaneously within one assay, limited only by the instrument scanning bandwidth. In the case of steroids, for example, in addition to the sensitivity that LC-MS/MS provides, it is also able to measure complete steroid profiles in one experiment, compared to one-at-a-time measurement performed in separate immunoassays. Additional evidence of this capability can be presented from LC-MS/MS assays used for the simultaneous analysis of multiple-drug panels, whereby as many as a few hundred of these drugs are identified and quantified in a single run [32].

Hence, it can be argued that one of the best features of LC-MS/MS is the multiplexing and high-throughput analyses of multiple analytes in patient samples. Multiplexed MRM-MS have become commonplace for tens to hundreds of analytes in a single assay, for example, such as the drug of abuse and pain panel assay.

19.4.4 Cost

The LC-MS/MS is markedly less expensive for daily operations once established in the clinical practice, but there is considerable capital cost for the platform, as well as significant cost for highly trained and professional personnel for assay development. However, LC-MS/MS, despite the long development time required, can take less time to offer an assay for clinical use than an immunoassay could accomplish. The latter requires lengthy time for targeted antibody development and selection as well as FDA approval for the market needs. LC-MS/MS assays, therefore, provide more timely support for emerging clinical needs to support patient care. Nonetheless, IAs are readily automated and more user friendly, whereas the LC-MS/MS assays still demand a significant amount of user attention with labor-intensive manual processes. Staff training remains a challenge for most laboratories. However, if the volume is right, the overall cost per assay on LC-MS/MS can be lower than some of the immunoassays. Manufacturers are working on FDA-approved kits to simplify the assay development time for LC-MS/MS which can potentially reduce the overall cost for the assay as well. Nonetheless, it is a tricky balance between the choice of the platforms and the cost. We believe that it is essential to put the patients' needs first when deciding the best platforms for clinical functions, regardless of the isolated assay cost for testing.

LC-MS/MS has been a well-established platform serving clinical diagnostic needs due to its unique advantages in specificity, sensitivity, multiplexing capabilities, as well as potential financial advantages. Due to the fact that most of the new biomarker discovery research has been on mass spectrometry-based "-omics" platforms, the current clinical applications of mass spectrometry provide opportunities to connect the discovery and translational research to enable the potential biomarkers to be seamlessly translated into clinical applications to directly serve patients' diagnosis and prognosis needs.

19.5 The role of clinical mass spectrometry in the analysis of traumatic brain injury

19.5.1 Traumatic brain injury—a brief overview

TBI results from mechanical impact to the brain, that is, during a concussion in contact sports such as boxing, martial arts, and football. The condition has also been diagnosed in subjects from cases of physical violence, vehicle accidents, and exposure to military activities. A sizable incidence of TBI also includes household accidents such as falling, bumping of the head, or even in the recurrent mishandling of infants and other humans during violent and domestic abuse. According to the CDC (https://www.cdc.gov/traumaticbraininjury/index.html) up to 2 million TBI incidents are reported in the United States annually, with 5% mortality, but five times as much hospitalization. Hence, TBI presents a massive disease burden to society, as well as the untold pain and suffering that comes with lowering of the quality of life to affected individuals.

Furthermore, in excess of 5 million subjects live with the effects of TBI, mostly from mild but chronically progressing cases of TBI. At much later stages of TBI, such as in chronic traumatic encelopathy (CTE) as experienced by military personnel, NFL athletes, and possibly boxers, some of the reported symptoms include irritability, temper, violent and suicidal tendencies, memory failures, tremors, as well as other negative behavioral and antisocial dispositions [59–62]. Most of these symptoms are often confused with other neurological disorders such as posttraumatic stress disorder (PTSD), Alzheimer's disease (AD), Parkinson's disease (PD), multiple sclerosis (MS), since many observable traits, clinical presentations, and biochemical expression are shared amongst these disorders [63]. However, TBI likely presents a unique phenotype in terms of the psychological and physiological profile.

The current guidelines for TBI diagnosis following the observation and/or suggestion of brain trauma include cognitive evaluations that are performed by a qualified neuropsychologist, which are based on several criteria including the Glasgow Coma Scale (GCS) and the Glasgow Outcomes Scale (GOS), excluding potential confounders such as drug use and other unrelated neurological stressors. In addition to the psychological evaluation, brain imaging can be recommended in order to rule out any intracranial damage, bleeding, and other lesions which may need immediate clinical attention. This imaging is usually performed using modern instrumental techniques such as computerized axial tomography (CAT or CT) scans, magnetic resonance imaging (MRI), positron emission tomography (PET), differential tensor imaging, and postmortem immunohistochemical (IHC) staining of sections.

Due to the inadequacy of diagnosing TBI, especially in subtle and mild but often recurrent cases, most TBI incidence may go largely undetected until the damage is very severe. In the past decades, very active clinical research on TBI diagnoses has taken place to search for rapid, easy, noninvasive, and cost-effective ways for early diagnosis and prognosis of TBI and particularly from the direct analysis of brain damage—related biomolecules such as neurospecific proteins, lipids, and small molecules [64–67]. Since such markers are released at the site during the onset of injury and should track predictably with disease progression in the brain and over time, they fulfill desirable attributes for good TBI biomarkers.

19.5.2 Current status of mass spectrometry-based traumatic brain injury research

19.5.2.1 Overview

Mass spectrometry has played an important role for biomarker discovery studies for TBI, as evident in literature from studies carried out in animal models and in large clinical cohorts around the world [68–74]. Numerous reviews summarize the enduring aspects of this TBI-related research and progressive developments thereof [64,65,75,76]. Briefly, mass spectrometry-based biomarker discovery has been used extensively in the uncovering of lipidomic, metabolomics, and proteomic markers that are associated with the phenotypes of acute and long-term TBI in animal models as well as in select clinical cohorts. Often, the studies in animal models preceded the validation of discovered candidate biomarkers and TBI signatures in real human patients. In other cases, studies in TBI patients themselves were the starting point of biomarker discovery which were later validated in independent patient cohorts. Fig. 19.5 shows a schematic of biomarker discovery for TBI in an animal model.

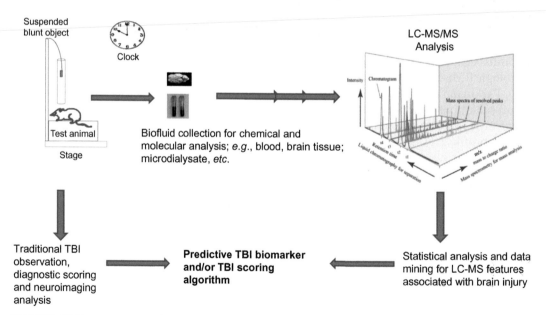

FIGURE 19.5   A schematic of biomarker discovery for TBI in an animal model is shown. Typically, a trained lab animal is immobilized on a stereotactic device and subjected to a timed and controlled impact from a falling blunt object. Thereafter, the traumatic brain injury is assessed on the live animal by traditional behavioral observation and MRI neuroimaging. The animal is eventually euthanized and blood and brain samples are collected for LC-MS/MS analysis.

Typically, a trained lab animal is immobilized on a stereotactic device, and subjected to a timed and controlled impact from a falling blunt object. Thereafter, the TBI is assessed in the live animal by traditional behavioral observation and MRI neuroimaging. The animal is eventually euthanized and blood and brain samples are collected for LC-MS/MS analysis to determine differential molecular signatures that may be associated with TBI.

Statistical approaches, cluster analysis, and multivariate analyses are used to evaluate the differential lipid, metabolite, and proteomic expression between TBI and control sets. From these studies, a wide variety of candidate biomarkers have been produced as shown in Tables 19.4 and 19.5, some of which represent differentially expressed molecules, and some of which are associated with scoring functions and algorithms used to diagnose TBI in real patient samples. LC-MS/MS functions as the major analytical tool to identify differentially expressed proteins or lipids or metabolites for potential biomarkers and to generate more targeted hypothesis for further research and study. We hereby discuss some selected examples of MS-based discovery work, starting with lipidomics and metabolomics studies, followed by neuroproteomics studies.

TABLE 19.4 Lipidomic and metabolomic candidates produced from biomarker discovery research are shown above. Their suggested pathophysiology is related to aberrant metabolism, mitochondrial failure and energy crisis, serial oxidative stress, dysregulated neurotransmitter pathways, and cell death.

Candidate biomarkers	Traumatic brain injury pathophysiology	Potential diagnostic utility
Sphingolipids	Aberrant lipid metabolism, neural damage	SL score
Glycophospholipids	Aberrant lipid metabolism, neural damage	Differential expression
Triglycerides	Aberrant lipid metabolism, neural damage, oxidative stress	Complex signatures
PUFAs and metabolites	Aberrant lipid metabolism, neural damage, oxidative stress	Saturation/Unsaturation/Peroxidation ratios
Glucocortisoids	Aberrant signaling	Complex metabolomic signatures
Neurotransmitters and amino acid metabolites	Aberrant neurosignaling, AA metabolism	Complex metabolomic signatures
Glutamate	Oxidative stress and metabolic syndrome	Complex metabolomic signatures; differential expression
Serum GSH and metabolites	Oxidative stress and metabolic syndrome	Complex metabolomic signatures; differential expression
2,3-bisphosphoglycerate (BPG)	Oxidative stress and metabolic syndrome	Complex metabolomic signatures; differential expression
Acrolein	Aberrant lipid metabolism, neural damage (stroke)	Complex metabolomic signatures; differential expression

TABLE 19.5   Protein candidates produced from neuroproteomic biomarker discovery research are shown above. Their suggested pathophysiology is related to mainly to cellular damage. The corresponding diagnostic utility and disease progression is often complex, dependent on proteomic expression and/or changes in the posttranslation modification, such as hyperphosphorylation and misfolding, etc.

Candidate biomarkers	Traumatic brain injury pathophysiology	Potential diagnostic utility
GFAP	Glial damage	Differential expression
S100β	Astroglial damage, blood–brain barrier	Differential expression
UCHL1	Neural cytoplasm	Differential expression
SPNA2 and fragments	Neural cytoplasm	Differential expression, PTM
NSE	Neural cytoplasm	Differential expression
MBP	Myelin, axon sheath	Differential expression, PTM
MAG	Myelin, axon sheath	Differential expression
MAP-Tau	Axonal injury, tangles, plaques	PTM, differential expression
TDP43	Axonal injury, tangles, plaques	PTM, differential expression
NF-L and NF-H	Axonal injury, tangles, plaques	Differential expression

19.5.2.2 Lipidomics and metabolomics in traumatic brain injury research

Sheth and coworkers [77] designed a murine model of TBI whereby the animals were subjected to controlled brain trauma using a translational device and analyzed postinjury for elevated levels of brain-related sphingolipids (SL) in the brain and plasma. The analysis was performed by hydrophilic interaction liquid chromatography (HILIC)–MS/MS on an LTQ-Orbitrap XL instrument. This analysis was augmented by brain imaging to collect complementary information on the graduated brain trauma, such as infarct size, lesion volume, etc. Having established correlation between lipidomic expression and TBI, an algorithm was then devised as the SL score based on the average of LC-MS/MS analyzed sphingolipid and ceramide SM 36:2 (a doubly unsaturated sphingomyelin with a 36-carbon chain (C_{36})) and Cer 42:1 (a singly unsaturated glucosyl ceramide with a 42-carbon chain (C_{42})) levels in the biofluid of the injured animal. This SL score was then validated against measurements in the plasma of a small population of TBI patients ($n = 14$) compared to a control group. This SL score tracked well with injury and lesion volume in human TBI patient with 80% diagnostic power compared to control.

In another study by Emmerich and coworkers [68], a military population returning from the Iraqi Operation Enduring Freedom tour ($n = 120$) was subjected within 30 days of return to TBI and PTSD screening, apolipoprotein-E (APOE ε4) genotyping, and plasma lipidomic profiling, which was performed using HILIC–MS/MS on an LTQ-XL MS. Statistical analysis was used to determine the MS-derived differential lipidomic expression for several classes of lipids between TBI vs. PTSD groups, APOE ε4 (+) versus APOE ε4 (−), as well as in stages of PTSD severity. In all the affected TBI as well as PTSD classes, lipidomic expression was markedly lower compared to controls. In addition, APOE ε4 (+) subjects had higher phospholipid expressions compared to the APOE ε4 (−) subjects.

This study used LC-MS/MS to posit that differential lipidomics coupled to genotyping of risk factors have a potential for use in clinical diagnostics of TBI in military personnel where PTSD may be a confounder. In a later study by Emmerich and coworkers [69], this statistically derived differential lipidomic profiling was used to track the longitudinal progression of mild-TBI (mTBI) in human subjects. A mice model with the corresponding injury protocol was used for the survey of the differential phospholipid profiling of mTBI compared to control and validated on human subjects. The lipidomic analysis was achieved on a HILIC-LTQ-XL platform and extracted traces were analyzed by an online lipidomic database using custom target lists. The trends in longitudinal phospholipid expressions observed in human subjects were similar to those observed in the animal model. In addition, phospholipid unsaturation and peroxidation were monitored to track suspected changes that occur in acute injury that may persist in the long term.

Lastly, a large metabolomics profiling study by Orešič et al. [78] was carried out using a patient population in Turku as a training model and an independent patient population in Cambridge, UK as a validation model. Briefly, both groups were evaluated, constituted, and stratified according to the GCS/GOS rules as mTBI, moderate TBI (modTBI), severe TBI (sTBI), and healthy controls with the Discovery/Validation comparisons as follows: 100/37 mTBI, 14/7 modTBI, 22/23 sTBI, and 28/27 of controls.

The mass spectrometry-based metabolomics profiling was carried on patient serum (30 μL) and brain microdialysate (100 μL), which were processed by protein crashing, derivatization, and GCxGC-TOFMS analysis against NIST metabolomics libraries. Principal component analysis and multivariate analysis were used, thereby resulting in 48 metabolites which were subsequently selected for use in the prediction of patient outcomes across the patient groups. This model was tested on the Cambridge validation set and found to perform with high accuracy (AUC = 0.84). Of these metabolites, a decanoic acid, octanoic acid, and 2,3-bisphosphoglycerate (2–3, BPG) were found to be particularly elevated in patients with poor outcomes. The study was used to posit that differential metabolite profiling is viable for use in predicting patient outcomes in a clinical setting.

These examples illustrated that small molecules, such as lipids and metabolic markers for TBI, present a very significant component of TBI translational research. These are related to the brain lipidome and metabolites, markers of energy and mitochondrial failure, serial oxidative stress, neurotransmitter pathways, and cell death (see summary in Table 19.4). Such metabolic markers include SL and other brain lipid metabolites, glucocorticoids, glutamate, neurotransmitter metabolites, glutathione (GSH), 2,3-bisphosphoglycerate (BPG), and acrolein, etc. These markers derived from the LC-MS/MS-based metabolomics research provide interesting opportunities toward clinical applications for TBI diagnosis and prognosis.

19.5.2.3 Neuroproteomics in TBI research

The earliest proteomics study in TBI research was carried out by Kobeissy and coworkers [71]. In that study, a rat TBI model was used and compared with a control to survey by shotgun proteomics the differential expression associated with incidence of TBI. Different brain slices from the harvested animals were processed by offline two-dimensional chromatographic separation using cation exchange chromatography and SDS-PAGE as the first and second dimensions. Thereafter, differentially expressed proteins observed by densitometry analysis of the gel bands were digested in-gel and analyzed by RPLC-MS/MS on a LCQ-Deca XP ion trap MS instrument (Thermo Electron). Several brain proteins shown to be differentially expressed in the shotgun proteomics experiment were further validated using a Western blot assay which confirmed cytoplasmic neuroproteins such as ubiquitin carboxyl-terminal hydrolase—L1 (UCH-L1), spectrin-alpha-II (SPNA-2) fragments, glyceraldehyde 3-phosphate dehydrogenase (GAPDH), microtubule-associated protein 2 A or 2B (MAP2A/B), and profillin as potential biomarker candidates.

Shortly thereafter, in a study by Haqqani and coworkers [70], a differential proteomics survey of six pediatric sTBI patients was performed in comparison to a control of a pooled serum of healthy patients. The patient and control samples were processed by the immunodepletion of globulin proteins followed by isotope-coded affinity tagging (ICAT) and gel-free LC-MS/MS analysis of strong-cation exchange (SCX) separated peptide fractions on a nano-LC-Q-TOF Ultima (Waters) MS instrument. Differential proteomic expression (ICAT heavy to light ratio >1.5 up or down) was observed for diverse proteins associated with the inflammatory and immune response.

Interestingly, in a published patent for the immunoassay detection of S100β in neurological conditions [79], 2D-SDS-PAGE coupled with LC-MS/MS was used in the speciation of various S100β isoforms, which included some from extracranial sources and others which are neurospecific. This was performed in order to characterize the form relevant to TBI. In-gel tryptic digestion of the S100β protein band followed by LC-MS/MS independently validated the isolated neural-specific isoform as S100β1 based on a unique isoform-specific peptide sequence.

In another targeted proteomics study, Ottens and coworkers [72] used a 1D-PAGE-LC-MS/MS strategy to analyze the TBI-dependent calpain degradation fragments of a lipid membrane—associated protein, myelin basic protein (MBP), in the brain slices of a mouse model of TBI. The brains of the animals were harvested 2 days after TBI, processed by SDS-PAGE and the isolated MBP bands, corresponding to proteolytic degradation isoforms were excised and in-gel digested using clostripain. For absolute quantification, internal standards (IS) were added which were deuterated analogues of five target peptides selective for the variable transcription of MBP. The RPLC-MS/MS analysis was then performed on a LCQ-Deca-XP ion-trap MS instrument to identify and quantify the variable protein fragments. All proteolytic fragments were analyzed and quantified to femtomole levels in tissue and in the cerebrospinal fluid of the injured animals and not in the naïve controls. This demonstrated the feasibility of isoform-specific and targeted quantitative proteomics in a TBI model while the isoform identification cannot be achieved by the Western blot analysis.

The global discovery as well as targeted neuroproteomic studies for TBI in animal models and patient samples showed similar promise comparable to lipidomics and metabolomics studies of TBI. Additional features in the proteomics studies included the targeted and isoform-specific analysis of potential TBI biomarkers, which can be very useful and provide higher specificity with disease phenotype and progression. This is analogous to other targeted neuroproteomics studies, such as a study by Friedrich and coworkers [80], which identified the enrichment of a potentially immunogenic and disease-related post-translation modification (PTM), the isoaspartate racemization in the MBP sequence in multiple sclerosis patients, as well as a study by Jin and coworkers [81] which reported on the citrullination profiling of several brain proteins including GFAP and MBP.

Targeted and isoform-specific proteomics is promising for TBI because a lot of the markers related to TBI pathophysiology may be significant in an isoform-dependent and/or perhaps not only expression-dependent manner, for example, neurospecific S100β1, p-Tau hyperphosphorylation, MBP degradation, and p-TDP43. These isoform and PTM-specific targeted proteomics can be used to distinguish unique TBI phenotypes from other toxic proteinopathies that are observed in AD and PD for example.

From the above studies, as well as in numerous reviews, it is worth noting that the major brain proteins that have advanced as the most promising for use in further validation and diagnostics studies, include GFAP, which is released into the CSF and circulation following glial injury, UCHL1, a cytoplasmic protein which is released from damaged neurons, MBP, a myelin sheath protein degraded in injury, SPDBs from cytosolic damage, and a neuron-specific calcium binding protein (S100β), which is released from astroglial cell breakdown and the blood−brain barrier (BBB), amongst many. These most promising biomarkers are summarized in Table 19.5.

19.6 New developments: FDA approval on the brain trauma indicator (Banyan BTI)

Following biomarker discovery and neuroproteomic research on TBI, some studies have progressed through clinical trials, and some have gone as far as producing commercial test kits. Nonetheless, only recently, has the FDA approved the first blood test related to TBI for clinical use, namely, the new Brain Trauma Indicator (Banyan BTI) (Banyan Biomarkers, Inc., Alachua, FL) [82,83]. This test was based on the success of the multicenter observation study (Evaluation of Biomarkers of TBI (ALERT-TBI; ClinicalTrials.gov Identifier NCT01426919)) conducted by Bazarian and coworkers [82] at 22 international clinical centers including 15 in the United States and seven in Europe. The test employs a chemiluminescent ELISA sandwich assay on a Synergy 2 Multi-mode Reader to provide a semiquantitative analysis of GFAP and UCH-L1 proteins in the serum of adult patients (18 years or older) collected within 12 h of injury and evaluated with a GCS value of 13−15 indicative of mTBI. A negative reading rules out a requirement for a CT scan for acute intracranial lesions. It is worth noting that the two validated protein markers out of the three initial candidates, viz., GFAP, UCH-L1, and S100β, came out of proteomics research [71,74,79]. In addition, while the immunoassay was eventually chosen for clinical diagnostics method, clinical mass spectrometry has also shown some promise in the translation stage as a good alternative platform for final validation and clinical diagnostics.

19.7 Future of clinical mass spectrometry in the diagnosis of traumatic brain injury

19.7.1 Challenges: from discovery research to the clinic

The remarkable progress in discovery research has provided unprecedented potentials in developing early diagnosis tools for TBI in a regular clinical setting to serve patient needs.

And yet, there are challenges in transitioning from the discovery to clinical practices.

According to Anderson and coworkers [84], the rate of FDA clearance for protein-related biomarkers has been about one test per year. Despite significant investments in biomarker discovery research, none of these FDA-approved markers were from the recent proteomics and metabolomics-based discovery research. This gap was attributed to many reasons and one of them is the lack of a systematic workflow and pipelines to translate the potential biomarkers to clinical applications through comprehensive clinical verifications and validations [84]. The lack of an efficient and productive pipeline is also a reflection of the communication/collaboration gap between researchers, and scientists from the translational research and clinical diagnostics fields, such as clinical chemists. The development of biomarker candidates to well-validated diagnostic markers—or a panel of markers for day-to-day clinical functions—requires preverification and validation, as well as clinical optimization steps which include the FDA approval at the end. The latter steps are all routine for people who are involved in routine clinical testing. From a technical perspective the challenges accrue from the lack of a powerful platform that is able to verify and validate hundreds of the potential markers in an effective manner, to narrow down to the last few candidates for further testing. Furthermore, the required number of samples for the validation process will accordingly increase to tens and hundreds as the number of markers narrows down to fewer and fewer. The scalability of the validation platform is of great significance for the success of the evaluation process. The ability of multiplexing for mass spectometry provides a great potential to fulfil that function.

Therefore the employment of targeted quantitative mass spectrometry is largely viewed as very promising technology for biomarker validation and clinical applications. The targeted mass spectometry approach provides opportunities to measure hundreds of marker candidates at once which helps to narrow the potential biomarkers systematically. The development of clinical proteomics assays, such as thyroglobulin, provided a tangible workflow and pipeline in analyzing proteins and peptides in clinical laboratories [57,85].

19.7.2 Opportunities: targeted mass spectrometry assays for traumatic brain injury biomarker validation and future clinical applications

To our knowledge, there are no published studies that demonstrate the utility of mass spectrometry for further marker validation and assay development for TBI research. Hence, here we explore the (in silico) opportunities to use targeted mass spectrometry for TBI biomarker validation and potential applications in the clinical field. An example of a bottom-up proteomics workflow is shown in Fig. 19.6, illustrating the elaborate sample preparation, biomarker enrichment/separation, and downstream MS analysis.

In Fig. 19.6, after the patient samples are collected and transported to the clinical lab, the workflow is depicted divided into four stages, namely protein purification, protease digestion, peptide enrichment, and LC-MS/MS analysis. The results are reported at the end. In this bottom-up workflow, peptides representing the protein of interest are the final analytes which are subject to the LC-MS/MS MRM analysis. The protein purification stage is to enrich protein(s) of interest or the potential biomarkers to be validated from the patient samples. The purification step will remove other interferences from the samples to increase the sensitivity and specificity of the assay. Protease digestion, typically involving

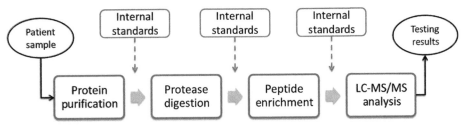

FIGURE 19.6   A representative schematic of a putative quantitative and clinical proteomics workflow.

trypsin, is put under desirable reaction conditions and used to digest the protein of interest to generate the peptides. The choice of peptides is essential so that the signature peptide(s) that uniquely identifies and presents the protein of interest will be enriched for further LC-MS/MS analysis.

Due to the quantitative nature of this assay, IS, which are stable isotope-labeled analogues of intact proteins or peptides, are required. Different strategies permit the IS to be added at different time points. It is preferred for the IS to be added as early as possible to help "monitor" the process. And yet, creating isotopically labeled proteins to be added during the protein digestion step can be cost prohibitive. Isotopically labeled peptides have been proven to be adequate for quantitative purposes and added before or after the peptide enrichment step. Other concerns such as IS availability and stability can also contribute to the experimental design. Nonetheless, it is essential to evaluate all the steps for ideal experimental conditions for protein enrichment, protease digestion conditions (type of proteases, duration, temperature, protease:protein ratio, etc.), choice of signature peptides, and enrichment conditions. In addition, HPLC running conditions and mass spectrometry MRM parameters for signature peptides are all important considerations for a reliable and robust clinical assay.

As an illustration, candidate markers (listed on Table 19.5 above) can be used to simulate the development of an MRM MS method for TBI biomarker validation. The accompanying Table 19.6 above shows an in silico list of TBI-related MRMs that can be generated. Here, Skyline was used to design a hypothetical multiplex assay for GFAP, UCHL1, Tau, NSE, MBP, and MAG (only MBP, ENOG, and UCHL1 are shown), whereby each protein could be identified by at least two tryptic peptides, each represented by at least two MRMs. In this example, 46 MRMs were generated from FASTA sequences for peptide precursors of charges (z) of +2 and +3. The MRMs were set to monitor the precursor ion b and y fragments, using reference LC-MS/MS spectra from a publicly accessible NIST database as a template. For MBP, [14]YLATASTMDHAR[25] ($C_{56}H_{90}N_{17}O_{19}S$, MW of 1336.5 Da)—a 12-mer tryptic peptide—obtained from the cleavage between the 13th and 26th residues, was used as an illustration (see Fig. 19.7 below).

Fig. 19.7 shows the in silico MS/MS spectrum (from a triply charged precursor, $M + 3H^{+}$ of m/z 446.22, z = 3) with many fragment ions appearing in the m/z range of 200—450. The top two MRMs (see highlighted in Table 19.6) were derived from the production of the most intense CID fragments as shown in the MS/MS spectrum. For example, the 446.2/249.6 transition for [14]YLATASTMDHAR[25] corresponds to the formation of the y4 + + fragment (D-H-A-R, in blue), whereas the 446.2/277.2 corresponds to the b2 + fragment (Y-L in red).

TABLE 19.6   Above shows an in silico list of TBI-related MRMs that can be generated. Here, Skyline was used to design a hypothetical multiplex assay for GFAP, UCHL1, Tau, NSE, MBP, and MAG (only MBP, ENOG, and UCHL1 are shown with the top two MBP peptides highlighted).

Compound group	Compound name	Precursor ion (m/z)	Product ion (m/z)	Ion name	Library rank
sp|P02686|MBP_HUMAN	YLATASTMDHAR	446.22	249.62	y4	1
sp|P02686|MBP_HUMAN	YLATASTMDHAR	446.22	277.15	b2	2
sp|P02686|MBP_HUMAN	YLATASTMDHAR	446.22	409.18	y7	3
sp|P02686|MBP_HUMAN	HRDTGILDSIGR	447.24	340.68	b6	2
sp|P02686|MBP_HUMAN	HRDTGILDSIGR	447.24	432.26	y4	3
sp|P02686|MBP_HUMAN	GFKGVDAQGTLSK	436.57	338.18	b7	2
sp|P02686|MBP_HUMAN	GFKGVDAQGTLSK	436.57	317.18	y6	3
sp|P09104|ENOG_HUMAN	DGKYDLDFK	367.51	409.21	y3	1
sp|P09104|ENOG_HUMAN	FAGHNFR	424.71	315.66	y5	1
sp|P09104|ENOG_HUMAN	DGKYDLDFK	367.51	404.18	b7	2
sp|P09104|ENOG_HUMAN	FAGHNFR	424.71	351.18	y6	2
sp|P09104|ENOG_HUMAN	DGKYDLDFK	367.51	294.18	y2	3
sp|P09104|ENOG_HUMAN	FAGHNFR	424.71	436.23	y3	3
sp|P09936|UCHL1_HUMAN	LGVAGQWR	443.75	358.7	y6	1
sp|P09936|UCHL1_HUMAN	FSAVALC[+57]K	448.24	235.11	b2	1
sp|P09936|UCHL1_HUMAN	LGVAGQWR	443.75	341.22	b4	2
sp|P09936|UCHL1_HUMAN	FSAVALC[+57]K	448.24	405.21	b4	2
sp|P09936|UCHL1_HUMAN	LGVAGQWR	443.75	270.18	b3	3
sp|P09936|UCHL1_HUMAN	FSAVALC[+57]K	448.24	420.23	y3	3

Obviously, more realistic MRMs can already be derived from peptides that were observed in the preexisting TBI neuroproteomics data, instead of hypothetical peptides.

Therefore targeted LC-MS/MS assays can be developed to validate potential TBI biomarkers for further validation and even clinical applications down the roads. They can be complementary to the new chemiluminescent ELISA sandwich assays, especially those that have already been developed for S100β, GFAP, and UCHL1. The case of S100β is particularly interesting because, whereas commercial assays for both UCHL1 and GFAP are now FDA approved in the United States, the S100β ELISA has not been equally successful. The protein has been known for a very long time to be present in TBI at higher concentrations than both GFAP and UCHL1, and it was at once considered to be a more promising prospect [70,86−90]. It is even more popular and commercialized internationally.

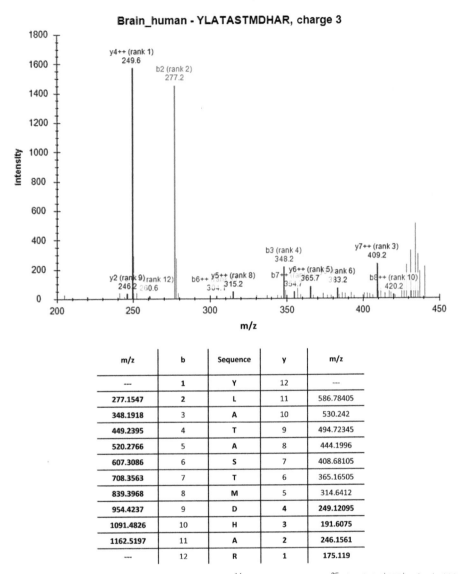

FIGURE 19.7 The hypothetical MS/MS spectrum for [14]YLATASTMDHAR[25], (with M[+]3H[+] of m/z 446.22, $z =$ 3), the 12-mer peptide of MBP highlighting the top 2 most intense peaks (shown in centroid), namely the y_4^{++} and b_2^+ product ions. The sequence annotation is shown on the right.

19.8 Summary

Mass spectrometry has been proven to be a very powerful platform in both clinical diagnostics and biomarker translational research. In clinical applications, it has provided unprecedented advantages over traditional technologies due to its high specificity,

VI. Analytical testing consideration

sensitivity, multiplexing capability, as well as its flexibility for laboratory developed testing due to its customized and unique requirements in individual labs. It has provided a great service for patients in newborn metabolic screening, drug of abuse testing, pain management, endocrine testing, microbiology organism identification, and others. The emerging developments in targeted mass spectrometry assays for analytes like thyroglobulin have paved the road for further implementation of proteins and peptides in clinical labs, which also have provided a workflow to expedite the validation process and clinical applications of new biomarkers for disease diagnosis and prognosis.

The immense value of mass spectrometry in biomarker translational research has been demonstrated by numerous publications for various disease conditions in the past decades and the recent developments in the "-omics" (proteomics, metabolomics, and lipidomics) research for TBI research. These include the now available BTI test amongst others, based on proteomic markers such as $S100\beta$, GFAP, UCHL1, etc., to diagnose some neurological condition related to TBI. However, the race still goes on toward the development of a comprehensive TBI test(s), which will diagnose mTBI to sTBI, in acute and longitudinal cases, across platforms, and which can lead to the successful monitoring of disease progression and therapy. We have explored the opportunity to develop LC-MS/MS targeted proteomics assays in silico for potential TBI biomarkers for their further validation and clinical applications. We believe that LC-MS/MS will certainly continue to play a pivotal role in this next phase of translational TBI research for TBI diagnosis and prognosis to bring more exciting news for the further advancement of clinical practice in this field.

References

[1] Thomson JJ. On the appearance of helium and neon in vacuum tubes. Science 1913;37(949):360–4.
[2] Aston FW. The story of isotopes. Science 1933;78(2010):5–6.
[3] Kondrat RW, Cooks RG. Direct analysis of mixtures by mass spectrometry. Anal Chem 1978;50(1):81A–92A.
[4] Tate JT, Smith PT. Ionization potentials and probabilities for the formation of multiply charged ions in the alkali vapors and in krypton and xenon. Phys Rev 1934;46(9):773–6.
[5] Munson MSB, Field FH. Chemical ionization mass spectrometry. I. general introduction. J Am Chem Soc 1966;88(12):2621–30.
[6] Barber M, et al. Fast atom bombardment of solids (F.A.B.): a new ion source for mass spectrometry. J Chem Soc Chem Commun 1981;7:325–7.
[7] Honig RE. Sputtering of surfaces by positive ion beams of low energy. J Appl Phys 1958;29(3):549–55.
[8] Inghram MG, Gomer R. Mass spectrometric analysis of ions from the field microscope. J Chem Phys 1954;22(7):1279–80.
[9] Macfarlane RD, Torgerson DF. Californium-252 plasma desorption mass spectroscopy. Science 1976;191:920–5.
[10] Whitehouse CM, et al. Electrospray interface for liquid chromatographs and mass spectrometers. Anal Chem 1985;57:675–9.
[11] Yamashita M, Fenn JB. Electrospray ion source. Another variation on the free-jet theme. J Phys Chem 1984;88(20):4451–9.
[12] Tanaka K, et al. Protein and polymer analyses up to mlz 100 000 by laser ionization time-of-flight mass spectrometry. Rapid Commun Mass Spectrom 1988;2(8):151–3.
[13] Fenn JB, et al. Electrospray ionization for mass spectrometry of large biomolecules. Science 1989;246:64–71.
[14] Karas M, Hillenkamp F. Laser desorption ionization of proteins with molecular masses exceeding 10,000 daltons. Anal Chem 1988;60:2299–301.
[15] Carroll DI, et al. Atmospheric pressure ionization mass spectrometry. Corona discharge ion source for use in a liquid chromatograph-mass spectrometer-computer analytical system. Anal Chem 1975;47:2369–73.

[16] Robb DB, Covey TR, Bruins AP. Atmospheric pressure photoionization: an ionization method for liquid chromatography—mass spectrometry. Anal Chem 2000;72:3653—9.

[17] Mellmann A, et al. Evaluation of matrix-assisted laser desorption ionization-time-of-flight mass spectrometry in comparison to 16 S rRNA gene sequencing for species identification of nonfermenting bacteria. J Clin Microbiol 2008;46(6):1946—54.

[18] Eigner U, et al. Performance of a matrix-assisted laser desorption ionization-time-of-flight mass spectrometry system for the identification of bacterial isolates in the clinical routine laboratory. Clin Lab 2009;55(7—8):289—96.

[19] Ilina EN, et al. Direct bacterial profiling by matrix-assisted laser desorption-ionization time-of-flight mass spectrometry for identification of pathogenic Neisseria. J Mol Diagn 2009;11(1):75—86.

[20] Nagy E, et al. Species identification of clinical isolates of Bacteroides by matrix-assisted laser-desorption/ionization time-of-flight mass spectrometry. Clin Microbiol Infect 2009;15(8):796—802.

[21] Seng P, et al. Ongoing revolution in bacteriology: routine identification of bacteria by matrix-assisted laser desorption ionization time-of-flight mass spectrometry. Clin Infect Dis 2009;49(4):543—51.

[22] Wang J, et al. Rapid determination of the geographical origin of honey based on protein fingerprinting and barcoding using MALDI TOF MS. J Agric Food Chem 2009;57(21):10081—8.

[23] Bessede E, et al. Matrix-assisted laser-desorption/ionization biotyper: experience in the routine of a University hospital. Clin Microbiol Infect 2011;17(4):533—8.

[24] Matsuyama Y. [Rapid microbial ID system based on MALDI TOF MS-MALDI biotyper-]. Rinsho Biseibutshu Jinsoku Shindan Kenkyukai Shi 2011;22(1—2):27—30.

[25] Saffert RT, et al. Comparison of Bruker biotyper matrix-assisted laser desorption ionization-time of flight mass spectrometer to BD phoenix automated microbiology system for identification of gram-negative bacilli. J Clin Microbiol 2011;49(3):887—92.

[26] Chaurand P, Caprioli RM. Direct profiling and imaging of peptides and proteins from mammalian cells and tissue sections by mass spectrometry. Electrophoresis 2002;23(18):3125—35.

[27] Chaurand P, et al. Proteomics in diagnostic pathology: profiling and imaging proteins directly in tissue sections. Am J Pathol 2004;165(4):1057—68.

[28] Longuespee R, et al. MALDI mass spectrometry imaging: a cutting-edge tool for fundamental and clinical histopathology. Proteom Clin Appl 2016;10(7):701—19.

[29] Stauber J, et al. MALDI imaging of formalin-fixed paraffin-embedded tissues: application to model animals of Parkinson disease for biomarker hunting. J Proteome Res 2008;7(3):969—78.

[30] Hoffman Ed. Tandem mass spectrometry: a primer. J Mass Spectrom 1996;31:129—37.

[31] Johnson JV, et al. Tandem-in-space and tandem-in-time mass spectrometry: triple quadrupoles and quadrupole ion traps. Anal Chem 1990;62(20):2162—72.

[32] Doyle RM. Screening and quantitative LC-MS/MS analysis of 495 drugs and their metabolites in urine on triple quadrupole and quadrupole orbitrap mass spectrometers. Society of Forensic Toxicologists (SOFT) Annual Meeting 2017. Boca Raton, FL, USA: Oxford Academic; 2017.

[33] Eneroth P, Haelstrom K, Ryhage R. Identification and quantification of neutral fecal steroids by gas-liquid chromatography and mass spectrometry: studies of human excretion during two dietary regimens. J Lipid Res 1964;5:245—62.

[34] Crawhall JC, et al. Beta-mercaptolactate-cysteine disulfide: analog of cystine in the urine of a mentally retarded patient. Science 1968;160(3826):419—20.

[35] Creveling CR, Kondo K, Daly JW. Use of dansyl derivatives and mass spectrometry for identification of biogenic amines. Clin Chem 1968;14(4):302—9.

[36] Crawhall JC, et al. Urinary phenolic acids in tyrosinemia. Identification and quantitation by gas chromatography-mass spectrometry. Clin Chim Acta 1971;34(1):47—54.

[37] Mamer OA, Crawhall JC, Tjoa SS. The identification of urinary acids by coupled gas chromatography-mass spectrometry. Clin Chim Acta 1971;32(2):171—84.

[38] Mamer OA, et al. Profiles in altered metabolism I—the organic acids accumulating in acute non-diabetic ketoacidosis associated with alcoholism. Biomed Mass Spectrom 1978;5(4):287—90.

[39] Kodo N, et al. Quantitative assay of free and total carnitine using tandem mass spectrometry. Clin Chim Acta 1990;186(3):383—90.

[40] Millington DS, et al. Tandem mass spectrometry: a new method for acylcarnitine profiling with potential for neonatal screening for inborn errors of metabolism. J Inherit Metab Dis 1990;13(3):321—4.

[41] Millington DS, et al. Application of fast atom bombardment with tandem mass spectrometry and liquid chromatography/mass spectrometry to the analysis of acylcarnitines in human urine, blood, and tissue. Anal Biochem 1989;180(2):331–9.

[42] Wilcken B, et al. Screening newborns for inborn errors of metabolism by tandem mass spectrometry. N Engl J Med 2003;348:2304–12.

[43] Brown HM, Pirro V, Cooks RG. From DESI to the MasSpec pen: ambient ionization mass spectrometry for tissue analysis and intrasurgical cancer diagnosis. Clin Chem 2018;64(4):628–30.

[44] Alexander J, et al. A novel methodology for in vivo endoscopic phenotyping of colorectal cancer based on real-time analysis of the mucosal lipidome: a prospective observational study of the iKnife. Surg Endosc 2017;31(3):1361–70.

[45] Balog J, et al. Intraoperative tissue identification using rapid evaporative ionization mass spectrometry. Sci Transl Med 2013;5(194). p. 194ra93.

[46] Guitton Y, et al. Rapid evaporative ionisation mass spectrometry and chemometrics for high-throughput screening of growth promoters in meat producing animals. Food Addit Contam Part A Chem Anal Control Expo Risk Assess 2018;35(5):900–10.

[47] Phelps DL, et al. The surgical intelligent knife distinguishes normal, borderline and malignant gynaecological tissues using rapid evaporative ionisation mass spectrometry (REIMS). Br J Cancer 2018;118(10):1349–58.

[48] St John ER, et al. Rapid evaporative ionisation mass spectrometry of electrosurgical vapours for the identification of breast pathology: towards an intelligent knife for breast cancer surgery. Breast Cancer Res 2017;19 (1):59.

[49] Verplanken K, et al. Rapid evaporative ionization mass spectrometry for high-throughput screening in food analysis: the case of boar taint. Talanta 2017;169:30–6.

[50] Eberlin LS. Analytical technologies to improve human health. Anal Chem 2018;90(7):4235.

[51] Garza KY, et al. Desorption electrospray ionization mass spectrometry imaging of proteins directly from biological tissue sections. Anal Chem 2018;90(13):7785–9.

[52] Porcari AM, et al. Multicenter study using desorption-electrospray-ionization-mass-spectrometry imaging for breast-cancer diagnosis. Anal Chem 2018;90(19):11324–32.

[53] Rockwood AL, Johnson-Davis KL. Mass spectrometry for clinical toxicology: therapeutic drug management and trace element analysis. Clin Lab Med 2011;31(3):407–28.

[54] McMillin GA, Johnson-Davis K, Dasgupta A. Analytical performance of a new liquid chromatography/tandem mass spectrometric method for determination of everolimus concentrations in whole blood. Ther Drug Monit 2012;34(2):222–6.

[55] Dasgupta A, Khalil SA, Johnson-Davis KL. Analytical performance evaluation of a new cobas tacrolimus assay on cobas e411 analyzer: comparison of values obtained by the CMIA tacrolimus assay and a liquid chromatography combined with tandem mass spectrometric method. Ann Clin Lab Sci 2016;46(2):204–8.

[56] McMahon LM, et al. High-throughput analysis of everolimus (RAD001) and cyclosporin A (CsA) in whole blood by liquid chromatography/mass spectrometry using a semi-automated 96-well solid-phase extraction system. Rapid Commun Mass Spectrom 2000;14(21):1965–71.

[57] Kushnir MM, et al. Measurement of thyroglobulin by liquid chromatography-tandem mass spectrometry in serum and plasma in the presence of antithyroglobulin autoantibodies. Clin Chem 2013;59(6):982–90.

[58] Herold DA, Fitzgerald RL. Immunoassays for testosterone in women: better than a guess? Clin Chem 2003;49 (8):1250–1.

[59] Ishibe N, Wlordarczyk RC, Fulco C. Overview of the institute of medicine's committee search strategy and review process for gulf war and health: long-term consequences of traumatic brain injury. J Head Trauma Rehabil 2009;24(6):424–9.

[60] Castellani RJ, Perry G. Dementia pugilistica revisited. J Alzheimers Dis 2017;60(4):1209–21.

[61] Corsellis JA, Bruton CJ, Freeman-Browne D. The aftermath of boxing. Psychol Med 1973;3(3):270–303.

[62] McKee AC, et al. Chronic traumatic encephalopathy in athletes: progressive tauopathy after repetitive head injury. J Neuropathol Exp Neurol 2009;68(7):709–35.

[63] Ling H, et al. Histological evidence of chronic traumatic encephalopathy in a large series of neurodegenerative diseases. Acta Neuropathol 2015;130(6):891–3.

[64] Adibhatla RM, Hatcher JF, Dempsey RJ. Lipids and lipidomics in brain injury and diseases. AAPS J 2006;8 (2):E314–21.

[65] Moghieb A, Mangaonkar M, Wang KKW. Mass spectrometry based translational neuroinjury proteomics. Transl Proteom 2013;1(1):65−73.

[66] Posti JP, et al. Metabolomics profiling as a diagnostic tool in severe traumatic brain injury. Front Neurol 2017;8:398.

[67] Wang HC, et al. The role of serial oxidative stress levels in acute traumatic brain injury and as predictors of outcome. World Neurosurg 2016;87:463−70.

[68] Emmerich T, et al. Plasma lipidomic profiling in a military population of mild traumatic brain injury and post-traumatic stress disorder with apolipoprotein E varepsilon4-dependent effect. J Neurotrauma 2016;33 (14):1331−48.

[69] Emmerich T, et al. Mild TBI results in a long-term decrease in circulating phospholipids in a mouse model of injury. Neuromolecular Med 2017;19(1):122−35.

[70] Haqqani AS, et al. Biomarkers and diagnosis; protein biomarkers in serum of pediatric patients with severe traumatic brain injury identified by ICAT-LC-MS/MS. J Neurotrauma 2007;24(1):54−74.

[71] Kobeissy FH, et al. Novel differential neuroproteomics analysis of traumatic brain injury in rats. Mol Cell Proteom 2006;5(10):1887−98.

[72] Ottens AK, et al. Proteolysis of multiple myelin basic protein isoforms after neurotrauma: characterization by mass spectrometry. J Neurochem 2008;104(5):1404−14.

[73] Ottens AK, et al. Post-acute brain injury urinary signature: a new resource for molecular diagnostics. J Neurotrauma 2014;31(8):782−8.

[74] Ren C, et al. Assessment of serum UCH-L1 and GFAP in acute stroke patients. Sci Rep 2016;6:24588.

[75] Ganau M, et al. Current and future applications of biomedical engineering for proteomic profiling: predictive biomarkers in neuro-traumatology. Med (Basel) 2018;5(1).

[76] Manek R, et al. Protein biomarkers and neuroproteomics characterization of microvesicles/exosomes from human cerebrospinal fluid following traumatic brain injury. Mol Neurobiol 2018;55(7):6112−28.

[77] Sheth SA, et al. Targeted lipid profiling discovers plasma biomarkers of acute brain injury. PLoS One 2015;10 (6):e0129735.

[78] Oresic M, et al. Human serum metabolites associate with severity and patient outcomes in traumatic brain injury. EBioMedicine 2016;12:118−26.

[79] Larner S, Patent US 2017/0176460A1: neural specific S100-beta for biomarker assays and devices for detection of a neurological condition. In: Banyan Biomarkers I, editor, United States: Banyan Biomarkers, Inc., 2017, p. 1−18.

[80] Friedrich MG, et al. Isoaspartic acid is present at specific sites in myelin basic protein from multiple sclerosis patients: could this represent a trigger for disease onset? Acta Neuropathol Commun 2016;4(1):83.

[81] Jin Z, et al. Identification and characterization of citrulline-modified brain proteins by combining HCD and CID fragmentation. Proteomics 2013;13(17):2682−91.

[82] Bazarian JJ, et al. Serum GFAP and UCH-L1 for prediction of absence of intracranial injuries on head CT (ALERT-TBI): a multicentre observational study. Lancet Neurol 2018;17(9):782−9.

[83] Samson K. In the clinic—traumatic brain injury: fda approves first blood test for brain bleeds after mild tbi/ concussion. Neurol Today 2018;18(12):12−18.

[84] Anderson NL, Ptolemy AS, Rifai N. The riddle of protein diagnostics: future bleak or bright? Clin Chem 2013;59(1):194−7.

[85] Hoofnagle AN, Wener MH. The fundamental flaws of immunoassays and potential solutions using tandem mass spectrometry. J Immunol Methods 2009;347(1−2):3−11.

[86] Calcagnile O, Undén L, Undén J. Clinical validation of S100B use in management of mild head injury. BMC Emerg Med 2012;12(13):1−6.

[87] Papa L, et al. GFAP out-performs S100beta in detecting traumatic intracranial lesions on computed tomography in trauma patients with mild traumatic brain injury and those with extracranial lesions. J Neurotrauma 2014;31(22):1815−22.

[88] Ercole A, et al. Kinetic modelling of serum S100b after traumatic brain injury. BMC Neurol 2016;16:93.

[89] Welch RD, et al. Ability of serum glial fibrillary acidic protein, ubiquitin C-terminal hydrolase-L1, and S100B to differentiate normal and abnormal head computed tomography findings in patients with suspected mild or moderate traumatic brain injury. J Neurotrauma 2016;33(2):203−14.

[90] Thelin EP, Nelson DW, Bellander BM. A review of the clinical utility of serum S100B protein levels in the assessment of traumatic brain injury. Acta Neurochir (Wien) 2017;159(2):209−25.

VI. Analytical testing consideration

20

Surface plasmon resonance

Daisuke Saito[1] and Takahito Nakagawa[2]

[1]Konica Minolta Healthcare Americas, Wayne, NJ, United States
[2]Konica Minolta, Tokyo, Japan

20.1 Introduction

The term surface plasmon resonance (SPR) may be unfamiliar to many, but its effects are part of daily life. For example, the stained-glass windows in the world's great cathedrals have remained vibrant over centuries as a result of SPR. Artisans in the Middle Ages recognized that mixing glass and metallic oxide under specific conditions would produce radiant stained-glass panels. Unknown to the artisans, this outcome was the result of plasmon resonance in the metallic oxide glass that they used. The specific refinement of this SPR is called localized SPR (LSPR), which is also familiar in commercially available home pregnancy tests. This application uses specifically prepared colloidal gold nanoparticles (NPs), which, in the presence of pregnancy hormones, cluster together to produce the color change, indicating pregnancy. This color modification is induced by plasmonic effects of the gold particles. Consider this analogy: a tone made by a violin reverberates within the instrument in order to be sustained. Similarly, SPR is sustained by the photon/particle interactions in the evanescent wave (EW) dancing between a metal and a dielectric surface (Fig. 20.1).

In short, SPR is the resonant oscillation of free electrons that occurs at the interface between negative (i.e., dielectric) and positive (e.g., metals) permittivity materials when stimulated by incident light. If the wave-vector component of the incident light that is oriented parallel to the interface matches the propagation constant of the surface plasmon wave, SPR then occurs. Most of the incident energy is coupled into the surface plasmon field, which results in shifts in the resonance angle and wavelength, along with changes in the intensity and phase of the reflected light [1]. There are a variety of configurations used to produce SPR, including prism-coupling, grating-coupling, and LSPR, using gold NPs as the conductive material. This chapter describes the evolution of these techniques as applied to SPR biosensors, assesses their advantages and disadvantages, and discusses their potential clinical applications to detect clinically important biomarkers in a variety of conditions that include cardiac disease and traumatic brain injury (TBI).

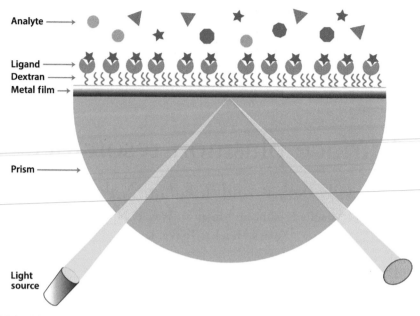

FIGURE 20.1   Illustration of surface plasmon resonance (SPR) stimulated by light at an interface of a dielectric and a conductive material. The amplification of the wave is traceable to SPR.

20.2 History

The stained glass in church windows has the same components as SPR-based sensors, which consist of a prism of glass or fine plastic, metal film, a light source, and a detector. In stained glass, the metallic-oxide-compound glass is the prism-plus-metal film that refracts natural light to our eyes, the detector.

It was not until the turn of the 20th century that researchers began to understand the mechanisms underlying the anomalies in light reflected from different dielectric surfaces [2] and to develop models to simulate this phenomenon [3]. And only in the 1940s were these theoretical concepts finally verified [4], with experimentation with light, metals, and prisms being accelerated.

During the 1950s the dielectric configuration of metal foils became a focus for SPR researchers, when Ritchie and colleagues demonstrated plasmon excitation in thin metal foils [5]. In 1968 a preliminary configuration of metal foil components such as silver and gold that would create an SPR model was proposed [6]. Later that year, Kretschmann and Raether subsequently modified the location of components in the metal foil material to produce a stable SPR platform with predictable characteristics. This Kretschmann–Raether configuration was a key invention that allowed the translation of SPR theory into an applied practical sensor [7].

Otto first demonstrated that the excitation occurs by metal-prism coupling in 1968 [6]. In Otto's configuration, when a light beam illuminates a prism at an angle greater than the critical angle (a "critical angle" is that at which total internal reflection would occur), the attenuated total internal reflection produces an EW at the base of the prism. A metal layer is then placed below the prism, in turn leaving a gap between the two. Subsequently, a sample liquid of lower refractive index than the prism is flowed into the gap. When the EW reaches the metal layer, the surface plasmon interacts with electromagnetic waves in the air or dielectric material to produce surface plasmon polaritons (SPPs) (Fig. 20.2A). The challenge with Otto's configuration was the difficulty of maintaining the optimal gap between the metal and the prism.

Kretschmann proposed a different model that overcame the gap problem in Otto's design. His pivotal configuration of SPR became the basic principle of today's commercially available products [7]. In Kretschmann's configuration, the metal film is evaporated onto the glass block. The light illuminates the glass block, and an EW penetrates through the metal film, with the plasmons being excited at the film's outer side. This demonstrated that the nonradiative mode excited by light can also radiate. Kretschmann's term for this phenomenon, "nonradiative surface plasma wave," was later replaced by the terminology SPP (Fig. 20.2B). Kretschmann's configuration eliminated the gap problem and made it possible to control the thickness and composition of the metal surface, thereby allowing for greater control, reproducibility, and improved detection.

Otto's and Kretschmann's configurations can be described by classical electromagnetism. The reflectance is a function of the angle of incidence θ, the relative permittivities of the metal $\varepsilon 1$, the dielectric medium $\varepsilon 0$, and angular frequency ω.

Significant technologic advances during the 1970s and 1980s in laser technology, optical systems, cameras, and in digital information modalities brought to the marketplace new

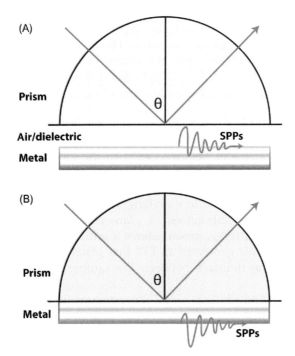

FIGURE 20.2 (A) Otto's configuration. (B) Kretschmann's configuration.

products such as video, CD, and DVD players, as well as miniaturized digital optical data formats. These advances made it easier to manufacture the basic components of the modern SPR sensors, which require a light source (p-polarized light) and an optical system, optical-coupling components (a prism, grating, waveguide, or optical fiber), an imaging optical system, and a photodetector such as a photodiode or a camera. Such improvements enabled precise design, stable quality, and bulk production of SPR-based sensor technology at an affordable cost. During this time, Biacore, AB (Uppsala, Sweden), which was later acquired by the General Electric Company, developed the first generation of SPR-based sensing products.

The first SPR immunoassay was proposed in 1983 by researchers in Sweden. Liedberg, Nylander, and Lundström adsorbed human immunoglobulin (IgG) onto a 600-angstrom silver film and used the assay to detect antihuman IgG in water solution [8]. SPR-based sensing products became commercially available in 1990. Today, a broad variety of SPR-based sensors from several manufacturers is available to researchers.

Existing techniques for biomarker detection, such as enzyme-linked immunosorbent assay (ELISA), require complex preparation steps, including a long incubation period that may last from several hours to days. The process often includes a series of washing and mixing steps that are labor-intensive and time-consuming [9]. Automated operation systems, such as the chemiluminescence enzyme immunoassay (CLEIA), make the immunoassay analysis clinically useful; however, they require sera or plasma as the assay sample. Therefore whole blood must first be centrifuged followed by analysis of the sample, which requires another process to complete [10].

SPR biosensors enable highly sensitive measurements of unlabeled interactions in real time with no destruction of original form and its function of materials. SPR-based sensors show promise for routine use in clinical settings to detect clinically important proteins in real time and with high sensitivity, without requiring labeled material. The advantages of SPR biosensors encompass the capability of using whole blood, the simple operation that finalizes an assay in about 10 minutes, the ability to check for multiple biomarkers in a single sample in one instrument, and the mobility (for example, use at point-of-care (POC), in military applications, or during disasters).

Since SPR's commercial introduction in the 1990s, it has been proven to be an effective technology in determining the binding of macromolecules in many bond types. This optical technique measures the refractive index changes of polarized light in the vicinity of thin metal layers (e.g., gold, silver, or aluminum films) in response to biomolecular interactions [11].

The factors necessary to produce SPR include the specific wavelength of incident light and the refraction indexes of metal and dielectric substances. A plane-polarized light beam entering the higher refractive index medium (glass prism) above a critical angle of incidence can undergo total internal refraction. This generates an EW that penetrates into the metal film to excite surface plasmons at the interface between the sample and the metal film [12].

The combined excitation of surface plasmon and photons yields electromagnetic waves in the air or dielectric material, which are entangled quasiparticles comprising both surface plasmons and photons [13]. These nonradiative electromagnetic surface waves propagate in a direction parallel to the negative permittivity/dielectric material interface. The wave is on the boundary of the conductor and the external medium, and any changes at this boundary, such as those caused by the adsorption of molecules on the conducting surface, will alter the SPR waves [14].

In SPR biosensors, ligand molecules are immobilized onto the sensor surface. A solution of analyte molecules is then flowed into contact with the surface, and binding of ligands and analytes occur. The SPR waves react very sensitively to the molecular structure of the medium adjacent to the metal—dielectric or metal—air interface. Changes due to biomolecular attachment interfere with the formation of plasmon, in turn altering the SPR waves [15].

By measuring the changes in the reflected light or by tracking the resonance angle shifts, the concentration of the analyte molecules in the sensing medium can be determined. The changes in the SPR angle, which is the angle of minimum reflectivity, can be determined by varying the incidence angle and recording the reflected light intensity during the biological binding reactions between various biomolecules [11].

The defined angle at which resonance occurs is determined by the refractive index of the material near the metal surface. Consequently, small changes in the reflective index of the sensing medium produced by ligand—analyte binding can restrict the formation of plasmon. By measuring the changes (dips) in the reflected light obtained on a detector, binding is noted. SPR is observed as a sharp dip in reflected intensity at a certain angle, which is dependent on the refractive index of the medium. This angle shifts when biomolecules bind to the surface and change the refractive index of the surface layer. The selectively accumulated ligand—analyte mass on the sensor chip changes the refractive index [12].

20.3 The sensorgram

As the analyte binds to the ligand, the accumulation of protein on the sensor surface causes an increase in refractive index. This refractive index change is measured in real time (sampling in a kinetic analysis experiment is taken every 0.1 s), and the result plotted as response units (RUs) versus time (termed a sensorgram). (Fig. 20.3) The sensorgram is a plot of the SPR angle against time and displays the real-time progress of the interaction at

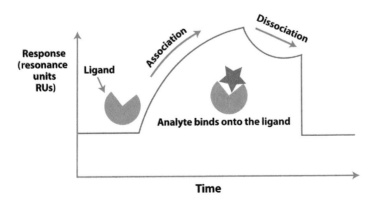

FIGURE 20.3 This refractive index change is measured in real time (sampling in a kinetic analysis experiment is taken every 0.1 s), and the result plotted as response units (RUs) versus time (termed a sensorgram).

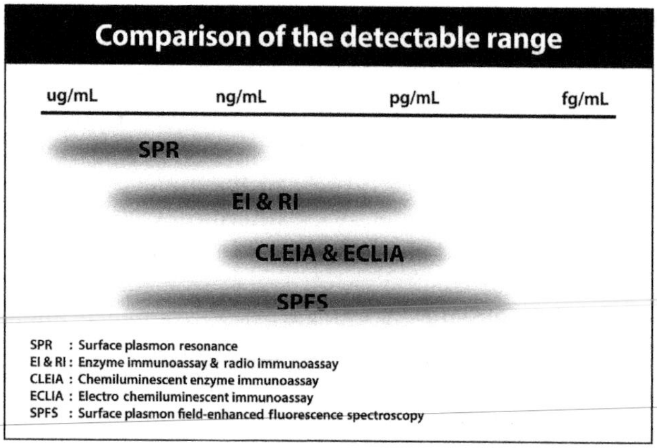

FIGURE 20.4 Comparisons of the detectable range for a biomolecule in blood for different assay methods.

the sensor surface. The signal is proportional to the amount of the bound molecule. The sensitivity of most SPR instruments is in the range of $10-0.01 \, pg/mm^{-2}$, which covers many molecules of clinical significance. For an instrument that uses light of 670 nm, $1 \, ng/mm^{-2}$ protein accumulation gives a signal of about 1000 RUs [16].

The main performance characteristics of SPR sensors include sensitivity, resolution, linearity, accuracy, reproducibility, and dynamic range. One of the challenges in SPR biosensors is to balance sensitivity and dynamic range. Sensitivity of an SPR sensor is the ratio of the change in sensor output to the change in the quantity to be measured (for example, the refractive index). The dynamic range is defined as the maximum possible signal level divided by the noise level, that is, when there is no light entering the system. A comparison of dynamic range and sensitivity of current and future immunoassays is depicted in Fig. 20.4.

The limit of detection (LOD) for SPR depends on a number of factors including the molecular weight, optical properties, and binding affinity of ligand to analyte molecules as well as the surface coverage of the probe molecule.

Sensitivity is critical when using different fluids where the index of refraction may be complicated by the presence of other molecules, for example, in human sera or cerebrospinal fluid (CSF), particularly for applications to detect protein markers such as markers for TBI. Because the blood–brain barrier inhibits the leakage of protein from the brain into the blood, the concentration of marker proteins in blood is low, making sensitivity a critical requirement for accurate detection and measurement.

20.4 Grating-coupled Surface plasmon resonance

Grating-coupled SPR (GC-SPR) is an alternative configuration to harness SPR using a thin metal grating deposited onto the prism or in place of the prism. The metal grating increases the interaction area for the sample and enhances the excitation of SPR. Since the grating pitch is larger than commonly used diffraction gratings, multiple SPR excitations traceable to several diffraction orders occur simultaneously. Grating-coupled sensors have

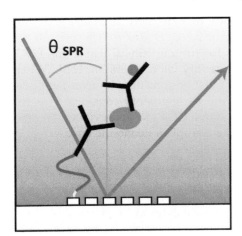

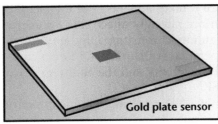

Gold plate sensor

FIGURE 20.5 Grating-coupled structures incorporated in compact frames are the basis for sensors in lab-on-a-chip technologies.

been developed on chips and show chip-to-chip reproducibility of assays with a resolution of 6×10^{-7} RU and an LOD of 1 nm.

Grating-coupled structures incorporated in compact frames are the basis for sensors in lab-on-a-chip technologies (Fig. 20.5) [17]. An advantage of using the grating-coupling excitation method is the fact that the prism is unnecessary. GC-SPR provides direct coupling between SPPs and the radiation modes, so inexpensive and disposable plastics can be mass produced by injection-molding techniques to serve as the substrates, allowing for more flexible configurations [16]. In addition, the use of GC-SPR eliminates the need for a washing process to remove unbound molecules because the binding of various molecules is reflected in different dips in the SPR reflectivity curve. Devices exploiting this method for immunosensing have been developed and consist of a substrate with a metal-coated grating structure termed a "plasmonic chip" [18]. Later in this chapter, the clinical applications of GC-SPR combined with fluorescent spectroscopy is described.

20.5 Surface plasmon resonance-based sensors

SPR-based sensors and instruments have been used in preclinical and clinical research since their discovery, such as for epitope mapping and binding, affinity ranking, fragment-based screening and monitoring, quantification, protein characterization, and validation. In each application, the requirements of functionality and instrumentation vary from high-speed and high-throughput bulk machines to extremely high-sensitive but time-consuming instrumentation.

Recent research has focused on SPR-based sensors for routine clinical use at the POC, for example, to determine cardiac troponin or to identify biomarkers for TBI. When designing for routine clinical use, a number of factors must be considered, including operability, footprint size, user-friendliness, and cost as well as regulatory considerations for US Food and Drug Administration (FDA) approvals and CE—the abbreviation for the French term for European Conformity—marking for the European Economic Area.

20.5.1 Localized surface plasmon resonance

The SPR signal is sometimes not large enough to detect analytes at the desired level for investigating small molecules. Instead, an LSPR effect may be employed by using gold NPs as a further signal amplification approach [19]. LSPR takes advantage of the fact that small changes in the thin overlayers on the metal surface strongly affect SPR resonance. The familiar home pregnancy test uses LSPR as an immunochromatography application. LSPR utilizes an ultrathin layer of NPs as its surface metal layer that respond to structures smaller than the wavelength of light. This allows high sensitivity and the ability to detect low concentrations from biological analytes such as CSF.

LSPR sensors rely on the high sensitivity of noble metal NPs to changes in the dielectric constant of the surrounding environment, such as adjustments produced when a ligand and an analyte bind. When substrate-selective polymer gels with gold NPs as the molecular recognition elements are used, swelling of the polymer gel is triggered by an analyte binding. This increases the distance between the gold NPs and the substrate, thereby causing the shift of an SPR dip [12].

LSPR occurs when the incident photon frequency is resonant with the collective oscillation of the conduction electrons in the metal NPs. When several NPs are positioned proximally, their dipole–dipole affinity excites multipole affinity, in turn producing an extremely strong SPR. The LSPR is dependent on the size, shape, interparticle spacing, and dielectric properties of the material as well as the dielectric properties of the local environment that surrounds the NPs [19].

Gold and silver NPs exhibit LSPR at visible as well as near-infrared frequencies, with sharp peaks in their spectral absorbance. SPR devices incorporating metallic nanostructures have the benefits of a small footprint for use in POC applications. They are readily integrated into an array format and can be manufactured at low cost to allow for one-time use and disposal. LSPR assays are not temperature-sensitive because LSPR sensing is based on a simple absorbance measurement and can be performed using typical laboratory equipment. Also, LSPR is a more rapid test as the sample spreads faster to the surfaces of the NPs than onto the metallic film [20].

LSPR technology based on silver NPs was used as a biosensor to detect amyloid-derived diffusible ligands (ADDLs) [19]. Amyloid β (Aβ), a peptide fragment derived from amyloid precursor protein, is recognized as a potential surrogate and diagnostic biomarker for Alzheimer's disease, the most common cause of dementia. ADDL is an oligomeric form of Aβ at 17−27 kDa, which requires a highly sensitive method for detection [21], suggesting a possible role for LSPR.

20.5.2 Surface plasmon resonance-MS

The combination of SPR and mass spectrometry (MS) uses SPR to amplify the signal for MS. SPR is used for protein detection and quantification, and MS provides the structural characterization of the proteins, revealing protein structure modifications that are not detected by SPR. Also referred to as biomolecular interaction analysis MS, early reports by Krone [22] and Nelson [23] demonstrated proof of principle that the combination of the two different modalities in one instrument could be used for real-time analysis. SPR-MS uses SPR to characterize the interactions between surface immobilized ligands and proteins on the SPR-sensor surface. This nondestructive process allows the proteins to be retrieved from the SPR-sensing surface for analysis to determine the identities of the bound proteins using MS [16].

20.5.3 Surface plasmon resonance imaging

A promising technology harnesses SPR in imaging applications. In SPR imaging (SPR-I) instruments, the SPR angles of many regions of interest may be monitored simultaneously by a camera, which optically images the sensor surface. For SPR-I, Kretschmann's configuration is used and a plane-polarized light with fixed angle is the incident light; a charge-coupled device camera is used for the detection of the reflected light [24]. This allows for the visualization of the whole biochip in real time. If the sensor surface is split into multiple sensing spots, then this multiarray format is capable of simultaneously monitoring hundreds of ligand/analyte bindings with the parallel support of a digital image that represents the intensity of binding in a color scale. The measurement areas can be accurately selected through direct image control to identify and reduce the nonspecific binding [25].

20.5.4 Surface plasmon field-enhanced fluorescence spectroscopy

Surface plasmon field-enhanced fluorescence spectroscopy (SPFS) is a derivative method from SPR that provides high sensitivity and wide dynamic range, making it an intriguing candidate for routine clinical or POC applications (Fig. 20.6). SPFS leverages the properties of SPR and enables lower limits of detection by labeling analyte molecules with fluorescent chromophores. The resonantly excited surface plasmon waves excite the fluorophores so that their emitted photons can be measured to maximize the sensitivity of detection [16]. Also see Fig. 20.4 for comparisons of SPFS dynamic range against other assay methods.

SPFS provides excellent LODs in an operationally simple manner because of the superior surface-selective enhanced fluorescence of this technique compared with conventional methods measured on a cover glass or a plastic plate. The origin of the enhanced fluorescence is the surface plasmon field under resonance conditions [26].

The most important component of SPFS is the sensor surface, which must be designed not only to enhance the generation of near-field light by making the angle of the prism precise, but also to provide a surface with high biocompatibility as a substrate for the ligand−analyte interactions being studied.

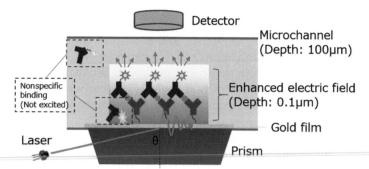

FIGURE 20.6 Surface plasmon field-enhanced fluorescence spectroscopy (SPFS) is a derivative method from SPR that provides high sensitivity and wide dynamic range, making it an intriguing candidate for routine clinical or point-of-care applications.

An innovation under development to solve these challenges is the creation of a disposable plastic sensor chip for SPFS-biosensing applications. Researchers have been successful in developing plastic chips that perform like glass prisms. Plastic sensor chips are less costly and can be mass produced with reliability and stability, making them attractive for commercial SPFS applications.

20.6 Biosensing applications of surface plasmon field-enhanced fluorescence spectroscopy

20.6.1 Cardiac troponin

SPFS has been investigated as a sensitive detection method for biomarkers such as cardiac troponin and D-dimer, which are important to clinicians. Cardiac troponin is a cardiospecific, highly sensitive marker for myocardial damage and is immediately released to the bloodstream during acute myocardial infarction (AMI). Sensitive detection of cardiac troponin is essential to rule out AMI. SPFS has been demonstrated to have a LOD of 0.62 ng/L for human troponin I, with an assay range of 0.62–500,000 ng/L using whole blood, plasma, or serum samples. Investigations have validated that analytical performance of SPFS (i.e., sensitivity, reproducibility, and linearity) were equivalent to a commercially available, fully automated immunoassay system widely used in today's laboratory setting [27].

20.6.2 D-dimer

D-dimer is another clinically important diagnostic marker for both pulmonary embolism (PE) and disseminated intravascular coagulation (DIC). The plasma level of D-dimer is nearly always increased in the presence of acute PE and in DIC [26]. DIC is a syndrome characterized by generally uncontrolled activation of the coagulation system with excess thrombin generation and consumptive coagulopathy. Normal D-dimer levels below a cutoff value of 500 μm/L can reliably rule out PE [26] and DIC [28]. Experimental studies have demonstrated utility for SPFS in this setting as it can reliably detect D-dimer in whole blood, plasma, or serum with a LOD of 0.52 to 50,000 ng/mL. This wide dynamic range allows this assay to rule out both PE and DIC [Konica Minolta. Data on file].

20.6.3 Traumatic brain injury-related biomarkers

Diagnosis of a mild TBI (mTBI) case is challenging, with over 90% of cases showing no anatomic abnormality in a computed tomography scan of the head, which may lead to missed diagnoses and lack of treatment. The American Congress of Rehabilitation Medicine defines mTBI as an acute injury resulting from mechanical force that impacts the head, and the criteria include additional subjective information (feelings of dizziness, confusion, disorientation, etc.) [29]. Therefore, introduction of an objective diagnostic test using blood-based biomarkers is needed for more reliable identification of mTBI.

A recent observational study known as HeadSMART in the emergency department examined the utility of blood-based biomarkers in the diagnosis of TBI [30]. A panel that included several potential biomarkers, including neurogranin (NRGN), neuron-specific enolase (NSE), and metallothionein 3 (MT3), was reported to improve diagnosis in patients with mTBI [31]. The simultaneous analysis of a panel encompassing multiple biomarkers is an advantage of assays based on SPR.

20.6.3.1 Glial fibrillary acidic protein

SPFS was evaluated in studies to detect GFAP, which is a brain-specific protein (50 kDa) released after TBI. SPFS showed sufficient sensitivity (LOD: 10 pg/mL) in a 10-minute assay, making it a good candidate for routine clinical use. However, recent studies have shown that GFAP also correlates with inflammation and hemorrhage and is an informative biomarker in moderate to severe TBI, but this protein is not sensitive in mild injury [32,33].

20.6.3.2 Neurogranin

An alternative biomarker for mTBI is NRGN, a small neuronal protein (78 amino acids, 7.6 kDa) that plays an important role in synaptic plasticity and cognitive function. NRGN has a potential as a circulating biomarker for acute TBI because of a small size that may enable it to cross an intact and/or damaged blood−brain barrier with relative ease [10].

A study by Yang and colleagues [10] measured NRGN in sera using ELISA. Median NRGN values were significantly higher among the TBI cases (0.18 ng/mL, interquartile range: 0.05−0.64 ng/mL) than non-TBI controls (0.02 ng/mL, IQR: 0.05−0.07 ng/mL). In the ELISA assay, which required a runtime of 3 hours (2 hours for the first antibody and 1 hour for the secondary antibody), the LOD for NRGN was 0.055 ng/mL and a limit of quantitation (LOQ) of 0.2 ng/mL [10], suggesting that a more sensitive test could provide more accurate results and a more rapid test could satisfy requirements for a clinically useful POC assay.

SPFS technology is being evaluated as a method to deliver a clinically useful way to assess NRGN more accurately and more rapidly than the complex and time-consuming ELISA methods. An SPFS assay requires only 10 minutes to complete and can detect NRGN at an LOD of 0.005 ng/mL (Fig. 20.7A). The LOQ for SPFS performed with

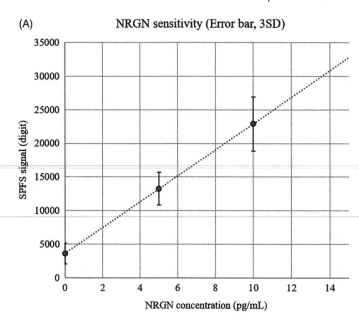

FIGURE 20.7 (A--B) Neurogranin (NRGN) sensitivity by surface plasmon field-enhanced fluorescence spectroscopy (SPFS).

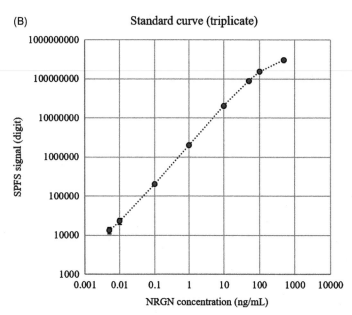

recombinant NRGN was 0.0146 ng/mL. In addition, the recovery without a blood sample matrix was 95.1%. In the whole blood sample, however, recovery was 93.7% at 0.01 ng/mL, which is near the LOQ, demonstrating the sensitivity of the SPFS signal even in dilute samples. SPFS results showed dramatically improved sensitivity over a wide five-digit dynamic range (0.005–500 ng/mL) compared with the performances on ELISA (Fig. 20.7B). These results suggest that an even more rapid SPFS test for NRGN is possible, which would have the potential for practical use in emergency clinical situations as a POC test.

SPFS has a further advantage over ELISA in that it does not require the use of biotinylated antibodies for binding but rather relies on chemical covalent bonding. The FDA has issued warnings that biotin in a patient sample may give false readings in ELISA [34].

20.6.4 Grating-coupled Surface plasmon field-enhanced fluorescence spectroscopy

Researchers have combined GC-SPR with SPFS to further improvement. The simplified GC-SPR optical setup does not require a prism, but rather uses a substrate with a metal-coated grating structure termed a "plasmonic chip" [18]. Using a sandwich immunoassay on a plasmonic chip combined with a fluorescent labeled marker system, researchers analyzed alpha-fetoprotein (AFP), with its measurement being important in two clinical settings. In pregnancy, AFP is measured in maternal blood or amniotic fluid as a screening test for certain developmental abnormalities. The serum AFP level is elevated in hepatocellular carcinoma, hepatoblastoma, and nonseminomatous germ cell tumors of the ovary and testis and is used as a biomarker to follow these diseases [35].

Tawa and colleagues used fluorescence immunosensing with a sandwich immunoassay on a plasmonic chip to measure known concentrations of AFP in solution. In this study, the LOD of AFP to 4 pg/mL (55 fM) was achieved, and AFP markers were detected in a wide concentration range of five orders of magnitude. The highly sensitive detection in the sandwich immunoassay suggests that the development of a plasmonic chip for clinical diagnosis of tumor markers by a blood test is promising [36].

20.7 Conclusion

The future is promising for the development of clinically valuable biosensors that detect biomarkers in blood, serum, or CSF for many conditions, including TBI at even the POC setting with SPR and its derivatives. As these biosensors become increasingly easy-to-use but also exquisitely sensitive across a wide dynamic range, their applications expand exponentially. Furthermore, the ability to manufacture inexpensive, reliable, and disposable miniaturized plasmonic chips satisfies the need for mobile applications at an accessible cost, making routine clinical applications possible.

References

[1] Deng S, Shijie P, Yu X. Phase-sensitive surface plasmon resonance sensors: recent progress and future prospects. Sensors 2017;17(12):2819.
[2] Wood RW. On a remarkable case of uneven distribution of light in a diffraction grating spectrum. London, Edinburgh, Dublin Philos Mag J Sci Ser 6 1902;4(21).

[3] Strutt JW. On the dynamical theory of gratings. Proc R Soc A 1907;79(532):399−416.

[4] Fano U. The theory of anomalous diffraction gratings and of quasi-stationary waves on metallic surfaces (Sommerfeld's waves). J Opt Soc Am 1941;31(3):213−22.

[5] Ritchie RH. Plasma losses by fast electrons in thin films. Phys Rev 1957;106(5):874−81.

[6] Otto A. Excitation of nonradiative surface plasma waves in silver by the method of frustrated total reflection. Z Für Phys A Hadron Nucl 1968;216(4):398−410.

[7] Kretschmann E, Raether H. Radiative decay of non radiative surface. Z Naturforsch 1968;23(a):2135−6.

[8] Liedberg B, Nylander C, Lunström I. Surface plasmon resonance for gas detection and biosensing. Sens Actuators 1983;4:299−304.

[9] Lin CC, Wang JH, Wu HW. Microfluidic immunoassays. J Lab Autom 2010;15(3):253−74.

[10] Yang J, Korley FK, Dai M, Everett AD. Serum neurogranin measurement as a biomarker of acute traumatic brain injury. Clin Biochem 2015;48(0):843−8.

[11] Nguyen HH, Park J, Kang S, Kim M. Surface plasmon resonance: a versatile technique for biosensor applications. Sensors. 2015;15(5):10481−510.

[12] Hodnik V, Anderluh G. Toxin detection by surface plasmon resonance. Sensors. 2009;9(3):1339−54.

[13] Kihm K, Cheon S, Park J, et al. Surface plasmon resonance (SPR) reflectance imaging: Far-field recognition of near-field phenomena. Opt Lasers Eng 2012;50(1):64−73.

[14] Zeng S, Baillargeat D, Ho HP, Yong KT. Nanomaterials enhanced surface plasmon resonance for biological and chemical sensing applications. Chem Soc Rev 2014;43(10):3426−52.

[15] Homola J, Yee SS, Gauglitzb G. Surface plasmon resonance sensors: review. Sens Actuators B: Chem 1999;54 (1−2):3−15.

[16] Schasfoort RBM. Handbook of surface plasmon resonance: edition 2. London: The Royal Society of Chemistry; 2017.

[17] Wang X, Zhan S, Huang Z, Hong X. Review: advances and applications of surface plasmon resonance biosensing instrumentation. Instrum Sci Technol 2013;41(6):574−607.

[18] Tawa K, Hori H, Kintaka K, Kiyosue K, Tatsu Y, Nishii J. Optical microscopic observation of fluorescence enhanced by grating-coupled surface plasmon resonance. Opt Exp 2008;16(13):9781−90.

[19] Zhao J, Zhang X, Yonzon CR, Haes AJ, Van Duyne RP. Localized surface plasmon resonance biosensors. Nanomedicine. 2006;1(2):219−28.

[20] Couture C, Zhaoa SS, Masson JF. Modern surface plasmon resonance for bioanalytics and biophysics. Phys Chem Chem Phys 2013;15(27):11190−216.

[21] Lambert M, Barlow A, Chromy B, et al. Diffusible, nonfibrillar ligands derived from Ab1−42 are potent central nervous system neurotoxins. Proc Natl Acad Sci USA 1998;95(11):6448−53.

[22] Krone JR, Nelson RW, Dogruel D, Williams P, Granzow R. BIA/MS: interfacing biomolecular interaction analysis with mass spectrometry. Anal Biochem 1997;244(1):124−32.

[23] Nelson RW, Krone JR. Surface plasmon resonance biomolecular interaction analysis mass spectrometry. 1. chip-based analysis. Anal Chem 1997;69(22):4363−8.

[24] Peng W, Liu Y, Fang P, et al. Compact surface plasmon resonance imaging sensing system based on general optoelectronic components. Opt Exp 2014;22(5):6174−85.

[25] Puiu M, Bala C. SPR and SPR imaging: recent trends in developing nanodevices for detection and real-time monitoring of biomolecular events. Sensors. 2016;16(6):870.

[26] Tawa K, Kondo F, Sasakawa C, et al. Sensitive detection of a tumor marker, α-fetoprotein, with a sandwich assay on a plasmonic chip. Anal Chem 2015;87(7):3871−6.

[27] Braga F, Aloisio E, Panzeri A, et al. Analytical validation of a highly sensitive point-of-care system for cardiac troponin I determination. Clin Chem Lab Med 2019;58(1):138−45.

[28] Perrier A, Desmarais S, Goehring C, et al. D-dimer testing for suspected pulmonary embolism in outpatients. Am J Respir Crit Care Med 1997;156(2 pt 1):492−6.

[29] Bates S, Takach Lapner S, Douketis J, et al. Rapid quantitative D-dimer to exclude pulmonary embolism: a prospective cohort management study. J Thromb Haemost 2016;14(3):504−9.

[30] Menon DK, Schwab K, Wright DW, Maas AI. Position statement: definition of traumatic brain injury. Arch Phys Med Rehab 2010;91(11):1637−40.

[31] Peters ME, Rao V, Bechtold KT, et al. Head injury serum markers for assessing response to trauma: design of the HeadSMART study. Brain Inj 2017;31(3):370−8.

[32] Peacock FW, Van Meter TE, Mirshahi N, et al. Derivation of a three biomarker panel to improve diagnosis in patients with mild traumatic brain injury. Front Neurol 2017;8:641.

[33] Lei J, Gao G, Feng J, et al. Glial fibrillary acidic protein as a biomarker in severe traumatic brain injury patients: a prospective cohort study. Crit Care 2015;19:362.

[34] Rozanski M, Waldschmidt C, Kunz A, et al. Glial fibrillary acidic protein for prehospital diagnosis of intracerebral hemorrhage. Cerebrovasc Dis 2017;43(12):76−81.

[35] (FDA) UFaDA. The FDA warns that biotin may interfere with lab tests: FDA safety communication. Safety Communications. November 28, 2017, <https://www.fda.gov/medicaldevices/safety/alertsandnotices/ucm586505.htm> [accessed 28.9.2018].

[36] Duffy MJ. Use of biomarkers in screening for cancer. Adv Cancer Biomarkers 2015;867:27−39.

21

Point-of-care testing for concussion and traumatic brain injury

Kent Lewandrowski

Department of Pathology, General Hospital, Boston, MA, United States

21.1 Introduction to point-of-care testing

Point-of-care testing (POCT) was defined by Nichols as laboratory testing performed close to the site of patient care [1]. Other names for POCT include ancillary testing, bedside testing, and decentralized testing [1]. Usually POCT is performed by nonlaboratory personnel on hospital inpatient units, outpatient clinics, and in the emergency department. Many POCT tests are also sold over the counter allowing patients to perform testing in their home with, or without, a physician's order [2].

The major advantage of POCT is that the test results are available immediately to facilitate rapid medical assessment and decisions concerning therapy. In many cases this improves the efficiency of medical care by eliminating delays that occur when testing is sent to a traditional centralized laboratory [2]. On the other hand POCT is usually more expensive on a unit cost basis than automated centralized laboratory testing. For this reason, it is important to demonstrate an improvement in outcomes when POCT is employed to justify the added incremental costs. There are essentially four types of outcomes that may be impacted by POCT.

1. Financial outcomes: By improving the efficiency of medical care the cost of POCT may be more than offset by reductions in the overall cost of the episode of care. For an example of this type of outcome see reference [3].
2. Medical outcomes: Rapid test results from POCT allows for immediate medical decisions which in some cases improves the quality or effectiveness of care. For an example of this type of outcome see reference [4].
3. Clinical operations outcomes: POCT may be employed to reduce or eliminate bottlenecks in an episode of care thus improving the efficiency of care or increasing the capacity of a clinical operation. For an example of this type of outcome see reference [3].

4. Patient/provider satisfaction: The availability of test results at the time of the clinical encounter may enhance patient/provider satisfaction. For an example of this type of outcome see reference [5].

Most POCT devices are designed for ease-of-use utilizing a minimum of intuitive steps to perform a test. Most devices are also designed to eliminate error-prone manual processes. Some devices also have software features to reduce or eliminate sources of operator errors such as the ability to lock out untrained users, forcing functions to ensure quality control (QC) is performed, the ability to detect and reject expired reagents, and other safety features [2]. Many POCT tests utilize samples that are easy to collect, such as capillary finger-stick whole blood, urine, and saliva. This eliminates the need for sample processing and the requirement for a skilled phlebotomist to obtain a venous blood sample. This is important because in many sites where POCT is performed, a phlebotomist is not readily available.

POCT tests usually take one of a few common configurations.

1. Single-use disposable visually read test strip or cartridge with a built-in QC indicator. This configuration yields a positive or negative qualitative result. An example of this configuration is a visually-read urine pregnancy test with a built-in QC.
2. Single-use test strip or cartridge with a reusable reader device producing either a qualitative or quantitative result. QCs may be built in to the cartridge or may be performed separately using additional test strips. These devices may be limited to testing a single analyte or may perform multitest panels or a menu of tests using different types of cartridges.
3. Multiuse devices employing a cartridge that can perform multiple tests or panels over the life of the cartridge. In some cases, QCs are run automatically by the device eliminating the need for testing separate QC samples.

Each of these configurations has certain advantages and disadvantages. The most optimal configuration depends on the individual test and how it is used. For example, a urine pregnancy test need only yield a positive or negative result. The test strip may be either visually read or inserted into a reader device. If the volume of testing is low it will be difficult to justify the cost of the reader, whereas in a higher volume setting the cost of the reader is spread out over a larger volume of tests. The reader eliminates the subjectivity of the visually read strip and allows for test results to flow electronically into the medical record. Visually read tests must be manually entered into the medical record which is time-consuming and error-prone.

21.2 Point-of-care testing for traumatic brain injury

According to the Centers for Disease Control and Prevention (CDC) "traumatic brain injury (TBI) is defined as a disruption in the normal function of the brain that can be caused by a bump, blow, or jolt to the head, or penetrating head injury [6]. Everyone is at risk for a TBI, especially children and older adults." Mild TBI is also called a concussion as defined by a Glasgow Coma Scale score of 13–15. TBI consumes considerable healthcare resources and presents potentially serious morbidity and mortality for those with head injuries. The CDC database lists the following causes of TBI: falls 40%, unknown/other 19%, struck by/against 16%, motor vehicle accident 14%, and assault 11%.

The CDC reports that in 2013 there were 2.8 million TBI-related visits to the emergency room in the United States of which there were 282,000 hospitalizations and nearly 50,000 deaths [6]. TBI is also a major issue for athletes and for the military, both for troops on active duty and those in training. Potential consequences of TBI include cognitive defects, impaired memory, motor, sensory, and neuropsychiatric sequelae.

TBI can be classified as mild or moderate to severe. The initial approach to TBI involves a history and physical examination with a thorough neurological examination including a Glasgow Coma Scale. If deemed clinically appropriate, a computed tomographic (CT) scan is performed to identify brain injury and/or bleeding. Overall 63% of patients with a possible TBI receive a head CT scan [7]. The vast majority of patients presenting to the ED with head injuries exhibit only mild symptoms and over 90% of CT scans prove to be negative [7]. This fact alone indicates a significant opportunity exists to improve diagnostic accuracy and reduce the costs of unnecessary CT scans. Further, in remote or resource-limited settings (including battlefields) CT scans may not be available such that the diagnosis must be made on clinical grounds alone.

Although clinical decision rules for determining which patients meet or do not meet criteria for a head CT have been developed (e.g., Canadian Head CT Scan Rule), one recent study reported that the use of the rule in an electronic decision support project did not reduce the number of CT scans in patients following mild TBI [7]. For this reason, an objective and reliable test for TBI would offer significant advantages.

Up until February, 2018 there were no Food and Drug Administration (FDA)-approved POCT or central laboratory blood tests for concussion and TBI. In 2016 the FDA approved a point-of-care electroencephalographic (EEG) device (Ahead 300 by Brainscope, Inc.) for the assessment of TBI. The device incorporates a disposable electrode headset with a hand-held smartphone technology and uses a proprietary algorithm to perform a multivariate classification utilizing linear and nonlinear EEG features along with clinical information (Fig. 21.1) [8]. In one study by Hack et al., the use of the device improved the predictive power for TBI as documented by positive computed tomographic findings (traumatic hematoma) when compared to loss of consciousness (LOC) alone or LOC plus amnesia. Reportedly the device improved the diagnostic receiver operator area under the curve by 83% and the odds ratio from 4.65 to 16.22. Other studies using quantitative EEG demonstrated that this technology was more specific for acute mild TBI than two current clinical decision rules (New Orleans Criteria, National Emergency X-Radiography Utilization Study II). Only the Canadian Head CT Rule was more specific albeit with low sensitivity (<50%) [9]. Another study reported that the brain function index (BFI) provided an objective marker of concussion and subsequent recovery [10].

In February 2018 the FDA approved a laboratory-based blood test from Banyan Biomarkers called the Banyan Brain Trauma Indicator that measures two blood-based biomarkers (ubiquitin C-terminal hydrolase L1(UCHL1) and glial fibrillary acidic protein (GFAP)) within 12 hours of brain injury. Test results are available in 3−4 hours. The company states that they expect to reduce this to less than 1 hour in the near future.

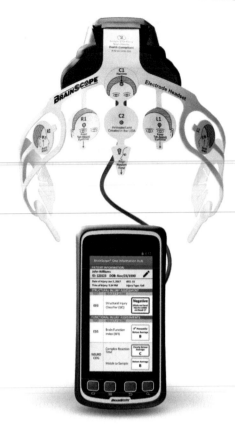

FIGURE 21.1 Brainscope, Inc. Ahead 300 point-of-care electroencephalographic device for the assessment of traumatic brain injury. The device incorporates a disposable electrode headset with a handheld smartphone technology.

Ultimately they plan to develop a handheld device that can be deployed in the field. The company recently partnered with Philips to jointly develop their test for use on the Philips Minicare I-20 handheld meter.

There are several other companies that are working on similar blood-based tests or on nonblood-based technologies. Some examples are listed below.

1. Biodirection, Inc. is developing a portable TBI blood test (Tbit) based on measurement of S100beta and GFAP. The device consists of a cartridge and a small reader device. Both of these biomarkers are released into the blood early following TBI. The device will use a finger-stick capillary blood sample as illustrated in Fig. 21.2.
2. Abbott Diagnostics is collaborating with Hennepin County Medical Center and the University of Minnesota to develop a TBI test utilizing GFAP and UCH-L1on their next-generation iSTAT Alinity analyzer.
3. ImmunArray is developing blood-based protein tests including multiple test panels to assess acute TBI and autoantibody tests to assess prognosis following established TBI.
4. Eye-tracking technology has been reported as a potential test for TBI [11]. One company, Oculogica, is developing an eye-tracking technology to detect concussions

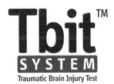

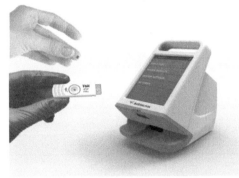

FIGURE 21.2 Biodirection, Inc. traumatic brain injury blood test device. The test utilizes a finger-stick blood sample and a single-use disposable test cartridge with a reader device.

and other brain injuries. The EyeBox device is reported to produce a result in less than 4 minutes.

5. Ko et al. [12] reported the development of a smartphone-enabled optofluidic device that can detect brain-derived exosomes in blood using an experimental mouse model for TBI. The device detects GluR2 positive exosomes in blood in 1 hour and is suitable for testing at the point-of-care.

A number of potential TBI biomarkers have been identified (Table 21.1). For a review of these see Dash et al. [13] and chapters on specific markers elsewhere in this book. Developing a blood test to detect brain injury is made more challenging by the fact that the biomarker must pass through the blood—brain barrier in sufficient quantity to be detected by an analytical device. In principle, a central laboratory test for TBI that either reduces unnecessary CT scans or improves diagnostic accuracy is theoretically possible. Assuming such a test can be developed with acceptable sensitivity and specificity, then several questions must be answered to determine if the test is appropriate for a POCT test.

1. Does the device have sufficient analytical sensitivity to detect very small concentrations of a biomarker in small sample volumes such as capillary finger-stick blood?
2. Can the test be configured into a POCT format such that it can be reliably performed and interpreted by nonlaboratory personnel?
3. Will the test require integrating the result with clinical findings or other data beyond the capabilities of nonmedical personnel?
4. In what clinical care settings will the POC test be performed?
5. What types of personnel would perform the testing?
6. Can test cartridges be designed to withstand a range of environmental extremes as controlled temperature storage facilities might not be readily available?

This is especially important for a test intended for use in the field outside of a healthcare facility.

TABLE 21.1   Potential biomarkers of traumatic brain injury.

Ubiquitin C-terminal hydrolase L1(UCHL1) and S100beta

Glial fibrillary acidic protein (GFAP)

Neurofilament light chain/neurofilament heavy chain

Tau

Brain-derived neurotrophic factor

Citrillinated G-fab

Neurogranin

Neuron specific enolase

Myelin basic protein

Inflammatory biomarkers

TABLE 21.2   Desirable design features of a point-of-care test for traumatic brain injury.

High diagnostic sensitivity and specificity when compared to clinical judgement alone

Rapid analytical time (≤15 min)

Single-use visually read or instrument-read cartridge

Cartridge reader device that is easy to use and has built-in design features to prevent operator errors

Ability for electronic interface to electronic medical record

Quality control built-in to the cartridge

Room temperature storage of consumables with a long shelf life

Consumables able to withstand environmental extremes

Finger-stick capillary blood sample

Acceptable cost of reader and consumables

7. Will the device be a visually read cartridge or a battery-operated reader device.
8. Can a use-case scenario be developed to justify testing outside of the central laboratory based on an analysis of the impact of the test on outcomes as described above.

Table 21.2 lists some of the desirable design features of a POCT test for TBI.

A key consideration for designing a POCT blood TBI test involves determining where the test would be performed (Table 21.3) and by what type of personnel. Many tests designed for the point-of-care are currently performed in a central laboratory mainly for economic or operational reasons [2]. For example, if a test is low volume it is very difficult to train and maintain competency for large numbers of nonlaboratory personnel such as occurs in a typical emergency department operating 24 hours per day, 7 days a week. Inventory management can also be problematic at the point-of-care especially if reagents

TABLE 21.3   Potential sites where a point-of-care test (POCT) for traumatic brain injury might be performed.

Central laboratory STAT test using a POCT device
Emergency department
Trauma center
Acute care clinic
Self-standing medical walk-in clinic (urgent care)
Ambulance
Military medical facility
Field location: Sporting event, resource limited or remote settings
Specialized settings (e.g., cruise ships)

require temperature control. As an alternative to POCT, samples can be sent within minutes to the central laboratory by courier or pneumatic tube and the test performed stat by qualified medical technologists. In most hospital emergency departments, the number of cases of TBI on any given day will probably not be large enough to justify testing at the point-of-care. The fact that a test is designed for POCT will usually mean that the test utilizes whole blood (eliminating sample processing), is rapid, and can be performed as needed one at a time (as opposed to batch testing). Where the test is physically performed, at the POC or centrally, does not matter so long as the result is immediately available.

On the other hand, some POC tests are designed to use a capillary finger-stick blood sample. In this case the test would typically be performed at the point-of-care regardless of the test volume. For clinical settings that do not have on-site STAT testing from a central laboratory, POCT is the only option. Many outpatient sites do not have on-site phlebotomy. In this case the ability to perform testing on a capillary blood sample is much more important as venous samples require personnel who are trained in phlebotomy.

21.2.1 Ease-of-use

Ease-of-use is essential to successful design of POC test devices. In the case of instrumented devices, the user interface with the device should be designed to ensure regulatory compliance under the clinical laboratory improvement amendment (CLIA-88) with minimal requirements for intervention by the operator. The use of required fields including operator identification, patient identification, date and time of the test, confirmation that QC has been performed, and confirmation that reagents are within their expiration date should be embedded in the user interface. The use of barcode scanners, RFID chips, and touchscreen technology should be employed to facilitate data transfer and to ensure accuracy of the information entered. Ideally the device would be interfaced to the institutional ADT system to cross-check the accuracy of patient-related data.

21.2.2 Testing by nonmedical personnel

A simple POCT test for TBI would present the potential for testing to be performed by nonmedical personnel outside of traditional medical facilities.

21.2.3 Use-case scenarios

As described above it is important to develop a use-case scenario to justify the cost of a laboratory test for TBI including one performed at the point-of-care. This can be based on the ability of the test to improve diagnostic accuracy or the ability of the test to impact the overall episode of care and improve operational efficiency.

1. Improved diagnostic accuracy: A recent study by Rowe et al. [14] reported that 16% of head injuries that met the World Health Organization criteria for concussion did not receive a diagnosis of concussion during their emergency department visit. Presumably some of these patients would not receive adequate follow-up or might resume normal activities prematurely. In addition, missed concussion may result in medical-legal liability if the patient experiences a poor outcome. If the TBI blood test proved more sensitive than clinical judgement alone a use-case scenario could be developed based on improved diagnostic accuracy. Establishing a diagnosis of concussion in certain patient populations may be difficult on clinical grounds (infants, elderly with impaired cognitive function, patients with language barriers, patients with drug or alcohol intoxication). A reliable blood-based test would be extremely helpful in these patients.

2. Impact on the overall episode of care: Over half of patients presenting with possible TBI receive a CT scan, the vast majority of which are negative. CT scans are expensive and take time to complete resulting in a prolonged emergency department length-of-stay. If the TBI blood test were sufficiently reliable such that many CT scans could be avoided the test could be justified based on economics alone based on its ability to impact emergency department length-of-stay and the overall cost of the episode of care.

3. In the field, outside of the hospital/emergency department a POC test for TBI could have several potential applications:

    a. Diagnosis or rule-out of TBI in remote or resource-limited settings: If the TBI test were sufficiently sensitive it could be used to rule out TBI thus avoiding the complex and expensive evacuation of the patient to an appropriate healthcare facility.

    b. Self-standing walk-in clinic or ambulance: A highly sensitive test for TBI could allow clinic staff or emergency medical technicians to rule out TBI and potentially avoid transfer to an emergency department. In these settings the test would need to turn positive or negative very shortly after the time of the head injury.

    c. Sporting events: Medical staff at sporting events could use the TBI test to rule out TBI thus allowing the patient to resume the sporting activity or to rule in TBI necessitating transfer to a medical facility. To be practical, as in (b) above, a definitive test result would need to be available very shortly after the injury

    d. Objective prognostic indicator: In the case of mTBI, it is the "second hit" that can result in markedly greater injury than the initial insult. Knowing which patients are at risk to a second impact injury would be optimal to today's subjective strategy (which is fraught by conflict of interest concerns of the participants). In patients who are required/likely to return to the TBI environment (e.g., soldiers, professional/ collegiate sports participants, police/firemen, etc.), an accurate and objective POC test for prognosis could identify patients in whom return to participation should be prevented.

References

[1] Nichols J. Point-of-care testing Chapter 1 In: Nichols J, editor. Point-of-care testing. New York: Marcel Dekker Inc; 2003. p. 1–30.

[2] Lewandrowski K. Point of care testing: an overview and look to the future. Clin Lab Med 2009;29:421–32.

[3] Crocker B, Lee-Lewandrowski L, Lewandrowski N, Baron J, Gregory K, Lewandrowski K. Implementation of point-of-care testing in an ambulatory practice of an academic medical center. Amer J Clin Pathol 2014;142:640–6.

[4] Cagliero E, Levina E, Nathan D. Immediate feedback of HbA1c levels improves glycemic control in type 1 and insulin-treated type 2 diabetic patients. Diabetes Care 1999;1785–9.

[5] Crocker B, Lee-Lewandrowski E, Lewandrowski N, Gregory K, Lewandrowski K. Patient satisfaction with point-of-care testing: report of a quality improvement program in an ambulatory practice of academic medical center. Clin Chem Acta 2013;424:8–11.

[6] <https://www.cdc.gov/traumaticbraininjury/data/index.html>.

[7] Szlosek D, Haydar S, Williams R, Jackson R, Hein C, Mick N, et al. The impact of an electronic best practice advisory on brain computed tomography ordering in an academic medical center. Am J Emerg Med 2017;35:1776–7.

[8] Hack D, Huff S, Curley K, Naunheim R, Sananwoy G, Prichep L. Increased prognostic accuracy of TBI when a brain electrical acyivity biomarker is added to loss of consciousness. Am J Emerg Med 2017;35:949–52.

[9] Ayaz S, Thomas C, Tolomello R, Mika V, Robinson D, Medado P, et al. Comparison of quantitative EEG to current clinical decision rules for head CT use in acute mild brain injury in the ED. Am J Emerg Med 2015;33:493–6.

[10] Brooks M, Jeffrey B, Prichep L, Samanoway D, Talavage T, Barr W. The use of an elctrophysiological brain function index in the evaluation of concussed atheletes. J Head Trauma Rehab 2018;33:1–6.

[11] Maruta J, Minah S, Sumit N, Mukherjee P, Jamshid G. Visual tracking synchronization as a metric for concussion screening. J Head Trauma Rehab 2010;25:293–305.

[12] <https://www.nature.com/articles/srep31215#discussion>.

[13] Dash P, Zhoa J, Hergenroeder G, Moore A. Biomarkers for the diagnosis, prognosis and evaluation of treatment efficacy for traumatic brain injury. Neurotherapeutics 2010;7:100–14.

[14] Rowe B, Eliyahu L, Lowes J, et al. Concussion diagnosis among adults presenting to three Canadian emergency departments: missed opportunities. Am J Emerg Med 2018; (published online March 20, 2018).

Further reading

<https://www.mayoclinic.org/diseases-conditions/traumatic-brain-injury/symptoms-causes/syc-20378557>.

Non-blood TBI biomarker strategy

Clinical risk factors of traumatic brain injury

L. Foerschner, K.-G. Kanz, Peter Biberthaler and Viktoria Bogner-Flatz

Department of Trauma Surgery, Klinikum rechts der Isar, School of Medicine, Technical University of Munich, Munich, Germany

22.1 Introduction

Traumatic brain injury constitutes a major factor for the development of disability in its survivors and thus displays a major economical and sociological burden [1,2]. In Germany approximately 270,000 patients are admitted to hospital with traumatic brain injury. Of those, 70,000 are not older than 16 years and 90% suffer from a light form of traumatic brain injury [3]. In the United States there are approximately 282,000 hospitalizations due to traumatic brain injury and of those 56,000 died, displaying around 30% of all trauma-related deaths in the United States, although the hidden number is thought to be much higher, as many patients did not receive medical care [4]. The incidence of traumatic brain injury also varies broadly depending on different countries. While New Zealand has the highest incidence with 811 per 100,000 incidence, traumatic brain injury is lowest in Western Europe with 7.3 per 100,000 [5]. A study in 2013 in the United States showed traumatic brain injury being most frequent in older patients with an age of ≥ 75 years (2232 per 100,000), followed by young patients aged 0−4 years (1591 per 100,000) and young adults between 15 and 24 years of age (1081 per 100,000) [4]. Furthermore, traumatic brain injury is more common among male (959 per 100,000) than female patients (811 per 100,000) [4]. Widespread mechanisms of traumatic brain injuries are accidents with motor vehicles (122 per 100,000), the impact of an object (142 per 100,000), or falls (413 per 100,000) [4]. Falls are also responsible for the increasing number of traumatic brain injuries as well as the increasing number of hospitalizations due to traumatic brain injury, especially in older patients [4]. Notably, causes of traumatic brain injury associated with death changed from accidents with motor vehicles to self-harming behavior in the last decade

[4]. Socioeconomic status is also a pivotal factor for traumatic brain injury, as lower socioeconomic status, drug usage, cognitive disorder, psychiatric disorder, and alcohol abuse are risk factors for traumatic brain injury [6,7]. Especially in adolescents, sport accidents also play a major role in traumatic brain injury [7].

There are many different classifications for traumatic brain injury. Especially clinical severity of traumatic brain injuries is addressed in these scores. The most frequently applied score for traumatic brain injury is the Glasgow Coma Scale (GCS) (Table 22.1) [8]. Here, traumatic brain injury can be classified into mild (GCS 15–13), moderate (GCS 12–9) or severe (GCS 8 or lower). The GCS is practical to use but also has limitations due to medical sedation, intoxication, or intubation in patients with low GCS score [9,10]. To overcome these limitations of the GCS, the Full Outline of UnResponsiveness (FOUR) score has been developed including an examination of the brainstem [11]. Whether this new score can be reproducibly used by nonneurologically trained staff is still a point of debate [11,12].

TABLE 22.1   Glasgow coma scale (GCS).

	Score
Eye opening	
Spontaneous	4
Response to verbal command	3
Response to pain	2
No eye opening	1
Best verbal response	
Oriented	5
Confused	4
Inappropriate words	3
Incomprehensible sounds	2
No verbal response	1
Best motor response	
Obeys commands	6
Localizing response to pain	5
Withdrawal response to pain	4
Flexion to pain	3
Extension to pain	2
No motor response	1
Total	

The GCS is scored between 3 and 15, 3 being the worst and 15 the best. It is composed of three parameters: best eye response (E), best verbal response (V), and best motor response (M). The components of the GCS should be recorded individually; for example, E2V3M4 results in a GCS score of 9. A score of 13 or higher correlates with mild brain injury a score of 9–12 correlates with moderate injury, and a score of 8 or less represents severe brain injury.

Neuroimaging is crucial in the identification of injuries associated with traumatic brain injury [13]. These injuries include subdural and epidural hematoma, subarachnoid and intraparenchymal as well as intraventricular hemorrhage, alongside fracture of the skull cerebral contusion and axonal damage with edema [13]. The Marshall scale and the Rotterdam scale are frequently used scores to classify traumatic brain injury [14]. The Marshall score ranks traumatic brain injury into four categories with a diffuse injury pattern and two categories with a located lesion (Table 22.2). It has a high predictive value for outcome and for risk of high intracranial pressure. The Rotterdam scale was developed to address the limitations of the Marshal score in multiple types of brain injury (Table 22.3).

Additionally, brain injury associated with traumatic brain injury can be divided into primary and secondary brain injury. Primary injury typically develops during the trauma due to mechanical force on intracranial structures. This can result in contusion and bleeding alongside with diffuse axonal damage and cerebral swelling. Patients with diffuse axonal damage from shearing stress present with deep coma. Intracranial pressure is within the normal range. CT is inferior to MRI imaging in the detection of diffuse axonal damage. The outcome is poor. Focal contusions are seen in the frontal and temporal area and can also lead to intraparenchymal bleeding to rupture of a vessel. Alongside with this, epidural hematomas are often associated with a skull fracture and injury of the middle meningeal artery and have a lenticular shape. Subdural hematomas result from rupture of a bridging vein and have a crescent appearance. Subarachnoid bleedings result from disruption of a pial vessel and are located in the interpeduncular space and the Sylvian fissures. Additionally, intraventricular bleeding is based on the rupture of subependymal veins.

In contrast to primary brain damage, secondary brain injury results from reactions of the body with molecular cascades, such as vasospasm with secondary ischemia, dysfunction of mitochondria, inflammation, electrolyte imbalance, apoptosis, and toxicity by neurotransmitters, similar to an acute ischemic stroke. In the end those mechanisms can lead to cerebral cell death, swelling, and increased intracranial pressure. The mechanisms of secondary brain damage are subject to ongoing studies; traumatic brain injury depicts a

TABLE 22.2   Marshall CT (computed tomography) classification of traumatic brain injury.

Category	Definition
Diffuse injury I (no visible pathology)	No visible intracranial pathology seen on CT scan
Diffuse injury II	Cisterns are present with midline shift of 0–5 mm and/or lesions densities present; no high or mixed density lesion >25 cm^3 may include bone fragments and foreign bodies
Diffuse injury III (swelling)	Cisterns compressed or absent with midline shift 0–5 mm; no high or mixed density lesion >25 cm^3
Diffuse injury IV (shift)	Midline shift >5 mm; no high or mixed density lesion >25 cm^3
Evacuated mass lesion V	Any lesion surgically evacuated
Nonevacuated mass lesion VI	High or mixed density lesion >25 cm^3; not surgically evacuated

Reproduced with permission from: Adelson PD, Bratton SL, Carney NA, et al. Guidelines for the acute medical management of severe traumatic brain injury in infants, children, and adolescents. Pediatr Crit Care Med 2003;4:S2. Copyright © 2003 Lippincott Williams & Wilkins.

VII. Non-blood TBI biomarker strategy

TABLE 22.3   Rotterdam CT (computed tomography) classification of traumatic brain injury.

Predicator value	Score
Basal cisterns	
Normal	0
Compressed	1
Absent	2
Midline shift	
No shift or shift ≤ 5 mm	0
Shift > 5 mm	1
Epidural mass lesion	
Absent	0
Present	1
Intraventricular blood or subarachnoid hemorrhage	
Absent	0
Present	1
Sum score	Total + 1

Reproduced with permission from: Mass AL, Hukkelhoven CW, Marshall LF, Steyerberg EW. Prediction of outcome in traumatic brain injury with computed tomographic characteristics: a comparison between the computed tomographic classification and combinations of computed tomographic predictors. Neurosurgery 2005;57:1173. Copyright © 2005 Lippincott Williams & Wilkins.

broad field of underlying mechanisms and risk factors which we aim to review and elucidate in this article.

22.2 Clinical risk factors in traumatic brain injury

22.2.1 Severity of traumatic brain injury and guideline-based treatment in high volume centers

For clinical management and further treatment of patients with traumatic brain injury, a standardized approach with assessment of risk factors defining further diagnostic steps and clinical care has improved over the last decades. Initially, clinical graduation of severity of traumatic brain injury is a crucial point. Here the GCS has emerged as a practical tool, by which traumatic brain injury is classified as mild (GCS 13–15), moderate (GCS 9–12), or severe (GCS < 9) [8,15]. Furthermore, standardization for treatment of patients is supported by numerous guidelines aiming to improve the outcome of the patient [16,17]. Despite this, most treatment algorithms are not based on well-designed randomized clinical trials but studies suggest improved outcome of patients with treatment in centers adhering to guidelines in conjunction with neurosurgical and neurointensive care unit support [18–20]. Tepas and coworkers therefore analyzed patients' between 16 and 64 years of age from 2000 until 2010 and found improved survival and quality of life after treatment in high volume centers (> 40/quarter of year) [21].

22.2.2 Cranial imaging in patients with traumatic brain injury

After admission and clinical examination as well as stabilization of vital functions, patients with traumatic brain injury should undergo cranial imaging depending on presence of risk factors. Noncontrast CT imaging detects cerebral edema, skull fractures, and intracranial hematomas. In cases of clinical aggravation of patients with traumatic brain injury, follow-up CT imaging is warranted. In the absence of aggravation, the repetition of a CT scan is not necessary in contrast to patients with intracranial hematoma without signs of aggravation who should receive a follow-up in 6 hours [22]. Here, current guidelines demand cranial CT imaging for patients with traumatic brain injury and coma, amnesia, reduced consciousness, neurological symptoms, vomiting, seizures, skull fracture, penetrating injury, loss of cerebrospinal fluid, or impaired coagulation function [17]. Cranial CT imaging should be evaluated in patients with unclear mechanisms of traumatic brain injury, severe headache, high energy trauma, or influence of drugs or alcohol [17].

22.2.3 Prehospital treatment — avoidance of secondary brain injury

In prehospital care of patients with traumatic brain injury, prevention of hypoxia and hypotension as risk factors for secondary brain injury are of significant importance [23,24]. Here, McHugh and colleagues investigated secondary brain injury due to hypoxia, hypotension, and hypothermia in a preclinical setting. They included seven phase III studies in their meta-analysis and found hypoxia (OR: 2.1 95% CI [1.7–2.6]), hypotension (OR: 2.7 95% CI [2.1–3.4]), and hypothermia (OR: 2.2 95% CI [1.6–3.2]) being significantly associated with poorer outcome of the patient after traumatic brain injury [24]. The pivotal role of systolic blood pressure (SBP) was further underlined in the study of Fuller et al. where they showed mortality after traumatic brain injury being six times higher with SBP <70 mmHg, three times higher with SBP <90 mmHg, doubled (SBP: <100 mmHg), and 1.5-fold increased with SBP <120 mmHg, respectively [25]. For initial resuscitation of low blood pressure randomized controlled trials did not show superiority of hypertonic fluids over normal saline concerning long-term neurological outcome or survival [26,27]. Additionally, airway management is of crucial relevance. Patients with GCS <9 or persistent oxygen saturation lower than 90% despite oxygen application should receive endotracheal intubation [28]. However, evidence for preclinical intubation is under debate [29]. A meta-analysis of van Elm et al. did not find a benefit from preclinical intubation (adjusted OR: 0.24–1.42) concerning in-hospital mortality, while Davis et al. even found decreased survival after prehospital intubation in moderate to severe traumatic brain injury (OR: 0.36; 0.32–0.42) [30,31]. On the other hand a randomized controlled trial from Australia showed improved long-term neurological outcomes after preclinical rapid sequence intubation (success rate of intubation 97%) after 6 months when compared with intubation in hospital in adult patients with severe traumatic brain injury (risk ratio, 1.28; 1.00–1.64; $P = .046$) [32]. Concerning prehospital intubation, despite well-trained personnel, avoidance of hypo- or hyperventilation and hemodynamic instability following raid sequence intubation should be granted. Furthermore, when intubation is necessary but cannot be achieved preclinical application of a supraglottic airway device should be evaluated.

22.2.4 In-hospital treatment — emergency department

For initial treatment of patients with severe traumatic brain injury adherence to the Advanced Trauma Life Support (ATLS) protocol should be considered. As in the preclinical setting airway management and stabilization of vital parameters are of special importance. Thus patients with a GCS <9 or impaired airway protection as well as SpO_2 lower than 90% with supplemented oxygen or clinical signs of cerebral herniation (e.g., abnormal posturing with flexed upper extremity and extended lower extremity, GCS 3–5, difference in pupils or failure of pupil constriction due to light) should receive endotracheal intubation. Here a PaO_2 of >60 mmHg should be aimed for alongside continuous measurement of heart rate, blood pressure, respiratory rate, including capnography, and temperature. Additionally, the patient has to be screened for further trauma adhering to the ATLS guideline and neurological status reevaluated frequently as worsening is often observed within the first hours after trauma. To this end, assessment of increased intracranial pressure should be performed and signs of cerebral herniation have to be addressed immediately [33]. Crucial signs of cerebral herniation include respiratory depression, unilateral or bilateral dilated and fixed pupils, pupillary asymmetry, abnormal posturing, and the "Cushing triad" (irregular respiration, hypertension, bradycardia). Here application of a monitoring device of intracranial pressure should be critically evaluated. In addition to that, evaluation of blunt cerebrovascular trauma, resulting from vertebral fractures or skull bases fractures injuring the carotid artery or the vertebral arteries, is mandatory. Cerebrovascular injury results in stroke at the time of trauma but may also be evident with a latency of up to days.

22.2.5 In-hospital treatment — emergency surgical intervention

The indication for neurosurgical interventions is commonly based on GCS and results of cranial imaging. Here, an epidural hematoma of >30 mL throughout all GCS scores as wells as patients with GCS ≤8 and anisocoria should be evacuated immediately [34]. On the other hand, epidural hematoma of <30 mL with midline shift <5 mm, <15 thickness, and GCS >8 is eligible for conservative treatment with follow-up by cranial imaging [34]. For intracerebral hemorrhage indication of evacuation is based on signs of a mass effect. These include obstructive hydrocephalus, brainstem compression, and fourth ventricle or basal cistern obliteration [35]. Furthermore intracerebral hemorrhage >50 mL should be evacuated [36]. Concerning subdural hematomas evacuation should be performed in patients with midline shift >5 mm or thickness of hematoma exceeding 10 mm [37]. Further indication for evacuation of subdural hematoma are GCS ≤8 or a decrease of ≥2 between trauma and admission as well as intracranial pressure exceeding 20 mmHg and dilated/fixed pupils. For penetrating injuries closure of the dura and superficial wound treatment are beneficial as well as application of broad-spectrum antibiotic substances to prevent infection. To this end, surgical treatment of depressed skull fractures exceeding the thickness of the cranium is recommended. Nonsurgical therapy is possible in patients with missing radiological or clinical signs of wound infection/contamination, dural penetration, or sinus involvement [38]. In cases of therapy refractory high intracranial-pressure surgical evacuation by craniectomy may be warranted.

22.2.6 Predictive factors for prognosis of outcome in traumatic brain injury

GCS is a crucial factor determining outcome after traumatic brain injury with a death rate of 30% in patients with GCS ≤ 8. McMillan et al. found in a case control cohort study of 767 patients, that survivors of traumatic brain injury have an increased risk of death from multiple causes for at least 13 years after the index hospitalization [39]. On the other hand, delayed neurologic recovery after nonpenetration severe traumatic brain injury with decompression craniectomy was observed. Here, high admission GCS (OR: 1.44, 1.07−1.96) and absence of nonevacuated intracerebral hematoma larger than 1 cm (OR: 6.67, 1.12−33.3) were significantly associated with chance of delayed neurological recovery after 6−18 months [40]. Furthermore, the there are several risk factors for determination of outcome after traumatic brain injury mainly driven by occurrence of medical complications as well as secondary cerebral insults. Here GCS at presentation, presence of cranial imaging abnormalities, age, pupillary dysfunction, FOUR score, extracranial and extracerebral trauma, hypotension, pyrexia, hypoxemia, high intracranial pressure, coagulopathy, and impaired cerebral perfusion are among the pivotal factors for poor outcome. Furthermore, brainstem injury or diffuse axonal damage on MRI have been shown to be associated with poor outcome [41,42]. Further predictors of poor outcome are elevated biomarkers, such as S-100βprotein, CSFα-synuclein, and NSE [43−45]. To this end, there are outcome prediction models for patients with traumatic brain injury, such as the CRASH model including GCS, age, pupils, extracranial injury, country and CT findings, as well as the IMPACT model with pupils, GCS motoric response, age alongside with CT imaging hypotension and hypoxemia, hemoglobin, and glucose levels [46,47].

References

[1] Schiller JS, et al. Summary health statistics for U.S. adults: National Health Interview Survey, 2010. Vital Health Stat 2012;10(252):1−207.

[2] Seifert J. Incidence and economic burden of injuries in the United States. J Epidemiol Commun Health 2007;61(10). p. 926-926.

[3] Rickels E. Diagnosis and treatment of traumatic brain injury. Chirurg 2009;80(2):153−62 quiz 163.

[4] Taylor CA, et al. Traumatic brain injury-related emergency department visits, hospitalizations, and deaths − United States, 2007 and 2013. MMWR Surveill Summ 2017;66(9):1−16.

[5] Li M, et al. Epidemiology of traumatic brain injury over the world: a systematic review. Austin Neurol Neurosci 2016;1(2) 1007., 2016.

[6] Liao CC, et al. Risk and outcomes for traumatic brain injury in patients with mental disorders. J Neurol Neurosurg Psychiatry 2012;83(12):1186−92.

[7] Ilie G, et al. Prevalence and correlates of traumatic brain injuries among adolescents. JAMA 2013;309 (24):2550−2.

[8] Teasdale G, Jennett B. Assessment of coma and impaired consciousness. Lancet 1974;304(7872):81−4.

[9] Stocchetti N, et al. Inaccurate early assessment of neurological severity in head injury. J Neurotrauma 2004;21(9):1131−40.

[10] Balestreri M, et al. Predictive value of Glasgow Coma Scale after brain trauma: change in trend over the past ten years. J Neurol Neurosurg Psychiatry 2004;75(1):161−2.

[11] Stead LG, et al. Validation of a new coma scale, the FOUR score, in the emergency department. Neurocrit Care 2009;10(1):50−4.

[12] Eken C, et al. Comparison of the Full Outline of Unresponsiveness Score Coma Scale and the Glasgow Coma Scale in an emergency setting population. Eur J Emerg Med 2009;16(1):29−36.

[13] Saatman KE, et al. Classification of traumatic brain injury for targeted therapies. J Neurotrauma 2008;25 (7):719—38.

[14] Marshall LF, et al. The diagnosis of head injury requires a classification based on computed axial tomography. J Neurotrauma 1992;9(Suppl. 1):S287—92.

[15] Foulkes MA, et al. The Traumatic Coma Data Bank: design, methods, and baseline characteristics. J Neurosurg 1991;75(Suppl.):S8—13.

[16] Carney N, et al. Guidelines for the management of severe traumatic brain injury, fourth edition. Neurosurgery 2017;80(1):6—15.

[17] Firsching R, Rickels E, Mauer UM, Sakowitz OW, Messing-Jünger M, Engelhard für DGAI K, Linn für DGNR J, Biberthaler für DGU P, Schwerdtfeger K, Leitlinie Schädel-Hirn-Trauma Im Erwachsenenalter.

[18] Patel HC, et al. Trends in head injury outcome from 1989 to 2003 and the effect of neurosurgical care: an observational study. Lancet 2005;366(9496):1538—44.

[19] Visca A, et al. Clinical and neuroimaging features of severely brain-injured patients treated in a neurosurgical unit compared with patients treated in peripheral non-neurosurgical hospitals. Br J Neurosurg 2006;20 (2):82—6.

[20] Brown JB, et al. Trauma center designation correlates with functional independence after severe but not moderate traumatic brain injury. J Trauma 2010;69(2):263—9.

[21] Tepas 3rd JJ, et al. High-volume trauma centers have better outcomes treating traumatic brain injury. J Trauma Acute Care Surg 2013;74(1):143—7 discussion 147-8.

[22] Brown CV, et al. Indications for routine repeat head computed tomography (CT) stratified by severity of traumatic brain injury. J Trauma 2007;62(6):1339—44 discussion 1344—5.

[23] Brain Trauma F, et al. Guidelines for the management of severe traumatic brain injury. I. Blood pressure and oxygenation. J Neurotrauma 2007;24(Suppl. 1):S7—13.

[24] McHugh GS, et al. Prognostic value of secondary insults in traumatic brain injury: results from the IMPACT study. J Neurotrauma 2007;24(2):287—93.

[25] Fuller G, et al. The association between admission systolic blood pressure and mortality in significant traumatic brain injury: a multi-centre cohort study. Injury 2014;45(3):612—17.

[26] Bulger EM, et al. Out-of-hospital hypertonic resuscitation following severe traumatic brain injury: a randomized controlled trial. JAMA 2010;304(13):1455—64.

[27] Cooper DJ, et al. Prehospital hypertonic saline resuscitation of patients with hypotension and severe traumatic brain injury: a randomized controlled trial. JAMA 2004;291(11):1350—7.

[28] Badjatia N, et al. Guidelines for prehospital management of traumatic brain injury 2nd edition. Prehosp Emerg Care 2008;12(Suppl. 1):S1—52.

[29] Gaither JB, et al. Balancing the potential risks and benefits of out-of-hospital intubation in traumatic brain injury: the intubation/hyperventilation effect. Ann Emerg Med 2012;60(6):732—6.

[30] von Elm E, et al. Pre-hospital tracheal intubation in patients with traumatic brain injury: systematic review of current evidence. Br J Anaesth 2009;103(3):371—86.

[31] Davis DP, et al. The impact of prehospital endotracheal intubation on outcome in moderate to severe traumatic brain injury. J Trauma 2005;58(5):933—9.

[32] Bernard SA, et al. Prehospital rapid sequence intubation improves functional outcome for patients with severe traumatic brain injury: a randomized controlled trial. Ann Surg 2010;252(6):959—65.

[33] Cadena R, Shoykhet M, Ratcliff JJ. Emergency neurological life support: intracranial hypertension and herniation. Neurocrit Care 2017;27(Suppl. 1):82—8.

[34] Bullock MR, et al. Surgical management of acute epidural hematomas. Neurosurgery 2006;58(3 Suppl.): S7—15 discussion Si—iv.

[35] Bullock MR, et al. Surgical management of posterior fossa mass lesions. Neurosurgery 2006;58(3 Suppl.): S47—55 discussion Si—iv.

[36] Bullock MR, et al. Surgical management of traumatic parenchymal lesions. Neurosurgery 2006;58(3 Suppl.): S25—46 discussion Si—iv.

[37] Bullock MR, Chesnut R, Ghajar J, Gordon D, Hartl R, Newell DW, et al. Surgical management of acute subdural hematomas. Neurosurgery 2006 Mar;58(3 Suppl.):S16—24 discussion Si-iv.

[38] Bullock MR, et al. Surgical management of depressed cranial fractures. Neurosurgery 2006;58(3 Suppl.): S56—60 discussion Si—iv.

[39] McMillan TM, et al. Death after head injury: the 13 year outcome of a case control study. J Neurol Neurosurg Psychiatry 2011;82(8):931—5.

[40] Ho KM, Honeybul S, Litton E. Delayed neurological recovery after decompressive craniectomy for severe nonpenetrating traumatic brain injury. Crit Care Med 2011;39(11):2495—500.

[41] Haghbayan H, et al. The prognostic value of mri in moderate and severe traumatic brain injury: a systematic review and meta-analysis. Crit Care Med 2017;45(12):e1280—8.

[42] Izzy S, et al. Revisiting grade 3 diffuse axonal injury: not all brainstem microbleeds are prognostically equal. Neurocrit Care 2017;27(2):199—207.

[43] Mondello S, et al. alpha-Synuclein in CSF of patients with severe traumatic brain injury. Neurology 2013;80 (18):1662—8.

[44] Mercier E, et al. Predictive value of S-100 beta protein for prognosis in patients with moderate and severe traumatic brain injury: systematic review and meta-analysis. BMJ 2013;346:f1757.

[45] Chabok SY, et al. Neuron-specific enolase and S100 BB as outcome predictors in severe diffuse axonal injury. J Trauma Acute Care Surg 2012;72(6):1654—7.

[46] Collaborators MCT, et al. Predicting outcome after traumatic brain injury: practical prognostic models based on large cohort of international patients. BMJ 2008;336(7641):425—9.

[47] Steyerberg EW, et al. Predicting outcome after traumatic brain injury: development and international validation of prognostic scores based on admission characteristics. PLoS Med 2008;5(8):e165 discussion e165.

Saliva biomarkers of traumatic brain injury

Šárka O. Southern[1], W. Frank Peacock[2] and Ava M. Puccio[3]

[1]Saliva Diagnostics Gaia Medical Institute, La Jolla, CA, United States [2]Emergency Medicine Baylor College of Medicine, Houston, TX, United States [3]Department of Neurosurgery, University of Pittsburgh, Pittsburgh, PA, United States

Our goal is to develop saliva tests for point-of-care (POC) diagnostics and prognostics of traumatic brain injury (TBI). Saliva holds a unique promise for TBI assessment. Saliva samples are noninvasive and can be easily and safely self-collected by adults and children in POC. The key technical challenges in developing saliva biomarkers of TBI are saliva handling, analytical assay and biomarker selection. This chapter describes innovative methods for saliva collection, assays and unbiased biomarker discovery that successfully identified new saliva biomarkers of TBI and post-concussion syndrome.

23.1 Biomarkers of traumatic brain injury

TBI is a leading cause of mortality and morbidity around the world, with increasing incidence [1−12]. Over 75% of TBI injuries are mild TBI (mTBI) [6]. mTBI is a significant public health concern because repetitive mTBI increases risk of the second impact syndrome and chronic neurocognitive pathologies such as chronic traumatic encephalopathy (CTE) [4,13,14]. Approximately one-third of mTBI patients experience persistent somatic, cognitive, and psychological or behavioral symptoms beyond the normal course of recovery. This condition is diagnosed as the postconcussion syndrome (PCS, ICD-10, adults and children) [15−19]. Adult patients that experience a decline in cognitive performance and function following a mTBI can be also diagnosed with the neurocognitive disorder due to TBI (NCDT, DSM-5) [20−25]. PCS and NCDT can lead to lifelong problems with a significant impact on the patient, family, society, and the economy [15−17,19−22,26−31]. Key symptoms include headache, dizziness, vision and hearing problems, cognitive deficits (loss of memory and executive function), fatigue, nausea, sleep disturbance, apathy, irritability, impulsivity, and aggression. Children are at higher risk for mTBI due to their developing coordination, changing head-to-body ratio, risk-taking behaviors, and broad participation in sports and play [8]. Long-term effects of PCS can affect the child's ability to function physically, cognitively, and psychologically [8,32–36]. Military service members have higher mTBI incidence than civilians (15%–23%) with estimated 316,000 mTBI reported between 2000 and 2018 by the Defense and Veterans Brain Injury Center (DVBIC). Military mTBI is different from the civilian mTBI in the manner of causation by explosive blasts and high cooccurrence with posttraumatic stress disorder (PTSD) [37–46]. The underlying pathophysiology of mTBI remains undetermined, and as a result there are currently no efficient diagnostic, prognostic, or therapeutic strategies available clinically [9,11,17,47].

Standard diagnostics of mTBI in the hospital are based on the American Congress of Rehabilitation Medicine (ACRM) and pediatric CDC/WHO diagnostic criteria relying on Glasgow Coma Scale (GCS) scores and head CT scan findings [8,9]. Advanced MRI has the potential to be more sensitive than CT but its high cost makes it prohibitive for routine use. At ≥3 months after injury, neurocognitive psychological (NP) tests are used to diagnose PCS and NCDT and the Glasgow Outcome Scale-Extended (GOS-E) test provides the gold standard measure of long-term global TBI outcome. Sports medicine takes a different approach to mTBI diagnostics. The Sport Concussion Assessment Tool (SCAT) 5 [48–54] is used to support diagnosis of concussion and the Immediate Postconcussion Assessment (IMPACT), Vestibular/Ocular Motor Screening (VOMS), and modified Balance Error Scoring System (mBESS) provide aid in decisions about return to work, school, and sports [48,50,52,55]. The standard practice has major weaknesses including subjective measures with low accuracy, slow and costly assessment, radiation risk of the head CT scan, no definitive diagnosis for patients with negative CT findings, potential for misdiagnosis, and inconsistent diagnostic methods in hospital and sports [56–58]. Many mTBI patients are not seeking any medical care [59]. As a result, a high percentage of mTBIs may go underdiagnosed or unidentified, increasing the risk of the second impact syndrome and CTE, and delaying treatment for PCS.

Biomarkers are emerging new tools for diagnostics and prognostics of TBI. Recent studies examined the use of brain-specific protein biomarkers in blood including UCHL-1, GFAP, NSE, S100b, Tau, and most recently, miRNAs [60–71]. Results showed potential for diagnosing acute mTBI and predicting long-term outcome after TBI. However, the clinical utility of these biomarkers is limited by several key factors: a short half-life (<48 h after injury) of UCHL-1 and GFAP (48 h after injury) prevents their use for detection of chronic TBI [65], invasive sample (blood or cerebrospinal fluid) is required, low concentration in the pg/mL range requires ultrasensitive laboratory assay, instability of miRNA during specimen freeze/thaw and room temperature handling [72] is not compatible with frozen samples from large clinical studies and a rapid diagnostic test (RDT) at POC settings.

A major barrier to advancing mTBI treatment and prevention is the inability to objectively and practically diagnose mTBI [5,8,9,11,17,48,52,53,55,60,64–67,73–84]. To close the technology gap, our team focused on saliva-based protein biomarkers of TBI that could be translated into a low-cost RDT for routine TBI diagnostics in POC, during sports, and at home.

TABLE 23.1   SRP biomarkers provide an innovative method for detecting systemic biological response to traumatic brain injury.

Biological effects of TBI		Homeostatic pathways	100 SRP biomarkers
Oxidative stress,glutamate release	1	Redox stress response	
Accumulation of toxic metabolites	2	Cellular detoxification Phase I/II	
Misfolded proteins and membranes	3	Protein chaperoning	
DNA damage, altered DNA methylation	4	DNA repair and modification	
Disrupted cell adhesion, cytoskeletal damage	5	Adhesion, cytoskeleton, exosomes	
Increased ATP production, metabolic changes	6	Cell cycle & energy metabolism	
Damaged cells	7	Apoptosis and autophagy	
Changes in hormones and neuropeptides	8	Neuroendocrine signaling	
Inflammation, chronic immune activation	9	Innate and specific immunity	
Gut microbiome changes	10	Microbiome stress response	
Disrupted transport of water/ions, cerebral edema	11	Osmotic stress response	

23.2 Stress response profiling: a new method for unbiased discovery of traumatic brain injury biomarkers

Saliva-based biomarkers of TBI described in this chapter were discovered using stress response profiling (SRP). SRP is a new patented method [85–90] for unbiased discovery of disease biomarkers. SRP uses an array of 100 biomarkers to measure persistent homeostatic perturbations associated with a specific disease. Results define the homeostatic pathway signature and identify candidate biomarkers of the disease. Table 23.1 shows links between the homeostatic pathways monitored by SRP biomarkers and systemic biological effects of TBI.

SRP biomarkers provide an innovative way to monitor TBI because they are independent predictors relative to standard indicators such as GCS and GOS-E scores, CT findings, and the known biomarkers in blood or CSF. SRP has been successfully applied to discover saliva biomarkers of diseases other than TBI, including heart failure, chronic pain and HIV, showing that the SRP method is innovative in a broad sense.

23.3 Homeostatic pathways monitored by stress response profiling biomarkers

A detailed description of SRP biomarkers and associated homeostatic pathways was published previously [85–90]. Each pathway is monitored by multiple SRP biomarkers to increase the sensitivity of disease detection. SRP biomarkers were selected to detect *persistent* homeostatic perturbations (i.e., chronic physiological stress) rather than acute effects because chronic physiological stress is a risk factor for disease development and progression. Individual biological pathways monitored by SRP biomarkers are summarized below.

23.3.1 Redox stress response

This pathway regulates levels of reactive oxygen and nitrogen species (RONS, e.g., superoxide, nitric oxide, carbon monoxide) through free radical-scavenging enzymes such as superoxide dismutases. RONS are essential cellular mediators but when in excess, they cause cellular dysfunction through peroxidation of lipids, protein aggregation, cell membrane damage, DNA lesions, mitochondrial dysfunction, and altered signal transduction. TBI is known to increase RONS while decreasing antioxidant enzymes leading to persistent oxidative and nitrosative stress.

23.3.2 Cellular detoxification

This pathway regulates Phase I and II cellular detoxification that provides defense against chemical threats to the cellular integrity. Phase I detox enzymes (e.g., cytochrome P450) oxidize, reduce, or hydrolyze endogenous metabolites (e.g., fatty acids, steroids) and foreign substances (drugs, alcohol, pesticides, and hydrocarbons). Phase II enzymes (e.g., glutathione-S-transferase, GST) modify xenobiotics to be more hydrophilic which increases their disposal, providing cellular resistance to hydrocarbons, heavy metals, and oxidants, including RONS generated by TBI.

23.3.3 Protein chaperoning

Protein chaperones (e.g. heat shock proteins such as Hsp70) fold newly synthesized polypeptides and refold misfolded proteins to prevent uncontrolled protein aggregation. Through hundreds of "client" proteins, chaperoning has a key role in multiple biological functions including cellular protection, metabolism, growth and development. Misfolded and aggregated proteins are the hallmark of neurodegenerative diseases including CTE. TBI promotes the accumulation and prion-like spread of misfolded protein aggregates that may propagate the changes induced by TBI. Hsp70 and its co-chaperones may play a direct role in TBI outcome by preventing the aggregation of Tau protein and facilitating the clearance of pTau through the proteasomal system.

23.3.4 DNA repair and modification

This pathway regulates multiple stages and mechanisms of DNA repair and epigenetic chromatin modification via DNA methylation and acetylation. Epigenetic modification is critical to normal genome regulation, development, and disease pathogenesis. DNA repair is closely linked with cell cycle control and apoptosis. DNA damage is ubiquitous and therefore the stability of the genome is under a continuous surveillance by multiple DNA repair mechanisms. DNA lesions are produced by free radicals during normal biological processes (e.g. DNA transcription and replication, metabolism and immunity), and and in response to injury and disease such as TBI and PCS.

23.3.5 Adhesion, cytoskeleton, extracellular matrix, and exosomes

This pathway regulates cellular interactions with the extracellular matrix, changes in cytoskeletal matrix including centrioles, kinetosomes, and other microtubule-organizing centers, and production of microvesicles including exosomes. These processes are essential for cellular survival, growth, metabolism, and motility, and also for the formation of microbial biofilms and microbial–host interactions. Exosomes and other microvesicles are biological nanoparticles that transfer specific molecular messages (microRNA, mRNA, proteins, and other biomolecules) between cells and remote tissues. Exosomes are secreted by most cells and circulate systemically through most body fluids including saliva. It was suggested that pathophysiological response to TBI might be mediated via systemic circulation of exosomes [91–94].

23.3.6 Cell cycle and energy metabolism

This pathway regulates the cell cycle and energy metabolism. In adult animal tissues, most cells do not cycle except for somatic stem cells involved in normal tissue turnover. Cell cycling is also arrested in starved cells and in cells with DNA or mitochondrial damage. A controlled increase in cell growth occurs during immune responses, wound healing, regeneration, and during developmental changes. Uncontrolled cell growth is associated with cancer. The key energy currency of the animal cell, ATP, is produced through oxidative phosphorylation of glucose in mitochondria. Loss of mitochondrial function can result in the excess fatigue and other symptoms common to almost every chronic disease. Systemic energy metabolism is controlled at the neuroimmunoendocrine level through hormones, cytokines, and growth factors. Dysregulation of systemic energy metabolism can be caused by infections (e.g., influenza and HIV), metabolic disorder (e.g., diabetes), or neurological disease such as TBI.

23.3.7 Apoptosis and autophagy

This pathway regulates the programmed cell death (apoptosis) and a self-catabolic process (autophagy). Apoptosis is increased during tissue remodeling, wound healing, and aging. During a disease, apoptosis can be increased within the diseased tissue (e.g., in psoriatic skin lesions) and also in remote tissues and biofluids (e.g., during HIV infection, soluble mediators trigger apoptosis in uninfected lymphocytes). Apoptosis can be also triggered by environmental stressors that cause mitochondrial damage (e.g., oxidative stress). Autophagy removes damaged somatic cells that do not turnover (e.g., cardiomyocytes), misfolded or aggregated proteins, damaged organelles, and intracellular pathogens. Both apoptosis and autophagy are activated after TBI and may play protective roles in the patient outcome.

23.3.8 Neuroendocrine signaling

This pathway is integrated with immunological signaling and regulates animal physiology and behavior. It involves a large number of mediators (hormones, neuropeptides, neurotransmitters) and cellular receptors produced by specialized tissues (glands and neural tissues), and also locally in peripheral tissues (e.g., skin and gut). In vertebrates, two signaling mechanisms are best known for providing initial responses to psychobiological stress: the limbic hypothalamic—pituitary—adrenal axis (HPA) via cortisol, and the sympathetic nervous system via catecholamines. However, chronic stress also activates many other neuroendocrine signaling pathways for sensing pain and anxiety, energy balance and metabolic, respiratory, circulatory, and reproductive status.

23.3.9 Immunity

This pathway regulates innate and specific immunity, defense mechanisms against biological threats to an organism's integrity such as injuries, tumors, and pathogenic microorganisms. Innate immunity provides a nonspecific defense to a variety of threats and dominates the initial defense phase. Specific immunity provides threat-specific defense through antibodies and lymphocytes. Both types of immunity are regulated through numerous specialized cells (e.g., hemocytes, phagocytes, natural killer cells, lymphocytes) and soluble mediators (e.g., agglutinins, antibodies, chemokines, cytokines and agglutinins). Increased immunity is beneficial when it is limited to a short-term and localized response (e.g., removal of bacterial infection). However chronic inflammatory response is harmful and may contribute to chronic disease such as PCS.

23.3.10 Microbial stress response

This pathway regulates stress responses in the microbiome and signaling between microorganisms and host cells. Commensal microbial biofilms are an integral part of animal and plant bodies and contribute to physiological homeostasis. In animals, microbial biofilms are primarily associated with the inner and the outer body surfaces (mucosal epithelium, mucosal fluids such as saliva and the skin) where they respond to environmental stressors outside the organism and microenvironmental conditions within host tissues and body fluids. During chronic physiological stress, increased signaling between microbial biofilms and host cells promotes protection of the organism through modulating the host's stress responses and immunity. Recent findings suggest that microbial alterations can influence the neurological system via the brain-gut axis, and systemic insults such as TBI may alter the gut microbiome, and changes in the microbiome may correlate with TBI severity and patient outcome [95—97].

23.3.11 Osmotic stress response

Osmotic stress response is triggered by water and electrolyte imbalance typically caused by dehydration. Given that water comprises approximately 70% of the cell content, osmotic stress can cause critical cell damage. The rapid change in the movement of water and ions across the cell membrane results in cell membrane distortion, protein aggregation and DNA damage. The initial cellular response to osmotic stress is the production of osmolytes (e.g., sorbitol and betaine) that stabilize molecular structures and prevent protein misfolding. Prolonged osmotic stress results in delayed cell cycle, DNA damage and apoptosis [98]. The increased osmotic stress response we have measured in TBI (see Figs 23.1 and 23.10) might be triggered by an abrupt water translocation between intra- and extracellular compartments in the brain driven by the mechanical force during a head injury.

23.4 Pathway signature of traumatic brain injury

Biomarker data from our clinical studies were translated into pathway signatures of acute mTBI and PCS. The pathway signature was constructed using a new algorithm to calculate the *pathway activation index* (Z) [90]. Z represents the cumulative change in all biomarkers associated with the pathway. Raw Z values are calculated from raw biomarker data to represent the relative magnitude of pathway activation in different disease conditions. Normalized Z values are calculated from normalized biomarker data (ratio to maximum value), to show preferentially activated pathways in each condition.

Pathway signatures of acute mTBI and PCS are shown in Fig. 23.1. Overall, Fig. 23.1 shows that multiple homeostatic pathways are activated in TBI. In PCS patients, pathway activation peaks at 3-6 months after injury, when postconcussion symptoms become persistent (see Fig. 23.1, early PCS, 3 months after injury). Multiple pathways stay activated across mTBI progression from acute to chronic stage (see Fig. 23.1, late and chronic PCS) suggesting that PCS is a systemic progressive disease in agreement with the clinical presentation of ongoing multifactorial symptomology.

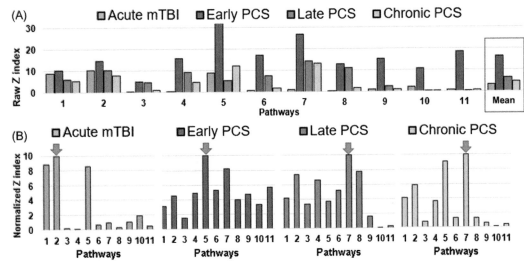

FIGURE 23.1 **Time-dependent evolution of pathway signatures during mTBI pathogenesis.** Acute mTBI: ≤48 h after injury. PCS, persistent postconcussion syndrome. Early, late, chronic PCS: 3−5, 6−9, 12−36 months after mTBI. Z index, a quantitative indicator of pathway activation. (A) Raw pathway profiles. (B) Normalized pathway profiles. Arrow indicates dominant pathway at each stage of mTBI pathogenesis. Pathways: 1, oxidative stress; 2, detoxification; 3, chaperoning; 4, DNA; 5, cell adhesion; 6, cell cycle; 7, apoptosis; 8, signaling; 9, immunity; 10, microbiome; 11, osmotic stress. Associations between SRP biomarkers and pathways are shown in Table 23.1.

Fig. 23.1A (raw profiles) shows that the pathway activation is highest during early PCS (3–6 months post injury). Fig. 23.1B (normalized profiles) shows time-dependent changes in dominant pathways during progression in PCS pathology. Pathway 2 (cellular detoxification) is preferentially activated in acute mTBI ($\leq$48 h after injury) suggesting increase in toxic metabolites. Pathway 5 (cell adhesion, cytoskeleton, extracellular matrix, exosomes) is preferentially activated in early PCS (3–6 months after injury) suggesting altered cell adhesion, damage to cytoskeleton and extracellular matrix, and increased secretion of exosomes. Pathway 7 (apoptosis, autophagy) is dominant in late and chronic PCS ($\geq$6 months after injury) suggesting a rise in irreversibly damaged cells.

The TBI pathway signature provides a novel insight into systemic TBI pathogenesis at the molecular level, and potentially identifies new targets for TBI treatment.

23.5 Saliva specimen for traumatic brain injury biomarkers

Saliva specimens have the potential to offer multiple advantages over blood for routine TBI testing including safe, easy self-collection at the POC. The main barrier to successful translation of saliva-based protein biomarkers into a rapid POC test is the lack of a saliva cartridge comparable in performance to commercial fingerprick blood cartridges that collect a standardized drop of specimen and rapidly translate it into a sample compatible with RDT. Presently available commercial devices for saliva collection do not provide saliva specimen with a high and reliable yield of analytically available protein biomarkers.

23.5.1 Standard saliva specimen

Currently, the standard saliva specimen is a cell-free fluid obtained by squeezing or centrifuging a cotton pad soaked in saliva, or by filtering whole saliva [99–104]. The weakness of this approach is the removal of cellular components of saliva, the main source of saliva biomarkers (see below). The cell removal is not standardized and consequently a variable amount of cellular biomarkers that leaks from ruptured cells into the saliva fluid contributes to the observed heterogeneity of the standard saliva specimen. The resulting biomarker concentration in the standard saliva specimen is typically very low (pg/mL) and requires ultrasensitive laboratory assays [99–104], which limits development of commercial RDTs based on the standard saliva specimen.

23.5.2 Whole saliva specimen

We were the first to show that saliva reproducibly contains numerous epithelial cells, monocytes, lymphocytes, and neutrophils [105,106], see Table 23.2 and Fig. 23.2.

Saliva cells are live and biologically functional as demonstrated by in vitro induction of stress response biomarkers in cultured saliva cells using heat shock or osmotic stress [89,107]. This new insight into saliva biology provided the basis for developing new methods for saliva handling and biomarker assays [86–90]. The key improvement of our methods is the standardized handling of saliva cells resulting in a high and reliable yield of

TABLE 23.2 Cellular composition of normal saliva in children and adults.

Cell concentration (cells/mL)	Infant	Child	Adult
	0.1 million	2.1 million	2.3 million
Cell type (%)			
Squamous epithelial cells	95−99	50−60	50−60
Neutrophiles	1−5	30−40	30−40
Monocytes	0.1−1	5−10	5−10
B and T lymphocytes	0.1	1−5	1−5
Bacteria and yeast	Not detected	Yes	Yes

Infant, 2−9 month of age. Child, 5−17 years of age. Adult, 18−75 years of age. Cell type was confirmed using immunochemical staining for specific antigens. Epithelial cells were positive for E-cadherin, EMA, and laminin. Monocytes were positive for CD68, T cells for CD3, and B cells for CD19.

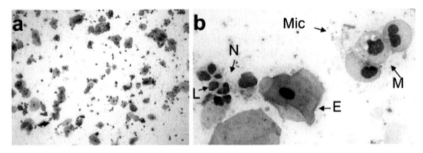

FIGURE 23.2 **Cellular composition of human saliva.** Whole saliva was stained with hematoxylin-eosin. (A) Saliva contains a high concentrations of cells. (B) Cell types present in saliva: epithelial cells (E), neutrophils (N), monocytes (M), lymphocytes (L), and microbial cells (Mic).

analytically available protein biomarkers. Saliva collected using our method has on average 12-fold higher concentration of detectable biomarkers and seven-fold lower variability in biomarker concentration compared to the standard specimen (cell-free saliva). This is a critical milestone for successful development of a rapid POC test.

23.5.3 Biomarker assays for whole saliva

The new insight into saliva cells as the main source of saliva biomarkers spurred the development of new assay methods for standardized measurement of saliva biomarkers in saliva cells as well as fluid. We have developed two new immunoassay methods: digital immunohistochemistry (IHC) and Western blot (WB). The methods were analytically validated for quantitative measurement of the core SRP panel of 100 biomarkers (Table 23.1).

Whole saliva is a complex biological specimen with highly modified proteins and a strong matrix effect compared to blood or urine [102,108−110]. Development of whole

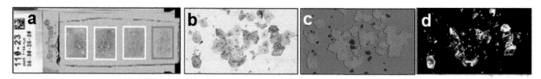

FIGURE 23.3   **Digital IHC of whole saliva.** (A) Digitized IHC slide with four saliva fields. Field 4 (green frame) selected for image analysis. (B) Mucin1 immunostain in epithelial cells (red signal). (C) Segmented image: red mask, epithelial cells; blue mask, leukocytes; cyan mask, saliva fluid. (D) Staining intensity map: white mask, Mucin1 signal.

saliva assays is therefore very challenging. To overcome the matrix effect, we had to substantially change sample preparation, assay chemistry, temperatures, and blocking procedures compared to standard IHC and WB assays.

The IHC assay measures biomarkers in the digital image of a standardized whole saliva sample fixed on a microscopy slide [102,108−110], see Fig. 23.3. Each assay run (120 slides) contains five control slides to monitor assay performance. Barcoded labels facilitate automated slide processing. Stained slides are digitized and images are analyzed using a high-speed automated image analysis algorithm. This is the first image analysis algorithm developed specifically for whole saliva. The mean total signal volume (duplicate saliva fields) provides the raw biomarker measurement. Recombinant protein standards spiked in the saliva matrix were used to construct standard curves to determine assay accuracy and specificity. The image analysis algorithm was analytically validated using standard curves for five reference biomarkers based on mean sensitivity of 10 pg/mL saliva, signal/noise ratio ≥ 10, CV = 16%, accuracy 97%, and 40-fold linear dynamic range.

To our knowledge, digital IHC and WB are the first quantitative biomarkers assays validated for whole saliva. The assay workflow is standardized, automated, and scalable to facilitate high-throughput when analyzing large sample sets from clinical studies. These new methods for saliva handling enabled measuring saliva isoforms of all 100 SRP proteins, many of which were not reported in saliva previously. This made possible the discovery of saliva-based biomarkers for TBI and PCS.

23.6 Saliva biomarkers of mild traumatic brain injury

N = 20 candidate biomarkers of acute mTBI and PCS were identified based on a study of N = 444 adult mTBI patients and controls. Acute mTBI patients were presenting to the emergency department (ED) within ≤ 48 h after injury (median 10 h). mTBI diagnosis was based on the ACRM diagnostic criteria: initial GCS score 13−15, loss of consciousness (LOC) 0−30 min, and verified posttraumatic amnesia (PTA) ≤ 24 h. The study included mTBI patients with positive and negative findings on the head CT scan. Controls were ED patients with general complains without a head injury. Chronic mTBI patients were hospital patients and military service members diagnosed with PCS at 3−36 months after injury. In addition to PCS symptomology, some patients had cognitive deficits and decline in

TABLE 23.3 Characteristics of candidate saliva biomarkers for acute mTBI and PCS. (A) Individual biomarkers. Shaded fields represent diagnostic accuracy less than 75%. (B) Composite biomarkers.

(A)

mTBI	Time after injury	B1	B2	B3	B4	B5	B6	B7	B8	B9	B10	B11	B12	B13	B14	B15	B16	B17	B18	B19	B20
									Diagnostic accuracy of individual biomarkers											
Acute	≤48h	88%	89%	92%	83%					84%	81%			94%		94%	80%				85%
PCS	3-6m		94%	99%		99%	95%	96%	94%	97%	94%	93%	92%	97%	94%	95%			94%	98%	
	6-9m			97%			81%			93%		90%		94%	90%	93%					
	12-36m			84%			80%	81%		91%		77%			89%						

(B)

mTBI	Time after injury	Composite biomarker	Diagnostic accuracy	Sensitivity	Specificity
		Diagnostic performance of composite biomarkers			
Acute	≤48h	B3-B14-B16	97%	100%	62%
PCS	3-36m	B3-B6-B15	98%	100%	66%

executive function consistent with a neurocognitive disorder due to TBI (NCDT). However, they were not formally diagnosed with NCDT because the DSM-5 definition of NCDT was not available at that time. Controls were civilian and military mTBI patients without persistent postconcussion symptoms at 3–12 months after mTBI. Healthy military volunteers provided control for exposure to repeated head injuries, physiological and psychological stress related to military training and deployment. Healthy civilians sampled on three consecutive days in the morning and afternoon defined the normal range of the TBI biomarker concentrations and the daily and diurnal biological variability.

Characteristics of the candidate mTBI biomarkers are shown in Table 23.3. Diagnostic accuracy, sensitivity, and specificity values for individual biomarkers across acute and chronic mTBI stages were determined using ROC analysis, see Table 23.3A. Most mTBI biomarkers had a diagnostic window limited to a specific time period after the injury, see Table 23.3. To overcome this problem, a *composite biomarker* (a biomarker panel) was selected to provide a high diagnostic accuracy for mTBI and PCS across a broad diagnostic window. The biomarker panel had to be small to allow translation into a RDT. Table 23.3B shows a model panel of five biomarkers meeting the requirements for diagnostic performance and RDT. To construct the model panel, independent predictors of acute and chronic mTBI were selected using stepwise multivariate logistic regression and multivariate ROC curve analysis.

Fig. 23.4 shows time-dependent changes in the concentration of the 20 candidate mTBI biomarkers (B1-B20) from acute mTBI to chronic PCS. The mean values (box) indicate that the biomarker level typically peaked during early PCS, 3–6 months after injury. The main challenge for achieving diagnostic power for chronic mTBI was to identify biomarkers that remained elevated in PCS patients at >6 months after injury.

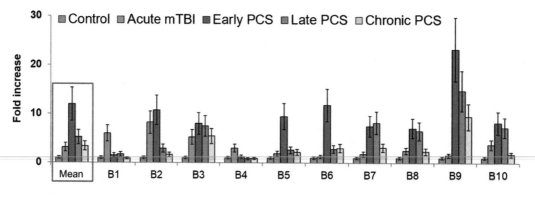

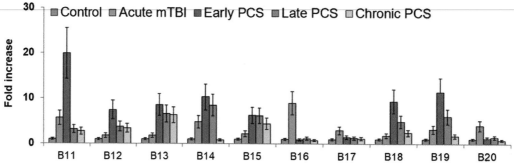

FIGURE 23.4   Time-dependent evolution of biomarkers profiles. Acute mTBI: ≤48 h after injury. PCS, persistent postconcussion symptoms. Early, late, chronic PCS: 3–5, 6–9, 12–36 months after mTBI. B1–B20, candidate biomarkers of mTBI and PCS, see Table 23.2.

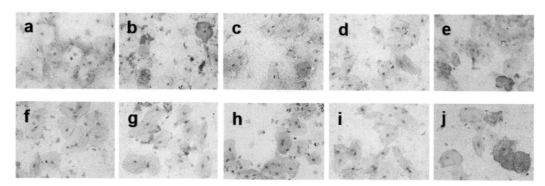

FIGURE 23.5   Acute mTBI biomarkers B3, B14 and B16. The biomarker protein was visualized in whole saliva using IHC assay with red label. (A–E) mTBI patient 10 h post injury. (F–J) control ED patient with a general complaint without head injury. (A and F) B3. (B and G) B14. (C and H) B16. (D and I) negative IHC control, no primary antibody. (E and J) reference saliva protein Mucin1. Original magnification ×400.

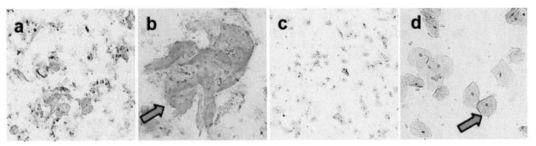

FIGURE 23.6 **PCS biomarker B6.** The biomarker protein was visualized in whole saliva using IHC assay with red label. (A–B), PCS patient at 4 months after mTBI. B6 is expressed strongly in epithelial cells and secreted to saliva fluid (arrow). (C–D), Healthy control. B6 is expressed weakly in epithelial cells (arrow) and not detectable in saliva fluid. Original magnifications: $\times 100$ (A, C) and $\times 400$ (B, D).

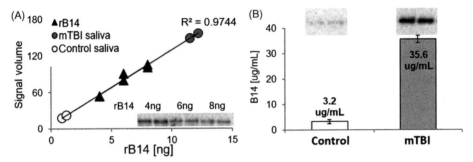

FIGURE 23.7 **Concentration of mTBI biomarker B14 in whole saliva.** The concentration of B14 protein was measured using digital ECL Western blot. (A) Standard curve was constructed using recombinant B14 protein. B14 was measured in pooled whole saliva samples from mTBI patients and controls. The calculated B14 concentration was accurate and reliable based on linearity of the standard curve ($R2 = 0.97$) and average $CV = 14\%$. (B) Comparison of B14 concentration in mTBI and control saliva. Error bars, standard deviation for duplicate samples.

The expression pattern of mTBI biomarkers in whole saliva was visualized in whole saliva cells and fluid using the IHC and WB assays described above. Figs. 23.5 and 23.6 show expression of three acute mTBI biomarkers (B3, B14, and B16) and one PCS biomarker (B6) in saliva. The concentration of these four biomarkers was strongly increased in TBI patients compared to controls. The IHC results show that the biomarkers are expressed within saliva cells and secreted from the cells into the saliva fluid. Within the saliva fluid, candidate mTBI biomarkers are concentrated in purified CD63-positive exosomes (data not shown). This offers a new insight into systemic physiological response to mTBI: cross-talk between brain and remote tissues including oral cavity might be mediated via systemic circulation of exosomes [91–94].

The saliva concentration of mTBI biomarkers was quantitatively measured using WB as illustrated in Fig. 23.7.

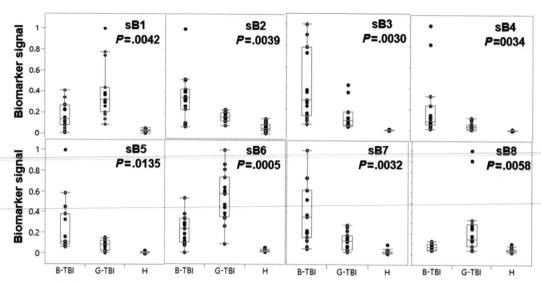

FIGURE 23.8   **Candidate saliva biomarkers of sTBI.** Expression levels of 6 candidate biomarkers sB1−sB6 are represented by box plots. The box represents 25th and 75th, line the 50th, and whiskers the 95th and 5th percentiles. Dots represent outliers. P value refers to the significance of difference between the TBI outcome groups. x axis labels: B-TBI, unfavorable outcome, G-TBI, favorable outcome; H, healthy control.

23.7 Saliva biomarkers of severe traumatic brain injury

Patients with moderate to severe TBI (sTBI) are likely to require emergency department (ED) visits, hospitalizations, rehabilitation and suffer long-term disability. Despite this large burden of disease and economical costs, there is unmet need for prognostic sTBI biomarkers to aid in individualized treatment decisions [60,64−67,73−84]. Our goal is to develop a commercial saliva test that will provide early and objective outcome prognosis for an individual patient using a noninvasive saliva sample in POC. This will potentially aid in treatment decisions, guide treatment efficacy and discharge disposition. To achieve the goal, we validated a new diagnostic specimen: saliva collected from comatose and intubated TBI patients.

N = 8 candidate biomarkers for prognostics of sTBI were identified based on the study of N = 91 adult sTBI patients and controls. Saliva samples were collected from comatose sTBI patients (GCS score 3−8) at 1−3 days after injury (the admission sample). Global outcome was classified using the gold standard approach, GOS-E scores at 6 months after injury [111]. Controls were ED patients without TBI and healthy volunteers. SRP profiling of saliva samples (see Table 23.1) identified 16 biomarkers based on > 3-fold difference in the concentration between sTBI with unfavorable vs. favorable 6 m outcome (GOS-E score 1-3 vs. 5-8).

Statistical analysis was performed using JMP Pro11 (SAS). The data was skewed so biomarkers were represented as the median (interquartile range) and nonparametric statistical tests were used. Fig. 23.8 compares biomarker levels in sTBI patients with favorable or unfavorable 6-month outcome, and controls. Biomarker levels were significantly different

TABLE 23.4   Characteristics of candidate biomarkers for sTBI prognostics. Prognostic accuracy for unfavorable global outcome (GOS-E score 1–3) was determined using ROC analysis. (A) Individual biomarkers sB1–8. (B) Composite biomarker (sB1 and sB7).

ROC analysis	sB1	sB2	sB3	sB4	sB5	sB6	sB7	sB8	Composite biomarker
Accuracy (%)	81	81	82	81	76	88	82	80	96
Sensitivity (%)	87	80	80	73	73	93	80	100	87
Specificity (%)	67	100	73	87	73	73	73	73	93
P value	.001	<.0001	.011	.001	.0025	<.0001	.0004	.0005	sB1.0001 sB7 <.0001

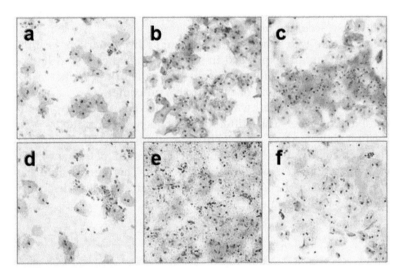

FIGURE 23.9 **sTBI biomarkers in saliva.** Digital sandwich IHC assay of whole saliva collected at admission. Biomarker signal was visualized using red label. (A–C) sB7 (Group 1, increased in unfavorable outcome). (D–E) sB1 (Group 2, increased in favorable outcome). (A and D) control ED patient with a general complaint without head injury. (B and E) sTBI patient with favorable outcome. (C and F) sTBI patient with unfavorable outcome. Original magnification × 400.

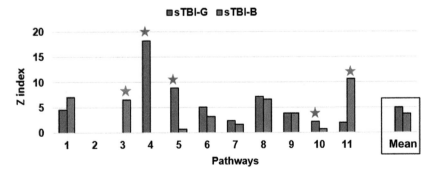

FIGURE 23.10   **Differences in pathway signatures of sTBI patients with favorable and unfavorable outcome.** Six-month global outcome, favorable (sTBI-G) or unfavorable (sTBI-B). Z index, a quantitative indicator of pathway activation calculated from admission saliva sample. Raw pathway profiles. The star indicates pathways that are significantly different between patients with favorable vs. unfavorable outcome. Pathways: 1, oxidative stress; 2, detoxification; 3, chaperoning; 4, DNA; 5, cell adhesion; 6, cell cycle; 7, apoptosis; 8, neuroendocrine signaling; 9, immunity; 10, microbiome; 11, osmotic stress. Associations between SRP biomarkers and pathways are shown in Table 23.1.

between the three groups (Kruskal—Wallis rank sum test, $P < .001$), see Fig. 23.8A. Median differences in biomarker levels between TBI patients with favorable (GOS-E 5—8) versus unfavorable (GOS-E 1—3) 6-month outcome were compared using Wilcoxon rank sum test. The difference between the outcome groups was significant ($P < .05$, see P values in the box plot). ROC analysis of the 16 biomarkers identified $N = 8$ candidate biomarkers with $\geq 80\%$ diagnostic and prognostic accuracy for sTBI and demonstrated the feasibility of using a composite biomarker (two biomarkers) to accurately predict sTBI outcome, see Table 23.4.

The candidate sTBI biomarkers formed two groups based on the correlation with outcome. Group 1 (sB2, sB3, sB4, sB5, sB7) had higher level in sTBI with unfavorable outcome (6m GOS-E score 1-3. Group 2 (sB1, sB6, sB8) had higher level in sTBI with favorable outcome (6m GOS-E score 5-8). This complementary trait makes groups 1 and 2 valuable as independent predictors that increase accuracy of sTBI prognostics.

The saliva expression pattern of the two groups of candidate sTBI biomarkers is illustrated in Fig. 23.9. The sTBI biomarkers are expressed in saliva epithelial cells and leukocytes. In acute sTBI, the biomarker expression in saliva cells and saliva fluid is increased, and the expression level correlates with favorable or unfavorable outcome.

Fig. 23.10 shows differences in the saliva pathway signature detected in sTBI patients with favorable and unfavorable outcome. The difference between these patients was detected already during the first days 3 days after sTBI (the admission saliva sample). This suggests an early difference in the molecular mechanism of sTBI pathogenesis in patients progressing toward unfavorable versus favorable outcome. This new insight has the potential to offer early prognostics for the individual patient, and aid in the discovery of new therapeutics for improving sTBI outcome.

23.8 Conclusions

Saliva shows a strong promise for biomarkers of TBI based on new methods for saliva handling, analysis, and biomarker discovery. These methodological advances identified new candidate biomarkers of mTBI and sTBI, and showed the feasibility of their use for diagnostics of acute mTBI and PCS, and prognostics of sTBI. If successfully validated, saliva biomarkers of TBI will break new ground by improving clinical management of TBI and advancing TBI treatments.

Future directions

The next steps in the development of saliva biomarkers for TBI comprise a rigorous clinical and analytical validation of the newly identified candidate biomarkers for mTBI diagnostics, PCS diagnostics and sTBI prognostics based on FDA guidelines. Qualified biomarkers will be translated into commercial RDTs for use in POC, sports and self-testing at home.

References

[1] McKinlay A, et al. An investigation of the pre-injury risk factors associated with children who experience traumatic brain injury. Inj Prev 2010;16:31–5. Available from: https://doi.org/10.1136/ip.2009.022483.

[2] Centers for Disease Control and Prevention. Report to congress on traumatic brain injury in the United States: epidemiology and rehabilitation. Atlanta, GA: National Center for Injury Prevention and Control; Division of Unintentional Injury Prevention; 2015.

[3] Centers for Disease Control. Traumatic brain injury in the United States: a report to Congress. Atlanta, GA: Centers for Disease Control and Prevention; 1999.

[4] Daneshvar DH, Goldstein LE, Kiernan PT, Stein TD, McKee AC. Post-traumatic neurodegeneration and chronic traumatic encephalopathy. Mol Cell Neurosci 2015;66:81–90. Available from: https://doi.org/10.1016/j.mcn.2015.03.007.

[5] Davis GA, et al. What is the difference in concussion management in children as compared with adults? A systematic review. Br J Sports Med 2017; bjsports-2016–097415.

[6] Bazarian JJ, et al. Mild traumatic brain injury in the United States, 1998–2000. Brain Inj 2005;19:85–91.

[7] Faul M, Xu L, Wald MM, Coronado VG. Traumatic brain injury in the United States: emergency department visits, hospitalizations and deaths 2002–2006. Atlanta, GA: Centers for Disease Control and Prevention, National Center for Injury Prevention and Control; 2010.

[8] Lumba-Brown A, Yeates KO, Sarmiento K, et al. Centers for Disease Control and Prevention Guideline on the Diagnosis and Management of Mild Traumatic Brain Injury Among Children JAMA Pediatr. 2018;172 (11):e182853. https://doi.org/10.1001/jamapediatrics.2018.2853.

[9] Kirkwood MW, et al. Management of pediatric mild traumatic brain injury: a neuropsychological review from injury through recovery. Clin Neuropsychol 2008;22:769–800. Available from: https://doi.org/10.1080/13854040701543700.

[10] McMahon P, et al. Symptomatology and functional outcome in mild traumatic brain injury: results from the prospective TRACK-TBI study. J Neurotrauma 2014;31:26–33. Available from: https://doi.org/10.1089/neu.2013.2984.

[11] Yeates KO, et al. Advancing concussion assessment in pediatrics (A-CAP): a prospective, concurrent cohort, longitudinal study of mild traumatic brain injury in children: protocol study. BMJ Open 2017;7:e017012. Available from: https://doi.org/10.1136/bmjopen-2017-017012.

[12] Levin HS, Diaz-Arrastia RR. Diagnosis, prognosis, and clinical management of mild traumatic brain injury. Lancet Neurol 2015;14:506–17. Available from: https://doi.org/10.1016/s1474-4422(15)00002-2.

[13] Adams JW, et al. Lewy body pathology and chronic traumatic encephalopathy associated with contact sports. J Neuropathol Exp Neurol 2018;77:757–68. Available from: https://doi.org/10.1093/jnen/nly065.

[14] Stern RA, et al. Long-term consequences of repetitive brain trauma: chronic traumatic encephalopathy. PM R 2011;3:S460–7. Available from: https://doi.org/10.1016/j.pmrj.2011.08.008.

[15] Dean PJ, O'Neill D, Sterr A. Post-concussion syndrome: prevalence after mild traumatic brain injury in comparison with a sample without head injury. Brain Inj 2011. Available from: https://doi.org/10.3109/02699052.2011.635354.

[16] Halbauer JD, et al. Neuropsychiatric diagnosis and management of chronic sequelae of war-related mild to moderate traumatic brain injury. J Rehab Res Dev 2009;46:757–96.

[17] Hung R, et al. Systematic review of the clinical course, natural history, and prognosis for pediatric mild traumatic brain injury: results of the International Collaboration on Mild Traumatic Brain Injury Prognosis. Arch Phys Med Rehabil 2014;95:S174–91. Available from: https://doi.org/10.1016/j.apmr.2013.08.301.

[18] King N, Crawford S, Wenden F, Moss N, Wade D. The rivermead post concussion symptoms questionnaire: a measure of symptoms commonly experienced after head injury and its reliability. J Neurol 1995;242:587–92.

[19] King NS, Kirwilliam S. Permanent post-concussion symptoms after mild head injury. Brain Inj 2011;25:462–70. Available from: https://doi.org/10.3109/02699052.2011.558042.

[20] The diagnostic and statistical manual of mental disorders. 5th ed American Psychiatric Association. American Psychiatric Publishing; 2013.

[21] Ganguli M, et al. Classification of neurocognitive disorders in DSM-5: a work in progress. Am J Geriatr Psychiat 2011;19:205–10.

[22] Sachdev PS, et al. Classifying neurocognitive disorders: the DSM-5 approach. Nat Rev Neurol 2014;10:634–42. Available from: https://doi.org/10.1038/nrneurol.2014.181.

[23] Lauterbach MD, Notarangelo PL, Nichols SJ, Lane KS, Koliatsos VE. Diagnostic and treatment challenges in traumatic brain injury patients with severe neuropsychiatric symptoms: insights into psychiatric practice. Neuropsychiat Dis Treat 2015;11:1601–7. Available from: https://doi.org/10.2147/NDT.S80457.

[24] Polinder S, et al. A multidimensional approach to post-concussion symptoms in mild traumatic brain injury. Front Neurol 2018;9. Available from: https://doi.org/10.3389/fneur.2018.01113.

[25] Cnossen MC, et al. Development of a prediction model for post-concussive symptoms following mild traumatic brain injury: a TRACK-TBI pilot study. J Neurotrauma 2017;34:2396–409. Available from: https://doi.org/10.1089/neu.2016.4819.

[26] Rao V, Koliatsos V, Ahmed F, Lyketsos C, Kortte K. Neuropsychiatric disturbances associated with traumatic brain injury: a practical approach to evaluation and management. SemNeurol 2015;35:64–82. Available from: https://doi.org/10.1055/s-0035-1544241.

[27] Willis AM, Williams JP, Sladkey JH, McClean JC. Management of mild traumatic brain injury, <http://www.psychiatrictimes.com/special-reports/management-mild-traumatic-brain-injury>; 2015.

[28] Cancelliere C, et al. Systematic search and review procedures: results of the International Collaboration on Mild Traumatic Brain Injury Prognosis. Arch Phys Med Rehabil 2014;95:S101–31. Available from: https://doi.org/10.1016/j.apmr.2013.12.001.

[29] Cancelliere C, et al. Systematic review of return to work after mild traumatic brain injury: results of the International Collaboration on Mild Traumatic Brain Injury Prognosis. Arch Phys Med Rehabil 2014;95:S201–9. Available from: https://doi.org/10.1016/j.apmr.2013.10.010.

[30] Cassidy JD, et al. Systematic review of self-reported prognosis in adults after mild traumatic brain injury: results of the International Collaboration on Mild Traumatic Brain Injury Prognosis. Arch Phys Med Rehabil 2014;95:S132–51. Available from: https://doi.org/10.1016/j.apmr.2013.08.299.

[31] Balu R. Inflammation and immune system activation after traumatic brain injury. Curr Neurol Neurosci Rep 2014;14:484. Available from: https://doi.org/10.1007/s11910-014-0484-2.

[32] Max JE, et al. Anxiety disorders in children and adolescents in the second six months after traumatic brain injury. J Pediat Rehab Med 2015;8:345–55. Available from: https://doi.org/10.3233/prm-150352.

[33] Max JE, et al. Psychiatric disorders in children and adolescents in the first six months after mild traumatic brain injury. J Neuropsychiat Clin Neurosci 2013;25:187–97. Available from: https://doi.org/10.1176/appi.neuropsych.12010011.

[34] Eastman A, Chang D. Return to learn: a review of cognitive rest versus rehabilitation after sports concussion, 2015;37(2), 235-44.

[35] Keightley ML, et al. Psychosocial consequences of mild traumatic brain injury in children: results of a systematic review by the International Collaboration on Mild Traumatic Brain Injury Prognosis. Arch Phys Med Rehabil 2014;95:S192–200. Available from: https://doi.org/10.1016/j.apmr.2013.12.018.

[36] Wade SL, et al. Problem-solving after traumatic brain injury in adolescence: associations with functional outcomes. Arch Phys Med Rehabil 2017;98:1614–21. Available from: https://doi.org/10.1016/j.apmr.2017.03.006.

[37] Wojcik BE, Akhtar FZ, Hassell LH. Hospital admissions related to mental disorders in U.S. Army soldiers in Iraq and Afghanistan. Mil Med 2009;174:1010–18.

[38] Wojcik BE, Stein CR, Bagg K, Humphrey RJ, Orosco J. Traumatic brain injury hospitalizations of U.S. army soldiers deployed to Afghanistan and Iraq. Am J Prev Med 2010;38:S108–16. Available from: https://doi.org/10.1016/j.amepre.2009.10.006.

[39] Eaton KM, et al. Prevalence of mental health problems, treatment need, and barriers to care among primary care-seeking spouses of military service members involved in Iraq and Afghanistan deployments. Mil Med 2008;173:1051–6.

[40] Hoge CW. Deployment to the Iraq war and neuropsychological sequelae. JAMA 2006;296:2678–9 author reply 2679–2680.

[41] Hoge CW. Suicide reduction and research efforts in service members and veterans-sobering realities. JAMA Psychiatry 2019. Available from: https://doi.org/10.1001/jamapsychiatry.2018.4564.

[42] Hoge CW, et al. Mild traumatic brain injury in U.S. Soldiers returning from Iraq. N Engl J Med 2008;358:453–63.

[43] Hoge CW, Warner CH, Castro CA. Mental health and the army. JAMA Psychiatry 2014;71:965−6. Available from: https://doi.org/10.1001/jamapsychiatry.2014.689.

[44] Vasterling JJ, et al. PTSD symptom increases in Iraq-deployed soldiers: comparison with nondeployed soldiers and associations with baseline symptoms, deployment experiences, and postdeployment stress. J Trauma Stress 2010;23:41−51.

[45] Schwab K, et al. Epidemiology and prognosis of mild traumatic brain injury in returning soldiers: a cohort study. Neurology 2017;88:1571−9. Available from: https://doi.org/10.1212/wnl.0000000000003839.

[46] Boyle E, et al. Systematic review of prognosis after mild traumatic brain injury in the military: results of the International Collaboration on Mild Traumatic Brain Injury Prognosis. Arch Phys Med Rehabil 2014;95: S230−7. Available from: https://doi.org/10.1016/j.apmr.2013.08.297.

[47] Lingsma HF, et al. Outcome prediction after mild and complicated mild traumatic brain injury: external validation of existing models and identification of new predictors using the TRACK-TBI pilot study. J Neurotrauma 2015;32:83−94. Available from: https://doi.org/10.1089/neu.2014.3384.

[48] Harmon KG, et al. American medical society for sports medicine position statement: concussion in sport. Br J Sports Med 2013;47:15−26. Available from: https://doi.org/10.1136/bjsports-2012-091941.

[49] Howell DR, et al. Identifying persistent postconcussion symptom risk in a pediatric sports medicine clinic. Am J Sports Med 2018;46:3254−61. Available from: https://doi.org/10.1177/0363546518796830.

[50] Iverson GL, et al. Factors associated with concussion-like symptom reporting in high school athletes. JAMA Pediatr 2015;169:1132−40. Available from: https://doi.org/10.1001/jamapediatrics.2015.2374.

[51] Karlin AM. Concussion in the pediatric and adolescent population: "Different Population, Different Concerns". PM R 2011;3:S369−79. Available from: https://doi.org/10.1016/j.pmrj.2011.07.015.

[52] McCrory P, et al. Consensus statement on concussion in sport—the 5th international conference on concussion in sport held in Berlin, October 2016. Br J Sports Med 2017.

[53] Davis GA, et al. The child sport concussion assessment tool 5th edition (child SCAT5): background and rationale. Br J Sports Med 2017;51:859.

[54] Echemendia RJ, et al. The sport concussion assessment tool 5th edition (SCAT5): background and rationale. Br J Sports Med 2017;51:848.

[55] McCrea M, et al. Role of advanced neuroimaging, fluid biomarkers and genetic testing in the assessment of sport-related concussion: a systematic review. Br J Sports Med 2017;51:919−29.

[56] Iverson GL. Misdiagnosis of the persistent postconcussion syndrome in patients with depression. Arch Clin Neuropsychol 2006;21:303−10. Available from: https://doi.org/10.1016/j.acn.2005.12.008.

[57] Wang Y, Chan RC, Deng Y. Examination of postconcussion-like symptoms in healthy university students: relationships to subjective and objective neuropsychological function performance. Arch Clin Neuropsychol 2006;21:339−47. Available from: https://doi.org/10.1016/j.acn.2006.03.006.

[58] Gaudet L, et al. P057: diagnosis for mild traumatic brain injury in three Canadian emergency departments: missed opportunities. CJEM 2017;19. Available from: https://doi.org/10.1017/cem.2017.259 S97-S97.

[59] Jagoda AS, et al. Clinical policy: neuroimaging and decisionmaking in adult mild traumatic brain injury in the acute setting. J Emerg Nurs 2009;35:e5−e40. Available from: https://doi.org/10.1016/j.jen.2008.12.010.

[60] Diaz-Arrastia R, et al. Acute biomarkers of traumatic brain injury: relationship between plasma levels of ubiquitin C-terminal hydrolase-L1 and glial fibrillary acidic protein. J Neurotrauma 2014;31:19−25. Available from: https://doi.org/10.1089/neu.2013.3040.

[61] Papa L, et al. Time course and diagnostic accuracy of glial and neuronal blood biomarkers GFAP and UCH-L1 in a large cohort of trauma patients with and without mild traumatic brain injury. JAMA Neurol 2016;73:551−60. Available from: https://doi.org/10.1001/jamaneurol.2016.0039.

[62] Welch RD, et al. Modeling the kinetics of serum glial fibrillary acidic protein, ubiquitin carboxyl-terminal hydrolase-L1, and S100B concentrations in patients with traumatic brain injury. J Neurotrauma 2017;34:1957−71. Available from: https://doi.org/10.1089/neu.2016.4772.

[63] Di Battista AP, et al. Blood biomarkers in moderate-to-severe traumatic brain injury: potential utility of a multi-marker approach in characterizing outcome. Front Neurol 2015;6:110. Available from: https://doi.org/10.3389/fneur.2015.00110.

[64] Albayram O, et al. Cis P-tau is induced in clinical and preclinical brain injury and contributes to post-injury sequelae. Nat Commun 2017;8:1000. Available from: https://doi.org/10.1038/s41467-017-01068-4.

VII. Non-Blood TBI biomarker strategy

[65] Rubenstein R, et al. Comparing plasma phospho tau, total tau, and phospho tau-total tau ratio as acute and chronic traumatic brain injury biomarkers. JAMA Neurol 2017;74:1063−72. Available from: https://doi.org/10.1001/jamaneurol.2017.0655.

[66] Wallisch JS, et al. Cerebrospinal fluid NLRP3 is increased after severe traumatic brain injury in infants and children. Neurocritic Care 2017;27:44−50. Available from: https://doi.org/10.1007/s12028-017-0378-7.

[67] Wang KK, et al. Plasma anti-glial fibrillary acidic protein autoantibody levels during the acute and chronic phases of traumatic brain injury: a transforming research and clinical knowledge in traumatic brain injury pilot study. J Neurotrauma 2016;33:1270−7. Available from: https://doi.org/10.1089/neu.2015.3881.

[68] Ji W, Jiao J, Cheng C, Shao J. MicroRNA-21 in the pathogenesis of traumatic brain injury. Neurochem Res 2018. Available from: https://doi.org/10.1007/s11064-018-2602-z.

[69] Hicks SD, et al. Overlapping microRNA expression in saliva and cerebrospinal fluid accurately identifies pediatric traumatic brain injury. J Neurotrauma 2018;35:64−72. Available from: https://doi.org/10.1089/neu.2017.5111.

[70] Pan Y-B, Sun Z-L, Feng D-F. The role of microRNA in traumatic brain injury. Neuroscience 2017;367:189−99. Available from: https://doi.org/10.1016/j.neuroscience.2017.10.046.

[71] Martinez B, Peplow P. MicroRNAs as diagnostic markers and therapeutic targets for traumatic brain injury. Neural Regen Res 2017;12:1749−61. Available from: https://doi.org/10.4103/1673-5374.219025.

[72] Glinge C, et al. Stability of circulating blood-based microRNAs—pre-analytic methodological considerations. PLoS One 2017;12:e0167969.

[73] Bell MJ, Adelson PD, Wisniewski SR. Challenges and opportunities for pediatric severe TBI-review of the evidence and exploring a way forward. Childs Nerv Syst 2017;33:1663−7. Available from: https://doi.org/10.1007/s00381-017-3530-y.

[74] Maas AIR, et al. Traumatic brain injury: integrated approaches to improve prevention, clinical care, and research. Lancet Neurol 2017;16:987−1048. Available from: https://doi.org/10.1016/s1474-4422(17)30371-x.

[75] Bell MJ, Kochanek PM. Traumatic brain injury in children: recent advances in management. Indian J Pediat 2008;75:1159−65. Available from: https://doi.org/10.1007/s12098-008-0240-1.

[76] Kochanek PM, et al. The potential for bio-mediators and biomarkers in pediatric traumatic brain injury and neurocritical care. Front Neurol 2013;4:40. Available from: https://doi.org/10.3389/fneur.2013.00040.

[77] Sarnaik A, et al. Age and mortality in pediatric severe traumatic brain injury: results from an international study. Neurocrit Care 2018. Available from: https://doi.org/10.1007/s12028-017-0480-x.

[78] Adams SM, et al. ABCG2 c.421 C > A is associated with outcomes after severe traumatic brain injury. J Neurotrauma 2018;35:48−53. Available from: https://doi.org/10.1089/neu.2017.5000.

[79] Korley FK, et al. Circulating brain-derived neurotrophic factor has diagnostic and prognostic value in traumatic brain injury. J Neurotrauma 2016;33:215−25. Available from: https://doi.org/10.1089/neu.2015.3949.

[80] McMahon PJ, et al. Measurement of the glial fibrillary acidic protein and its breakdown products GFAP-BDP biomarker for the detection of traumatic brain injury compared to computed tomography and magnetic resonance imaging. J Neurotrauma 2015;32:527−33. Available from: https://doi.org/10.1089/neu.2014.3635.

[81] Nwachuku EL, et al. Time course of cerebrospinal fluid inflammatory biomarkers and relationship to 6-month neurologic outcome in adult severe traumatic brain injury. Clin Neurol Neurosurg 2016;149:1−5. Available from: https://doi.org/10.1016/j.clineuro.2016.06.009.

[82] Au AK, et al. Autophagy biomarkers beclin 1 and p62 are increased in cerebrospinal fluid after traumatic brain injury. Neurocrit Care 2017;26:348−55. Available from: https://doi.org/10.1007/s12028-016-0351-x.

[83] Au AK, et al. Cerebrospinal fluid levels of high-mobility group box 1 and cytochrome C predict outcome after pediatric traumatic brain injury. J Neurotrauma 2012;29:2013−21. Available from: https://doi.org/10.1089/neu.2011.2171.

[84] Au AK, et al. Brain-specific serum biomarkers predict neurological morbidity in diagnostically diverse pediatric intensive care unit patients. Neurocrit Care 2018;28:26−34. Available from: https://doi.org/10.1007/s12028-017-0414-7.

[85] Southern SO. Health test for a broad spectrum of health problems. US Patent No. 10,317,416 (Issued June 11, 2019); 2019.

[86] Southern SO. Health test for a broad spectrum of health problems. European Patent EP 2 660 596 B1, EPO Application No. 13 165 830.4 (Issued November 30, 2018); 2018.

[87] Southern SO. Health test for a broad spectrum of health problems. US Patent No. 9,874,573 (Issued January 18, 2018); 2018.

[88] Southern SO. Health test for a broad spectrum of health problems. US Patent No. 9,176,149 (Issued November 3, 2015); 2015.

[89] Southern SO. Health test for a broad spectrum of health problems. US Patent No. 8,771,962 (Issued July 8, 2014); 2014.

[90] Southern SO. Systems and methods for analyzing persistent homeostatic perturbations. US Patent No. 8,518,649 (Issued August 27, 2013); 2013.

[91] Andrews AM, Lutton EM, Merkel SF, Razmpour R, Ramirez SH. Mechanical injury induces brain endothelial-derived microvesicle release: implications for cerebral vascular injury during traumatic brain injury. Front Cell Neurosci 2016;10:43. Available from: https://doi.org/10.3389/fncel.2016.00043.

[92] van der Vos KE, Balaj L, Skog J, Breakefield XO. Brain tumor microvesicles: insights into intercellular communication in the nervous system. Cell Mol Neurobiol 2011;31:949–59. Available from: https://doi.org/10.1007/s10571-011-9697-y.

[93] Zhang Y, et al. Effect of exosomes derived from multipluripotent mesenchymal stromal cells on functional recovery and neurovascular plasticity in rats after traumatic brain injury. J Neurosurg 2015;122:856–67. Available from: https://doi.org/10.3171/2014.11.jns14770.

[94] Levy E. Exosomes in the diseased brain: first insights from in vivo studies. Front Neurosci 2017;11:142. Available from: https://doi.org/10.3389/fnins.2017.00142.

[95] Sundman MH, Chen NK, Subbian V, Chou YH. The bidirectional gut-brain-microbiota axis as a potential nexus between traumatic brain injury, inflammation, and disease. Brain Behav Immun. 2017;66:31–44.

[96] Nicholson SE, Watts LT, Burmeister DM, et al. Moderate Traumatic Brain Injury Alters the Gastrointestinal Microbiome in a Time-Dependent Manner. Shock. 2019;52(2):240–248.

[97] Urban RJ, Pyles RB, Stewart CJ, Ajami N, Randolph KM, Durham WJ, et al. Altered Fecal Microbiome Years after Traumatic Brain Injury. J Neurotrauma. 2020;37(8):1037–1051. doi: https://doi.org/10.1089/neu.2019.6688. Epub 2020 Jan 17.

[98] Burg MB, Ferraris JD, Dmitrieva NI. Cellular response to hyperosmotic stresses. Physiol Rev. 2007;87(4):1441–1474. doi: https://doi.org/10.1152/physrev.00056.2006.

[99] Chiappin S, Antonelli G, Gatti R, De Palo EF. Saliva specimen: a new laboratory tool for diagnostic and basic investigation. Clin Chim Acta 2007;383:30–40.

[100] Malamud D. Saliva as a diagnostic fluid. BMJ 1992;305:207–8.

[101] Malamud D. Saliva as a diagnostic fluid. Dent Clin North Am 2011;55:159–78. Available from: https://doi.org/10.1016/j.cden.2010.08.004.

[102] Miller CS, et al. Current developments in salivary diagnostics. Biomark Med 2010;4:171–89.

[103] Streckfus CF, Bigler LR. Saliva as a diagnostic fluid. Oral Dis 2002;8:69–76.

[104] Yan W, et al. Systematic comparison of the human saliva and plasma proteomes. Proteom Clin Appl 2009;3:116–34. Available from: https://doi.org/10.1002/prca.200800140.

[105] Southern S., Southern P. (2002) Cellular Mechanism for Milk-Borne Transmission of HIV and HTLV. In: Davis M.K., Isaacs C.E., Hanson L.Å., Wright A.L. (eds) Integrating Population Outcomes, Biological Mechanisms and Research Methods in the Study of Human Milk and Lactation. Advances in Experimental Medicine and Biology, vol 503. Springer, Boston, MA.

[106] Southern SO. Milk-borne transmission of HIV. Characterization of productively infected cells in breast milk and interactions between milk and saliva. J Hum Virol 1998;1:328–37.

[107] Southern SO. Saliva proteomics of human dehydration. Final Technical Report. US Army Research Institute of Environmental Medicine Contract No: W911QY09P0333 2009.

[108] Oppenheim FG, Salih E, Siqueira WL, Zhang W, Helmerhorst EJ. Salivary proteome and its genetic polymorphisms. Ann N Y Acad Sci 2007;1098:22–50. Available from: https://doi.org/10.1196/annals.1384.030.

[109] Helmerhorst EJ, Zamakhchari M, Schuppan D, Oppenheim FG. Discovery of a novel and rich source of gluten-degrading microbial enzymes in the oral cavity. PLOS One 5 2010;e13264. Available from: https://doi.org/10.1371/journal.pone.0013264.

[110] Walt DR, et al. Microsensor arrays for saliva diagnostics. Ann N Y Acad Sci 2007;1098:389–400. Available from: https://doi.org/10.1196/annals.1384.031.

[111] Jennett B, Snoek J, Bond MR, Brooks N. Disability after severe head injury: observations on the use of the Glasgow Outcome Scale. J Neurol Neurosurg Psychiatry 1981;44:285–93. Available from: https://doi.org/10.1136/jnnp.44.4.285.

Digital neurocognitive testing

Karina M. Soto-Ruiz, MD

Comprehensive Research Associates, Houston, TX, United States

Clinicians have utilized neurocognitive testing across a wide variety of pathologies for several decades. They have traditionally been performed by trained staff utilizing no more than pen and paper while interacting with the patient. Through ample research, some assessments have come to be regarded as globally accepted gold standards that can identify or detect a deficit or impairment after head injuries.

Cognitive function evaluation is oftentimes broken down into cognitive domains, some of them being the following:

- Instant verbal memory (VBM)
- Delayed VBM
- Attention
- Focus
- Impulse control
- Spatial memory
- Emotional identification
- Information processing
- Processing speed
- Working memory
- Executive function
- Flexible thinking

Technology has slowly but surely found its way into neurocognitive testing with several research institutes around the globe undertaking the task of adapting and transforming existing tests into digital platforms, which are gaining widespread acceptance across the medical field [1].

Traditional neurocognitive (also known as neuropsychological) testing standards are defined by the American Academy of Clinical Neuropsychology and the National Academy of Neuropsychology. These organizations released a position paper with recommendations on appropriate standards and conventions for computerized neuropsychological assessment devices [2]. The position paper includes standards for the psychometric development issues, especially with regards to reliability and validity. They included the need for device makers to be clear on their labeling and claims to include how a normative database (if applicable) was obtained, the intended patient population on which the device was tested, and who can administer the test.

The administration of these test digitally:

Advantages
- It can reduce total test administration time allowing the clinician more time to discuss results and next steps with the patients.
- It could be administered by nonspecialist staff, allowing the clinician to focus on other aspects of patient care.
- Provides a more precise measure of time-dependent tasks.
- By automating test interpretation and scoring; it removes the potential for human error and rater-specific variance.
- It eliminates administrator bias.
- Maximizes data accuracy.
- They are less expensive.
- Can be administered simultaneously, making them practical in group-sports settings.
- Provides information instantly
- The time reduction and process automation can also help streamline clinical research studies, allowing neurocognitive assessments and follow-ups to be done in a timely and cost-effective manner by decreasing the amount of time and resources allocated to neurocognitive assessments.

Disadvantages
- Internet connectivity might be necessary, limiting where tests can be administered.
- Data transmitted electronically requires specific security measures and is vulnerable.
- Infrastructure, and sometimes, special equipment is needed, this can incur additional costs and also limit the areas where tests can be administered as well as the administration logistics (i.e., can only do one test at a time instead of multiple).

Reliability is an issue for most tests and becomes increasingly relevant with computerized neurocognitive testing for concussion due to the potential for serial administration. This has led to an increased relevance of the *reliable change index* (RCI), which estimates the magnitude of differences in scores necessary to suggest a true change. Ideally, an athletes' score shouldn't change between testing periods if no injury occurred; yet this occurs on most of the available tests [3].

Software is considered Software as a Medical Device (SaMD), if it meets the definition of the International Medical Device Regulators Forum (IMDRF), which states "software intended to be used for one or more medical purposes that perform these purposes without being part of a hardware medical device" [4].

They are overseen and regulated by the Food and Drug Administration (FDA) and will be subjected to premarketing and postmarketing regulatory controls if they are labeled, promoted, or used in a manner set forth in the Federal Food Drug & Cosmetic (FD&C) Act as "intended for use in the diagnosis of disease or other conditions, or in the cure, mitigation, treatment, or prevention of disease, in man or other animals" [5].

Any software or program that advertises or claims to be a digital or computerized neurocognitive test would fall under one of the definitions previously mentioned.

Digital cognitive tests available (in alphabetical order):

ANAM—the automated neuropsychological assessment metrics

www.vistalifesciences.com/anam-intro

This is a library of computer-based tests that were initially developed in the 1980s and 1990s through the Department of Defense. It has been used both for research and in clinical use by the military and prestigious institutions, such as NASA and the FAA. It currently includes 22 tests that can be grouped into flexible or standardized batteries, with a broad spectrum of applications [6]:

- Two-choice reaction time (RTI)
- Code substitution—learning, immediate or delayed
- Demographics/history module
- Effort measure
- Go/No-Go
- Grammatical reasoning
- Logical relations—symbolic
- Manikin
- Matching grids
- Matching to sample
- Math processing
- Memory search
- Mood scale
- Posttraumatic stress assessment
- Procedural RTI
- Pursuit tracking
- Running memory continuous performance test (CPT)
- Simple RTI
- Sleep scale
- Spatial processing—sequential and simultaneous
- Standard continuous performance task
- Stroop
- Symptoms scale
- Switching
- Tapping
- Tower puzzle

With such a modular, customizable test, despite the hundreds of research articles published, it is challenging to know what set of tests were used for a particular study. This makes reproducibility, sensitivity, and specificity hard to pinpoint. They do state it takes an average of 20–25 minutes to complete and it can be administered on a laptop or desktop computer with a MS Windows operating system and a USB-connected mouse. It has been described, depending on the tests used a sensitivity that ranges from 6% to 23.8% within 24 hours of injury [7]. Finally, there is an ANAM—Sports medicine battery (ASMB) developed and validated to be used for patients with head injuries from contact sports [8].

BrainCheck Inc

www.braincheck.com

BrainCheck is the result of 20 years of research conducted at the Eagleman Laboratory for Perception and Action at Baylor College of Medicine, where they turned gold-standard cognitive tests into interactive mobile games. It is registered with the FDA as a class II medical device. It can be done on an iPad, iPhone, or desktop computer, takes on average 10 minutes to complete and can compare patient's results to their individual baseline if available and to a normative population database of >40,000 controls with an age range of 10—99 years [9].

They have two products:

1. BrainCheck memory—created for seniors; and
2. BrainCheck Sport—created to evaluate several aspects of mild traumatic brain injury (mTBI).

The tests on BrainCheck sport are:

- Coordination test
- It measures a patient's static and dynamic balance. The patient holds the tablet out in front at arm's length and tilts it as appropriate. This test requires the use of an iPad or iPhone.
- Digit symbol substitution
- Flanker test
- Stroop effect
- Trails making A and B
- Immediate and delayed recall

The cognitive domains measured are:

- Processing speed and accuracy
- Stimuli response
- Impulse control
- RTI
- Measuring of cognitive inhibition
- Visual search speed
- Mental flexibility
- Executive function
- Immediate and delayed recall

A composite score is created to discriminate patients with traumatic brain injury while minimizing false positives. This metric provided a sensitivity of 83% and specificity of 87% [10].

Cambridge Neuropsychological Test Automated Battery

www.cambridgecognition.com

Originally developed at the University of Cambridge, it has been used in clinical trials for over 15 years. There are several batteries fine-tuned for a wide variety of pathologies. For head injury research, they have a battery with the following tests [11]:

- Paired associated learning (PAL)
- RTI
- Spatial working memory (SWM)
- Multitasking test (MTT)
- One touch stockings of Cambridge (OTS)

They evaluate the following domains:

- Episodic memory
- Executive function
- Processing speed
- Multitasking and planning

It takes about 33 minutes to complete. It can be administered without the need of an internet connection [12]. The CANTAB research suite contains a normative database from healthy individuals aged 4–90 years and spans four different estimated IQ bands. It is built into the software for some but not all tests, allowing researchers to accurately calculate standardized scores from subjects' raw test scores.

CNS–Vital signs

www.cnsvs.com

This is an in-office neurocognitive test that assesses a broad spectrum of brain function with over 50 computerized clinical and quality rating instruments. It was created to establish baseline and then longitudinally track patients [13].

Their core test is called CNS-VS BRIEF CORE, it consists of seven subtests:

- VBM
- Visual memory (VIM)
- Finger tapping (FFT)
- Symbol digit coding (SDC)
- Stroop test (ST)
- Shifting attention test (SAT)
- CPT.
- They evaluate the following domains:
- Composite memory
- VBM
- VIM
- Executive function
- Processing speed
- Psychomotor speed
- RTI
- Complex attention
- Cognitive flexibility
- Simple visual attention
- Motor speed.

VII. Non-blood TBI biomarker strategy

These tests were normalized with a sample size of 1662 controls from ages 8 to 89. Normal was defined as individuals with no active medical conditions, no history of neurological or psychiatric disorders, and not on any psychotropic medications.

There is also an extended version developed for brain and behavioral specialists that includes the following tests:

- Test for perception of emotions (POET);
- Nonverbal reasoning (NVRT); and
- Four-part CPT (FPCPT).
- They evaluate:Social acuity, reasoning, sustained attention, and working memory.

CNS also has the VSX—TBI—concussion toolbox/test to assess patients after a head injury. This includes the neurocognitive test and rating scales that can be used to help track symptoms and behavior longitudinally.

It's performed on a laptop or desktop computer via a web-based software application. To administer, a computer, monitor, and keyboard are needed. They also offer a special keyboard, that while it's not necessary it is suggested that it might make testing a better experience for patients [14]. A medical office assistant can initiate the test, and a child with a fourth-grade reading level can take the test battery unassisted [15].

Cogstate

www.cogstate.com

Founded in 1999 [16] in Australia, it is a company dedicated to measuring cognition to guide decision-making in clinical trials, research, and healthcare and brain injury, with sensitivity and specificity ranges of 69%—96.6%, and 86.9%—91.5% [17], respectively. It assesses several cognitive domains including:

- Memory
- Working memory,
- Delayed recall
- Executive function
- Attention and learning
- Verbal, visual, and PAL
- Emotional recognition
- Psychomotor function.

In July 2017 they received notification from the FDA that the cognitive assessment COGNIGRAM met the requirements necessary to market and commercially distribute in the United States as a Class II Exempt Medical Device.

The COGNIGRAM test, an abbreviated version, is self-administered and is intended to aid in measuring cognition in patients 6—99 years of age. It can be administered via iPad or computer, and takes an average of 12—15 minutes to complete [18].

A single study of their battery found 100% sensitivity to sport-related concussion, but only 50.8% specificity [17]. A different study found, within 24 hours of injury, a sensitivity of 60.3%, dropping to 20.8%—26.7% at 8 days postinjury [7].

C3Logix

www.c3logix.com

Developed at the Cleveland Clinic in Ohio, this test has several modules besides a neurocognitive component, which allows for a customizable, 15-minute, assessment tool. All modules are performed on an iPad and include:

1. The Graded Symptom Checklist; a standardized checklist that allows symptoms self-reporting on a 1–6 scale,
2. The Standard Assessment of Concussion (SAC); an industry assessment that is part of the SCAT3 tool for the assessment of concussion,
3. The Balancing Error Scoring System (BESS); which is done by securing the iPad to the patient's waist and uses its gyroscope and accelerometer calibrated to match the Natus NeuroCom Balance System to be able to record a subject's movements parameters by collecting biomechanical data to quantify postural stability.
   - The iPad is secured to a belt provided by the company.
4. It assesses visual acuity by utilizing a Snellen Eye Chart from 40 in. or 1 m [19].

The cognitive domains of the neurocognitive component are:

- Cognitive process speed
- Working memory and focus
- Fine motor movement
- Planning
- Sequencing
- Set-shifting

Research has suggested their multimodal approach to assessing patients after head injuries could be effective [20,21].

Defense Automated Neurobehavioral Assessment
www.danabrainvital.com

The DANA software was developed by AnthroTronix, a company founded in 1999. It runs as a mobile application on Android and iOS devices, they include cognitive and psychological test batteries [22,23].

They have three configurations [24,25]:

1. DANA Brain Vital [24] is an FDA-cleared, 5-minute outcome measure designed to provide information on cognitive efficiency. It consists of three tests:
   a. Simple RTI, procedural RTI, and go/no go
   b. The cognitive domains evaluated are:
      i. Pure RTI
      ii. Executive function
      iii. Sustained attention
      iv. Impulsivity
2. DANA Standard is a 25-minute test (on average), that can be used as a follow up to DANA Brain Vital. It consists of cognitive tests and psychological surveys including a standard test battery that has been validated with over 2000 individuals. The tests included are:
   a. Simple RTI
   b. Code substitution

c. Procedural RTI

d. Spatial processing

e. Go/no go

f. Matching to sample

g. Memory search (Stenberg)

h. Simple RTI a second time

i. Patient health questionnaire (PHQ8)

j. Insomnia severity index (ISI)

   The cognitive domains they evaluate are:

   i. Pure RTI

   ii. Visual scanning

   iii. Attention

   iv. Learning and immediate recall

   v. Executive function

   xvi. Visuospatial analytic ability

   xvii. Sustained attention and impulsivity

   xviii. Learning and short-term memory

   xix. Working memory

3. DANA Modular can be configured to include any combination of individual cognitive and psychological tests.

There is also a DANA version developed for the Department of Defense that is currently available only on Android devices.

Immediate Post-Concussion Assessment and Cognitive Testing

www.impacttest.com

Created in 2002, they released their first product called ImPACT. In August of 2016 they became the first concussion-specific medical device to receive FDA de novo clearance as a computerized cognitive assessment aid for concussion for both ImPACT and ImPACT pediatric. They recommend a baseline test to document the brain function of a patient, and if they suffer a head injury, administer the postinjury test to help guide treatment and next steps [26]. To administer a test, specific training is required and provided by the company.

In June 2017 they obtained FDA clearance for ImPACT Quick Test. According to their website, as of August 2018, over 16 million tests of ImPACT have been administered [26,27].

They have three tests:

1. ImPACT pediatric—for patients ages 5–11, it can be administered on a computer or laptop as long as the screen is at least 12 in. in size.
2. ImPACT—for patients 12–59 years of age, it can be administered on a computer or laptop as long as the screen is at least 12 in. in size.
3. ImPACT quick test—for patients ages 12–70. It is advertised as a "removal from activity" support tool that takes 5–7 minutes to complete, it doesn't replace ImPACT [26]. It includes an assessment of symptoms. It must be administered on an iPad, the screen must be at least 9 in. in size.

The cognitive domains they evaluate are:

- RTI
- Visual and VBM capacity
- Speed of mental processing
- Executive functions

There is ample research with this product and, depending on the publication, sensitivity ranges from 55% to 91.4%, while specificity ranges from 69.1% to 89.4% [28–30].

King-Devick
www.kingdevicktest.com
They have several products, all are administered on either an iPad or Android tablet or a laptop computer.

1. The K-D RAP King-Devick reading acceleration program—advertised as a learning tool for children.
2. The KDt King-Devick monitoring—for assessing and monitoring eye movement disorders.
3. The K-D Balance—has been FDA 510(k) cleared to assess vestibular dysfunction.
4. The King-Devick in association with Mayo Clinic—advertised as a sport sideline test after a potential head injury has occurred.

The King-Devick in association with Mayo Clinic, is a 2-minute rapid number naming assessment in which an individual quickly reads aloud single digit numbers and evaluates:

- Impairments of eye movements
- Attention
- Language function.

It does not use normative data, instead the subject is always compared to their personal baseline. Patients 10 years and younger must recheck their baselines every 6 months. Subjects over 10 years of age need to have their baselines reestablished annually.

It should take a patient older than 14 years of age less than 60 seconds to complete, it might take longer if reading disabilities are present or if there are learning disabilities and attention disorders, such as ADHD, which underscores the importance of recognizing individual performance [31].

With sensitivity and specificity documented to range from 86% to 90%, and 90% to 91%, respectively [32,33], special considerations must be made for patients with learning disabilities and attention disorders, such as ADHD, as slower performances by them have been reported [34].

Savonix
www.savonix.com
Created in 2014, this product delivers a set of digitized neurocognitive tests via Android and iOS mobile operating systems. It is supported by a web-based data dashboard and takes 30 minutes to complete. It was designed for touchscreens and tracks swipes, taps, draws, and scrolls. It takes 30 minutes to complete. They have data on over 4500 patients from the United States and Asia.

The cognitive domains they evaluate are:

- Instant VBM
- Delayed VBM
- Attention
- Focus
- Impulse control
- Spatial memory
- Emotion identification
- Information processing
- Working memory
- Executive function
- Flexible thinking.

According to their website they are preparing their results for publication [35].

There are ample options to choose from. It is important to consider the patient population to whom the tests would be administered, as well as the environment. These can include the sideline of a sports game, a clinician's outpatient office, or a hospital setting (e.g., an emergency department). It is important to find the best fit, both in terms of user friendliness for each of the patients and the staff administering the tests, as well as the physical space constraints applicable to the test. Finally, while accessing their platforms and administering these tests will incur an additional expense, it is worth noting that these procedures are reimbursed by some insurance companies.

References

[1] Harmon KG, Drezner JA, Gammons M. Endorsed by the National Trainers' Athletic Association and the American College of Sports Medicine, et al American Medical Society for Sports Medicine position statement: concussion in sport. Br J Sports Med 2013;47:15—26.

[2] Bauer RM, Iverson GL, Cernich AN, Binder LM, Ruff RM, Naugle RI. Computerized neuropsychological assessment devices: joint position paper of the American Academy of Clinical Neuropsychology and the National Academy of Neuropsychology. Arch Clin Neuropsychol 2012;27(3):362—73. Available from: https://doi.org/10.1093/arclin/acs027.

[3] Farnsworth II JL, Dargo L, Ragan BG, Kang M. Reliability of computerized neurocognitive tests for concussion assessment: a meta-analysis. J Athletic Train 2017;52(9):826—33.

[4] <http://www.imdrf.org/docs/imdrf/final/technical/imdrf-tech-131209-samd-key-definitions-140901.pdf>.

[5] <https://www.fda.gov/medical-devices/classify-your-medical-device/product-medical-device>.

[6] <http://vistalifesciences.com/anam-intro>.

[7] Nelson LD, LaRoche AA, Pfaller AY, et al. Prospective, head-to-head study of three computerized neurocognitive assessment tools (CNTs): reliability and validity for the assessment of sport-related concussion. J Int Neuropsychol Soc 2016;22(1):24—37. Available from: https://doi.org/10.1017/S1355617715001101.

[8] Cernich A, Reeves D, Sun W, Bleiberg J. Automated neuropsychological assessment metrics sports medicine battery. Arch Clin Neuropsychol 2007;22(Suppl_1):S101—14. Available from: https://doi.org/10.1016/j.acn.2006.10.008.

[9] <https://braincheck.com/science>.

[10] Yang S, Flores B, Magal R, Harris K, Gross J, Ewbank A, et al. Diagnostic accuracy of tablet-based software for the detection of concussion. PLoS One 2017;12(7):e0179352. Available from: https://doi.org/10.1371/journal.pone.0179352.

[11] <https://www.cambridgecognition.com/cantab/test-batteries/traumatic-brain-injury/>.

[12] <https://www.cambridgecognition.com/cantab/technology>.

[13] <https://www.cnsvs.com/ClinicalPractice.html>.

[14] <https://www.cnsvs.com/FAQs.html>.

[15] Thomas Gualtieri C, Johnson LG. Reliability and validity of a computerized neurocognitive test battery, CNS vital signs. Arch Clin Neuropsychol 2006;21(7):623–43. Available from: https://doi.org/10.1016/j.acn.2006.05.007.

[16] <https://www.cogstate.com/clinical-practice/concussion/>.

[17] Louey AG, Cromer JA, Schembri AJ, Darby DG, Marruf P, Makdissi M, et al. Detecting cognitive impairment after concussion: sensitivity of change from baseline and normative data methods using the CogSport/Axon cognitive test battery. Arch Clin Neuropsychol 2014;29(5):432–41. Available from: https://doi.org/10.1093/arclin/acu020.

[18] <https://www.cogstate.com/cogstate-receives-positive-fda-notification-regarding-medical-device-regulatory-submission/>.

[19] <https://www.c3logix.com/carrick/?>.

[20] Makwana B, Xu X(M). C3Logix assessment of neuropsychological performance in athletes and nonathletes. Appl Neuropsych: Adul 2019;0(0):1–7.

[21] Borges A, Raab S, Lininger M. A comprehensive instrument for evaluating mild traumatic brain injury (mtbi)/concussion in independent adults: a pilot study. Int J Sports Phys Ther 2017;12(3):381–9.

[22] <http://www.danabrainvital.com/about-us/>.

[23] <http://www.danabrainvital.com/technology/>.

[24] <https://www.anthrotronix.com/our-work/mhealth/>.

[25] Spira JL, Lathan CE, Bleiberg J, Tsao JW. The impact of multiple concussions on emotional distress, postconcussive symptoms, and neurocognitive functioning in active duty United States marines independent of combat exposure or emotional distress. J Neurotrauma. 2014;31(22):1823–34. Available from: https://doi.org/10.1089/neu.2014.3363.

[26] <https://impacttest.com/about/>.

[27] <https://www.fda.gov/news-events/press-announcements/fda-allows-marketing-first-kind-computerized-cognitive-tests-help-assess-cognitive-skills-after-head>.

[28] Schatz P, Sandel N. Sensitivity and specificity of the online version of ImPACT in high school and collegiate athletes. Am J Sports Med 2013;41(2):321–6. Available from: https://doi.org/10.1177/0363546512466038.

[29] Schatz P, Pardini JE, Lovell MR, Collins MW, Podell K. Sensitivity and specificity of the ImPACT test battery for concussion in athletes. Arch Clin Neuropsychol 2006;21(1):91–9. Available from: https://doi.org/10.1016/j.acn.2005.08.001.

[30] Resch JE, Brown CN, Schmidt J, et al. The sensitivity and specificity of clinical measures of sport concussion: three tests are better than one. BMJ Open Sport Exer Med 2016;2:e000012. Available from: https://doi.org/10.1136/bmjsem-2015-000012.

[31] <https://kingdevicktest.com/products/concussion/sideline-concussion-screening/>.

[32] Dhawan PS, Leong D, Tapsell L, et al. King-Devick Test identifies real-time concussion and asymptomatic concussion in youth athletes. Neurol Clin Pract. 2017;7(6):464–73. Available from: https://doi.org/10.1212/CPJ.0000000000000381.

[33] Galetta KM, Liu M, Leong DF, Ventura RE, Galetta SL, Balcer LJ. The King-Devick test of rapid number naming for concussion detection: meta-analysis and systematic review of the literature. Concussion 2015;1(2):CNC8. Available from: https://doi.org/10.2217/cnc.15. Published 2015 Sep 10.

[34] Mrazik M, et al. King Devick computerized neurocognitive test scores in professional football players with learning and attentional disabilities. J Neurol Sci 2019;399:140–3.

[35] <https://www.savonix.com/science-2/>.

Electroencephalographic as a biomarker of concussion

Jerald H. Simmons[1,2] and Harry Kerasidis[3]

[1]Comprehensive Sleep Medicine Associates, Houston, TX, United States [2]Sleep Education Consortium, Houston, TX, United States [3]Chesapeake Neurology Associates, Center for Neuroscience at Calvert Health, Prince Frederick, MD, United States

25.1 Why should electroencephalographic be considered for use as a biomarker of concussion?

Electroencephalographic (EEG) activity can be thought of as a vital sign of the brain. The changes in the electrical signals generated from the brain can provide insight into cerebral function that other technologies such as CT, fMRI, and serum-based markers cannot provide. As opposed to MRI and CT scans, for example, which characterize anatomy, EEG characterizes real-time neuronal activity, down to the millisecond level. EEG is the best method to date, that can be practically utilized on a large scale, to capture ongoing neurophysiological activity of the brain, in a cost-efficient manner. Though this capability offers a vast potential for analyzing detailed real-time central nervous system activity, only recently has improved computer-based analysis of the data allowed neurophysiologists to tap beyond the surface of the information that exists in the EEG signal. Therefore, although presently EEG is often thought of as a secondary-level technology when evaluating a patient who has sustained a concussive injury, present advances may soon make EEG the most useful tool for both the acute assessment and the ongoing monitoring in these clinical situations.

Assessing the brain using EEG signals can be limited by the state of the brain at the time of the assessment. To illustrate this important point, comparison is made with the well-established protocols for assessing the electrical activity of the heart using the EKG signal. The optimal method for assessing the EKG is with 12 leads strategically placed on the limbs and chest, which allows for proper characterization of the electrical fields generated by the heart as it goes through a repeated series of events, with each cardiac cycle. Since the heart always performs the same sequence of events, the EKG signal is relatively easy to interpret, and very specific correlations have been established between abnormal EKG waveforms and pathology of the heart. However, many abnormalities of the heart may go undiagnosed if the heart is only assessed in a resting state. Therefore patients in whom there is a concern, such as coronary artery disease, need to have their heart stressed by exercising on a treadmill, to trigger ischemic abnormalities, in the form of ST wave changes. Without stressing the heart such abnormalities frequently go undetected. The brain, which is several magnitudes more complex than the heart, similarly may not produce a detectable abnormal EEG pattern from an underlying abnormality until specific testing conditions are used that make the abnormality evident. Routine EEGs typically utilize activation maneuvers such as hyperventilation, or the presentation of strobe lights, to attempt eliciting abnormalities. However, it may require performance of cognitive tasks to unmask subtle abnormalities, such as those associated with concussions. Controlling the conditions of such testing is problematic. Nonetheless, as enhanced methods of signal processing are developed, the opportunity to extract clinically significant results from the EEG is becoming more feasible.

There are many theories regarding the functional organization of the brain. However, to date, there is clearly a consensus that an organized configuration exists in the cortex that differs in various cortical regions, to provide optimal performance of the specific tasks, unique to each region. For example, cortical regions involved with integrating sounds in the temporal lobe are structurally configured differently than those involved in primary visual perception on the visual cortex of the occipital lobe. Cortical regions communicate with each other to perform complex tasks. The connectivity between adjacent regions is different than those involving regions at a distance. Subcortical structures provide modulatory processes that bring these different cortical events into concert together, thus achieving a highly sophisticated output of human activity.

The EEG signal, as measured from the scalp is the summation of billions of small electrical currents in the brain, with the largest amplitude coming from the relatively large pyramidal neurons in the cortex, and also from deeper structures in the subcortical regions. There is a reduction of resolution in the electrical signal measured on the scalp caused by the distance between the scalp and the brain tissue, as well as the density and electrical properties of the bone and tissue in between. However, even with the reduction of resolution, there still exists a tremendous amount of information within the EEG signal recorded at the scalp. Extracting that information has been the challenge within the field of clinical neurophysiology. What is clear is that visual inspection of the EEG, which has been the main method of clinical use, has important but limited value.

Studies looking at interrater reliability have found limited correlation between reviewers performing visual inspection of the EEG with low correlation scores [1]. Using computers to perform signal processing allows for better standardization and statistical assessments, beyond what can be obtained by visual inspection alone. Below, we give examples of how basic visual inspection method of EEG is reliably used, but then we will explain how computer-assisted analysis can extract more information from the EEG data. Then we will present examples of how current state-of-the-art EEG analysis methods can be used in clinical practice. In general, as it is with many physiological tests, it is important to place the information derived by these EEG techniques in the proper clinical context of the patient being evaluated. Placing test results in the proper clinical context is always necessary, and not limited to EEG interpretations. For example, on MRI scans, a finding of increased T2 signal in cerebral white matter regions is not specific to one pathologic process and has a differential that can range from ischemic small vessel vascular disease to demyelination or even transient post migraine changes. So clinical correlation is imperative to arrive at the proper conclusion. So too is the case for abnormal EEG findings, including those from computerized quantitative EEG techniques. These findings need to be placed in context of the clinical setting in which they occur so as to utilize the information properly.

25.2 Standard clinical electroencephalographic using visual inspection

Historically, routine EEGs, performed by all hospitals and many neurologists, consist of 18–20 electrodes, placed on the scalp in a systematic fashion referred to as the 10–20 placement system [2] (Fig. 25.1) and the data is reviewed by visual inspection. The data is typically displayed in 10-second increments on either a large page of paper or across a computer screen. Each vertical line of the EEG represents the difference in electrical potential between two inputs, such as two different electrodes on the scalp. There are a variety of configurations combining the electrodes over the scalp. Each configuration can emphasize the electrical field of the EEG in a particular fashion. Each configuration is referred to as a montage. An anterior to posterior bipolar montage is described in Fig. 25.2. Typically, several montages are used on each EEG study in order to characterize the electrical fields of the EEG. This method is most useful in identifying abnormal events associated with seizures, such as spikes and sharp waves. Visual inspection is still thought to be the best method of identifying robust seizure abnormalities such as the 3-Hz spike and wave pattern seen in a patient during a primary generalized seizure. The eye can clearly identify

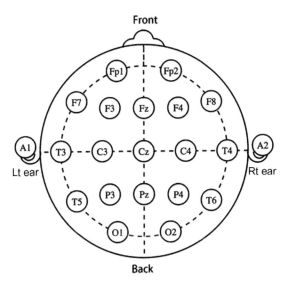

FIGURE 25.1 Figure shows the different electrode positions that comprise the International 10–20 electrode placement system with each electrode labeled. Even numbers on the right, odd on the left, midline designated with a "z." The letters F, C, T, P, and O designate Frontal, Central, Temporal, Parietal, and Occipital regions respectively.

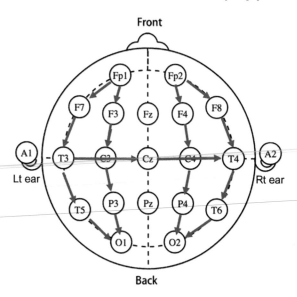

Front

Back

FIGURE 25.2   The figure shows the configuration of the anterior to posterior bipolar montage. Arrows depict the referencing of each channel with the first input of the channel being represented by the origin of the arrow and the second input of the channel being the termination point of the arrow. The EEG output from the montage can be seen in Fig. 25.3 which consists of EEG displayed using this same bipolar montage.

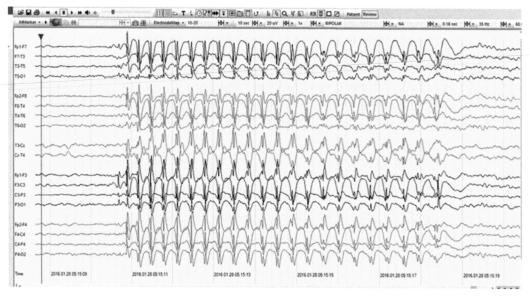

FIGURE 25.3   The figure displays 10 s of EEG in the anterior to posterior bipolar montage containing a 7-s generalized seizure with a typical 3-s spike and wave pattern as is seen with primary generalized seizures. However, close inspection demonstrates a focal onset around the F3 (left frontal) electrode about 200 ms before it becomes generalized. This type of focal onset is not an uncommon finding in primary generalized epilepsy.

this abnormal pattern and distinguish it from artifact. An example of this obvious abnormality is seen in Fig. 25.3 from a patient sitting still, staring off, unresponsive for a few seconds while having a 7-second seizure.

Though the waveform patterns witnessed in some pathological events (such as the seizure pattern shown in Fig. 25.3 above) are easily discernable to a trained eye, the use of visual inspection to determine subtle changes in the underlying rhythmic activity is not as sensitive as the computerized statistical methods discussed later in this chapter. Since most neurologists performing EEG limit their analysis to visual inspection and because of the limitation of visual inspection, EEG has not been widely used in concussion assessment. When there is a concern of postconcussive epilepsy, visual inspection is adequate. Visual assessment is still held as the gold standard in determining a diagnosis of seizures.

Even when a seizure has occurred, in most cases, the routine EEG will be read as normal when performed hours to days after the acute event. There is a low likelihood of capturing a seizure event, or epileptiform abnormality, during an EEG performed hours or days after the clinical event. Any background abnormalities, such as slowing of the normal rhythms, that may be present are not readily discernable by visual analysis. Figs. 25.4 and 25.5 are demonstrations of a patient who developed seizures from a right temporal lobe abnormality following a head injury. Both Figs. 25.4 and 25.5, are of the same segment of EEG data but displayed using two different montages. When present to a dramatic degree,

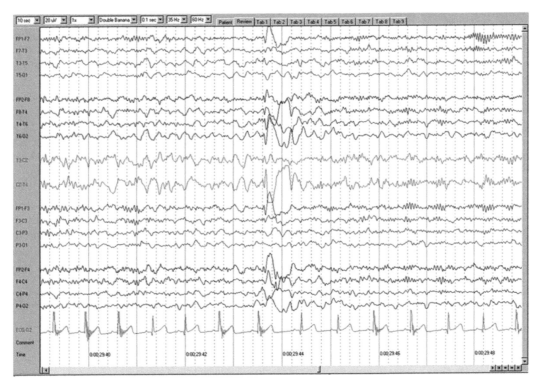

FIGURE 25.4   The figure is a display of 10 s of EEG with the bipolar montage with a small spike and sharp wave on the right side that is picked up in the adjacent left frontal polar electrode. Identifying the maximal amplitude of this event is difficult with this montage on this occasion. The event represents an epileptiform abnormality. To help characterize the event, the same data is displayed in Fig. 25.5 using an averaged reference montage where each channel has the same reference input, which is the average of all the electrodes.

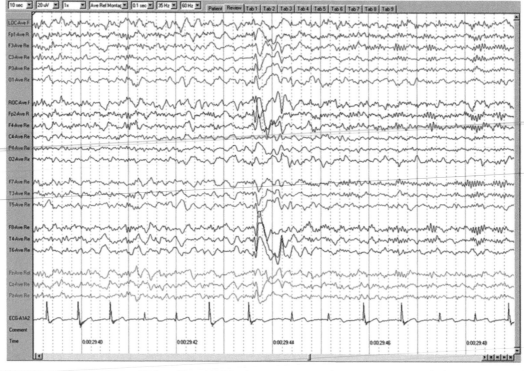

FIGURE 25.5 The figure displays 10 s of EEG using an average reference montage. With this montage, each channel has a unique electrode as input one and an average of all of the electrodes as input two. This allows for a direct comparison of all electrodes since they all have the same second input (referred to as the reference). This is the same EEG data as in Fig. 25.4 but displayed with a different montage. With this montage it can be seen that the epileptiform discharge is mainly in the temporal region and involves the adjacent right frontopolar region.

like in this case, there is a visually discernable event in the EEG pattern that is relatively easily identified. With this type of EEG finding it is common that a structural abnormality may be identified on an MRI as well. However, electrical abnormalities of this magnitude are not always present when an injury has occurred, and more subtle abnormalities may be present that are difficult to extract from the EEG.

Below is a list of clinical situations where visual inspection of EEG is very useful.

> To provide evidence of seizure like (epileptiform) discharges.
> To identify slow background rhythms associated with encephalopathy.
> To demonstrate focal slowing consistent with a focal abnormality of the brain.
> To identify sleep and characterize the different features of different sleep stages.
> To identify the presence of specific pathologic discharges associated with certain clinical conditions (example, triphasic waves in metabolic encephalopathy).

There are reports of changes in the EEG immediately following a concussion, consisting of slowing of the posterior dominant rhythm and diffuse increased theta activity that typically clears within hours of the injury [3], but obtaining the EEG in this acute setting is not currently a practical reality.

Visual inspection of the EEG has not proven to be very useful in the assessment of concussion. As a result, most clinicians involved in the diagnosis and management of concussion do not resort to EEG testing as part of their protocol. This limitation results from the insensitivity provided by visual inspection.

25.3 Evoked potentials

With the development of computers, signal processing of the EEG data has taken many new directions. One such method is referred to as evoked potentials or EP for short. EPs are obtained by presenting stimuli and time-locking the acquisition of the EEG to the presentation of the stimuli. The EEG data from each presentation of the stimuli is put into an array and then the arrays are averaged such that the output, or result, is an averaged waveform that represents the brain processing of the stimulus. The concept behind this is that activity not related to the processing of the stimulus is in essence "random." With repetitive stimuli presentation, the random activity cancels out, leaving the waveform that corresponds to the processing of the stimulus. There are many forms of EPs as described below.

25.3.1 Brain stem auditory evoked potentials

Brain stem auditory EPs otherwise known as brain stem auditory evoked response or BAERs have been extensively utilized in the medical field and illustrate the power of EPs. BAERs are elicited by headphones presenting a click sound to the patient. The voltages at the scalp from the click stimulus are very small in relation to the other "random" EEG activity that is simultaneously present. This can be stated as a low signal-to-noise ratio and therefore requires thousands of click stimuli to be averaged in order to eliminate the random EEG (noise) and obtain a clean brain stem EP (signal). The different components of the signal relate to generators in specific anatomical regions in the brain stem, relating to auditory processing. From a time frame perspective, the main waveforms I–V occur within 10 ms from the time of the click as the neuronal impulse from the click travels through the brain stem. While some reports claim initial delayed responses in wave I–V intervals in 27%–46% of concussed patients [4], BAER have not been widely utilized as part of the assessment battery. Furthermore, BAERs have not been found to have any prognostic value in patients sustaining a concussive injury [5]. However, in traumatic brain injury in which there is clear brain stem damage or damage to the cochlear vestibular apparatus or 8th CN then the BAERs can confirm an abnormality and be tracked as part of the recovery process. An example of a BAER, listing the different wave components and associated anatomy, is seen in Fig. 25.6.

25.3.2 Visual evoked potentials

Visual EPs are elicited by either a repeated flash, presented by goggles or a reversing checkerboard pattern displayed on a computer monitor, with each stimulus being

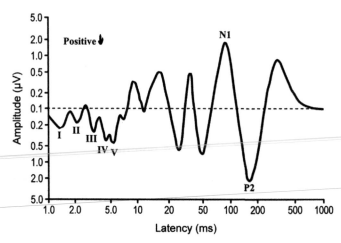

FIGURE 25.6 Figure showing wave forms of a normal Brain stem Auditory Evoked Potential (BAEP). Each wave is associated with electrical generators along the auditory pathway: Wave I—distal acoustic nerve; Wave II—proximal acoustic nerve; Wave III—superior olive and projections to the lateral lemniscus; medial nucleus of trapezoid body; Wave IV—most likely the lateral lemniscus; Wave V—high pontine or lower midbrain structures: probably the lateral lemniscus, inferior colliculus, or a combination. The mid-latency N1P2 complex originates from primary sensory cortex processing in the primary auditory cortex of the temporal lobes with other supporting centers within the temporal lobes.

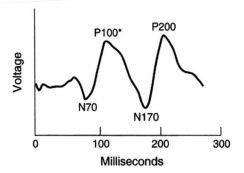

FIGURE 25.7 Figure illustrating a normal visual evoked potential waveform. The earlier waveforms (N70, P100) arise from generators in the primary visual cortex in the occipital lobe. The N1P2 complex arises from generators in the association cortex in the occipital-parietal and occipital-temporal regions.

generated by a reverse of each block of the checkerboard from white to black or black to white. The electrical signal generated by the visual stimulus is larger than with the click stimulus used for BAERs and as a result the signal-to-noise ratio is higher than with BAER. For VEPs hundreds of stimuli are required in order to generate a clean VEP signal as compared to thousands of stimuli with BAERs. VEP are rarely abnormal in cases of concussion. As in BAEP, an abnormal VEP would suggest a structural abnormality and a corresponding finding on MRI scans may be identified as well but not always [6]. Examples of VEP are displayed in Fig. 25.7 with the labeling of associated anatomical structures.

25.3.3 Cognitive evoked potentials/event related potentials

Cognitive EPs, otherwise known as event related potentials or ERPs, consist of cognitive recognition tasks and time-locking the collection of the EEG to the presentation of an event, which is the stimulus. The averaged signal corresponds to the presentation of the stimuli used in the test in which the patient or subject is recognizing a unique feature of the stimulus, which requires cognitive processing, and thus is the basis for the term cognitive EPs. ERPs typically have a much higher signal-to-noise ratio and therefore less stimuli are needed to be averaged in order to obtain a clean signal. Averaging 30–50 stimuli will typically provide a stable clean waveform. Cognitive EPs have been found to be associated with concussion-related dysfunction and may ultimately prove to be one of the better EEG measures to be used as a biomarker of concussion. However, ERPs have been met with a lot of controversy within the medical field, in spite of having great relevance for patients with concussion.

Of the different types of cognitive EPs, the P300 is the most widely understood and utilized. To generate a P300, the patient is presented two different types of stimuli, such as a high tone and a low tone. The EEG responses to each type of stimuli are averaged separately. One of the stimuli is presented less frequently and randomly intermixed with the frequent stimuli. For example, a low tone is presented frequently and intermixed within these are high tones, randomly interspersed. Only one stimulus is presented at a time and the interval between stimuli is at least 1 second, such that there is no overlap of signal presentation while still processing the prior stimulus. Typically, the less frequent stimulus is presented about 20%–30% of the time and it is referred to as the "oddball" stimulus, whereas the other stimulus is referred to as the "frequent" stimulus. It takes about 30 "oddball" stimuli to obtain a clean response.

What is obtained from this type of testing is a significant difference between the "oddball" and "frequent" stimulus at about 300 ms after the presentation of the stimulus. This difference is a positive waveform referred to as the P300. The P300, also referred to as the P3, has been subdivided into two components, P3a and P3b. There is a consensus that P3a relates to the attention level and the incoming perception of a unique stimulus, whereas P3b is associated with a decision process or memory updating associated with the unique stimulus.

The beauty of the P300 oddball paradigm is the variety of stimuli that may be used to evoke the P300 response. In its simplest form, the stimuli can be tones of different frequencies with a common low-pitched tone and the rare occurrence of the target high-pitched tone. The task can be more complex and cognitively driven. For example, the stimuli can be single words visually presented on a computer screen, with the target being contextually defined words, such as words that represent the animals "dog" or "cat." This provides a useful tool to evaluate for specific cognitive functions, related to specific anatomic regions of the brain involved in such processing.

The N400 is a negative potential occurring 400 ms after the presentation of an incongruent word within a sentence. This potential is related to semantic processing and is maximal over the parietal regions lateralized to the left with an important contribution from the left temporal lobe [7]. Another well-described event-related potential is the N170, a negative potential occurring 170 ms after the presentation of pictures of faces depicting the expression of various emotions. The source of this potential has been localized to the superior and middle temporal lobes [8]. Mismatch negativity (MMN) is yet another well-documented event-related negative potential occurring between 150 and 250 ms after an unexpected stimulus. The auditory MMN is localized to the frontal lobes, lateralized to the right.

Many research groups investigating the P3 just report a single amplitude, not subdividing into the subcomponents. Nonetheless, the P3 has been identified as an EEG phenomenon that represents higher level cerebral functioning that relates to processing of unique sensory stimuli that is in contrast to other stimuli of which the brain has become habituated. From a conceptual standpoint, it would make sense that the P3 would be more sensitive in identifying cerebral dysfunction associated with disruption of networks within the brain such as what occurs from concussions. An example of a P300 is shown in Fig. 25.8.

The majority of studies of event related potential and concussion have looked at the P300 potential, but most are limited to small sample sizes and most do not have a preconcussion baseline for comparison. A review of the literature was published by Rapp et al. in 2015 consisting of 97 ERP studies in traumatic brain injury [9]. Their review demonstrated that P3 latency seems to be the most sensitive electrophysiologic measure to distinguish between normal and concussed groups. In contrast to these results, a study not included in the previous review was reported by Francois Dupuis et al. in which P300 was evaluated in a small study of college athletes. The study consisted of 10 nonconcussed athletes, 10 with concussions

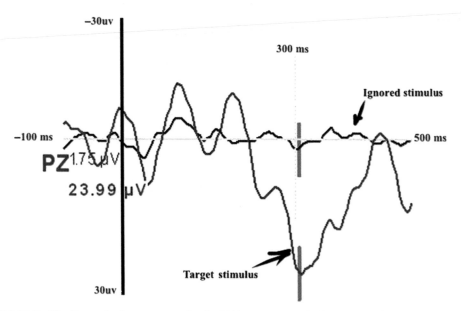

FIGURE 25.8 The figure displays an example of a P300 cognitive evoked potential. There are two waveforms displayed. One is the wave corresponding to the more frequently presented nontarget, or ignored stimulus, and the other wave corresponds to the less frequently presented, target stimulus. It can be clearly seen that at about 300 ms following the stimulus, the target stimulus produces a large positive voltage (down) deflection which represents the P300. This wave is not present with the ignored (nontarget) stimulus.

between 1 month and 2 years prior to testing with no current symptoms, and a third group with concussions between 1 week and 6 months prior to testing who had postconcussive symptoms at the time of testing. Their study demonstrated that the symptomatic group demonstrated a lower amplitude of the P300 where all other objective tests failed to distinguish between groups [10]. This finding of decreased amplitude is not unique. Duncan et al. found that the P300 had a reduced amplitude in individuals who had sustained closed head injuries [11,12]. Other studies claim an association between depression scores following injury positively correlated with decreased P300 amplitudes [13].

25.4 Spectral analysis

Although quantitative analysis of features of the EEG such as amplitude and frequency have been performed since the days of paper polygraphs, it was not until the development of computer technology and the digitization of the EEG signal in the 1960s and early 1970s that allowed for advanced mathematics to be applied to EEG analysis in a practical fashion. One such method, referred to as fast Fourier transformation (FFT) provided a quantifiable measure of the EEG for different frequency bands. The output data from the FFT is reported as "power" of the signal. The FFT analysis of EEG typically provides the power of the EEG signal for delta (0.5–4 Hz), theta (4–8 Hz), and alpha (8–13 Hz). The beta band is variably defined as ranging from 13 to 30 Hz by some authors and 13–40 Hz by others. Similarly, the gamma band is defined as either above 30 or 40 Hz. Frequencies between 30 and 35 Hz make up a borderline band that is variably categorized as high-beta by some authors and gamma by others. For the purpose of this chapter we will refer to this band as beta-gamma.

Transforming the EEG into numerical output representing the amount of activity in each of the frequency bands through FFT allowed for statistical analysis to be performed more readily, making EEG research quantifiable. Prior to this, only visual inspection was performed, with less accuracy in the analysis and most of the activity within the EEG signal was not objectively assessed.

Frequency analysis of the EEG has been successfully utilized in a number of clinical venues, with well-established results. One example is in the operating room for patients undergoing carotid endarterectomy surgery. The patients are monitored for ischemia of the brain using intraoperative EEG with FFT in a method called compressed spectral arrays [14]. The asymmetric slowing of the EEG is easily identified giving the surgeon important guidance during critical parts of the surgical procedure. Ongoing FFT and compressed spectral array monitoring also has been demonstrated to be useful in the ICU setting in comatose patients as far back as the 1970s [15]. Acute ischemia in the ICU can also be identified using these techniques [16,17].

For concussion, it would be very advantageous if the EEG could be used in a simplified fashion to provide identification of when a concussion has occurred. Studies specifically evaluating the utility of spectral analysis have been reviewed and published by Rapp et al. in 2015 in which they included both peer-reviewed and nonpeer-reviewed studies on QEEG in mTBI. They identified 25 studies that presented direct statistical evidence of QEEG as a discriminator for mTBI. Of these, 15 used spectral analysis as a measure to compare injured from normal controls. The most prevalent finding amongst these studies was an increase in delta, theta, and beta power and a decrease in alpha power. It is important to point out that several groups also reported that when they did the statistical analysis of the entire frequency band (from 0.5 to 50 Hz) without breaking the data into the subbands, there were no statically significant differences identified [18–20]. This points to the importance of setting up the data analysis method properly in order to identify the specific features within the EEG data that become altered by mTBI. Otherwise the mTBI changes can be drowned out by the multiplicity of events that are simultaneously occurring within the brain.

Thatcher et al. [21] reported a discriminant analysis function (discussed later in the chapter) that they developed from recordings performed 3–8 days after injury. One of the characteristic changes associated with mild traumatic brain injury (mTBI) includes reduction of alpha power in the posterior head regions, similar to what other researchers have found.

The FFT actually functions as a filter of the data so that specific frequency data can be characterized, quantified, and statistically analyzed, thus comparing apples with apples. Additionally, the data can be assessed in a variety of ways, mainly consisting of the absolute power of the signal at each frequency band and the relative power of each band. This is an important distinction, as in any given individual there may be conditions that would lead to an increase or decrease in the signal. For example, if the skull were unusually thin, then the amplitude of the EEG would be higher than normal, but when compared to all the other frequency bands, the relative power distribution would be normal. It is customary to present the FFT data in both absolute power and relative power. Relative power is a representation of a particular band as a percentage of all of the activity in all bands.

With the explosion of computer technology in the 1980s came faster, cheaper, and more readily available computers allowing for the development of commercially available digital EEG analysis products which included features such as brain mapping and database comparisons [22].

Flat maps characterizing the layout of the scalp were first used by Duffy in a technique he labeled brain electrical activity mapping or BEAM, for short [22]. Fig. 25.9 is an example of a patient's EEG displayed in flat maps broken down into frequency bands. In the top row is the absolute power at each frequency band. The power of the EEG is reported in uV Sq units. In the second row is the relative power of each frequency band reported as a percentage of the total power of all bands.

Duffy then implemented a technique in which statistical maps display an individual's EEG data compared to an age-matched control population in a technique called *significant probability mapping* [23]. With this method, a map of Z-scores characterize regions that are higher or lower than the mean of a control population. This method of data reduction allows for large amounts of information to be conveyed in a simplified fashion. The problem with this type of data reduction is that it can be misleading when segments of EEG signals that have artifact are included into the analysis. Without visually inspecting the raw EEG segments used in QEEG analysis, erroneous conclusions may be derived. The commercialization of EEG devices that perform QEEG analysis such as topographic mapping must be viewed cautiously. Such tools require skilled users such that segments of the recording that represent artifacts can be excluded from the recording so that erroneous conclusions are not derived. In order to prevent erroneous conclusions, it is imperative that only qualified individuals with the proper knowledge of EEG perform the initial

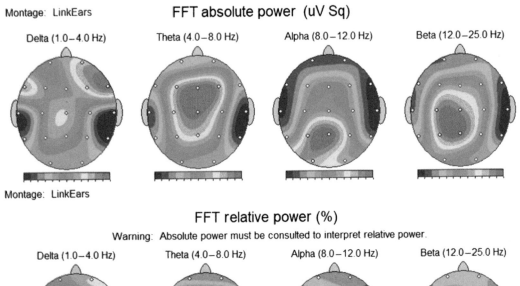

Montage: LinkEars

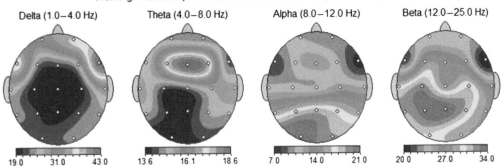

FIGURE 25.9   The figure is a display of flat head maps that show the distribution on the scalp of the different frequency bands. The top row is absolute power which is reported in millivolts squared (uV Sq). The second row is a display of relative power which is reported as a percentage of the total power. In both of the display methods, dark blue represents the lowest values and dark red represents the highest values. This is an example of a normal individual. Bright colors in this format do not represent an abnormality.

analysis of the recording, so as to make sure that data is collected properly and only artifact-free data segments are collected and used for analysis.

With the development of statistical mapping of EEG came the expansion of normative databases including the NYU database, University of Maryland database, and the Russian Human Brain Institute database, to name a few [24,25].

Subsequently, cross-validation studies brought added validity to the concept of clinical applications of QEEG to cross-cultural populations, exemplified by E. Roy John's cross-validation between a Swedish normative database and a normal population of children growing up in Harlem, New York [25,26].

Fig. 25.10 demonstrates Z-score maps displaying the regions and frequency bands that deviate from a normal age-matched control group to a statistically significant degree. It can be seen that the data is normal. However, a similar analysis in Fig. 25.11 is from a 74-year-old male patient after a right middle cerebral artery stroke which is not normal.

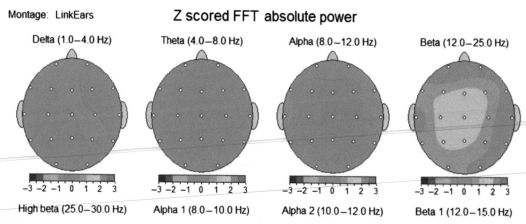

Montage: LinkEars

Z scored FFT absolute power

| Delta (1.0–4.0 Hz) | Theta (4.0–8.0 Hz) | Alpha (8.0–12.0 Hz) | Beta (12.0–25.0 Hz) |

High beta (25.0–30.0 Hz)   Alpha 1 (8.0–10.0 Hz)   Alpha 2 (10.0–12.0 Hz)   Beta 1 (12.0–15.0 Hz)

FIGURE 25.10 The figure is an example of significant probability mapping with Z-scores displayed over the scalp. In this configuration, green represents a Z-score of zero. As the colors progress to blue, the Z-scores become further deviated below the mean of a control population. On the other end of the spectrum, as the colors progress to red, the Z-scores become further deviated above the mean of the control group. This is from the same individual as in Fig. 25.9 in which the absolute and relative power maps were displayed. It can be seen that this individual has normal EEG power spectral analysis.

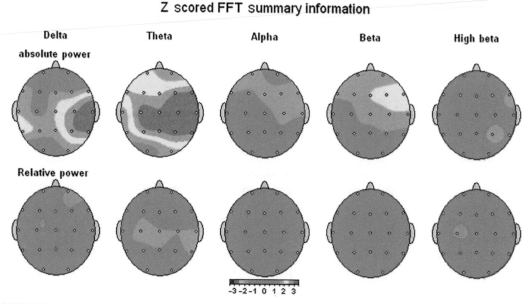

Montage: LinkEars   EEG ID: 1.NaHeAsse_EC

Z scored FFT summary information

| Delta | Theta | Alpha | Beta | High beta |

absolute power

Relative power

FIGURE 25.11 The figure displays two-dimensional surface Z-scored maps (significant probability mapping) from a 74-year-old male after right middle cerebral artery stroke. Maps demonstrate excess delta slow activity consistent with cerebral dysfunction due to the stroke injury. There is a more generalized increased theta activity, lateralized to the right, consistent with a more diffuse cortical dysfunction. The routine visual inspected EEG was read as normal.

25.5 3D electroencephalographic mapping—standardized low-resolution electromagnetic tomographic activity

The development of magnetoencephalography (MEG) has opened the door to more elaborate measurements of brain activity that provide information on the generator depth. The magnetic flux associated with an electrical current is a field that is perpendicular to direction of current. Therefore the current generated by neurons within the brain produces a magnetic field, that if measured, provides data that points to the depth of the current generator. The magnetic flux is extremely small in magnitude and measuring this MEG signal requires elaborate equipment that is costly, requires very stringent recording conditions in a shielded room and is not a practical method to be implemented on a large scale. With the new millennium came revolutionary analysis that took advantage of the direct relationship between electric and magnetic activity using inverse solution models that provided three-dimensional (3D) maps approximating the source within the brain that generated the EEG activity measured on the scalp surface. Of the different approaches, the most widely utilized, developed by Pascual-Marqui, is known as standardized low-resolution tomographic electromagnetic activity (sLORETA) [27]. This discovery came about by combining simultaneous measurements of MEG and EEG in subjects in whom MRI scans were also obtained. Calculations were carried out to characterize the relationship between these different data sets. The result of sLORETA analysis provides a reasonable approximation of the current source within the brain by only measuring the EEG from a full complement of 18 standard EEG electrode sites in accordance with the 10–20 system (as shown in Fig. 25.2). Conceptually, this could be thought of as a similar measurement to that provided by MEG, but with using only a relatively inexpensive EEG system, in a less stringent recording environment. The 3D images consist of thousands of voxels, each depicting the magnitude of current at that 3D location, referred to as current source density. The resulting 3D images of voxel data depict a specific quality of the current source data, such as frequency band when FFT is performed or direct magnitude if ERPs data averaging is performed [27,28].

Studies have been done to assess the ability of sLORETA to localize changes in cerebral activity to those from fMRI with complementary results supporting the use of sLORETA for localization of cerebral activity [29,30].

Because of the strength provided by sLORETA analysis in identifying cerebral activity, groups developed normative databases that could be used to provide Z-score analysis with age-matched controls resulting in 3D maps where each voxel represents a Z-score. To have a meaningful assessment, data from normal controls were collected in a similar condition, typically with two data sets from each individual used in the control group. One for awake, relaxed with eyes open, and the other while awake, relaxed with eyes closed. A minimum of 1 minute of artifact-free raw EEG is used from each individual for each condition (eyes open and eyes closed). Studies evaluating the stability of this type of analysis in normals over a 30-day period provided reproducible results [31].

The sLORETA Z-score analysis produces a 3D image of regions in which an individual differs from controls in a particular EEG feature (i.e., delta frequency). Fig. 25.12 displays a sLORETA EEG image at 8.2 Hz demonstrating an increased current source density

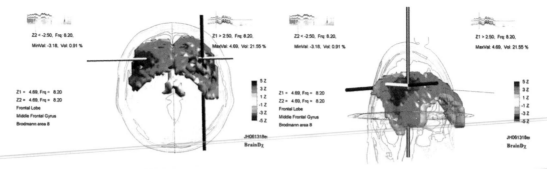

FIGURE 25.12 sLORETA Z-score 3D images in which areas of red are more than 2.5 standard deviations above the mean of an age-matched control population, all collected with eyes closed awake. The cross bars depict the maximal point in which there was alpha 4.6 SD above the mean. The image to the right is with the head looking forward in a skewed angle and the image to the left is viewing the head from above looking down with the front at the top of the image.

activity bilaterally in the frontal regions with Z-scores beyond 4 SD above the mean in a patient in whom the routine EEG that was read as normal with visual inspection and also normal flat map FFT statistical probability mapping in the alpha band. Like other methods of QEEG, special care needs to be placed on not including in the analysis EEG segments that contain artifacts or may be collected when the patient is in a different recording condition, such as eyes open when comparing to eyes closed. When correctly collected, our view is that this method of EEG analysis holds great promise in the future of concussion assessment and management. It has become common practice to use sLORETA normal databases for a variety of assessments and clinical purposes [26,32–36].

A relatively recent study utilizing sLORETA with cognitive EPs, using a high-resolution electrode placement of 256 electrodes in asymptomatic college athletes with prior concussion compared to nonconcussed controls, found that the concussed group demonstrated a higher magnitude P300 in the left inferior parietal gyrus with a delayed latency. They speculate that the increased amplitude is the result of compensatory recruitment of additional neuronal networks needed to overcome the deficiencies that resulted from the concussions [34]. As more studies are performed using sLORETA or similar methods that provide activity in localized brain regions, similar findings may be demonstrated that cannot be recognized by routine scalp/flat map analysis methods.

Kerasidis et al. studied the EEGs of 40 high school athletes (20 male) shortly after concussion injury using sLORETA current source density analysis. Delta, theta, and alpha activity was increased in both genders with no statistical gender difference. Beta activity was increased in females but not males, where beta activity tended to be reduced in comparison to the age-matched norm. The beta-gamma band activity (30–35 Hz) was increased in both genders, however, the proportion of gray matter volume contributing to this increase was twice as much in females than in males (60% in females, 30% in males) [32,33]. This increase in beta and beta-gamma activity is paradoxical, being the opposite of what is seen in adults who have reduced beta and beta-gamma activity. The authors hypothesize that these differences are related to differences in stage and rate of maturation of the adolescent brain, as corroborated by structural MRI studies of adolescent maturation, with males having more prominent age-related gray matter decreases and white matter volume and corpus callosal area increases compared with females. The elevation of beta-gamma activity is relatively widespread and, although persistent, varies in location over time. This may reflect that this activity is a compensatory mechanism for physiologic changes and dysfunction induced by concussion-related trauma.

Repeat EEGs were recorded after these athletes had clinically recovered, that is, being cognitively back to baseline and symptom-free at full exertion after a period of progressive exertion, as defined by several internationally recognized guidelines [37–39]. The repeat QEEG sLORETA findings demonstrated a trend towards normalization, although there was a persistence of elevated activity in delta, theta and alpha activity. There was also a persistence diffuse elevation of beta-gamma activity and diffuse reduced beta activity. These results suggest that there are persistent physiologic changes after clinical resolution of concussion in high school athletes. The clinical relevance and implications of these findings need to be studied further.

25.6 Discriminant analyses methods

Researchers have been seeking a methodology in which a combination of variables can be identified that would specifically characterize a specific clinical condition. This has been referred to as discriminant analysis. In 1989 Thatcher reported that the combination of an increase in EEG signal coherence with a decrease in the signal transmission (phase) between the frontal and frontal–temporal regions, along with a decrease in the power difference between the anterior and posterior cortical regions and a reduced alpha power in the posterior regions, could discriminate between normal and those with mild head trauma. He reported discriminant accuracy up to 96% [21]. Although the reduced alpha power is a finding that has been repeatedly reported in association with mTBI, the other EEG measures have not been consistently reported and there is still no consensus as to clinical guidelines of how discriminant analysis can be used. Nonetheless, Thatcher reported a high capability to discriminate between normals and those with mTBI using his combination of variables. Intuitively, it is reasonable that this type of method would increase the reliability of identifying an abnormality, but it is not clear how specific the analysis would be in differentiating from other neurologic conditions such as multiinfarct cerebral vascular disease or demyelinating conditions such as multiple sclerosis with large cerebral lesions.

A novel approach using a discriminant analysis of specific EEG segments that are time-locked to the presentation of stimuli has been developed by Reches and colleagues in what they call brain network activation (BNA) analysis. The testing conditions are similar to those of ERPs with an oddball stimulus randomly presented infrequently, but they use multiple types of analysis methods on the time-locked data segments, such as signal averaging, frequency analysis, phase analysis, etc. They then use cluster analysis to identify discriminants specific to a particular clinical group, such as mTBI. Independent of the mTBI work, they demonstrated changes in BNA analysis in a group of subjects given scopolamine, suggesting an ability to identify cholinergic specific changes in the EEG. Their methodology is not open for others to evaluate without the use of their system, which is currently in the process of commercialization. The BNA analysis method is reported to identify and track subjects with traumatic brain injuries and in published reports the authors describe how their BNA measure can be used clinically to track the progress of patients with TBI [40].

In 2017 Hanley et al. presented a multiinstitutional study of 720 patients presenting to the emergency department following head trauma who were evaluated by an EEG system designed for quick EEG assessment applied by emergency department personnel. The system consisted of a subset of the 10−20 electrodes, and used a proprietary discriminant analysis method hypothesized to identify patients with acute brain lesions, such as small cerebral hemorrhages. The study included only those individuals with Glasgow Coma Scales scores of 12−15 in whom injury was within 72 hours of presentation. They assessed their discriminant function to those of CT scans. They report a sensitivity of correctly identifying an individual with a positive or negative CT scan of 92.3% and negative predictive value (NPV) of 96.0%. Using ternary classification (likely CT + , equivocal, likely CT −) they demonstrated enhanced sensitivity to traumatic hematomas (≥1 mL of blood), 98.6% (95% CI = 92.6%−100.0%), and NPV of 98.2% (95% CI = 95.5%− 99.5%) [41].

25.7 Practical application of electroencephalographic in the clinical setting

The evaluation of individuals acutely after a suspected concussive event is often complicated by the lack of objective independent measures to assess the individual and establish a diagnosis. With sports, this is further complicated by conflicts of interest and underreporting of symptoms in athletes. Many assessment tools have recently been developed to address this issue but more reliable objective assessments using physiologic measures would dramatically help to confirm the presence and help assess the severity of a concussion injury. Quantitative EEG analysis adds an additional layer of objective assessment of cerebral injury but currently is not practically administered in the acute setting. However, QEEG analysis is useful in the initial office postinjury evaluation to document electrophysiologic abnormalities that can be presumed related to the trauma, in a previously asymptomatic individual. Studies have demonstrated acute changes in quantitative EEG analysis that correlated with the severity of the injury symptoms and resolution of the abnormalities paralleled symptomatic and cognitive recovery [42]. Increasing reports of using QEEG to identify and track mTBI over time during the period of recovery are appearing in the literature [32,33,36,42−44].

With improved EEG application techniques, there may soon be a strong argument for performing baseline QEEGs prior to the start of each season, just as other types of testing are currently being performed. The baseline EEG can be used as a template for comparative purposes should a potential injury occur. Statistical comparisons can be made to the individual's own baseline EEG to determine new abnormalities due to the trauma. These changes can be tracked over time as the individual recovers from the concussion and undergoes physiologic changes as outlined in recent studies [45−47].

Research is still needed to identify the variables most relevant to return to normal activity and return to gameplay in injured athletes and it is here that EEG may come to play as a cost-effective, practical, reliable tool for tracking the changes following a mTBI event.

Using QEEG as part of an assessment battery in patients in a clinical setting is currently being done in practice. Below are two clinical examples of how this is carried out.

25.7.1 Case #1

LR was a 41-year-old woman who slipped on ice falling backwards, striking her occiput. She did not lose consciousness. She complained of pain in the occiput, nausea, and dizziness at the time of her injury. Over the next week she suffered daily headaches in the occipital regions, disequilibrium, light and sound sensitivity. She had no prior history of migraines. She saw her primary care provider, and subsequently was referred for neurologic evaluation. Detailed neurologic examination was normal. Computerized neurocognitive testing demonstrated average (50%) performance in all domains. Her first EEG was recorded within a week of her injury. Routine visual inspection of this EEG was unremarkable. Quantitative EEG analysis included spectral flat maps with absolute power, relative power, and z-score comparisons against an age-matched normative database. Fig. 25.13 displays the z-score flat maps of both absolute and relative power in the eyes closed, awake condition. Z-score absolute power maps demonstrate increased delta/theta activity in the temporal regions, right parietal and right occipital regions. sLORETA 3D current source density Z-score analysis comparisons to the age-matched norms demonstrated increased delta activity in the temporal lobes, occipital lobes, and right parietal lobe, increased theta activity in the right parietal lobe, and reduced beta activity in the midline frontal lobes displayed in Fig. 25.14, first row (EEG 1 Delta).

She began neurofeedback after 4 months of persistent symptoms. Neurofeedback therapy is a form of biofeedback which monitors EEG in real time during the therapy sessions to guide operant conditioning feedback by rewarding specific EEG features during the session. In LR's case the neurofeedback reward was designed to provide rewards when her EEG activity demonstrated reduced delta/theta activity and increased beta activity in the regions of interest guided by the QEEG, including the temporal lobes, occipital lobes, and right parietal lobe. She completed 20 sessions in 8 weeks, after which she reported dramatic improvement of symptoms, estimating she was 85% back to normal. Repeat QEEG demonstrated a marked improvement in delta excess and beta deficit with persistent increased delta activity in the right temporal lobe, and reduced beta activity in the midline frontal lobes. This was not clearly identified on the 2D spectral map (Fig. 25.13 row 2/EEG 2) but was seen using the sLORETA analysis. The delta band sLORETA maps are displayed in Fig. 25.14, second row/EEG 2 Delta. She completed another 10 sessions of neurofeedback over the next 2 months focused on the remaining regions of interests that showed EEG deregulation (right temporal and midline frontal lobes). At follow-up 10 months after injury she experienced occasional headaches, less than once per month, with complete resolution of all other concussion-related symptoms. Computerized neurocognitive testing demonstrated performance in the top quartile in comparison to her peers. QEEG showed complete resolution of the excess delta activity and only a small region of

EEG 1

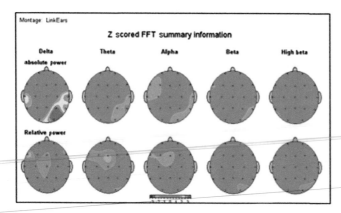

EEG 2

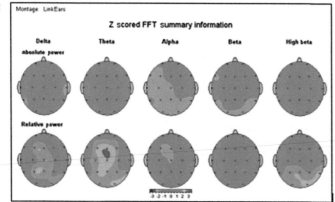

EEG 3

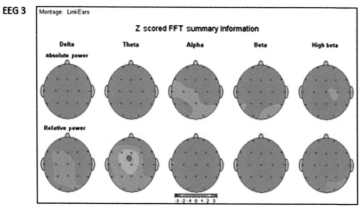

FIGURE 25.13 EEG1: 41-year-old woman, 3 days after slip and fall injury on ice, striking the occiput. The first EEG done within 1 week of injury (EEG 1) surface 2D maps demonstrate increased delta/theta activity in the right occipital, parietal, and bilateral temporal regions. EEG2: Quantitative EEG analysis surface 2D maps 4 months after injury with marked improvement of signs and symptoms of concussion "85% back to normal" demonstrate resolution of the increased delta activity. EEG3: Quantitative EEG surface 2D analysis 10 months after injury demonstrates normal quantitative mapping.

reduced beta activity in the left frontal lobe remained (Fig. 25.13, third row/EEG 3 and Fig. 25.14, third row EEG 3 delta). Figs. 25.15 and 25.16 display sLORETA abnormalities that resolved in theta and beta bands, respectively, in this same patient.

EEG 1 Delta

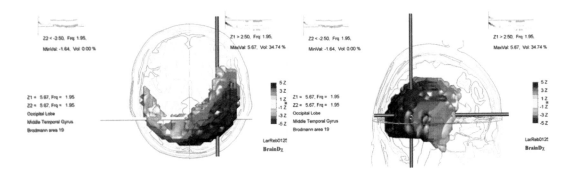

EEG 2 Delta

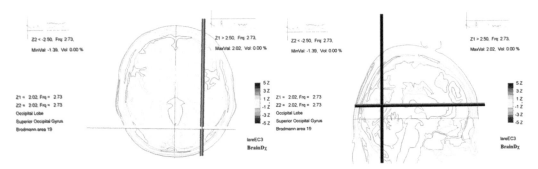

EEG 3 Delta

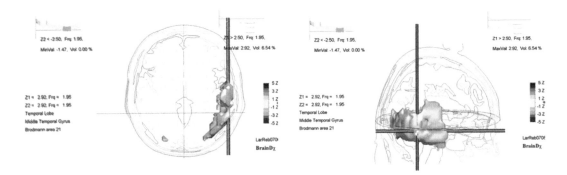

FIGURE 25.14   EEG 1: sLORETA 3D current source density analysis demonstrates Z-score 3D maps of band activity. The top row EEG 1 delta sLORETA maps display an increase in delta band activity in the temporal lobes, occipital lobes, and right parietal lobe. EEG 2 delta sLORETA maps taken 4 months later demonstrate marked improvement of the increased delta activity with a residual region of increased delta activity in the right temporal lobe. The third row, EEG 3 delta, taken 10 months following injury, demonstrate resolution of the increased delta activity.

EEG 1 Theta

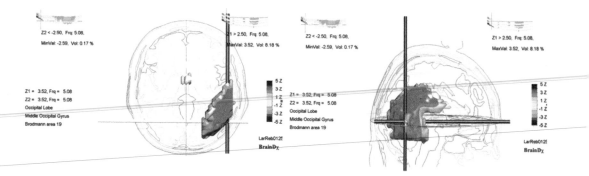

EEG 2 Theta

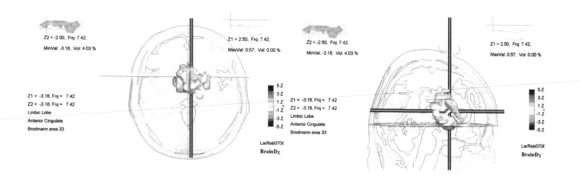

EEG 3 Theta

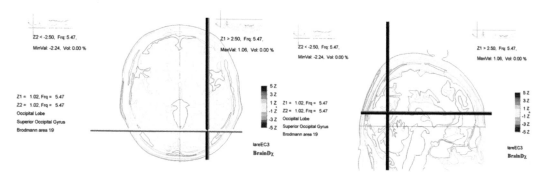

FIGURE 25.15   The figure showing a similar progressive improvement in the theta band abnormality, with increased theta activity in the right temporal lobe, resolving by the second EEG.

EEG 1 Beta

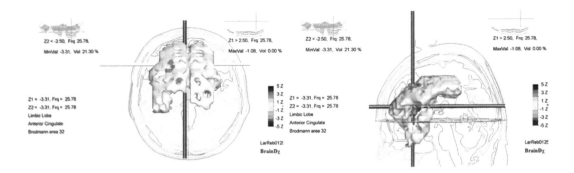

EEG 2 Beta

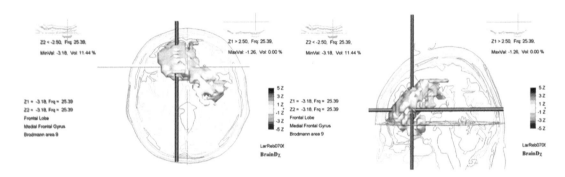

EEG 3 Beta

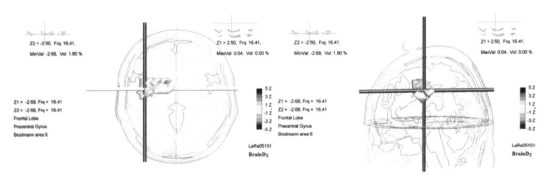

FIGURE 25.16   Figure demonstrating abnormally reduced beta band activity in the frontal regions following the injury that progressively improved at 4 and 10 months.

25.7.2 Case #2

JS was a 16-year-old female cheerleader who was stunting during practice when a flyer fell on her head causing a flexion—extension "whiplash" injury. Immediate symptoms included nausea, light-headedness, vertigo, pulsatile headache, vertigo, light and sound sensitivity. Later she developed constant daily headaches that rate mild to severe, trouble sleeping, extreme fatigue, personality and emotional changes, blurred vision, problems focusing, problems trying to find the right words to say, or forgetting what words mean. Prior to the injury she was an A—B student at a college prep school. She complained of feeling off-balance while going from sitting to standing or walking up or down stairs. She had a previous history of two concussions in the previous 2 years. Detailed neurological examination was normal. Vergence testing demonstrated 6 diopter weakness of convergence compared to normal. Computerized neurocognitive testing demonstrated broad impairment of multiple cognitive domains. Vestibular autorotation test was consistent with peripheral vestibular dysfunction. Her first EEG was recorded 8 days after injury while still symptomatic. Routine visual inspection of the EEG was normal. Quantitative surface 2D flat maps failed to demonstrate any abnormalities on Z-score analysis (Fig. 25.17). On the contrary, sLORETA 3D current source density Z-score analysis demonstrated increased delta activity in the temporal lobes bilaterally and left frontal lobe (Fig. 25.18), increased beta and gamma (25–35 Hz) activity in the left frontal, temporal, and parietal lobes (Fig. 25.19). Concussion management included relative rest until symptom free, nutritional supplements, trazodone to help with sleep, and neurofeedback with operant conditioning feedback, rewarding normalization of delta, beta, and gamma activity in the regions of deregulation identified on the sLORETA QEEG stated above. The neurofeedback utilized real-time instantaneous comparisons to the normative database (live Z-score training, LZT) [36,48].

After 10 sessions over 10 weeks, her headaches had subsided to occasional and only to a mild degree of pain, her vision and vertigo had improved, and her school performance returned to straight As. Vergence testing normalized. She remained symptom-free through a five-step progressive exertion program. Repeat computerized neurocognitive testing showed a return to the 90th percentile performance. Repeat EEG demonstrates a marked reduction of the excess delta activity (Fig. 25.18), and modest reduction of excess beta and gamma activity on sLORETA Z-score analysis (Fig. 25.19). However, in spite of resolution of her clinical signs and symptoms of concussion there was still some degree of residual EEG abnormality with increased beta-gamma activity. This is the same finding as stated in the work presented by Kerasidis suggesting that this increased beta-gamma activity may reflect a compensatory process occurring to overcome the physiologic changes and dysfunction induced by concussion related to the mTBI [32,33].

25.8 Future directions of electroencephalographic technologies in the field of concussion identification and management

The information embedded within the EEG signal, if extracted properly and processed correctly, can provide insight that can be utilized clinically way beyond other type of

EEG 1

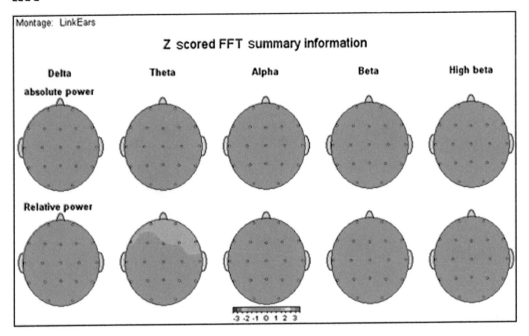

EEG 2

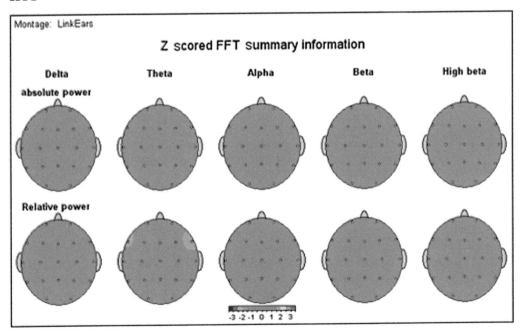

FIGURE 25.17 Figure displays surface 2D quantitative analysis performed 8 days after concussion injury, which fails to demonstrate any significant variation from the age-matched normative database (top rows/EEG 1) and again with the second EEG recorded 64 days after injury (bottom rows/EEG 2).

EEG 1 Delta

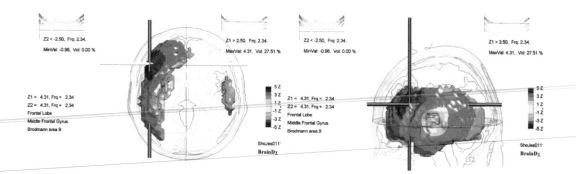

EEG Delta

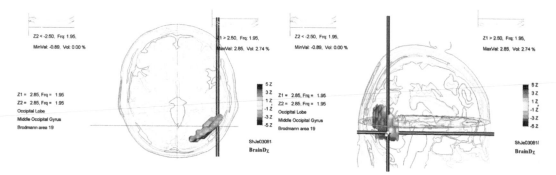

FIGURE 25.18   Figure displays sLORETA EEG data. The top row/EEG 1 is of sLORETA 3D current source density analysis, recorded 8 days after injury. This demonstrates increased delta activity in the left frontal, left temporal, and, to a lesser extent, the right temporal lobe. The bottom row/EEG 2 is of similar sLORETA 3D maps, recorded after symptom resolution at 64 days after injury. This demonstrates a marked reduction of the increased delta activity confined to a small region in the right occipital lobe.

signals, such as magnetoencephalography, that are not feasible to be implemented in a large-scale fashion in a multitude of settings. Using the advanced signal processing methods described above, present progress suggests that we will soon be able to use QEEG to identify mTBI in the acute setting and track clinical progress in a routine fashion. The EEG will be viewed as a vital sign of the brain, as it should. The reliance of qualitative assessment that can deviate tremendously between clinicians will no longer be an issue. Collecting data in the acute setting, from the side line of the football field, or from the scene of an accident, will become commonplace as electrode and cap technologies improve. Data will be transmitted immediately to a remote center for analysis and clinical guidance will be given based on the results of the assessment. These concepts are not new.

EEG 1 Delta

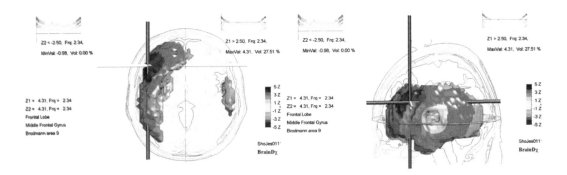

EEG Delta

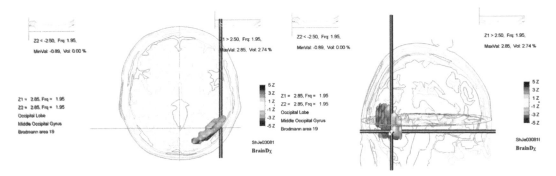

FIGURE 25.19   Figure displays sLORETA 3D current source density analysis in the beta-gamma band. The top row/EEG 1 beta-gamma, taken 8 days after injury, demonstrates increased beta-gamma activity in the left frontal, temporal, and parietal lobes. The bottom row/EEG 2 beta-gamma, taken after clinical resolution of concussion symptoms at 64 days postinjury, demonstrates improvement with reduction of the gray matter volume generating increased beta-gamma activity in the right occipital, parietal, and mesial temporal lobes.

Simmons and colleagues [49] were granted funding by the NIH in 1997 to explore method of EEG acquisition and remote transmission using wireless technologies. Ahead of its time, the grant looked to explore how EEG could be used in the acute setting by EMTs out in the field. Now with the miniaturization of the electrical components and the vast extension of cellular data transmission technologies, the incorporation of EEG in the acute clinical evaluation is much more realistic than it was in 1997. We anticipate that as this text becomes published and read, updated editions will have more extensive coverage of EEG technologies, as these become more readily available, verified, and incorporated as common assessment and treatment tools for patients with concussions.

References

[1] Azuma H, Hori S, Nakanishi M, Fujimoto S, Ichikawa N, Furukawa T. An intervention to improve the inter-rater reliability of clinical EEG interpretations. Psychiat Clin Neurosci 2003;57:485–9.

[2] Jasper HH. The ten-twenty electrode system of the international federation. Electroencephalogr Clin Neurophysiol 1958;10:371–5.

[3] Nuwer M, Hovda D, Schrader L, Vespa P. Routine and quantitative EEG in mild traumatic brain injury. Clin Neurophysiol 2005;116(9):2001–25.

[4] Fenton G. The postconcussional syndrome reappraised. Clin Electroencephalogr 1996;27(4):174–82.

[5] Schoenhuber R, Gentilini M, Orlando A. Prognostic value of auditory brain-stem responses for late postconcussion symptoms following minor head injury. J Neurosurg 1988;68(5):742–4.

[6] Kothari R, Bokariya P, Singh S, Singh R. A comprehensive review on methodologies employed for visual evoked potentials. Scientifica (Cairo) 2016;2016:9852194.

[7] Kutas M, Hillyard SA. Reading senseless sentences: brain potentials reflect semantic incongruity. Science 1980;207:203–8.

[8] Hinojosa J, Mercado F, Carretié L. N170 sensitivity to facial expression: a meta-analysis. Neurosci Biobehav Rev 2015;55:498–509.

[9] Rapp P, Keyser D, Albano A. Traumatic brain injury detection using electrophysiological methods. Front Hum Neurosci 2015;9:11.

[10] Dupuis F, Johnston M, Lavoie M, et al. Concussions in athletes produce brain dysfunction as revealed by event-related potentials. NeuroReport 2001;11:4087–92.

[11] Duncan CC, Kosmidis MH, Mirsky AF. Event–related potential assessment of information processing after closed head injury. Psychophysiology 2003;40:45–59.

[12] Duncan CC, Kosmidis MH, Mirsky AF. Closed head injury-related information processing deficits: an event-related potential analysis. Int J Psychophysiol 2005;58:133–57.

[13] Gosselin N, Bottari C, Chen JK, Huntgeburth SC, De Beaumont L, Petrides M, et al. Evaluating the cognitive consequences of mild traumatic brain injury and concussion by using electrophysiology. Neurosurg Focus 2012;33(6).

[14] Tempelhoff R, Modica P, Grubb R, et al. Selective shunting during carotid endarterectomy based on two-channel computerized electroencephalographic/compressed spectral array analysis. Neurosurgery 1989;24(3):339–44.

[15] Bricolo A, Turazzi S, Faccioli F, Odorizzi F, Sciaretta G, Erculiani P. Clinical application of compressed spectral array in long-term EEG monitoring of comatose patients. Electroencephalogr Clin Neurophysiol 1978;45(2):211–25.

[16] Nuwer M. Assessment of digital EEG, quantitative EEG, and EEG brain mapping: report of the American Academy of Neurology and the American Clinical Neurophysiology Society. Neurology 1997;49(1).

[17] Vespa PM, Nuwer MR, Juhasz C, et al. Early detection of vasospasm after acute subarachnoid hemorrhage using continuous EEG Monitoring. Electroencephalogr Clin Neurophysiol 1997;103(6):607–15.

[18] Gosselin N, Lassonde M, Petit D, Leclerc S, Mongrain V, Collie A, et al. Sleep following sport-related concussions. SleepMed 2009;10:35–46. Available from: https://doi.org/10.1016/j.sleep.2007.11.023.

[19] Haglund Y, Persson HE. Does Swedish amateur boxing lead to chronic brain damage. 3. A retrospective clinical neurophysiological study. Acta Neurol Scand 1990;82:353–60. Available from: https://doi.org/10.1111/j.1600-0404.1990.tb03316.x.

[20] Coutin-Churchman B, Anez Y, Uzcategui M, Alvarez L, Vergara F, Mendez LO, et al. Quantitative spectral analysis of EEG in psychiatry revisited: drawing signs out of numbers in a clinical setting. Clin Neurophysiol 2003;114:2294–306. Available from: https://doi.org/10.1016/S1388-2457(03)00228-1.

[21] Thatcher R, Walker R, Gerson I, Geisler F. EEG discriminant analyses of mild head trauma. Electroencephalogr Clin Neurophysiol 1989;73(2):94–106.

[22] Duffy FH, Burchfiel JL, Lombroso CT. Brain electrical activity mapping (BEAM): a method for extending the clinical utility of EEG and evoked potential data. Ann Neurol 1979;5(4):309–21.

[23] Duffy FH, Bartels PH, Burchfiel JL. Significance probability mapping: an aid in the topographic analysis of brain electrical activity. Electroencephalogr Clin Neurophysiol 1981;51(5):455–62.

[24] Thatcher R, Walker R, Biver C, North D, Curtin R. Quantitative EEG normative databases: validation and clinical correlation. J Neurother 2003;7(3–4):87–121. Available from: https://doi.org/10.1300/J184v07n03_05.

[25] John E. Neurometrics: clinical applications of quantitative electrophysiology. Hillsdale, NJ; New York: L. Erlbaum Associates Distributed by the Halsted Press Division, Wiley; 1977. ISBN 9780470992722.

[26] Thatcher R, Lubar J. History of the scientific standards of QEEG normative databases. introduction to quantitative EEG and neurofeedback advanced theory and applications. Academic Press; 2009. Chapter 2.

[27] Pascual-Marqui R. Review of methods for solving the EEG inverse problem. Int J Bioelectromagn 1999;1 (1):75−86.

[28] Pascual-Marqui R. Standardized low resolution brain electromagnetic tomography (sLORETA): technical details. Method Find Exp Clin Pharmacol 2002;24D:5−12.

[29] Cannon R, Kerson C, Hampshire A. sLORETA and fMRI detection of medial prefrontal default network anomalies in adult ADHD. J Neurother 2011;15(4):358−73.

[30] Vitacco D, Brandeis D, Pascual-Marqui R, Martin E. Correspondence of event-related potential tomography and functional magnetic resonance imaging during language processing. Hum Brain Mapp 2002;17:4−12.

[31] Cannon R, Baldwin D, Shaw T, et al. Reliability of quantitative EEG (qEEG) measures and LORETA current source density at 30 days. Neurosci Lett 2012;518(1):27−31.

[32] Kerasidis H, Ims D. sLORETA quantitative EEG analysis demonstrates persistent EEG changes beyond clinical recovery from sport concussion in high school athletes: a volumetric study. Abstract presented at the annual meeting of the American Academy of Neurology Sport Concussion Conference; 2017.

[33] Kerasidis H, Ims D, Rector S. Gender differences in quantitative volumetric analysis shortly after sport concussion in high school athletes. Abstract presented at the annual meeting of the American Academy of Neurology Sport Concussion Conference; 2018.

[34] Ledwidge P, Molfese D. Long-term effects of concussion on electrophysiological indices of attention in varsity college athletes: an event-related potential and standardized low-resolution brain electromagnetic tomography approach. J Neurotrauma 2016;33(23):2081−90.

[35] Thatcher R, North D, Biver C. Evaluation and validity of a LORETA normative EEG database. Clin EEG Neurosci 2005;36(2):116−22.

[36] Thompson M, Thompson L, Reid-Chung A. Treating postconcussion syndrome with LORETA Z-score neurofeedback and heart rate variability biofeedback: neuroanatomical/neurophysiological rationale, methods, and case examples. Biofeedback 2015;43(1):15−26.

[37] Giza CC, Kutcher JS, Ashwal S, Barth J, Getchius TSD, Gioia GA, et al. Summary of evidence-based guideline update: evaluation and management of concussion in sports: report of the guideline development subcommittee of the American Academy of Neurology. Neurology 2013;80(24):2250−7.

[38] Broglio S, Cantu R, Gioia G, et al. National athletic trainers' association position statement: management of sport concussion. J Athl Train 2014;49(2):245−65.

[39] Mccrory P, Meeuwisse WH, Aubry M, Cantu B, Dvorak J, Echemendia RJ, et al. Consensus statement on concussion in sport the 4th international conference on concussion in sport held in Zurich, November 2012. Clin J Sport Med 2013;23(2):89−117.

[40] Reches A, Kutcher J, Elbin R, et al. Preliminary investigation of brain network activation (BNA) and its clinical utility in sport-related concussion. Brain Inj 2017;31(2):237−46.

[41] Hanley D, Prichep L, Bazarian J. Emergency department triage of traumatic head injury using a brain electrical activity biomarker: a multisite prospective observational validation trial. Acad Emerg Med 2017;24 (5):617−27.

[42] McCrea M, Prichep L, Powell M, Chabot R, Barr W. Acute effects and recovery after sport-related concussion: a neurocognitive and quantitative brain electrical activity study. J Head Trauma Rehabil 2010;25 (4):283−92.

[43] Duff Jaques. The usefulness of quantitative EEG (QEEG) and neurotherapy in the assessment and treatment of post-concussion syndrome. Clin EEG Neurosci 2004;35(4):198−209.

[44] Barr W, Prichep L, Chabot R, Powell M, McCrea M. Measuring brain electrical activity to track recovery from sport-related concussion. Brain Inj 2012;26(1):58−66.

[45] Giza CC, Hovda DA. The new neurometabolic cascade of concussion. Neurosurgery 2014;75(Suppl. 4): S24−33.

[46] Wright AD, Jarrett M, Vavasour I, et al. Myelin water fraction is transiently reduced after a single mild traumatic brain injury—a prospective Cohort study in Collegiate hockey players. PLoS One 2016;11:e0150215.

[47] Wang Y, Nelson LD, LaRoche AA, et al. Cerebral blood flow alterations in acute Sports-Related concussion. J Neurotrauma 2015;10:1—36.

[48] Koberda L. Z-Score LORETA neurofeedback as a potential therapy in cognitive dysfunction and dementia. J Psychol Clin Psychiatry 2015;1(6):00037.

[49] NIH SBIR Contract # NS72370-000, rest technologies, Chris Mann, Jerald Simmons, continuous EEG monitoring methodologies, awarded; 1997.

Further reading

Cao C, Slobounov S. Alteration of cortical functional connectivity as a result of traumatic brain injury revealed by graph theory, ICA, and sLORETA analyses of EEG signals. IEEE Trans Neural Sys Rehab Eng 2010;18(1).

Lavoie M, Dupuis F, Johnston K, et al. Visual P300 effects beyond symptoms in concussed college athletes. J Clin Exp Neuropsychol 2004;26(1).

Mendez C, Hurley R, Lassonde M, et al. Mild traumatic brain injury: neuroimaging of sports-related concussion. J Neuropsychiatry Clin Neurosci 2005;17(3):297—303.

Pascual-Marqui R, Esslen M, Kochi K, Lehmann D. Functional imaging with low resolution brain electromagnetic tomography (LORETA): a review. Method Find Exp Clin Pharmacol 2002;24C:91—5.

Pascual-Marquia R, Lehmanna D, Koenig K, et al. Low resolution brain electromagnetic tomography (LORETA) functional imaging in acute, neuroleptic-naive, first-episode, productive schizophrenia. Psychiat Res Neuroimag 1999;90(3):169—79.

Reches A, Levy-Cooperman N, Laufer I, Shani-Hershkovitch R, Ziv K, Kerem D, et al. Brain Network Activation (BNA) reveals scopolamine-induced impairment of visual working memory. J Mol Neurosci 2014;54(1):59—70.

Neuropsychological testing

*Jeffrey Brennan[1], Kevin K. Wang[2,3], Richard Rubenstein[4],
Claudia S. Robertson[5] and Harvey Levin[5,6]*

[1]University of Texas School of Public Health, Houston, TX, United States [2]University of
Florida, Gainesville, FL, United States [3]Brain Rehabilitation Research Center, Malcom Randall
VA Medical Center, Gainesville, FL, United States [4]Downstate Medical School, Brooklyn, NY,
United States [5]Neurosurgery Department, Baylor College of Medicine, Houston, TX, United
States [6]Michael E. DeBakey Veterans Affairs Medical Center, Houston, TX, United States

26.1 Neuropsychological tests

Traumatic brain injuries (TBI) produce lasting mental effects that inhibit the patient's quality of life. It is imperative to test patients for neuropsychological outcomes in order to guide treatment. In addition to these tests, fluid biomarkers that are known to significantly correlate with outcome measures can aid in diagnosing damage resulting from TBI. Four domains of neuropsychological testing were considered: (1) memory; (2) processing speed; (3) executive function; and (4) mood, including posttraumatic stress disorder (PTSD) and postconcussive syndrome (PCS).

Table 26.1 summarizes four primary outcome categories that are assessed after a TBI event to determine the neuropsychological functioning of the patient. These tests extend biomarker sampling by directly assessing the outcome domains most likely to be impaired by a TBI event. Tests that were included in the table are frequently used in clinical practice and research; they are also NINDS common data elements. Supplemental tests, which can be more expensive, time-consuming, or complex, can be given to the patient contingent on their initial test performance.

However, neuropsychological tests have notable limitations such as the effects of the patient's mood, medications, fatigue, and other factors that affect performance. Administration of neuropsychological tests should be supervised by a licensed clinical neuropsychologist who is also qualified to interpret the results. It may also be appropriate to administer more than a single test to evaluate a domain such as memory or processing

Biomarkers for Traumatic Brain Injury
DOI: https://doi.org/10.1016/B978-0-12-816346-7.00026-9

TABLE 26.1   Core neuropsychological assessments of patient outcome for TBI.

Test	Description	Measurement	Time (min)
Memory			
Brief Visuospatial Memory Test—Revised (BVMT) [1]	Patient is asked to recall the design and location of six geometric figures both immediately and after 25 min. Patient is then given a new grid of figures and asked which were in the original set.	Number of designs recalled (three separate trials)	45
Rey Auditory Verbal Learning Test (RAVLT) [2]	Patient is given 15 words and is required to recall them in any order both immediately and after a long delay (usually 20 min).	Percent of words remembered (averaged over five trials)	15
Processing speed			
Trail Making Test Part A (TMT-A) [3]	Patient is asked to draw lines that connect 25 numbers in numeric order on a piece of paper.	Number of seconds to complete	5–10
Wechsler Adult Intelligence Scale IV: Processing Speed Index (WAIS-IV) [4]	Patient is asked to quickly fill in symbols and pattern match symbols.	Score averaged between both subsets and adjusted for age	10
Executive function			
Controlled Oral Word Association Test (COWAT) [5]	Patient is given a letter from the alphabet and asked to say as many words that they can think of which start with that letter.	Number of words spoken which conform to the rules (e.g., no proper nouns). Measures verbal fluency and executive function	5
Wechsler Adult Intelligence Scale IV: Complete (WAIS-IV) [4]	Patient is given a battery of 10 subtests that are used to measure general intelligence.	Score on each subtest	45
Delis-Kaplan Executive Function System: Color Word Interference (Stroop Test) [6]	Patient reads words for colors that do not match the printed color of the word (interference condition) and the time taken is compared to a control condition in which the words match the color of the font.	Number of seconds to complete	7–10
Trail Making Test Part B (TMT-B) [3]	Patient connects numeric and alphabetical circles in ascending order, alternating between numbers and letters.	Number of seconds to complete	5
Mood, Postconcussion symptoms, and posttraumatic stress disorder symptoms			
Patient Health Questionnaire-9 (PHQ-9) [7]	Patient identifies the frequency with which they experience symptoms consistent with depression.	Sum of responses (frequency of depressive symptoms) to questionnaire	3
Center for Epidemiologic Studies Depression Scale (CES-D) [8]	Patient identifies the frequency with which they experience symptoms consistent with depression.	Sum of responses (frequency of depressive symptoms) to questionnaire	5

(Continued)

TABLE 26.1 (Continued)

Test	Description	Measurement	Time (min)
PTSD checklist for DSM-5 (PCL-5) [9]	Patient self-completes questionnaire that assesses PTSD symptoms based on DSM-5 definitions.	Sum of responses (strength of PTSD symptoms) to questionnaire	5
Rivermead Post-Concussion Symptoms Questionnaire (RPQ) [10]	Patient self-completes questionnaire that assesses severity of postconcussion symptoms as compared to preinjury.	Total score: sum of responses; cluster scores for cognitive, somatic, and emotional symptoms	5

speed, but this decision must be balanced by other considerations such as patient fatigue. Screening of auditory and visual abilities is also advised to avoid confounds by sensory deficits; even subtle motor deficits or incoordination could also affect the results.

Another limitation that especially affects self-report measures includes the impact of patient effort on the validity of the results. This can be assessed by using measures of symptom validity and effort. In many studies and clinical practice, data are used only when the patient passes tests of validity and effort. Despite these limitations, self-report tests offer the benefit of reduced costs and improved accessibility when compared to tests that need to be administered by a licensed interpreter. For these tests, it is important to consider the length of the assessment and whether an electronic version is available for accessibility. Most of the self-report tests also require both a neuropsychologist to interpret the results and a trained technician to administer them. Finally, normative data tables are used by clinical neuropsychologists to transform raw scores to standard scores which correct for age, education, and sex.

26.2 Memory

After a TBI event, the frontal and temporal lobes of a patient's brain are often injured. Afterward, patients have experienced impairments in both their verbal memory (which involves tasks focusing on the recall and recognition of verbal information) as well as their visual memory (which involves tasks relating to pattern recognition or picture memory) [11]. In severe cases, this impairment can last for years after the brain injury, surpassing other TBI-related cognitive impairments. Memory is a complex and multifactorial aspect of cognition. In order to accurately assess a patient's memory, a battery of different tests may be conducted depending on the context of use (e.g., clinical trial versus rehabilitation planning). The Brief Visuospatial Memory Test—Revised (BVMT) and Rey Auditory Verbal Learning Test (RAVLT) represent two introductory level tests to be used in the initial screening for memory loss following TBI. While together they do not provide a comprehensive understanding of patient memory, they provide a baseline of both the verbal and visual memory performance of the patient.

26.2.1 Brief Visuospatial Memory Test

The revised version of the BVMT was constructed by Benedict et al. in 1996, and aims to assess the visuospatial memory of a patient through pattern recognition. Patients are presented with a grid of shapes and asked to recreate them after the grid is removed from view. In addition to this test of immediate recall, patients are also asked to perform a delayed recall 25 minutes later. The third test presents a new grid of patterns to patients, who must then identify which ones were in the original set [1]. This test requires a trained practitioner to administer and a neuropsychologist to interpret. Despite its relative complexity compared to other questionnaires, the BVMT lacks the ability to effectively assess memory impairment. A study of 109 veterans found that the revised BVMT had a sensitivity of 0.31, a specificity of 0.92, and an area under the curve of 0.7 [12]. This study was replicated with 80 veterans, and Bailey et al. were unable to replicate these findings, citing that cognitive impairment and processing speed inhibited test performance too much to be considered useful, a finding first identified by Tam and Schmitter-Edgecombe in 2013 [13,14]. Researchers should take this into consideration, as well as patient age when administering this test. In Benedict's revision of the BVMT, single trial recall scores were found to be significantly associated with patient age [1].

26.2.2 Rey Auditory Verbal Learning Test

The RAVLT targets verbal memory performance. Auditory verbal learning is used as a proxy for generalized cognitive functioning. The sensitivity and specificity of this test among TBI patients varies by number of trials, with a study of 68 patients identifying a maximal area under the curve in trial V with a sensitivity of 0.735 and a specificity of 0.434. Results were found to be significantly correlated with age as well [15]. Like many neuropsychological tests, patient effort confounds RAVLT performance and should be evaluated. One performance validity indicator used to assess patient effort in the RAVLT is the embedded performance validity indicator (EPVI). This indicator was found to have a high sensitivity but low specificity for assessing patient effort [16]. While this measure can be used, it will likely produce a large number of false positive results (where patients will be flagged as exhibiting inadequate effort when in reality their effort is sufficient). Other, more widely used measures of effort and symptoms validity can be found on the NINDS website.

26.3 Processing speed

The associations between cognitive processing speed and TBI are well documented. Processing speed refers to the time it takes to complete tasks and react to stimuli. Patients who have suffered a TBI are more likely to process information slower compared to those who have not [11,17]. The Trail Making Test Part A (TMT-A) and Wechsler Adult Intelligence Scale IV: complete (WAIS-IV) processing speed index (PSI) are two core tests used for assessing processing speed, but do not represent the full range of options available.

26.3.1 Trail Making Test Part A

The paper version of the Trail Making Test Part A prompts a patient to draw a single, uninterrupted line between 25 numbered circles placed randomly on a piece of paper. While most commonly used in pediatric TBI, this test can be used with patients of all ages. Despite its relative simplicity, this test requires a trained administrator for timing patient performance and a neuropsychologist to interpret. Education and age are known to be confounders for this test, with education having a larger effect in the variation of test performance [18]. The ability for TMT-A to accurately assess a patient's processing speed is well documented, and the methodology of the test has changed over time. New studies have found that a computerized version of the test reduces variability in test scores resulting from inconsistencies in how the paper test is administered and timed. The computerized version was found to have better reliability and sensitivity compared to the paper test in a study of 165 subjects [19]. Although sensitivity is improved, the administration of a computer-based test introduces the confounder of previous computer usage, as patients with less familiarity will tend to move the mouse slower between points.

26.3.2 Wechsler Adult Intelligence Scale IV processing speed index

The WAIS-IV PSI is a subtest of the complete WAIS-IV intelligence assessment. This score has been found to significantly correlate with injury severity, and is able to discriminate between severe TBI patients and patients without TBI [20]. In addition, PSI scores can also serve as an embedded validity indicator for the complete test, with a cutoff of 79 resulting a low sensitivity (0.23–0.56) but very high specificity (0.92–0.98) [21].

26.4 Executive function

The following neuropsychological tests focus on assessing a patient's executive function, and involve completing more complex tasks and synthesizing elements of working memory, attention, organization, and flexibility. TBI patients tend to perform poorly on these assessments compared to healthy controls [22].

26.4.1 Controlled Oral Word Association Test

The Controlled Oral Word Association Test (COWAT) is a simple expressive language test that assesses the patient's ability to rapidly retrieve and verbally communicate words (verbal fluency); it also taps semantic memory when the category fluency measure is used. A version of the semantic memory test alternates strategies recalling exemplars of categories and is more sensitive to executive function. However, the phonemic (initial letter) word fluency version is sensitive to expressive language impairment. The phonemic version (COWAT) can be scored in a number of ways—the easiest of which is to sum the number of valid words said within a time period. However, additional scoring methods have been used, such as the types of word clusters and hard switches [23]. In a study of 108 undergraduates, the COWAT was found to correlate with performance on the color word interference test, but not most other tests for executive function [24]. Further, COWAT and the semantic memory version (see color-word interference test below) represent one of multiple domains of executive function. If a study or clinical trial is focusing on executive function, other neuropsychological tests are also needed. Retest reliability for the total word count was 0.84.

26.4.2 Wechsler Adult Intelligence Scale IV Complete

The complete WAIS-IV intelligence test is comprised of multiple indices: the working memory index, the PSI, the perceptual organization index, verbal comprehension index, and the full scale IQ. Together, this battery of assessments has been found to provide an accurate summary of an adult patient's intelligence, but performance may be affected by factors mentioned above [25].

26.4.3 1D-KEFS color word interference

The color word interference test comprises several subtests that assesses the executive function of a patient. This test is found to have high specificity in the detection of TBI as well as PCS [26,27]. A study of 77 patients found that the color word interference test had a sensitivity of 0.29 and a specificity of 0.95 for performance validity [28].

26.4.4 Trail Making Test Part B

Part B of the Trail Making Test has patients switch between numbered circles and letter-coded symbols. This assesses executive function in the patient, with most patients performing part B much slower than they can complete part A [29]. Completion time for part B is a sensitive and valid indicator of executive function. Age and education confounder affect the scores of part B as well. As in part A, variability in scores can be reduced through the use of a computerized version of the test [19]. Although Trail Making Test Part B (TMT-B) assesses executive function, there is a correlation coefficient of 0.73 between the two parts of the test [29].

26.5 Mood, postconcussive syndrome, posttraumatic stress disorder tests

26.5.1 Patient Health Questionnaire-9 and Center for Epidemiologic Studies Depression Scale

Beyond essential outcomes of memory and processing speed, TBI has also been found to significantly correlate with depression. Osborn et al. identified a prevalence of depression between 27% and 38% following TBI in adult patients [30]. Similar to other TBI outcomes of memory loss and cognition impairment, depression can be debilitating for the patient and inhibit their ability to heal. The most commonly used tests for depression include the Patient Health Questionnaire-9 (PHQ-9) and Center for Epidemiologic Studies Depression Scale (CES-D). The PHQ-9 is a self-administered, short neuropsychiatric test that is most commonly used to quickly assess the depressive status of a patient. The CES-D expands the questionnaire by asking additional information on the patient's frequency of positive emotions (happiness, enjoyment of life). Both of these tests produce a score which correlates with the severity of the patient's depression [7,8].

Score ranges for the PHQ-9 are broken into the following: minimal depression (0–4); mild depression (5–9); moderate depression (10–14); moderately severe depression (15–19); and severe depression (20–27). The most commonly used and sensitive cutoff point for a depression diagnosis is 10 or higher [7]. Donders and Pendery found that PHQ-9 scores >9 have a sensitivity of 91.7 and a specificity of 60.2 for predicting a major depression diagnosis [31]. Fann et al. also found the PHQ-9 to be valid and reliable, with a sensitivity of 0.93, specificity of 0.89, and a Pearson's correlation of 0.76 for test–retest reliability [32]. Overall, the PHQ-9 offers the primary advantage of being a powerful and brief screening survey to direct further patient treatment. Because of the test's brevity, there are elements of depression which are not directly assessed, and should be analyzed in a supplemental test or interview for patients with high PHQ-9 scores. Another consideration is whether the patient had any psychiatric conditions prior to TBI, which Donders and Pendery found to be the most significant confounder for elevated PHQ-9 Scores [31].

The CES-D has 20 items that target four factors of depression: depressed affect, positive affect, somatic activity, and interpersonal activity [8]. Similar to the PHQ-9, patients are asked to report how frequently they experience each symptom over the course of the week. Possible scores for this test range from 0 to 60, with each question having a weight between 0 and 3, depending on the severity of the response. The validity of the CES-D is also well-established, with strong correlations to other depression inventories, such as the Beck depression inventory [33]. One study of 336 patients who experienced TBI in the military found that the CES-D had a sensitivity of 0.897 and specificity of 0.826 when a cut point for depression was set at a score of 18 or higher. Other studies for civilian populations found the ideal cut point for a depression diagnosis to be set at a score of >15 [34,35].

26.5.2 PTSD checklist for DSM-5

The PTSD checklist for DSM-5 (PCL-5) assesses PTSD symptoms in patients following TBI, with each question targeting a factor of the DSM-5. Like the PHQ-9, the PCL-5 is a brief assessment used as a screening tool for patients who may have PTSD. In a study population of 471 undergraduate students, the PCL-5 was found to have an internal consistency alpha statistic of 0.94, and a retest reliability Pearson's r squared of 0.66 [36]. One important consideration when assessing PTSD is the performance validity of the patient, as poor performance in a word memory test could result in poor performance for subsequent cognitive tests [37].

26.5.3 Rivermead Post-Concussion Symptoms Questionnaire

The Rivermead Post-Concussion Symptoms Questionnaire (RPQ) is a 16-item questionnaire with a score range of 0 to 64. Each response is weighted equally that ranges from 0 (symptom not experienced) to 4 (symptom experienced severely) [10]. Although the RPQ has been found to be a valid and reliable assessment, researchers have identified that the utility of the test improves when the questions are split into two categories (the RPQ-13 and the RPQ-3) [38]. The scores for each section are then summed separately instead of together. Eyres et al. found the RPQ-13 to have retest reliability of 0.89 for the RPQ-13 and a retest reliability of 0.72 for the RPQ-3 (headaches, dizziness, and nausea) [38]. This was substantiated by Lannsjö et al., who also found that summing all dimensions of the RPQ into a single score resulted in poor validity, citing that the test assessed more than one single cognitive domain [39].

26.6 Biomarkers

Although the most commonly used outcome measurement studied in relation to biomarkers is the Glasgow outcome score extended (GOSE), studies have been conducted that relate biomarker levels to the outcomes of neuropsychological tests. Given the validity of neuropsychological tests in measuring specific aspects of TBI outcome, knowing which biomarkers correlate with test findings is informative for health practitioners in the treatment of their patient.

26.6.1 Glial fibrillary acidic protein

Glial fibrillary acidic protein (GFAP) is a classical biomarker recognized for its remarkable specificity compared to other biomarkers in predicting TBI [40]. Several mouse model studies have been conducted to assess functional outcomes after TBI. Increases in GFAP level correlate with inhibited spatial learning, as evidenced by decreased performance in maze trials [41–43]. Human trials focusing on TBI outcome and GFAP have been conducted, and GFAP was found to be significantly associated with Glasgow outcome score (GOS) [44]. There is currently a lack of studies in the literature that assess the relationship of GFAP to neuropsychological outcomes in human patients.

26.6.2 Ubiquitin C-terminal hydrolase L1

Ubiquitin C-terminal hydrolase L1 (UCH-L1) has been found to have a mechanical association with learning and memory [45]. Levels of UCH-L1 correlate with performance on tests of working memory (spatial span test), visual memory (complex figure test), and RAVLT. The biomarker, however, does not significantly correlate with many other neuropsychological assessments, including TMT-A, TMT-B, Stroop Test, and COWAT [46]. Overall, there is a gap in the literature regarding the relation of UCH-L1 to neuropsychological findings, and additional tests need to be done to test the work of Dey et al.

26.6.3 Tau

In a mouse model, reducing serum tau resulted in improved memory and spatial learning among mice subjected to mTBI [47]. However, cleaved tau remains a poor predictor of PCS, as it has been found to not correlate with Rivermead Post-Concussion Questionnaire performance [48,49]. Similar to GFAP and UCH-L1, there is a lack of research conducted specifically on the relationship between tau levels and neuropsychiatric test performance.

26.6.4 Neuron-specific enolase

In pediatric populations, neuron-specific enolase (NSE) significantly correlates with measures of outcome (GOS), IQ, and socialization (as measured by the Vineland adaptive behavior scale) [50,51]. NSE also correlates with neurocognitive dysfunction, including executive function and attention [52].

26.6.5 S-100β

S-100β is a classic biomarker for detecting TBI. As such, there exists a wealth of studies on the relationship between S-100β levels and various neuropsychological tests. S-100β lacks utility in detecting PCS, as the biomarker was found to not be correlated with Rivermead Post-Concussion Questionnaire scores [49]. In a review of 18 studies, Townend and Ingebrigtsen found that S-100β does not appear to significantly correlate with tests of cognition or memory (including the Stroop color test), but does, in general, correlate with postinjury disability [53,54]. Although S-100β is specific for TBI, it lacks specificity compared to both GFAP and NSE [40]. Since the relation of S-100β to various outcome measures is heterogeneous, other biomarkers appear to have better utility for this task [55–57].

26.6.6 Brain-derived neurotrophic factor

Brain-derived neurotrophic factor (BDNF) is a novel serum biomarker that has been used in studies of memory and depression. A study of 113 patients identified that this biomarker is negatively correlated with PHQ-9 scores at 12 months [58]. Reduced levels of BDNF are associated with increased PHQ-9 scores (which reflect a greater severity of depression). The same study also assessed the relationship between BDNF and a cognitive composite score. This score comprised Trails Making Test A, the Wechsler Adult Intelligence Scale-R, Controlled Oral Word Association, Trails Making Test B, and Color Word Interference tests, among others. BDNF was found to positively correlate with the memory composites at 6 and 12 months. Additional studies in mouse models have also found a correlation between BDNF and short-term as well as long-term memory performance, establishing the mechanism for this interaction [59]. In addition to a correlation with neuropsychological outcomes, a decrease in BDNF also correlates with TBI injury severity [60].

26.7 Conclusion

As blood biomarker research continues to grow and biomarkers are clinically implemented as a diagnostic tool, it is crucial for the relationship between biomarkers and neuropsychological tests to be understood. In instances of strong correlation, biomarker levels can be used in the consideration of valid test performance, and may also indicate the need for additional testing. Despite a substantial amount of research existing on the relation between blood biomarkers and neuropsychological findings, there are many combinations of biomarkers and test outcomes that have not yet been studied. Biomarkers especially in need of additional research in this regard include GFAP, UCH-L1, and tau.

Acknowledgment

Preparation of this chapter and the research described were supported by NINDS grant #- U01NS086090, TRACK-TBI (PI: Geoff Manley, MD, PhD).

Subject

The relation of fluid biomarkers to neuropsychological functioning as determined by commonly used neuropsychological tests.

References

[1] Benedict RHB, Schretlen D, Groninger L, Dobraski M, Shpritz B. Revision of the brief visuospatial memory test: studies of normal performance, reliability, and validity. Psychol Assess 1996;8(2):145–53. Available from: https://doi.org/10.1037/1040-3590.8.2.145.

[2] Rey A. L'examen psychologique: Dans les cas d'encephalopathie traumatique (Les problemes). Arch Psychol 1941;28:286–340.

[3] Reitan RM, Wolfson D. The Halstead-Reitan neuropsychological test battery. The neuropsychology handbook: behavioral and clinical perspectives. New York, NY, US: Springer Publishing Co; 1986. p. 134–60.

[4] Wechsler DA. Wechsler adult intelligence scale. 4th ed. San Antonio, TX: Psychological Corporation; 2008.

[5] Benton AL, de Hamsher SK, Sivan AB. Multilingual aplasia examination. 2nd ed. Iowa City, IA: AJA Associates; 1983.

[6] Delis DC, Kaplan E, Kramer JH. Delis–Kaplan Executive Function System (D-KEFS): examiner's manual. San Antonio, TX: The Psychological Corporation; 2001.

[7] Kroenke K, Spitzer RL, Williams JBW. The PHQ-9. J Gen Intern Med 2001;16(9):606–13. Available from: https://doi.org/10.1046/j.1525-1497.2001.016009606.x.

[8] Radloff LS. The CES-D Scale: a self-report depression scale for research in the general population. Appl Psychol Meas 1977;1(3):385–401. Available from: https://doi.org/10.1177/014662167700100306.

[9] Weathers FW, Litz BT, Keane TM, Palmieri PA, Marx BP, Schnurr PP. The PTSD checklist for DSM-5 (PCL-5); 2013. Available from: https://www.ptsd.va.gov/professional/assessment/adult-sr/ptsd-checklist.asp.

[10] King NS, Crawford S, Wenden FJ, Moss NE, Wade DT. The Rivermead Post Concussion Symptoms Questionnaire: a measure of symptoms commonly experienced after head injury and its reliability. J Neurol 1995;242(9):587–92.

[11] Vakil E. The effect of moderate to severe traumatic brain injury (TBI) on different aspects of memory: a selective review. J Clin Exp Neuropsychol 2005;27(8):977–1021. Available from: https://doi.org/10.1080/13803390490919245.

[12] Sawyer RJI, Testa SM, Dux M. Embedded performance validity tests within the Hopkins Verbal Learning Test—Revised and the Brief Visuospatial Memory Test—revised. Clin Neuropsychologist 2017;31(1):207–18. Available from: https://doi.org/10.1080/13854046.2016.1245787.

[13] Bailey KC, Soble JR, Bain KM, Fullen C. Embedded performance validity tests in the Hopkins Verbal Learning Test—revised and the Brief Visuospatial Memory Test—revised: a replication study. Arch Clin Neuropsychol 2018;33(7):895–900. Available from: https://doi.org/10.1093/arclin/acx111.

[14] Tam JW, Schmitter-Edgecombe M. The role of processing speed in the Brief Visuospatial Memory Test—Revised. Clin Neuropsychol 2013;27(6):962–72. Available from: https://doi.org/10.1080/13854046.2013.797500.

[15] Schoenberg MR, Dawson KA, Duff K, Patton D, Scott JG, Adams RL. Test performance and classification statistics for the Rey Auditory Verbal Learning Test in selected clinical samples. Arch Clin Neuropsychol 2006;21(7):693−703. Available from: https://doi.org/10.1016/j.acn.2006.06.010.

[16] Poreh A, Tolfo S, Krivenko A, Teaford M. Base-rate data and norms for the Rey Auditory Verbal Learning Embedded Performance Validity Indicator. Appl Neuropsychol Adult 2017;24(6):540−7. Available from: https://doi.org/10.1080/23279095.2016.1223670.

[17] Madigan NK, DeLuca J, Diamond BJ, Tramontano G, Averill A. Speed of information processing in traumatic brain injury: modality-specific factors. J Head Trauma Rehab 2000;15(3):943−56.

[18] Periáñez JA, Ríos-Lago M, Rodríguez-Sánchez JM, et al., Trail making test in traumatic brain injury, schizophrenia, and normal ageing: sample comparisons and normative data, Arch Clinic Neuropsychol 2007;22(4):433−47. https://doi.org/10.1016/j.acn.2007.01.02.

[19] Woods D, Wyma J, Herron T, Yund E. The effects of aging, malingering, and traumatic brain injury on computerized trail-making test performance. PLoS One 2015;10(6):e0124345. Available from: https://doi.org/10.1371/journal.pone.0124345.

[20] Carlozzi NE, Kirsch NL, Kisala PA, Tulsky DS. An examination of the Wechsler Adult Intelligence Scales, Fourth Edition (WAIS-IV) in individuals with complicated mild, moderate and severe traumatic brain injury (TBI). Clin Neuropsychol 2015;29(1):1−17. Available from: https://doi.org/10.1080/13854046.2015.1005677.

[21] Erdodi LA, Abeare CA, Lichtenstein JD, Tyson BT, Kucharski B, Zuccato BG, et al. Wechsler Adult Intelligence Scale-Fourth Edition (WAIS-IV) processing speed scores as measures of noncredible responding: the third generation of embedded performance validity indicators. Psychol Assess 2017;29(2):148−57. Available from: https://doi.org/10.1037/pas0000319.

[22] Mozeiko J, Le K, Coelho C, Krueger F, Grafman J. The relationship of story grammar and executive function following TBI. Aphasiology 2011;25(6−7):826−35. Available from: https://doi.org/10.1080/02687038.2010.543983.

[23] Abwender DA, Swan JG, Bowerman JT, Connolly SW. Qualitative analysis of verbal fluency output: review and comparison of several scoring methods. Assessment 2001;8(3):323−38. Available from: https://doi.org/10.1177/107319110100800308.

[24] Ross TP, Calhoun E, Cox T, Wenner C, Kono W, Pleasant M. The reliability and validity of qualitative scores for the controlled oral word association test. Arch Clin Neuropsychol 2007;22(4):475−88. Available from: https://doi.org/10.1016/j.acn.2007.01.026.

[25] Iverson GL, Holdnack JA, Lange RT. Chapter 10—Using the WAIS−IV/WMS−IV/ACS following moderate-severe traumatic brain injury. In: Holdnack, JA, Drozdick, LW, Weiss, LG, Iverson, GL, editors. WAIS-IV, WMS-IV, and ACS; 2013. p. 485−544. https://doi.org/10.1016/B978-0-12-386934-0.00010-9.

[26] Cicerone KD, Azulay J. Diagnostic utility of attention measures in postconcussion syndrome. Clin Neuropsychol 2002;16(3):280−9. Available from: https://doi.org/10.1076/clin.16.3.280.13849.

[27] Simpson A, Schmitter-Edgecombe M. Intactness of inhibitory attentional mechanisms following severe closed-head injury. Neuropsychology 2000;14(2):310−19. Available from: https://doi.org/10.1037/0894-4105.14.2.310.

[28] Guise BJ, Thompson MD, Greve KW, Bianchini KJ, West L. Assessment of performance validity in the Stroop Color and Word Test in mild traumatic brain injury patients: a criterion-groups validation design. J Neuropsychol 2014;8(1):20−33. Available from: https://doi.org/10.1111/jnp.12002.

[29] Sánchez-Cubillo I, Periáñez JA, Adrover-Roig D, Rodríguez-Sánchez JM, Ríos-Lago M, Tirapu J, et al. Construct validity of the Trail Making Test: role of task-switching, working memory, inhibition/interference control, and visuomotor abilities. J Int Neuropsychol Soc 2009;15(3):438−50. Available from: https://doi.org/10.1017/S1355617709090626.

[30] Osborn AJ, Mathias JL, Fairweather-Schmidt AK. Depression following adult, non-penetrating traumatic brain injury: a meta-analysis examining methodological variables and sample characteristics. Neurosci Biobehav Rev 2014;47:1−15. Available from: https://doi.org/10.1016/j.neubiorev.2014.07.007.

[31] Donders J, Pendery A. Clinical utility of the Patient Health Questionnaire-9 in the assessment of major depression after broad-spectrum traumatic brain injury. Arch Phys Med Rehab 2017;98(12):2514−19. Available from: https://doi.org/10.1016/j.apmr.2017.05.019.

[32] Fann RJ, Bombardier CH, Dikmen S, Esselman P, Warms CA, Pelzer E, et al. Validity of the Patient Health Questionnaire-9 in assessing depression following traumatic brain injury. J Head Trauma Rehab 2005;20(6):501−11. Available from: https://doi.org/10.1097/00001199-200511000-00003.

[33] Bush BA, Novack TA, Schneider JJ, Madan A. Depression following traumatic brain injury: the validity of the CES-D as a brief screening device. J ClPsychol Med Sett 2004;11(3):195–201. Available from: https://doi.org/10.1023/B:JOCS.0000037613.69367.d4.

[34] Kennedy JE, Reid MW, Lu LH, Cooper DB. Validity of the CES-D for depression screening in military service members with a history of mild traumatic brain injury. Brain Inj 2019;0(0):1–9. Available from: https://doi.org/10.1080/02699052.2019.1610191.

[35] Lewinsohn PM, Seeley JR, Roberts RE, Allen NB. Center for Epidemiologic Studies Depression Scale (CES-D) as a screening instrument for depression among community-residing older adults. Psychol Aging 1997;12(2):277–87.

[36] Conybeare D, Behar E, Solomon A, Newman MG, Borkovec TD. The PTSD Checklist—Civilian version: reliability, validity, and factor structure in a nonclinical sample. J Clin Psychol 2012;68(6):699–713. Available from: https://doi.org/10.1002/jclp.21845.

[37] Wisdom NM, Pastorek NJ, Miller BI, Booth JE, Romesser JM, Linck JF, et al. PTSD and cognitive functioning: importance of including performance validity testing. Clin Neuropsychol 2014;28(1):128–45. Available from: https://doi.org/10.1080/13854046.2013.863977.

[38] Eyres S, Carey A, Gilworth G, Neumann V, Tennant A. Construct validity and reliability of the Rivermead Post-Concussion Symptoms Questionnaire. Clin Rehab 2005;19(8):878–87. Available from: https://doi.org/10.1191/0269215505cr905oa.

[39] Lannsjö M, Borg J, Björklund G, Af Geijerstam J-L, Lundgren-Nilsson A. Internal construct validity of the Rivermead Post-Concussion Symptoms Questionnaire. J Rehab Med 2011;43(11):997–1002. Available from: https://doi.org/10.2340/16501977-0875.

[40] Honda M, Tsuruta R, Kaneko T, Kasaoka S, Yagi T, Todani M, et al. Serum glial fibrillary acidic protein is a highly specific biomarker for traumatic brain injury in humans compared with S-100B and neuron-specific enolase. J Trauma Acute Care Surg 2010;69(1):104. Available from: https://doi.org/10.1097/TA.0b013e3181bbd485.

[41] Ferguson S, Mouzon B, Paris D, Aponte D, Abdullah L, Stewart W, et al. Acute or delayed treatment with anatabine improves spatial memory and reduces pathological sequelae at late time-points after repetitive mild traumatic brain injury. J Neurotrauma 2016;34(8):1676–91. Available from: https://doi.org/10.1089/neu.2016.4636.

[42] Marschner L, Schreurs A, Lechat B, Mogensen J, Roebroek A, Ahmed T, et al. Single mild traumatic brain injury results in transiently impaired spatial long-term memory and altered search strategies. Behav Brain Res 2019;365:222–30. Available from: https://doi.org/10.1016/j.bbr.2018.02.040.

[43] Broussard JI, Acion L, Jesús-Cortés HD, Yin T, Britt JK, Salas R, et al. Repeated mild traumatic brain injury produces neuroinflammation, anxiety-like behaviour and impaired spatial memory in mice. Brain Inj 2018;32(1):113–22. Available from: https://doi.org/10.1080/02699052.2017.1380228.

[44] Nylén K, Öst M, Csajbok LZ, Nilsson I, Blennow K, Nellgård B, et al. Increased serum-GFAP in patients with severe traumatic brain injury is related to outcome. J Neurol Sci 2006;240(1):85–91. Available from: https://doi.org/10.1016/j.jns.2005.09.007.

[45] Guo Y-Y, Lu Y, Zheng Y, Chen X-R, Dong J-L, Yuan R-R, et al. Ubiquitin C-terminal hydrolase L1 (UCH-L1) promotes hippocampus-dependent memory via its deubiquitinating effect on TrkB. J Neurosci 2017;37(25):5978–95. Available from: https://doi.org/10.1523/JNEUROSCI.3148-16.2017.

[46] Dey S, Gangadharan J, Deepika A, Kumar JK, Christopher R, Ramesh SS, et al. Correlation of ubiquitin C terminal hydrolase and S100β with cognitive deficits in young adults with mild traumatic brain injury. Neurol India 2017;65(4):761. Available from: https://doi.org/10.4103/neuroindia.NI_884_15.

[47] Cheng JS, Craft R, Yu G-Q, Ho K, Wang X, Mohan G, et al. Tau reduction diminishes spatial learning and memory deficits after mild repetitive traumatic brain injury in mice. PLoS One 2014;9(12). Available from: https://doi.org/10.1371/journal.pone.0115765.

[48] Ma M, Lindsell CJ, Rosenberry CM, Shaw GJ, Zemlan FP. Serum cleaved-tau does not predict postconcussion syndrome after mild traumatic brain injury. Am J Emerg Med 2008;26(7):763–8. Available from: https://doi.org/10.1016/j.ajem.2007.10.029.

[49] Bazarian JJ, Zemlan FP, Mookerjee S, Stigbrand T. Serum S-100B and cleaved-tau are poor predictors of long-term outcome after mild traumatic brain injury. Brain Inj 2006;20(7):759–65. Available from: https://doi.org/10.1080/02699050500488207.

[50] Beers SR, Berger RP, Adelson PD. Neurocognitive outcome and serum biomarkers in inflicted versus non-inflicted traumatic brain injury in young children. J Neurotrauma 2007;24(1):97−105. Available from: https://doi.org/10.1089/neu.2006.0055.

[51] Berger RP, Hayes RL, Richichi R, Beers SR, Wang KKW. Serum concentrations of ubiquitin C-terminal hydrolase-L1 and αII-spectrin breakdown product 145 kDa correlate with outcome after pediatric TBI. J Neurotrauma 2011;29(1):162−7. Available from: https://doi.org/10.1089/neu.2011.1989.

[52] Herrmann M, Curio N, Jost S, Grubich C, Ebert A, Fork M, et al. Release of biochemical markers of damage to neuronal and glial brain tissue is associated with short and long term neuropsychological outcome after traumatic brain injury. J Neurol, Neurosurg, Psychiatr 2001;70(1):95−100. Available from: https://doi.org/10.1136/jnnp.70.1.95.

[53] Stapert S, de Kruijk J, Houx P, Menheere P, Twijnstra A, Jolles J. S-100B concentration is not related to neurocognitive performance in the first month after mild traumatic brain injury. Eur Neurol 2005;53(1):22−6. Available from: https://doi.org/10.1159/000083678.

[54] Townend W, Ingebrigtsen T. Head injury outcome prediction: a role for protein S-100B? Injury 2006;37 (12):1098−108. Available from: https://doi.org/10.1016/j.injury.2006.07.014.

[55] Pleines UE, Morganti-Kossmann MC, Rancan M, Joller H, Trentz O, Kossmann T. S-100β reflects the extent of injury and outcome, whereas neuronal specific enolase is a better indicator of neuroinflammation in patients with severe traumatic brain injury. J Neurotrauma 2001;18(5):491−8. Available from: https://doi.org/10.1089/089771501300227297.

[56] Ryb GE, Dischinger PC, Auman KM, Kufera JA, Cooper CC, Mackenzie CF, et al. S-100β does not predict outcome after mild traumatic brain injury. Brain Inj 2014;28(11):1430−5. Available from: https://doi.org/10.3109/02699052.2014.919525.

[57] Waterloo K, Ingebrigtsen T, Romner B. Neuropsychological function in patients with increased serum levels of protein S-100 after minor head injury. Acta Neurochir 1997;139(1):26−31 discussion 31-32.

[58] Failla MD, Juengst SB, Arenth PM, Wagner AK. Preliminary associations between brain-derived neurotrophic factor, memory impairment, functional cognition, and depressive symptoms following severe TBI. Neurorehabil Neural Repair 2016;30(5):419−30. Available from: https://doi.org/10.1177/1545968315600525.

[59] Alonso M, Vianna MRM, Depino AM, Souza TME, Pereira P, Szapiro G, et al. BDNF−triggered events in the rat hippocampus are required for both short- and long-term memory formation. Hippocampus 2002;12 (4):551−60. Available from: https://doi.org/10.1002/hipo.10035.

[60] Kalish H, Phillips TM. Analysis of neurotrophins in human serum by immunoaffinity capillary electrophoresis (ICE) following traumatic head injury. J Chromatogr B, Anal Technol Biomed Life Sci 2010;878 (2):194−200. Available from: https://doi.org/10.1016/j.jchromb.2009.10.022.

Outpatient risk stratification for traumatic brain injury

Zubaid Rafique and Rodmond Singleton

Emergency Medicine, Baylor College of Medicine, Houston, TX, United States

According to current Centers for Disease Control (CDC) data on traumatic brain injuries (TBI), about 2.5 million patients present to emergency departments in the United States every year and are diagnosed with TBI. It contributes to an estimated third of all injury-related deaths in the United States with an estimated economic cost of US$76.5 billion [1]. TBIs can lead to a range of short- and long-term sequelae including diminished cognitive function, impaired motor and sensory function and emotional lability, depression, anxiety, and aggression [1]. TBIs exist along a spectrum from mild to severe and include nonintracranial hemorrhage like concussion and cerebral contusion to brain hemorrhage and diffuse axonal injury (DAI) [2,3].

Eighty percent of patients with a head trauma who seek emergent care are treated and released; less than 10% suffer from an intracranial injury identified on CT and less than 1% require neurosurgical intervention [4]. Emergency medicine physicians (EPs) have the challenging task of determining which of these patients who do not have discrete ICH on CT imaging have associated significant intracranial trauma that, nonetheless, requires acute and long-term care. In accordance with Advanced Trauma Life Support (ATLS) and Advanced Pediatric Life Support (PALS) guidelines, EPs should also evaluate any patient with trauma for clinical evidence of surgical trauma [5]. The majority of these patients who present with mild TBI have a clear clinical presentation indicating the presence of TBI including nausea, dizziness, syncope, headache, and emesis.

Due to the importance of readily identifying patients who require neurosurgical intervention, several risk stratification tools have been developed for clinical use in identifying patients with head injuries who may have ICH. As standard practice, EPs make use of well-validated clinical decision tools like the Canadian CT Head Rule (CCHR) and the New Orleans Criteria to assist in determining which patients with head trauma will likely benefit from computed tomography (CT) imaging. The diagnostic imaging of choice for assessment of TBIs in the emergency department is the noncontrast CT of the head given its high sensitivity and specificity for epidural hematomas, subdural hematomas, and cranial fractures [6]. These tools take into consideration GCS score, age, mechanism of injury, clinical symptoms, evidence of trauma, and memory loss [7]. In its validation trial, the CCHR was 100% sensitive and 76.3% specific for detecting injuries that required neurosurgical intervention [8]. There have been multiple validation studies comparing the CCHR and NOC with varying results, but overall the NOC was found to also be 100% sensitive for significant intracranial injuries but with a much lesser specificity of around 25% [9] (Figs. 27.1 and 27.2).

For pediatric patients, EM physicians often employ clinical decision-making tools like the Pediatric Emergency Care Applied Research Network (PECARN) Pediatric Head Injury algorithm that assists in safely ruling out the presence of clinically significant TBI in children with GCS scores less than or equal to 14. This includes those that would require neurosurgical intervention without the need for computed tomography [10]. PECARN takes into account the patient's age, GCS, signs of altered mental status or basilar skull fracture, history of loss of consciousness, severe headache, and mechanism of injury. PECARN has been externally validated in multiple studies boasting a sensitivity of 100% and specificity of 55%. Many studies have demonstrated that PECARN has led to beneficial outcomes and more cost-effective care in the ED [11]. Other risk stratification tools have been developed including Canadian Assessment of Tomography for Childhood Head Injury (CATCH) rule and the Children's Head Injury Algorithm for the Prediction of Important Clinical Events (CHALICE) rule, however PECARN and CATCH are most commonly utilized in the emergency setting. The CATCH is used in

Canadian CT head trauma rule (CCHR)	
CT Head Rule is only required for patients with minor head injuries with any one of the following	
High-Risk (for Neurosurgical Intervention)	*Signs of basal skull fracture:
1. GCS score <15 at 2 h after injury	• Hemotympanum,
2. Suspected open or depressed skull fracture	• "raccoon" eyes,
	• CSF otorrhea or rhinorrhea,
3. Any sign of skull fracture*	• Battle's sign
4. Vomiting ≥ 2 episodes	
5. Age ≥ 65 years	‡Dangerous Mechanism:
Medium Risk (for brain injury)	• Pedestrian struck by motor vehicle
6. Amnesia (of events) before impact ≥ 30 min	• Occupant ejected from motor vehicle
7. Dangerous mechanism‡	• Fall from elevation ≥ 3 feet or 5 stairs
Exclusion Criteria: if present, CCHR does not apply	
• GCS < 13	
• Age < 16 years	
• Taking blood thinners or bleeding disorder	

FIGURE 27.1 Canadian CT head rule [4].

New orleans head CT rule
• Headache
• Vomiting
• Age > 60 years
• Alcohol or drug intoxication
• Persistent anterograde amnesia
• Visible trauma above clavicle
• Seizure
Recommend CT head if GCS of 15 and one of the above findings after minor head trauma

FIGURE 27.2 New Orleans head CT Rule [8].

patients up to 16 years old with minor head injury with GCS of at least 13 with injury sustained with the past 24 hours and considers presence of suspected skull depression or fracture, history of worsening headache, irritability, signs of basilar skull fracture, presence of "boggy" hematoma, and mechanism [8]. While both PECARN and CATCH were found to be effective in determining the necessity of computerized brain tomography for children with minor blunt head trauma, PECARN proved to be more useful for emergency centers because of its higher sensitivity of 100% [12]. In one prospective study designed to evaluate the diagnostic accuracy of these pediatric clinical decision rules and physician judgment for identifying ciTBIs in children with minor head injuries who present to the ED, only physician practice and PECARN identified all clinically important TBIs, with PECARN being slightly more specific at 62%. CHALICE was not very sensitive (84%) but was the most specific (85%) of all rules while CATCH had poor sensitivity and had the least specificity of all modalities of 91% and 41%, respectively [13] (Fig. 27.3).

An accurate history and physical examination are paramount in making prompt diagnosis of concussion in the emergency department. Important elements of the history include the mechanism of injury elicited from the patient, family members, and emergency response personnel, the presence of seizures, loss of consciousness, deterioration in mental status, vomiting, or history of previous neurological intervention [10]. Other critical historical elements include drug or alcohol use, anticoagulant use, and the presence of a bleeding diathesis. Elements of the physical examination are integral in increasing diagnostic sensitivity and risk stratification of TBI and completion of a focused neurological examination is paramount. Focused attention is paid to establishing a GCS score, evaluating pupils, cognitive function, as well as motor and cerebellar function. Performing serial neurological exams allow the clinician to recognize clinical deterioration [14]. The remaining portion of the physical exam focuses on findings that raise the suspicion for clinically significant intracranial injuries, including evidence of basilar skull fracture, spinal cord injury, and carotid or vertebral artery dissection. Some of the physical findings that are concerning for basilar skull fractures include hemotympanum, periorbital ecchymosis (Raccoon sign), CSF rhinorrhea, or ottorhea (Halo sign) [15]. Bony spinal tenderness, paresthesia, incontinence, weakness, and priapism can be indicative of spinal cord injuries as well [16]. Reviewing the relevant elements of the physical exam is important because the majority of the concussion assessment tools rely heavily on the clinician's ability to incorporate these findings.

Comparison of Canadian CT and New Orleans Criteria

FIGURE 27.3 Sensitivities and specificities for need for neurosurgical intervention in patients with GCS score of 15 [8].

	Sensitivity	Specificity
Canadian CT head rule	100%	76.3%
New Orleans criteria	100%	12.1%

Despite greater recognition of the causal link between sports-related injuries and clinically significant TBIs, establishing standardized diagnostic criteria for concussions has proven to be challenging. It is now known that there is greater susceptibility to sustaining repeat concussions and that subsequent concussions occur with less force and take longer to recover, so timely identification on the field and in the ED is critical. Furthermore, the diagnosis of concussion continues to be ill-defined with at least three different consensus statements put forth by specialty organizations [17]. Most notable among them are definitions offered by the Concussion in Sport Group (CISG), American Academy of Neurology (AAN), and the American Medical Society for Sports Medicine (AMSSM) [18].

CISG: concussion is a complex pathophysiological process affecting the brain, induced by traumatic biomechanical forces caused by a direct blow to the head, face, neck, or elsewhere in the body with an impulsive force transmitted to the head resulting in rapid onset of short-lived neurological impairment.

AAN: concussion is a trauma-induced alteration in mental status that may or may not involve loss of consciousness but is characterized by confusion and amnesia that occur rapidly after injury.

AMSSM: concussion is a pathophysiological process affecting the brain induced by direct or indirect biomechanical forces.

The complete definition from CISG and AMSSM incorporates neuroimaging findings while that from AAN does not. Of note, the AAN uses the terms concussion and mTBI interchangeably while the CISG considers concussion as a subset of TBI [17].

Prior to the emergence of current protocols and decision tools, determination of athletes who had concussions was largely devoid of empirical evidence given the paucity of literature devoted to the field theretofore. Despite the enormous progress in TBI research, reliance on the clinical evaluation is critical for diagnosis. The Sports Concussion Assessment Tool (SCAT-5) is the most recent revision of the sports concussion evaluation tool designed for use by healthcare professionals. It is a revision of the SCAT-3 (first published in 2013) that was based on a systematic review of the literature at the time of its creation by an expert panel during the 5th International Consensus Conference on Concussion in Sport in 2016 [19]. This standardized tool involves a rapid on-field assessment for signs of concussion after first aid and emergency care is administered. The immediate assessment includes noting observable "red flag" signs, evaluating memory, determining GCS, and evaluating the cervical spine. The off-field assessment involves obtaining a history and physical, comprehensive symptom evaluation, neurological screening, and cognitive screening. The original SCAT was created in 2004 and subsequent iterations were based upon review of the literature that was current at that time of their revisions. In 2012 with the creation of the SCAT-3, a separate clinical decision tool was created for children under the age of 13 as previous versions were determined to not be age-specific and appropriate for younger concussed patients [20]. The current Child SCAT-5 includes various modifications but some notable changes were the removal of modified Maddocks and orientation questions which were found to lack reliability and changes to the Rapid Neurological Screen (RNS) assessment. The modified Maddocks questions were adapted to be more appropriate for reliability and usefulness in young children and included these items: "Where are we now?"; "Is it before or after lunch?"; "What did you have last lesson/class?"; and "What is your teacher's name?" [20].

The Balance Error Scoring System (BESS) was originally developed to assess balance but has become a supplementary tool to evaluate for concussion. The exam consists of a calculation performed by adding one error point for each error during six different 20-second tests. The patient is evaluated while executing balance exercises in a double leg stance (feet together), a single leg stance, and a tandem stance (nondominant foot in back), both on a soft and firm surface [21]. The utility of the BESS derives from its ability to detect balance deficits in participants with concussions by assessing effects of mild head injury on static postural stability [21]. According to one systematic review by Bell et al., BESS has moderate to good reliability to assess static balance. Low to moderate levels of interobserver reliability have also been reported but with good correlation with other measures of balance [21]. A modified BESS has also been incorporated into the SCAT-5 as a subscale for balance [19].

Studies demonstrating that individuals with TBI often have oculomotor dysfunction have given rise to other formal tools for diagnosing concussion. Symptoms of oculomotor dysfunction include diplopia, difficulty following targets, and loss of reading speed and duration, given that visual function utilizes a large portion of the brain's pathways. As a result, the King–Devick Test (KD) has been proposed as another concussion screening test in some settings [22]. It has been used as a screening tool in a variety of contact sports. The KD utilizes rapid number testing to detect the presence of concussion. It uses a timed vision-based measure that requires the integration of eye movements and number identification. A meta-analysis demonstrated that the KD test was able to detect concussions with great sensitivity (86%) and specificity (90%) [23]. However, a recent prospective cohort study was performed in the UK that compared the KD test's ability to detect concussion in elite English Rugby players. It was compared alongside the World Rugby HIA-1 screening tool and was found to have limited accuracy as a standalone screening test with a sensitivity and specificity of 93% and 33%, respectively [24].

Because in many cases, mild cognitive deficits may persist after the common neurological signs of brain injury have passed, computerized concussion assessment tools have been developed. These tests demonstrate advantages over standard "paper and pencil" neurocognitive test batteries which were designed to detect gross, acute cognitive changes in a singular event [25]. The practical advantages of the computer-based testing approach are infinite randomized forms, standardized self-administration, rapid testing, internet-based delivery, and centralized data storage, analysis, and reporting [25]. The ImPACT, CogSport, and ANAN computer-based testing batteries incorporate baseline and postinjury testing used to diagnose and determine when return to play is prudent. These tests have demonstrated good diagnostic efficiency for detecting concussion-related cognitive impairment [26].

Despite the development of these concussion assessment tools, notable limitations of the current concussion tests include the lack of a standardized definition of concussion and that the testing pathways rely so heavily on clinical opinion and symptom reporting by athletes. These issues make accurate recognition and prospective validation of concussion assessment tools difficult. Athletes are also incentivized to not actually disclose the extent of their disability for multiple reasons, including financial incentive, stoicism inherent in sports culture, and fear of being excluded from play. Variability in education and communication skills also limit the ability of some athletes to articulate their symptoms limiting the utility of these tests [26]. Some resources discuss the role of ceiling effects in highly educated athletes, which results from the limitation in the range of assessment scores in that they are incapable of detecting meaningful functional changes at the upper or lower ends of the scale. For example, if an individual has achieved a maximum preinjury score, more subtle deficits will go undetected resulting in many occult TBIs going undiagnosed [27].

Many of the limitations presented with current subjective symptom-based testing have been outlined and are driving efforts to identify more sensitive and objective metrics for identifying concussion. Significant progress has been made in the search of biomarkers for mild TBI, with a focus on markers for neuronal, axonal, oligodendrocyte, astroglial, and blood—brain barrier injury [28]. Current research suggests that blunt forces causing linear and rotational accelerations of the brain lead to microscopic neuronal shearing with a transient hypermetabolic state that, when paired with alterations in cerebral blood flow and autoregulation, results in the clinical symptoms of mild TBI [29]. Several proteins have been identified that are released from injured central nervous system (CNS) structures and have a potential role as serum biomarkers in patients with mild TBI [28]. The research is robust in this field and a complete itemization of potential markers is beyond the scope of this text. Development of these markers is critical in identifying individuals at high risk of long-term sequelae of mild TBI, differentiating between repetitive mild TBI and chronic neurological symptoms, and developing strategies to prevent chronic disease [28].

Despite the development of reliable conventional and computer-based neurocognitive testing, the diagnosis and clinical assessment of concussion remains challenging. In addition to the variability in clinical presentation and the absence of a reliable direct biomarker of injury and recovery, the evolution of concussion symptoms is unpredictable, complicating the clinical assessment. While some athletes demonstrate the symptoms and signs of concussion immediately following impact, in many the symptoms evolve over minutes, and in some, over days [30]. Accurate and rapid diagnosis of concussion has important implications given our understanding about postconcussive syndrome, CTE, and other irreversible neurological sequelae associated with missed and delayed diagnosis, as well as premature return to activities which could further exacerbate insults. However, the current diagnostic modalities lack the sensitivity and specificity to rapidly diagnose mild TBI leaving much room for further research and investigation. In addition, the variable definitions for concussions complicate the research process and the ability to apply data derived from the various studies to clinical practice.

References

[1] Taylor C, Bell J, Breiding M, Xu L. Traumatic brain injury-related emergency department visits, hospitalizations, and deaths-United States, 2007 and 2013. Morbidity and Mortality Weekly Report; 2013. Available at https://doi.org/10.15585/mmwr.ss6609a1.

[2] Wright DW, Merck L. Head trauma In: Tintinalli JE, ed.,. Tintinalli's Emergency Medicine: A Comprehensive Study Guide. 8th edition. New York: McGraw-Hill; 2016.

[3] Tator CH. Concussions and their consequences: current diagnosis, management and prevention. CMAJ: Can Med Assoc J 2013;185(11):975−9.

[4] Stiell IG, Wells GA, Vandemheen K, Clement C, Lesiuk H, Laupacis A, et al. The Canadian CT head rule for patients with minor head injury. Lancet. 2001;357:1391.

[5] Vos PE, Alekseenko Y, Battistin L, Ehler E, Gerstenbrand F, Muresanu DF, Potapov A, Stepan CA, Traubner P, Vecsei L, von Wild K. Mild traumatic brain injury. Eur J Neurol 2012;19:191−8.

[6] Shetty VS, Reis MN, Aulino JM, Berger KL, Broder J, Choudhri AF, et al. ACR Appropriateness criteria head trauma. J Am Coll Radiology 2016;668−79.

[7] Smits M, Dippel DW, de Haan GG, Dekker HM, Vos PE, Kool DR, et al. External validation of the Canadian CT head rule and the New Orleans criteria for CT scanning in patients with minor head injury. JAMA. 2005;1519−25.

[8] Stiell IG, Clement CM, Rowe BH, Schull MJ, Brison R, Cass D, et al. Comparison of the Canadian CT head rule and the New Orleans criteria in patients with minor head injury. JAMA. 2005;1511−18.

[9] Haydel MJ, Preston CA, Mills TJ, Luber S, Blaudeau E, DeBlieux PM. Indications for Computed Tomography in Patients with Minor Head Injury. N Engl J Med July 2000;343:100−5.

[10] Kuppermann N, Holmes JF, Dayan PS, Hoyle Jr. JD, Atabaki SM, Holubkov R, et al. Identification of children at very low risk of clinically-important brain injuries after head trauma: a prospective cohort study. Lancet 2009;1160−70 October.

[11] Nishijima DK, Yang Z, Urbich M, Holmes JF, Zwienenberg-Lee M, Melnikow J, et al. Cost-effectiveness of the PECARN rules in children with minor head trauma. Ann Emerg Med 2015;72−80 January.

[12] Bozan O, Aksel G, Kahraman HA, Giritli Ö, Eroğlu SE. Comparison of PECARN and CATCH clinical decision rules in children with minor blunt trauma. Eur J Trauma Emerg Surg 2017;1−7.

[13] Easter JS, Bakes K, Dhaliwal J, Miller M, Caruso E, Haukoos JS. Comparison of PECARN, CATCH and CHALICE rules for children with minor head injury: a prospective cohort study. Ann Emerg Med 2014;145−52.

[14] Davis DP, Serrano JA, Vilke GM, Sise MJ, Kennedy F, Eastman AB, et al. The predictive value of field versus arrival glasgow coma scale score and TRISS calculations in moderate-to-severe traumatic brain injury. J Trauma-Inj Infect Crit Care 2006;985−90 May.

[15] Gardner AJ, Shores EA, Batchelor J, Honan C. Diagnostic efficiency of ImPACT and CogSport in concussed rugby union players WHo have not undergone baseline neurocognitive testing. Appl Neuropsychol Adult 2012;90−7.

[16] Phang SY, Whitehouse K, Lee L, Khalil H, McArdle P, Whitfield PC. Management of CSF leak in base of skull fractures in adults. Br J Neurosurg 2016;596−604.

[17] McCrory P, Feddermann-Demont N, Dvořák J, Cassidy JD, McIntosh A, Vos PE, et al. What is the defintion of sports-related concussion: a systematic review. Br J Sports Med 2017;877−87.

[18] Cochrane GD, Owen M, Ackerson JD, Hale MH, Gould S. Exploration of the US men's professional sport organization concussion policies. Pysician Sports Med 2017;178−83.

[19] Echemendia RJ, Meeuwisse W, McCrory P, Davis GA, Putukian M, Leddy J, et al. The Sport Concussion Assessment Tool 5th Edition (SCAT5): background and rationale. Br J Sports Med 2017;848−50.

[20] Davis GA, Purce L, Schneider KJ. The Child Sport Concussion Assessment Tool 5th Edition (Child SCAT5): background and rationale. Br J Sports Med 2017;859−61.

[21] Bell DR, Guskiewicz KM, Clark MA, Padua DA. Systematic review of balance error scoring system. Sports Health 2011;287−95.

[22] Ciuffreda KJ, Kapoor N, Rutner D, Suchoff IB, Han ME, Craig S. Occurrence of oculomotor dysfunctions in acquired brain injury: a retrospective analysis. Optometry 2007;155−61.

[23] Galetta KM, Liu M, Leong DF, Ventura RE, Galetta SL, Balcer LJ. The King-Devick test of rapid number naming for concussion detection: meta-analysis and systematic review of the literature. Concussion 2016.

[24] Fuller GW, Cross MJ, Stokes KA, Kemp SPT. King-Devick consussion test performs poorly as a screening tool in elite rugby union players: a prospective cohort study of two screening tests versus a clinical reference standard. Br J Sports Med 2018.

[25] Collie A, Darby D, Maruff P. Computerised cognitive assessment of athletes with sports related head injury. Br J Sports Med 2001;297–302.

[26] Costello DM KAOTSS. Sport-related concussion -potential for biomarkers to improve acute management. J Clin Neurosci 2018.

[27] Hall KM, et al. Assessing traumatic brain injury outcome measures for long-term follow-up of community-based individuals. Arch Phys Med Rehabil 2001;367–74.

[28] Zetterberg HBK. Fluid biomarkers for mild traumatic brain injury and related conditions. Nat Rev Neurol 2016;563–74.

[29] Barkhoudarian G. The molecular pathophysiology of concussive brain injury. ClSports Med 2011;33–48.

[30] Makdissi M, Davis G, McCrory P. Clinical challenges in the diagnosis and assessment of sports-related concussion. Neurology 2015;2–5.

Peptidomics and traumatic brain injury: biomarker utilities for a theragnostic approach

Hamad Yadikar[1,2,3], *George A. Sarkis*[1,4,5], *Milin Kurup*[1], *Firas Kobeissy*[1,6,7] *and Kevin K. Wang*[1,7]

[1]Departments of Emergency Medicine, Psychiatry, Neuroscience and Chemistry, University of Florida, Gainesville, FL, United States [2]Department of Biological Sciences, Faculty of Science, Kuwait University, Safat, Kuwait [3]Department of Chemistry, University of Florida, Gainesville, FL, United States [4]Department of Chemistry, Faculty of Science, Alexandria University, Alexandria, Egypt [5]Department of Biological Engineering, Massachusetts Institute of Technology, Cambridge, United States [6]Faculty of Medicine, American University of Beirut Medical Center, Beirut, Lebanon [7]Brain Rehabilitation Research Center, Malcom Randall VA Medical Center, Gainesville, FL, United States

28.1 Introduction

Proteomics is known as the "next step after genomics," specifically functional genomics. Although the DNA is relatively a steady component, the proteome produces sophisticated and interactive networks that continuously change. Mutations can alter genotype and, therefore might detect susceptibility to a disorder, while proteins identify a phenotype, and it could represent a pathogenic pathway. Thus proteomics is appropriate for the definition of disease development, representing the actual condition and its advancement. In the various components of an organ, at distinct phases of its life cycle, and responding to external variables such as pathology, one organism has a different protein expression and processing. As an example, a genome with less than 30,000 genes was discovered to produce over 300,000 proteins.

Low-molecular-weight peptides and proteins (less than 15 kDa) extend the unpredictability in this research area. Peptides that are specific breakdown products generated from high-molecular-weight proteins by posttranslational processing can become biologically active compounds. Such protein precursors hold out different biological functions that are dormant before being triggered by varying proteolytic actions. Many peptides are produced as potent chemicals to act as secondary messenger molecules. Peptidomics is the qualitative and quantitative study of entire sets of peptides, which are controlled under distinct biological conditions; this process helps us to understand the molecular mechanism of proteins such as tau.

When conducting peptidomic research, the first issue that needs to be addressed is choosing which type of sample to sue for analysis. Too many proteins and peptides are present within the blood plasma to be assigned as an optimal target. Cerebrospinal fluid (CSF) has shifted our concentration as it is possible now to access the laboratory TBI models and human biofluid. CSF is an ultrafiltrate of plexus, from choroid plexus, and is used to assess the health state of the blood–brain barrier (BBB) [1–3]. Also, the choroid plexus continually produces and secretes proteins and peptides into CSF.

There is a wide variety of challenging and distinct goals in neurotrauma studies. The implementation of peptidomics may be envisaged as a useful technique for discovering efficient neuroprotective multitarget approaches, gaining more significant perspectives into full recovery and rehabilitation, or for the improvement of neurochemical screening to advance the traditional protocols. Peptidomics is also used to identify biomarkers, which could, for example, imply occurrences of injury to neurons or glial cells. Biomarkers obtained from peptidomics might suggest an associated TBI occurrence and may then be used as a tool for medical treatment, pathophysiological perspectives, and thus a stronger comprehension of the disease. Both unpredictability and the variability of human TBI assessments are the challenges for basic research. The systemic evaluation of neurochemical cascades by human peptidomics can be an unsolicited starting point because of a variety of affecting factors such as the severity of the trauma, secondary injury, preexistent comorbidity, age, gender, and side effects of therapy. Thus experimental animal models with structured initial conditions and defined trauma are much more appropriate for exploring the capabilities and effectiveness of peptidomics.

28.2 Peptidome in biofluids as biomarkers

A biomarker has specific characteristics that are used as a reporter to measure standard biological processes, pathological processes, or response to therapeutic intervention. Neurodegeneration following TBI results in tau detachment from the microtubule, elevating the levels of tau and tau-BDP in biofluids. Research interests are increasing in analyzing biofluids such as CSF, plasma, or serum tau as a biomarker for TBI and chronic traumatic encephalopathy.

28.3 Serum

For mTBI diagnosis, prognosis, return to play/duty evaluations, a quantifiable measure like a serum biomarker is required. mTBI is challenging to diagnose due to the lack of noninterventional diagnostic tools. Serum biomarkers are currently clinically used to diagnose other pathologies, such as cardiac troponin for myocardial infarction, and lipase for pancreatitis. Increased tau serum levels were observed in experimental animal TBI and human TBI [4,5]. Serum tau direct escape mechanisms include direct release via BBB opening, ventricular wall damage, release via the glymphatic system, or more complex intracellular transport via macrophages or microglia phagocytosis. In human TBI, the elevation of tau serum levels might be associated with injury severity and have been reported to reach the highest levels within two days after the injury [6]. A study has shown that cleaved-tau (c-tau) is elevated in serum after severe TBI; however, more prospective studies are needed to establish a definite conclusion [7].

28.4 Cerebrospinal fluid

CSF is a viscous fluid that covers the brain and spinal cords and offers mechanical support, regeneration resource storage, metabolites flow, and controlling functions of the central nervous system (CNS). The source of CSF peptides is derived from either the blood filtrate or brain tissue [8]. However, the invasive aspect of sampling leaves it unsuitable for overall testing of healthy subjects or subjects with neurodegenerative disorders [9,10]. Due to blood biomarkers performing poorly in the detection of acute mTBI, researchers are starting to look to the example of Alzheimer's disease (AD) research [5]. Since CSF is available in experimental models of TBI and from humans, researchers moved into analyzing it. The choroid plexus actively synthesizes and secretes proteins and small peptides into the CSF.

CSF has a biomarker diagnostic potential in tauopathies of AD [11]. In severe TBI, increased levels of CSF total tau and phosphorylated tau continue to rise beyond two days and reach the maximum levels between 5 and 15 days after the injury [11−14]. Moreover, CSF sample studies following severe TBI have shown increases in c-tau isoforms levels postinjury, suggesting that proteolytic enzymes play a critical role in neuropathological processes contributing to mortality and morbidity [15−18]. Tau concentration in CSF increases during the acute phase of severe head trauma, which is beneficial in determining the stage of prognosis. Ultrasensitive analytical methods, such as Quanterix digital Simoa assay platform, allow single-molecule detection and facilitate the analysis of plasma tau levels [19−21].

28.5 Plasma

After centrifugation, the plasma is the fluid supernatant portion of the blood without the tissues or cells. To obtain plasma, blood should be collected with anticlotting agents such as EDTA, citrate, or heparin to reduce cell clotting. A study has shown that comparing phosphorylated plasma tau and phosphorylated tau/total tau ratio offers an efficient and consistent way as a diagnostic and prognostic biomarker compared to total tau alone, revealing elevations among patient with chronic TBI [19]. As of now, the biggest hindrance toward the use of plasma in diagnostic/therapeutic peptidomic tests is the emergence of artificial peptides breakdown products during plasma collection, making it challenging to isolate the peptides from the actual disorder [22]. Furthermore, the attachment of some peptides to receptor proteins (e.g., albumin) should be prevented to obtain full peptide retrieval in blood peptidome research.

28.6 Urine

The urine peptidome might be another attractive source for biomarker discovery because of the low complexity compared to plasma peptidome and the noninvasive nature of urine collection. Since 70% of the urine proteome originates from the urinary tract [23,24], the use of urine for investigation of neurodegenerative disorders might be neglected. Although far from the brain or the cerebrospinal region, traces of peptides are detectable. Many experiments have already shown that urine proteome are involved with neurological disorders, revealing the potential value of urine peptidome analysis and the introduction of neurodegenerative disease diagnostic assays [25–27]. The enhanced sensitivity of mass spectrometers and the creation of a standardized, versatile, and cost-effective protocol for sample preparation are the limiting factors for success in urine peptidome analysis.

28.7 Saliva

The appeal of using saliva for diagnostics is the straightforwardness and the noninvasive nature of the technique. Saliva is a bodily fluid naturally produced by the human body containing enzymes that contribute to nutrition metabolism, lubricating the oral cavity, and protecting from infectious diseases. The current advancement in mass spectrometric techniques has opened the door to exploring biomarkers for TBI in saliva. Studies on saliva proteome have shown their involvement in neurodegenerative diseases, including AD and Parkinson's disease [28]. A proteomic study showed that tau is present in the saliva [29]. However, saliva peptidome is complicated and inconsistent. Nutrient digestion happens as quickly as the enzymes reach the mouth opening, and endogenous peptides are overshadowed with exogenous peptides. Other prior-analytical factors are sex, age, nutrition, and metabolic cycles which all have an effect on saliva protein diversity [10,30–32].

28.8 Tissue

The proteomic analysis of tissue homogenate is well-established, has a dynamic range, and is conventional compared to the analysis of proteome from plasma, urine, and serum. A wide variety of biomarkers linked to neurodegenerative diseases in animal and human samples can be investigated using MALDI (matrix-assisted laser desorption/ionization), and ion-mobility mass spectrometry (IM-MS).

28.9 Tear

The noninvasive nature of sample collection of tears encouraged scientists that peptidomics assessment could be helpful for a wide variety of clinical uses. As well as the primary role of tears as eye moisturizer, tears can prevent diseases, and act as an eye shield. While not expected originally, the tear peptidome is indeed very complicated. The peptidome makeup of tears could represent the physiological state of the surrounding tissue [33]. While the variability of tears compositions throughout the day seems to be small, a notable variability between individuals adds even more difficulty to the assessment. Studying tear peptidome mainly focuses on characterizing tear peptides which are normally digested since these are bioactive peptides and therefore can perform particular functions that are not assigned to the initial parent protein, including antimicrobial action, or cell signaling [33]. One study observed significant changes in tear flow levels, overall tear protein content, AD-specific chemical barrier, and possible biomarkers mixture of lipocalin-1, dermcidin, lysozyme-C, and lacritin [34].

28.10 Microvesicles and exosomes

An emerging field is the study of microvesicles and exosomes (MV/E) in CSF and blood after TBI [35]. Exosomes and microvesicles are membrane-enclosed particles (0−100 nm in diameter) produced from organisms (healthy or diseased) into the extracellular fluid. They compromise separate proteins or miRNA materials transmitted under a specific condition or disorder. For instance, TBI patient plasma has a distinct array of protein disclosed by a mass-based approach [36]. A study found the MV/E produced in TBI individuals includes high concentrations of several protein biomarkers [spectrin breakdown products (SBDP)], synaptophysin, UCH-L1, and GFAP [37]. Tau-embedded exosomes may be a stronger therapeutic method for acute TBI patients at the danger of creating chronic traumatic encephalopathy [38].

28.11 Fractionation and separation

Most of the procedures for peptide separation and extraction are well documented but are continuously under application development. Fundamental methods for separating protein, enriching, and handling samples are derived from studies in the 1950s to 1970s, which focused mostly on enzymes. However, several advances in analytical techniques, mainly evolved with proteomics in mind, also advocate for innovative peptidomic methods and protocols.

The use of LC-MS in both proteomics and peptidomics has become a routine application. This was accomplished by reducing column diameters from 1 mm to capillary LC columns with a diameter of 75 μm, causing quite a decrease in flow speed and sample quantity [39]. Separation with pressure above 1000 bar (UPLC) is now possible with innovative chromatographic instruments of two or fewer micrometers in diameters.

Therefore separation times with similar sensitivity are now much faster, typically used to boost throughput, and are now the standard LC technology for peptide analysis. An appealing option for the use of chromatography is the pairing of capillary electrophoresis (CE) to MS [40,41,42]. Several dedicated teams have optimized the use of CE-MS for human fluid clinical specimens [9,23].

28.12 Peptide identification and data analysis

One of the main challenges in peptidomics research is the incomplete proteome database of existing and speculated proteins. The identification of a peptide algorithm depends on the occurrence of an identical or homologous amino acid sequence of the protein being screened [43]. The initial strategy now used is to enable a "no-enzyme specificity" choice to scan the protein database, which searches in all potential peptide combinations taking into consideration any protein cleavage sites. The unbiased search will contribute to enormous computational complexity and will require more time and bandwidth. Newer search engines are now much quicker than traditional versions, such as Morpheus [44], or MSFragger [45], and Peptigram [46] that can tackle these issues. By using these softwares, a specific mass spectrum is searched against several potential candidates peptides, which are unlikely to be detected in the actual sample, thus lowering the false positive detection rates and increasing the stringency for valid peptide identifications.

Another strategy is to build a directory containing recognized and expected target proteins to boost recognition yields [43,47−49]. This is only plausible if the sample includes only natural proteolytic peptides, reinforcing the significance of sample processing and peptide concentration in peptidomics. Another stringent strategy is to permit only biologically active peptides in a database corresponding to the targeted proteins. This is accomplished by choosing only proteins containing cleavage domains in the analyzed sample for discovered proteases and peptidases. Several proteolytic peptides will be unidentified with this strategy because of the presence of alternative spectra that originate from other modifications of the same peptide in the database (e.g., altered N- or C-terminal modifications). An option to explore these "modified peptides" is to use the six-frame translation of the whole genome incorporating ETD and CID to enhance confidence in gathering data against all of the available reading frames, possibly using RNA-seq as in proteogenomics research.

28.13 Peptidomic approach for discovery of novel proteolytic peptides in traumatic brain injury

Peptidomics is described as the research of the whole array of naturally generated peptides in groups of distinct environments, including qualitative and quantitative comparison with the biological process to unravel mechanisms. In recent promising findings for biomarker discovery [50,51]. Peptidomics have recently been employed as a tool for studying human body fluids; of particular interests are blood plasma, serum, urine, saliva, and CSF [52]. Natural endogenous peptides have potent biochemical functions in respiratory, cardiovascular, endocrine, inflammatory, and nervous systems. Most neurons have biologically active peptides together with conventional neurotransmitters. In neurodegenerative disorders, biologically active neuropeptides are implicated in the neuropathology [10,53].

Several peptidomics studies characterizing CSF and blood plasma supplied alternative strategies for biomarker diagnosis, which showed increased sensitivity to endogenous peptide alterations not evidenced by standard proteomics approaches [10,54]. Valuable information is lost when the samples of proteins are digested artificially with trypsin in proteomics quantification on the measurement of tryptic peptides. Therefore from an analytical standpoint, studying endogenous peptides decreases sources of inconsistencies, is less expensive, and decreases sample preparation time, which are critical factors for building the basis for clinical biomarker research and routine work.

Ultrafiltration of HMW proteins, which make up most of the CSF protein pool (e.g., albumin and immunoglobulins), can enrich the natural proteolytic peptides. This ultrafiltration step enriches LMW peptides for identification by LC-MS (Fig. 28.1). The potential identified peptides can be assessed using software programs that implement different approaches for characterizing and sequencing, which then can be correlated with peptides that are found in neurodegenerative disorders and peptides of special interests (i.e., potential biomarkers) [26,32,53,55—58].

Unfortunately, several potential biomarker candidates published in peptidomics studies could not be validated further. Human TBI has a sophisticated and heterogenic clinical presentation. Influencing factors that complicate peptidomics are distribution and severity of the trauma, preresuscitation secondary injury, the different time-point of the injury, preexisting and confounding comorbidity, and side effects of the treatment. Technological variances for biomarker discovery approaches should be less than 10% to expect a decent probability of detection with sets of clinical samples. The most important variable, however, is not the identification, but the quality and quantity of the clinical specimens being

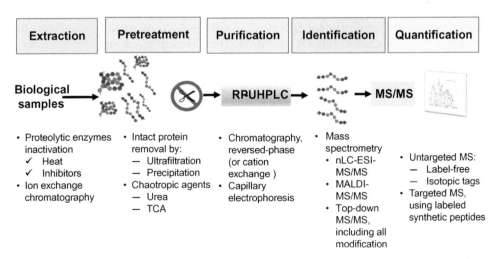

FIGURE 28.1   Workflow for the commonly used peptidomics analytical process which is divided into five major steps comprising different types of methods.

examined and the experimental layout [26,56,59–61]. Thus experimental models with controlled conditions and trauma are more informative as a starting point to explore the possibilities and the power of peptidomics. Using peptidomics for TBI research has been rare so far. To the best of our knowledge, there are no reports about systematic peptidomic study with experimental or human patients with TBI.

28.14 Current mass spectrometric peptidomic technologies

Mass spectrometry technology has undertaken a tremendous development since the invention of biopolymer ionization. All critical parameters of mass spectrometry have been improved dramatically, including ionization, quantification, resolution, time needed for sample MS, and identification methods, driven by innovation in analytical chemistry. The development of micro- and nanoelectrospray achieved a considerable increase in the sensitivity of ESI-MS, allowing the analysis of mass spectra from samples of femtomolar to picomolar concentrations of peptides. Nanoelectrospray ionization has become the standard platform in peptidomics. MALDI-MS studies also delivered similar sensitivity with a high-throughput screening for hundreds of samples, allowing a new way of assaying peptides [62].

The use of tandem MS (MS/MS) was another major pivotal breakthrough for the identification of peptides and from which emerged the ideas of peptidomics. Chemical derivatization of peptides was overcome by using the mass spectrometric methodology known as collision-induced dissociation (CID) for sequencing peptides. The combination of nano-LC-ESI-MS/MS and CID delivered more robust data without the need of extra chemical sample preparation and significantly improved throughput and speed of peptide fragmentation and sequencing processes. N-terminal chemical sequencing still complements these methods for proteolytic peptide or neuropeptide discovery [52].

Electron transfer dissociation (ETD) is another applied technique that transfers a "soft" electron from singly charged anthracene anions to multiply protonated peptides to trigger fragmentation, avoiding vibrational energy as in CID [63]. Another technique is the higher energy collisional dissociation (HCD), specific to the Orbitrap mass spectrometer, in which fragmentation occurs external to the trap. One advantage of HCD is that it does not suffer from the low mass cutoff of resonant-excitation and therefore is used for isobaric tag-based quantification as reporter ions can be observed [64]. The combination of HCD and ETD was effectively used for peptidomics experiments. The development of the Orbitrap mass analyzer provided a further increase in the quality of MS/MS data analysis by substantially increasing the resolution, mass accuracy, and speed for thousands of peptides identification [65].

Peptide extraction is mostly overrun with metabolites and other nonpeptide molecules in clinical samples. The wide variety of singly charged molecules interruption can interfere with the identification of peptide ions, creating a challenge. Also, lipids and metabolites can occupy the binding sites on the chromatographic columns (occasionally irreversibly). Although not yet commonly used, MS workflows may include IM-MS and asymmetric high-field waveform-ion mobility spectrometry (FAIMS). The gas-phase electrophoretic methods used in these instrumentations allows one to discriminate and isolate molecules depending on their charge, molecular mass, and mobility [66]. Thus gas-phase electrophoretic methods allow the separation based on structure, coeluting contaminants (e.g., metabolites), or low abundance of chemical interference [67]. It further enables peptide isomers to be separated, or the characterization of peptide posttranslational modifications.

Quantitative measurement of peptide samples is one of the most challenging tasks in peptidomics, especially in different physiological circumstances. The techniques of peptide quantitation most frequently used are label-free (isobaric) and label-based (isotopic) [49,68−70]. Targeted techniques might also be used to achieve absolute quantitation outcomes.

28.15 Concluding remarks

Peptidomics is a small growing field governed by several specialized groups compared to proteomics. Since tauopathy is a hallmark of several neurodegenerative diseases, using a peptidomic approach to study tau in TBI is possible today, given the technological advancement of liquid chromatography and mass spectrometric instrumentations over the last decade. Using a peptidomic technique allows the extraction, separation, enrichment, quantification, and characterization of natural neurotoxic proteolytic peptides of interest. The analytical technologies are now universally available to researchers interested in studying tau peptidome in TBI. Studying tau peptidome in TBI and other chronic neurodegenerative diseases might provide critical insight into the disease occurrence and development that can serve as biomarker utilities for clinical intervention. The development of this methodology can be groundbreaking for future diagnosis and possibly lead to a new prognosis tool for mTBI and severe TBI patients.

References

[1] Agoston DV, Shutes-David A, Peskind ER. Biofluid biomarkers of traumatic brain injury. Brain Inj 2017;31 (9):1195−203.
[2] Huff T, Dulebohn SC. Neuroanatomy, cerebrospinal fluid. StatPearls Publishing; 2017. 2017/11/29.
[3] Yuan X, Desiderio DM. Human cerebrospinal fluid peptidomics. J Mass Spectrom 2005;40(2):176−81.
[4] Pashtun S, Thomas L, Dilek I, Asser K, Kaj B, Yelverton T, et al. Serum tau fragments predict return to play in concussed professional ice hockey players. <https://homeliebertpubcom/neu>; 2016.
[5] Gabbita SP, Scheff SW, Menard RM, Roberts K, Fugaccia I, Zemlan FP. Cleaved-tau: a biomarker of neuronal damage after traumatic brain injury. J Neurotrauma 2005;22(1):83−94.
[6] Anada RP, Wong KT, Jayapalan JJ, Hashim OH, Ganesan D. Panel of serum protein biomarkers to grade the severity of traumatic brain injury. Electrophoresis. 2018.
[7] Pandey S, Singh K, Sharma V, Pandey D, Jha RP, Rai SK, et al. A prospective pilot study on serum cleaved tau protein as a neurological marker in severe traumatic brain injury. Br J Neurosurg 2017;31(3):356−63.
[8] Spector R, Robert Snodgrass S, Johanson CE. A balanced view of the cerebrospinal fluid composition and functions: focus on adult humans. Exp Neurol 2015;273:57−68.
[9] Holtta M, Zetterberg H, Mirgorodskaya E, Mattsson N, Blennow K, Gobom J. Peptidome analysis of cerebrospinal fluid by LC-MALDI MS. PLoS One 2012;7(8):e42555.
[10] Magalhães B, Trindade F, Barros AS, Klein J, Amado F, Ferreira R, et al. Reviewing mechanistic peptidomics in body fluids focusing on proteases. Proteomics. 2018;e1800187.
[11] Buerger K, Teipel SJ, Zinkowski R, Blennow K, Arai H, Engel R, et al. CSF tau protein phosphorylated at threonine 231 correlates with cognitive decline in MCI subjects. Neurology. 2002;59(4):627−9.

[12] Liu MC, Kobeissy F, Zheng W, Zhang Z, Hayes RL, Wang KK. Dual vulnerability of tau to calpains and caspase-3 proteolysis under neurotoxic and neurodegenerative conditions. ASN Neuro 2011;3(1):e00051.

[13] Hampel H, Buerger K, Zinkowski R, Teipel SJ, Goernitz A, Andreasen N, et al. Measurement of phosphorylated tau epitopes in the differential diagnosis of Alzheimer disease: a comparative cerebrospinal fluid study. Arch Gen Psychiatry 2004;61(1):95–102.

[14] Hampel H, Goernitz A, Buerger K. Advances in the development of biomarkers for Alzheimer's disease: from CSF total tau and Abeta(1-42) proteins to phosphorylated tau protein. Brain Res Bull 2003;61(3):243–53.

[15] Ferreira A, Afreen S. Methods related to studying tau fragmentation. Methods Cell Biol 2017;141:245–58.

[16] Olivera-Santa Catalina M, Caballero-Bermejo M, Argent R, Alonso JC, Cuenda A, Lorenzo MJ, et al. Hyperosmotic stress induces tau proteolysis by caspase-3 activation in SH-SY5Y cells. J Cell Biochem 2016;117(12):2781–90.

[17] Park SY, Tournell C, Sinjoanu RC, Ferreira A. Caspase-3- and calpain-mediated tau cleavage are differentially prevented by estrogen and testosterone in beta-amyloid-treated hippocampal neurons. Neuroscience. 2007;144(1):119–27.

[18] Krishnamurthy PK, Mays JL, Bijur GN, Johnson GV. Transient oxidative stress in SH-SY5Y human neuroblastoma cells results in caspase dependent and independent cell death and tau proteolysis. J Neurosci Res 2000;61(5):515–23.

[19] Rubenstein R, Chang B, Yue JK, Chiu A, Winkler EA, Puccio AM, et al. Comparing plasma phospho tau, total tau, and phospho tTau-total tau ratio as acute and chronic traumatic brain injury biomarkers. JAMA Neurol 2017;74(9):1063–72.

[20] Mielke MM, Hagen CE, Xu J, Chai X, Vemuri P, Lowe VJ, et al. Plasma phospho-tau181 increases with Alzheimer's disease clinical severity and is associated with tau- and amyloid-positron emission tomography. Alzheimers Dement 2018.

[21] Massaro AN, Wu YW, Bammler TK, Comstock B, Mathur A, McKinstry RC, et al. Plasma biomarkers of brain injury in neonatal hypoxic-ischemic encephalopathy. J Pediatr 2018;194:67–75 e1.

[22] Aristoteli LP, Molloy MP, Baker MS. Evaluation of endogenous plasma peptide extraction methods for mass spectrometric biomarker discovery. J Proteome Res 2007;6(2):571–81.

[23] Krochmal M, Kontostathi G, Magalhães P, Makridakis M, Klein J, Husi H, et al. Urinary peptidomics analysis reveals proteases involved in diabetic nephropathy. Sci Rep 2017;7(1):15160.

[24] Zhao M, Li M, Yang Y, Guo Z, Sun Y, Shao C, et al. A comprehensive analysis and annotation of human normal urinary proteome. Sci Rep 2017;7(1):3024.

[25] Watanabe Y, Hirao Y, Kasuga K, Tokutake T, Semizu Y, Kitamura K, et al. Molecular network analysis of the urinary proteome of Alzheimer's disease patients. Dement Geriatr Cogn Dis Extra 2019;9(1):53–65.

[26] Sigdel TK, Nicora CD, Qian WJ, Sarwal MM. Optimization for peptide sample preparation for urine peptidomics. Methods Mol Biol 2018.

[27] An M, Gao Y. Urinary biomarkers of brain diseases. Genomics Proteom Bioinforma 2015;13(6):345–54.

[28] Farah R, Haraty H, Salame Z, Fares Y, Ojcius DM, Said Sadier N. Salivary biomarkers for the diagnosis and monitoring of neurological diseases. Biomed J 2018;41(2):63–87.

[29] Shi M, Sui YT, Peskind ER, Li G, Hwang H, Devic I, et al. Salivary tau species are potential biomarkers of Alzheimer's disease. J Alzheimers Dis 2011;27(2):299–305.

[30] Amado F, Lobo MJ, Domingues P, Duarte JA, Vitorino R. Salivary peptidomics. Expert Rev Proteom 2010;7(5):709–21.

[31] Amado F, Calheiros-Lobo MJ, Ferreira R, Vitorino R. Sample treatment for saliva proteomics. Adv Exp Med Biol 2019;1073:23–56.

[32] La Barbera G, Capriotti AL, Cavaliere C, Ferraris F, Montone CM, Piovesana S, et al. Saliva as a source of new phosphopeptide biomarkers: development of a comprehensive analytical method based on shotgun peptidomics. Talanta. 2018;183:245–9.

[33] Azkargorta M, Soria J, Acera A, Iloro I, Elortza F. Human tear proteomics and peptidomics in ophthalmology: toward the translation of proteomic biomarkers into clinical practice. J Proteom 2017;150:359–67.

[34] Kallo G, Emri M, Varga Z, Ujhelyi B, Tozser J, Csutak A, et al. Changes in the chemical barrier composition of tears in Alzheimer's disease reveal potential tear diagnostic biomarkers. PLoS One 2016;11(6):e0158000.

[35] Sowers JL, Wu P, Zhang K, DeWitt DS, Prough DS. Proteomic changes in traumatic brain injury: experimental approaches. Curr Opin Neurol 2018;31(6):709–17.

[36] Ercole A, Magnoni S, Vegliante G, Pastorelli R, Surmacki J, Bohndiek SE, et al. Current and emerging technologies for probing molecular signatures of traumatic brain injury. Front Neurol 2017;8:450.

[37] Manek R, Moghieb A, Yang Z, Kumar D, Kobessiy F, Sarkis GA, et al. Protein biomarkers and neuroproteomics characterization of microvesicles/exosomes from human cerebrospinal fluid following traumatic brain injury. Mol Neurobiol 2018;55(7):6112–28.

[38] Lucke-Wold BP, Turner RC, Logsdon AF, Bailes JE, Huber JD, Rosen CL. Linking traumatic brain injury to chronic traumatic encephalopathy: identification of potential mechanisms leading to neurofibrillary tangle development. J Neurotrauma 2014;31(13):1129–38.

[39] Raida M, Schulz-Knappe P, Heine G, Forssmann WG. Liquid chromatography and electrospray mass spectrometric mapping of peptides from human plasma filtrate. J Am Soc Mass Spectrom 1999;10(1):45–54.

[40] Jorgenson JW. Capillary liquid chromatography at ultrahigh pressures. Annu Rev Anal Chem (Palo Alto Calif) 2010;3:129–50.

[41] Figeys D, Aebersold R. High sensitivity analysis of proteins and peptides by capillary electrophoresis-tandem mass spectrometry: recent developments in technology and applications. Electrophoresis. 1998;19 (6):885–92.

[42] Monton MR, Terabe S. Field-enhanced sample injection for high-sensitivity analysis of peptides and proteins in capillary electrophoresis-mass spectrometry. J Chromatogr A 2004;1032(1–2):203–11.

[43] Costa EP, Menschaert G, Luyten W, De Grave K, Ramon J. PIUS: peptide identification by unbiased search. Bioinformatics. 2013;29(15):1913–14.

[44] Gemperline DC, Scalf M, Smith LM, Vierstra RD. Morpheus spectral counter: a computational tool for label-free quantitative mass spectrometry using the Morpheus search engine. Proteomics. 2016;16(6):920–4.

[45] Kong AT, Leprevost FV, Avtonomov DM, Mellacheruvu D, Nesvizhskii AI. MSFragger: ultrafast and comprehensive peptide identification in mass spectrometry-based proteomics. Nat Methods 2017;14(5):513–20.

[46] Manguy J, Jehl P, Dillon ET, Davey NE, Shields DC, Holton TA. Peptigram: a web-based application for peptidomics data visualization. J Proteome Res 2017;16(2):712–19.

[47] Falth M, Skold K, Norrman M, Svensson M, Fenyo D, Andren PE. SwePep, a database designed for endogenous peptides and mass spectrometry. Mol Cell Proteom 2006;5(6):998–1005.

[48] Falth M, Svensson M, Nilsson A, Skold K, Fenyo D, Andren PE. Validation of endogenous peptide identifications using a database of tandem mass spectra. J Proteome Res 2008;7(7):3049–53.

[49] Verdonck R, De Haes W, Cardoen D, Menschaert G, Huhn T, Landuyt B, et al. Fast and reliable quantitative peptidomics with labelpepmatch. J Proteome Res 2016;15(3):1080–9.

[50] Sasaki K, Sato K, Akiyama Y, Yanagihara K, Oka M, Yamaguchi K. Peptidomics-based approach reveals the secretion of the 29-residue COOH-terminal fragment of the putative tumor suppressor protein DMBT1 from pancreatic adenocarcinoma cell lines. Cancer Res 2002;62(17):4894–8.

[51] Sato K, Sasaki K, Akiyama Y, Yamaguchi K. Mass spectrometric high-throughput analysis of serum-free conditioned medium from cancer cell lines. Cancer Lett 2001;170(2):153–9.

[52] Dallas DC, Guerrero A, Parker EA, Robinson RC, Gan J, German JB, et al. Current peptidomics: applications, purification, identification, quantification, and functional analysis. Proteomics. 2015;15(0):1026–38.

[53] Verhaert PDEM. The bright future of peptidomics. Methods Mol Biol 2018;1719:407–16.

[54] Arapidi G, Osetrova M, Ivanova O, Butenko I, Saveleva T, Pavlovich P, et al. Peptidomics dataset: blood plasma and serum samples of healthy donors fractionated on a set of chromatography sorbents. Data Brief 2018;18:1204–11.

[55] Agyei D, Tsopmo A, Udenigwe CC. Bioinformatics and peptidomics approaches to the discovery and analysis of food-derived bioactive peptides. Anal Bioanal Chem 2018.

[56] Kanlaya R, Thongboonkerd V. Quantitative peptidomics of endogenous peptides involved in TGF-β1-induced epithelial mesenchymal transition of renal epithelial cells. Cell Death Discov 2018;4:9.

[57] Li L, Andrén PE, Sweedler JV. Editorial and review: 29th ASMS Sanibel conference on mass spectrometry-peptidomics: bridging the gap between proteomics and metabolomics by MS. J Am Soc Mass Spectrom 2018;29(5):801–6.

[58] Sheng B, Larsen LB, Le TT, Zhao D. Digestibility of bovine serum albumin and peptidomics of the digests: effect of glycation derived from α-dicarbonyl compounds. Molecules. 2018;23(4).

[59] Di Meo A, Pasic MD, Yousef GM. Proteomics and peptidomics: moving toward precision medicine in urological malignancies. Oncotarget. 2016;7(32):52460–74.

[60] Betz BB, Jenks SJ, Cronshaw AD, Lamont DJ, Cairns C, Manning JR, et al. Urinary peptidomics in a rodent model of diabetic nephropathy highlights epidermal growth factor as a biomarker for renal deterioration in patients with type 2 diabetes. Kidney Int 2016;89(5):1125−35.

[61] Menschaert G, Vandekerckhove TTM, Baggerman G, Schoofs L, Luyten W, Criekinge WV. Peptidomics coming of age: a review of contributions from a bioinformatics angle. J Proteome Res 2010;9(5):2051−61.

[62] Schrader M, Schulz-Knappe P, Fricker LD. Historical perspective of peptidomics. EuPA Open Proteom 2014;3:171−82.

[63] Syka JE, Coon JJ, Schroeder MJ, Shabanowitz J, Hunt DF. Peptide and protein sequence analysis by electron transfer dissociation mass spectrometry. Proc Natl Acad Sci USA 2004;101(26):9528−33.

[64] Chiva C, Sabido E. HCD-only fragmentation method balances peptide identification and quantitation of TMT-labeled samples in hybrid linear ion trap/orbitrap mass spectrometers. J Proteom 2014;96:263−70.

[65] Scigelova M, Makarov A. Orbitrap mass analyzer—overview and applications in proteomics. Proteomics. 2006;6(Suppl. 2):16−21.

[66] Harvey SR, Macphee CE, Barran PE. Ion mobility mass spectrometry for peptide analysis. Methods. 2011;54 (4):454−61.

[67] Pai PJ, Cologna SM, Russell WK, Vigh G, Russell DH. Efficient electrophoretic method to remove neutral additives from protein solutions followed by mass spectrometry analysis. Anal Chem 2011;83(7):2814−18.

[68] Anand S, Samuel M, Ang CS, Keerthikumar S, Mathivanan S. Label-based and label-free strategies for protein quantitation. Methods Mol Biol 2017;1549:31−43.

[69] Gunawardena HP, O'Brien J, Wrobel JA, Xie L, Davies SR, Li S, et al. QuantFusion: novel unified methodology for enhanced coverage and precision in quantifying global proteomic changes in whole tissues. Mol Cell Proteom 2016;15(2):740−51.

[70] Wilkes E, Cutillas PR. Label-free phosphoproteomic approach for kinase signaling analysis. Methods Mol Biol 2017;1636:199−217.

Autoantibodies in central nervous system trauma: new frontiers for diagnosis and prognosis biomarkers

Firas H. Kobeissy[1,2,3], Fatimah Ahmad[1,*], Abdullah Shaito[4,*],
Hiba Hasan[1], Samar Abdel Hady[1,5], Leila Nasrallah[4],
Nour Shaito[1,4], Houssein Hajj Hassan[4], Kazem Zibara[6],
Hamad Yadikar[7], Zhihui Yang[2,3], Ayah Istanbouli[2] and
Kevin K. Wang[2,3]

[1]Department of Biochemistry and Molecular Genetics, Faculty of Medicine, American
University of Beirut, Beirut, Lebanon [2]Departments of Emergency Medicine, Psychiatry,
Neuroscience and Chemistry, University of Florida, Gainesville, FL, United States
[3]Brain Rehabilitation Research Center, Malcom Randall Veterans Affairs Medical Center
(VAMC), Gainesville, FL, United States [4]Department of Biological and Chemical Sciences,
Lebanese International University, Beirut, Lebanon [5]Faculty of Medicine, Alexandria
University, Alexandria, Egypt [6]Biology Department, Faculty of Sciences, Lebanese University,
Beirut, Lebanon [7]Department of Biological Sciences, Faculty of Science, Kuwait University,
Safat, Kuwait

29.1 Introduction

The central nervous system (CNS) trauma or traumatic CNS injuries refer to traumatic brain injury (TBI) and spinal cord injury (SCI). In CNS trauma, a mechanical impact leads to neural and molecular pathophysiological responses. Both types of injuries have complex underlying pathophysiological processes that are still not completely elucidated due to the

* Equal contribution.

heterogeneity of brain injury itself; despite the overwhelming research that has addressed them over the years.

TBI is considered one of the most pervasive healthcare issues worldwide, with a considerable socioeconomic burden. TBI is associated with serious progressive complications and long-term impairments and disabilities. Sixty nine million individuals are estimated to suffer from TBI each year [1]. Annually, about 1.7 million Americans sustain a TBI, 52,000 of which result in death [2–4]. TBI, categorized as focal or diffuse, is caused by sudden brain trauma, often a blow or jolt to the head resulting in hypoxia, intoxication, or vascular injuries of the cerebrum among other insults [5]. TBI has an immediate primary injury phase that represents the physical damage caused by the impact which is associated with challenging therapeutic modalities. The primary injury can lead to a latent injurious signaling cascade referred to as the "secondary injury" including edema, intracranial hypertension, ischemia, excitotoxicity, mitochondrial and metabolic dysfunction, oxidative stress, delayed axonal injury, inflammation, and cell death [5,6]. Furthermore, it has been shown that a subset of TBI patients (around 15%) may end up with persistent and serious latent TBI complications including cognitive and behavioral deficits as well as neuropsychiatric and movement disorders. The secondary injuries stemming from TBI are regarded as risk factors for the development of other neurodegenerative disorders including Alzheimer's disease (AD), Parkinson's disease, and chronic traumatic encephalopathy (CTE) [7,8].

SCI has similar causes as TBI, and is usually due to traumas sustained by physical impacts including road traffic accidents, falls as well as contact sports. In 2016 the National SCI Statistical Center reported a total of 282,000 patients living with SCI in the United States, alone. Similar to TBI, SCI has different severity levels and it proceeds through several phases [9]. During the SCI primary injury phase, patients suffer from a spinal shock, in the form of urinary incontinence and respiratory/circulatory disruptions and these currently are the main SCI therapeutic targets. Spinal trauma can lead to a temporary reduction or total loss of most or all of the spinal reflexes below the injury level. The secondary injury phase, during which patients gradually recover from the spinal shock, takes place within few days following the primary injury. Finally, SCI patients may advance to the chronic phase of SCI where they show signs of delayed neurologic symptoms including neuropathic pain [10,11].

Currently, there are no diagnostic approaches that can identify the subset of TBI patients who will eventually develop chronic complications. As a result, latent TBI manifestations have proven to be a treatment challenge. Therefore there are few efficient therapies targeted against the latent manifestations of TBI [12–16]. In recent years, biological molecular signature markers, referred to as "biomarkers," have stood out as promising prognostic and diagnostic tools that can predict neurological outcomes of CNS trauma [7,8,10,16–18].

Biomarkers of a specific disease can be diagnostic, prognostic, or even predictive. The Food and Drug Administration (FDA), defines biomarkers as a "characteristic that serves as an objective indicator of normal biological processes, pathogenic processes, or response to an exposure or intervention, including therapeutic interventions" [19]. The National Institute of Health (NIH) proposes five phases for the evaluation of biomarkers: (1) discovery using genomics or proteomics, (2) developing an assay that is portable and reproducible, (3) measuring sensitivity and specificity, (4) affirming the measurement in a large cohort, and (5) determining the risks and benefits of using the new diagnostic biomarker [20]. This five-step process was later refined into a three-step process by the National Institute of Medicine: (1) analytical validation (2) qualification and (3) utilization [21].

Early used biomarkers, such as protein and gene biomarkers, had the limitation of low specificity and sensitivity [22]; hence, the immediate need to find other types of biomarkers in the field of brain trauma. Recently, microRNAs and autoantibodies have emerged as novel classes of biomarkers in this field and are now under intense investigation for their potential capabilities as personalized biomarkers.

Here, we highlight the potential use of autoantibodies as candidate biofluid (blood and CSF) diagnostic biomarkers and discuss their potential roles in the secondary progression as well as the underlying pathology of CNS injury. These autoantibodies are orchestrated by the imbalance in the CNS—immune system cross talk as will be discussed later.

29.2 The immunological events following central nervous system injury

It has been long thought that our nervous system is an immunoprivileged entity where the immune cells are not in direct proximity to our neural cells. However, immune cells are normal dwellers of the CNS and can confer neuroprotection during CNS injury [23]. In fact, CNS injury results in the early activation of complex immunological reactions that profoundly support the spontaneous brain regenerative processes like neovascularization, axonal sprouting, and neurogenesis, leading to recovery from injury. It is demonstrated that early immune activation (within minutes) post-CNS injury provides neuroprotective effects and that the modulation of innate and adaptive immune responses is a fundamental part of the regenerative processes. However, the degree of recovery may be dependent on the mode of these immunological mechanisms, as discussed [24].

Following CNS injury, there is an activation of a cascade of events that includes the release of inflammatory mediators whose effects are observed at chronic time points postinjury. This cascade begins with initial signaling events and changes at the injury site, including instantaneous damage and even death of neural cells. The damaged cells release damage-associated molecular patterns (DAMPs). Then the cascade progresses to include innate and adaptive immune responses. DAMPs signal to resident immune cells via toll-like receptors (TLRs). This primes and activates resident microglia and astrocytes at the site of injury leading to their morphological changes as well as secretion of proinflammatory mediators. This immune activation is followed by the recruitment of peripheral immune cells that traffic through the damaged blood—brain barrier (BBB) during the acute posttraumatic period [23,25]. This cascade is detailed below.

29.2.1 Initial signaling

The immune system has evolved to respond quickly to brain injuries and can participate in the repair process, as well. Also, it can respond to the death of self-cells causing an inflammatory response in the absence of infection, the so-called sterile inflammatory response or "sterile inflammation." This response is an essential physiological response to brain injury and is the first step on the road of restoration of homeostasis in the brain [26–28]. This process involves key mediators, such as:

1. Danger signals:
    Brain injury activates the innate immune system via the release of specific molecules referred to as DAMPs that encompass alarmins. Examples of alarmins include HMGB1, S100 proteins, adenosine triphosphate (ATP), DNA or RNA, interleukin 1α (IL-1α), and heat shock proteins (HSPs) [29]. Following TBI, a sterile immune reaction is triggered through the release of alarmins to maintain homeostasis. DAMPs signaling is triggered when DAMPs are recognized by the TLRs and their coreceptors, such as the scavenger receptors SCARF1 and CD36. Studies have shown that scavenger receptors play a crucial role in the clearance of debris and apoptotic cells in the CNS; therefore they are considered as potential therapeutic targets in a variety of CNS conditions, especially TBI [27,28].

2. Inflammasomes:
    Inflammasomes are cytosolic multiprotein complexes involved in the initiation of the innate immune response and usually are expressed by myeloid cells. Inflammasomes initiate the immune activation responses via the release of proinflammatory cytokines. Interleukin-1β (IL-1β), a proinflammatory cytokine, is a major player in triggering the TBI-induced inflammatory cascade [30]. Also, post-TBI amplification of the initial tissue damage is mediated by inflammasome-induced cell destruction [31]. The nucleotide-binding domain (NOD)-like receptor protein 1 (NLRP1)-inflammasome assembly is enhanced by the TBI where the therapeutic neutralization of the cortical NLPR1 inflammasome reduced the activation of the innate CNS inflammatory response. Interestingly, neutralization of the NLRP1 inflammasome reduced the brain lesion size at 3 days post fluid percussion injury [32]. However, Brickler et al. found no effect of NLPR1 knockout on the histopathology or motor control improvement in a mouse controlled cortical impact (CCI) model of TBI [33]. Of interest, NLRP3 inflammasome is a regulator of caspase-1 activation, and IL-1β and IL-18 maturation and secretion [34]. NLRP3 expression increases in the cortex of rats following TBI [35]. Interestingly, a small molecule inhibitor of the NLRP3 inflammasome alleviates the neuroinflammatory response post-TBI [36]. These findings indicate that the blockade of inflammasome activation signaling might serve a neurotherapeutic target in TBI.

29.2.2 Microglial activation

Microglia, the primary resident immune cells of the CNS, are usually among the first responders to any intraparenchymal injury and participate in restoring CNS homeostasis following injury [37]. Microglia proliferation following TBI is induced by the release of paracrine or autocrine factors, such as brain-derived neurotrophic factor (BDNF), macrophage colony-stimulating factor (M-CSF), neurotrophin 3 (NT-3), and IL-1 [28,38]. Microglia have major immune functions including phagocytosis mediated by the recognition of UDP released from dead cells by the P2Y6 receptor on activated microglia [39,40], and maintenance of the BBB integrity and CNS barrier structures such as the glial limitans and vasculature [39,41]. These functions suggest that microglia can be neuroprotective after brain injury. Recent studies are interested in investigating the role of microglia in CNS trauma taking into consideration the effects of age and gender on the inflammatory response and the functional outcomes following injury [42–44]. However, microglia functions during TBI and SCI depend on their activation states, which result in different phenotypic and functional responses. Initial microglial activation is neuroprotective as discussed above, but chronic microglia activation can further contribute to the later tissue damage following injury and can potentially lead to neurodegeneration due to the continued release of proinflammatory mediators by microglia [25,45,46]. It has been shown that IFN-γ cytokine secreted by Th1 T helper cells, can lead to the transformation of resting microglia into M1 microglia which produce proinflammatory cytokines. Conversely, IL-4 and IL-13 cytokines derived from Th2 T helper cells can induce the transformation of microglia cells into the M2 phenotype which can facilitate phagocytosis of cell debris, tissue repair, and support the survival of neurons [47,48]. Therapies that can shift the balance between the different activation phenotypes of microglia may be used to enhance CNS repair following TBI [25,49].

29.2.3 Peripheral innate immune activation

Following CNS injury, the disrupted BBB permits the leakage of inflammatory cytokines, complement proteins, and debris into the periphery outside the brain; thus activating the peripheral innate immune response. Following CNS injury, a remarkable increase in the number of leukocytes and neutrophils in the peripheral circulation around the CNS is noticed. Neutrophils are usually the first cells to infiltrate the CNS following injury. There is evidence of the infiltration of neutrophils into the CNS parenchyma near the site of injury [50,51].

29.2.4 Adaptive immunity in traumatic brain injury and spinal cord injury

TBI can induce both components of adaptive immunity: cell-mediated immunity (primarily mediated by activated memory effector T lymphocytes or regulatory T cells) and humoral immunity (mediated by B-lymphocytes that are responsible for the production of antibodies following activation by an antigen).

The role of T cells in TBI pathogenesis is not entirely clear. T cell-mediated immunity can mediate either destructive or homeostatic effects [28]. Activated T cells are recruited to the CNS after an injury [52,53], and a significant number of T cells infiltrate the pericontusional cortex, but not the hippocampus or thalamus. These T cells continue to increase in number until at least 7 days following CCI in mice [30]. In a closed head injury model, there was no difference between wild-type and Rag1-deficient mice that lack mature T and B cells, with respect to injury severity and neurological impairment for up to 7 days after head injury. These findings may suggest that adaptive immunity plays little role in early TBI pathogenesis; however, caution must be taken when looking at injury type, severity, and animal model [54]. Similar results were obtained by Weckbach et al. using Rag1 knockout mice using weight drop injury model of TBI. They concluded that the absence of adaptive immunity had no effect on neurological outcomes, BBB integrity, pro- or antiapoptotic mediators, hippocampal architecture, or astroglial activation [55]. In accordance, inhibition of the T cell migration to the brain post-TBI did not provide any protection from TBI but reduced posttraumatic inflammation by reducing the numbers of neutrophils and macrophages/microglia after one day of injury [55]. Furthermore, CD4 + T cells adoptively transferred into Rag1$^{-/-}$ mice that underwent aseptic cerebral injury exacerbated the lesion size and number of apoptotic cells [56]. Besides, it has been shown that the adoptively transferred effector T cells, rather than naïve T cells, show a more extensive brain injury [56].

In addition, it has been shown that during the early acute phases of TBI or SCI there is immunosuppression, which can cause excessive extracranial infections. Yang et al. suggested that TBI contributes to immunosuppression through sympathetic nervous system activation, via impairing CD4 + and CD8 + T cell functions by upregulation of the immune checkpoint molecule PD-1 [49]. Also, the antiviral immune responses post-SCI were reduced in mice due to impairment of T cell infiltration and effector functions [57]. Interestingly, autoreactive T cells targeted to CNS self-antigens [such as myelin basic protein (MBP)] can be neuroprotective after SCI [54,58].

29.2.5 Role of autoimmunity

B cells as immune cells act as antigen-presenting cells as well as antibody secreting cells [59,60]. To ensure proper development, B cells undergo two types of selection: negative-selection to eliminate overreactive lymphocytes, whereas positive selection keeps the "sub-threshold" stimulation of lymphocytes to identify self/host antigens and increase sensitivity to foreign antigens [61]. The process of positive selection is significant when the threshold level has exceeded an abnormal condition of autoimmunity [61].

Autoinflammation and autoimmunity are two immune pathways implicated in the progression of the secondary injury following CNS injury [62−66]. Autoimmunity occurs when an adaptive immune response develops against self-antigens. The self-antigens activate autoreactive B cells that, in turn, differentiate into plasma cells producing autoantibodies. The nature and degree of this activation determine whether the response is beneficial or detrimental to recovery [63].

In one study by Lopez-Escribano et al., it was shown that serum taken from acute TBI patients would induce leukemic cell apoptosis coupled with autoantibody secretion, which was attributed to TBI-induced cell death mechanism which may be potential sources of self-antigen presentation that can produce autoantibodies [67]. In fact, TBI causes BBB disruption and thus facilitates the release of intracellular proteins or their digested fragments from TBI-damaged cells/tissues into the cerebrospinal fluid (CSF) or bloodstream. Consequently, an autoimmune response is triggered, leading to the production of autoantibodies targeted against brain-specific antigens as depicted in Fig. 29.1.

According to previous studies, TBI-evoked autoimmunity could have either pathogenic or protective roles in the brain. "Natural" autoantibody responses are considered beneficial since they activate intracellular repair pathways [68]. An example is the natural IgM autoantibodies that can clear apoptotic cells and enhance remyelination and neurite outgrowth, as shown in mouse models of multiple sclerosis [68]. One study suggests that

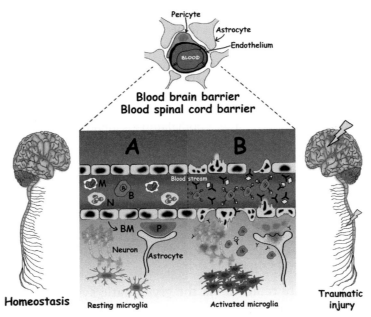

FIGURE 29.1 **Activation of the immune responses leading to autoantibodies production following CNS injury.** (A) Without CNS injury, the blood−brain/spinal cord barriers are intact and the autoantigens are protected by the CNS immune privilege. (B) Following CNS trauma, there will be a disruption of the blood−brain/spinal cord barriers. CNS-specific proteins are released to the periphery and are no longer protected by the CNS immune privilege. The CNS-specific proteins act as autoantigens that will be recognized by overactivated B cells leading to the production of autoantibodies. This leads to abnormal immune responses which involve the excessive release of cytokines and inflammatory mediators that increase vascular permeability and further disrupt the BBB. Recent neurotherapeutic approaches target overreactive B cells to reduce the damage caused by autoantibodies. For this purpose, autoantibodies are being investigated as diagnostic/prognostic biomarkers, neurotherapeutic targets, or as neurotoxic mediators that may exacerbate the injury. *B*, B cells; *BM*, basement membrane; *M*, macrophage; *N*, neutrophils; *P*, pericytes.

naturally occurring IgG autoantibodies bind specifically to dying neurons and may participate in phagocytosis and removal of the injured neurons following a cortical lesion [69]. Interestingly, another study supports the concept of "beneficial autoimmunity" by showing that autoreactive T cell responses against myelin self-antigens were associated with improved neuronal survival and functional recovery in murine models of CNS injury [70]. However, it was shown that SCI-induced autoantibodies can bind nuclear antigens as well, including DNA and RNA, exacerbating postinjury neuropathology [71].

Furthermore, T cells interact with autoantibodies by secreting cytokines that synergize with autoantibodies to cause cell damage [6]. There exist various factors that influence autoantibody production post-TBI, for example, the lesion location, the severity of primary injury, and time postinjury [6].

In CNS injury, several proteins have been identified as a potential source for autoantibodies, including the neuron-specific UCHL1 protein, axon-specific microtubule-associated Tau protein, glial-specific GFAP/GBDP, S100B, and peroxidredoxin 6 as well as MBP and glutamate receptors [72–75]. It has been reported that increased levels of autoantibodies against glial protein S100B are present in football players with repeated concussions [76]. Other studies have revealed the production of autoantibodies specific to other brain proteins such as MBP, GFAP, peroxiredoxin 6, and glutamate receptors [77–79]. Also, antipituitary antibodies were found in patient serum several years after head trauma [80,81]. In fact, hypothalamic-pituitary autoimmunity seems to contribute to TBI-induced pituitary damage and is associated with an increased risk of onset/persistence of posttraumatic hypopituitarism (PTHP) [82]. The antihypothalamus antibodies (AHA) and antipituitary antibodies (APA) [22] show remarkable associations between these antibodies and head trauma [81,83]. High titers of APA and AHA were associated with hypopituitarism even after 5 years post-TBI [80]. SCI-induced autoantibodies have also been reported, including autoantibodies against GFAP, MBP, and S100β [71,84,85]. Further studies are necessary to evaluate the role of autoimmunity, particularly the role of autoantibodies as "beneficial" and neuroprotective products of the immune system, or "detrimental" products that can exacerbate the CNS injury.

29.2.6 Neurotoxic waste removal via the glymphatic system is impaired posttraumatic brain injury

Considering the brain is in a constant state of metabolic activity then a waste removal system must exist by which extracellular proteins are cleared. As demonstrated recently, the solutes and cellular components in the brain interstitium move toward the CSF [86]. Astrocytes that support and protect neurons were long thought to have a role in facilitating changes in blood flow as well as removal of waste from the brain [87,88]; nevertheless, the exact mechanism is still underinvestigated. It was discovered that an efficient paravascular macroscopic waste clearance system exists to eliminate metabolites and soluble proteins including amyloid-β from CNS interstitium. It utilizes networks of periarterial and perivenous conduits coupled with aquaporin-4 (AQP-4) water channels found mainly on perivascular astroglial endfeet where subarachnoid CSF enters the brain rapidly, along the paravascular spaces surrounding the penetrating arteries, which then exchanges these components with the surrounding interstitial fluid. It was therefore named as the glymphatic system owing to the involvement of glia cells and its resemblance to the lymphatic system [86,89,90]. It is known that the BBB and the glymphatic system complement each other to maintain a well-balanced, healthy microenvironment for neurons [90,91]. Of interest, this system is most efficient during resting states. The efficiency of clearance of the waste by the glymphatic system via exchange of CSF with interstitial fluid increases by 70% in the sleeping brain. It was suggested that the restorative function of sleep may be related to the enhanced removal of potentially neurotoxic waste products [92]. It should be noted that sleep disturbance is commonly reported post-TBI and this seems to play a role in the accumulation of neurotoxic waste products in the interstitial space [93–95].

Following TBI, the waste clearance performed by the glymphatic system is altered. After TBI, the glymphatic system function is reduced by ∼60%, with this impairment persisting for at least 1 month postinjury [96]. This system was found to be affected at the acute phase following mTBI which reduced the efficacy of the system to remove waste [97]. In addition, it was shown that the knockout of AQP-4 (1) accentuated the glymphatic system dysfunction as evidenced by impairment of paravascular CSF−ISF exchange and interstitial solute clearance, and (2) exacerbated neurodegeneration along with development of neurofibrillary pathology. The absence of the AQP-4 gene reduced the amyloid-beta clearance by 55% [96]. In TBI patients, relocalization of AQP-4 channels away from astrocycic endfeets combined with astroglial scars, inflammation, the buildup of proteinaceous neurotoxic waste products [cleaved tau (C-tau), p-tau and beta-amyloid (Aβ)], and astrocytic proteins (GFAP and S100B), are thought to contribute to glymphatic system dysfunction [96,98,99]. These findings highlight the role of the glymphatic system in protecting from neurodegenerative disorders, attributed to faulty aggregation of proteins, and that accumulation of these neurotoxic waste products increases the risk of neurodegenerative disorders that are mostly associated with repetitive TBI like AD [100] and CTE [101].

29.2.7 Autoantibodies as biomarkers in central nervous system trauma

The role of autoantibodies in TBI has been questioned for more than 40 years [102,103]. As previously mentioned, TBI causes a breach in the BBB coupled with the activation of injurious pathways (e.g., excitotoxicity, apoptosis, necrosis, etc.) leading to neural cell injury. The BBB is a dynamic network of specialized capillary endothelial cells that separates the brain from the circulating blood and restricts the transport of molecules and solutes, thus contributing to the brain's immune privilege [6]. The blood−spinal cord barrier (BSCB) is considered to be the functional equivalent to the BBB. Both share similar structural building blocks that provide a specialized microenvironment for the cellular constituents [104]. BBB and BSCB integrity can be compromised by several local and systemic factors, including trauma, activation of circulating leukocytes, and molecular mediators that affect vascular permeability [104,105].

Following an injury, molecular components (DNA, lipids, proteins, receptors) of injured cells, are released through the disrupted BBB, into the peripheral circulation, as shown in Fig. 29.1. The adaptive immune system (B and T lymphocytes) recognizes these as nonself-antigens, inducing an autoimmune response. Autoantibodies, produced by B cells, may represent putative long-term biomarkers, that may be correlated to the severity of the injury. Autoantibodies can also serve as prognostic disease indicators that may act as potential neurotherapeutic targets, as discussed later.

29.2.8 List of identified autoantibodies

A list of several autoantigens and their corresponding autoantibodies have been identified and characterized in different human pathologies, including CNS injury, as shown in Table 29.1 (see Fig. 29.2 for illustration) [115].

A list of these neural proteins implicated in TBI and considered as a major source for autoantibodies includes MBP, GFAP, S100β, α7 ACR, GluR1 and NR2A, AHA, APA.

TABLE 29.1   A concise list of autoantibodies reported following TBI/SCI studies.

	Antibody	TBI/SCI	References
Human studies	Acetylcholine receptor	TBI	[106]
	Peroxiredoxin 6	Mild−moderate TBI	[79]
	Antinuclear antibodies	Severe TBI	[67]
	Glial fibrillary acidic protein	Mild−severe, severe TBI/SCI	[77,85]
	Glutamate receptors GluR1 and NR2a	Mild−severe, mild TBI	[78,106−108]
	Myelin basic protein	Severe TBI/SCI	[77,84,109,110]
	S100B	Mild repeated TBI/SCI	[7,76,111,112]
	Hypothalamus	TBI	[83,113]
	Pituitary	Mild−severe, mild repeated TBI	[81,83,113]
Animal studies	Myelin basic protein	Experimental TBI/SCI	[84,114]
	Peroxiredoxin 6	Experimental TBI	[79]
	Antinuclear antibodies (possibly glutamate receptors)	Experimental SCI	[71]

SCI, Spinal cord injury; *TBI*, traumatic brain injury.

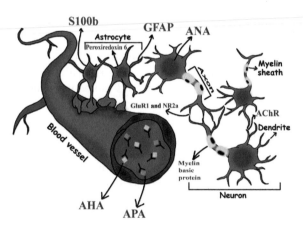

FIGURE 29.2   **Autoantigens that have been implicated in human CNS injury.** These include the AHA, APA, MBP, GluR1, NR2A, GFAP, ANA, and S100B autoantigens.

29.2.8.1 Myelin basic protein

MBP was the among the first identified brain self-antigenic target of autoimmunity [109]. MBP is involved in the process of myelination of nerves in the nervous system. Elevated levels of anti-MBP autoantibodies have been reported in human TBI [77]. Also, MBP autoantibodies have been identified in CSF from TBI patients, and their concentration strongly correlated to the severity of injury on the first day after TBI [110]. MBP autoantibody also increased in experimental SCI, at the level of T8, as was detected by immunohistochemistry. It was also present in the in sera from acute phase of SCI patients [84].

29.2.8.2 GFAP

Damage to CNS astrocytes, in conjunction with compromised BBB or BSCB, causes the release of GFAP and its breakdown products (BDPs) into the peripheral circulation [116]. In an interesting study, the presence of GFAP-BDPs in circulation was associated with TBI. The influx of these molecules triggers an autoimmune response characterized by the production of autoantibodies specific to this protein. TBI patients showed an average 3.77-fold increase in the levels of anti-GFAP autoantibody from early to late time points postinjury with elevated circulating IgG autoantibodies against brain proteins with molecular weight 38–50 kDa. The results revealed that the 38–50 kDa autoantigen was in fact GFAP with its associated breakdown products. In addition, the same study showed that GFAP autoantibodies can enter living astroglial cells in culture and compromise their survival [77]. In addition, significantly increased anti-GFAP levels were detected in the plasma of patients with acute SCI and were correlated with SCI-associated neuropathic pain [85].

29.2.8.3 S100β protein

S100β, a calcium binding protein in the brain, is another astrocyte-specific protein. The S100β protein levels, in serum and CSF, were correlated with TBI incidence and severity of injury [117–123]. S100β autoantibody can also be used as a CNS injury biomarker. Studies have shown that S100β autoantibodies are seen in both repeated mild TBI as well as single major TBI [76]. Long-lasting autoimmune responses, generating S100β autoantibodies, have been suggested to be associated with various adverse CNS injury outcomes, including prolonged postconcussive symptoms, early cognitive decline, CTE, and dementia of the Alzheimer's type [76,124–127]. Analysis of serum samples from 67 football players revealed that the number of subconcussive head impacts and serum levels of S100β autoantibody were positively correlated with the future risk for cognitive deficits [76]. Interestingly, it was demonstrated that the antibodies against S100β were present 48 hours following SCI [111]. Further research is needed to assess the role of S100β autoantibodies as a specific marker for sports-related concussions and as a risk factor for the development of postconcussive symptoms, impaired recovery, and long-term complications.

29.2.8.4 Acetylcholine receptor (α7 ACR)

Another candidate neural autoantigen is α7-subunit of acetylcholine receptor (α7 ACR). Signal transduction following binding the receptor supports neuronal plasticity and suppresses the secretion of proinflammatory cytokines like TNF-α [128,129]. Blood serum levels of α7 ACR autoantibodies against several fragments of ACR were measured in children with different severities of TBI. The results showed that the level of autoantibodies to different fragments of ACR is proportional to the severity of trauma in the first week of the insult [106]. These findings highlighted the hypothesis that an inflammatory reaction is activated coupled with the disruption of the BBB intensifies the leakage of structural neuronal components into the peripheral circulation leading to the production of autoantibodies against them.

29.2.8.5 Peroxiredoxin 6

Peroxiredoxin 6 enzyme, an antioxidant, is a protein that is highly expressed in astrocytes and it acts as a target for TBI-induced autoantibodies. Peroxiredoxin 6 is of special interest as it represents a putative TBI biomarker that was identified using autoimmune profiling approach [79]. A study showed that peroxiredoxin 6 was highly expressed in human traumatized cerebral cortex and the circulating levels of peroxiredoxin 6 were elevated fourfold over control values in serum, 4−24 hours following mild to moderate TBI [79].

29.2.8.6 Glutamate receptors (GluR1 and NR2A)

Serum levels of autoantibodies against AMPA glutamate receptors (GluR1 subunit) and NMDA glutamate receptor (NR2A subunit) were examined in 60 children, aged 7−16 years, with chronic posttraumatic headache at 6 and 12 months following trauma. Titers of autoantibodies to GluR1 subunit and largely NR2A subunit were found to be higher in children that exhibited neurological symptoms. These symptoms were suggested to be due to hypoxic brain lesions, with evidence of hyperstimulation of NMDA glutamate receptors, increased BBB permeability, and an overreactive autoimmune response post-TBI [78]. In this study, it was found that the anti-NMDA receptor antibodies, in children, appear to correlate with the development of seizure disorders postbrain injury [78]. Importantly, this antibody was reported in several studies addressing TBI [106,107]. Mice with a mid-thoracic spinal contusion injury had elevated serum levels of autoantibodies that were found to bind to CNS proteins, nuclear antigens and neuronal antigens [71].

29.2.8.7 Other personalized autoantigens

In addition to the above brain neuronal and glial target antigens, antibodies against the hypothalamic-pituitary axis proteins have been reported [82,83]. In encephalitis associated with severe status epilepticus, GABA receptor antibodies have been studied and identified as a potential target for directed therapy [130]. Additionally, antibodies against NMDA receptors have been associated with cytotoxic T cell activity in paraneoplastic encephalitis [131]. The involvement of APA in the TBI-induced hypopituitarism was investigated 3 years after acute TBI. It was found that the risk of hypopituitarism increased in APA positive patients 3 years post-TBI as assessed in the sera [81]. This finding was even evident post sports-related chronic repetitive head trauma. AHAs were detected in 21.3%, and APAs were detected in 22.9% of the boxers, but in none of the healthy controls [83]. To get valuable clinical information, we believe that measuring the levels of these autoantibodies, taking into consideration the contribution of other markers, is essential.

29.2.9 Evaluation of autoantibodies as central nervous system injury biomarkers

The current experimental and clinical status for autoantibodies as CNS injury biomarkers requires further investigation to correlate the presence of a specific autoantibody with a specific CNS injury, and how this specific autoantibody modulates the functions of CNS cells or leads to the development of CNS dysfunction. In reality, the data to support the direct contribution of autoantibodies to the progression of neuropathologies, in patients with trauma, is scarce.

A more rigorous clinical studies should address the following points in the area of CNS injury autoantibodies field: (1) identification of the pattern of autoantibody expression levels in different phases posttrauma, in correlation to clinical outcomes; (2) increasing the knowledge about autoimmunity activation post-TBI; (3) identification of a diagnostic and prognostic autoantibodies baseline level prior to injury in order to evaluate degree of the damage and possible injury outcomes; (4) identification of new CNS-specific antigens; (5) specifying the relation between a specified autoantibody and a phenotype; and finally (6) accounting for age or sex as factors influencing autoantibody production [132]. The latter point is essential as autoimmune responses vary with sex and age. For example, in a study investigating age-related autoimmunity, older patients have shown more autoreactive antibodies in their sera, and they had reduced regulatory T cells because of thymic regression but more circulatory T4 cells [133]. Nonetheless, another study has shown that younger patients are more likely to produce autoantibodies against neuronal antigens after brain injury [70].

29.3 Activation of B cells exacerbates secondary central nervous system injury

Currently, most data indicate that the activation of B cells post-CNS trauma can lead to further injury-associated impairments that increase tissue damage and disturb neurological recovery. In TBI models, mice devoid of B cells could regain locomotion better and have reduced pathological manifestations compared to wild-type mice, with antibody-producing B cells and IgG in their CSF [134]. Also, it was shown that myelin damage at the site of CNS injury provokes the release of MBP autoantibodies that, in turn, could result in secondary injury impairments [53]. In fact, B cells and their secreted antibodies contribute to CNS inflammation, in addition to the systemic pathologies post-CNS trauma. Some of the systemic and organ-related disturbances, including increased oxidative metabolism in human blood neutrophils and monocytes [135], damage to the lungs and kidneys, and increased inflammatory signaling, have been attributed to autoantibodies secretion [136,137]. CNS injury permits the entry of environmental pathogens, including bacteria and viruses, and increases the permeability of the intestine leading to commensal bacterial translocation from the gut into the blood [138]. This influx of bacteria induces the activation of B cells through the TLRs; hence, enhancing the neuroinflammatory reactions post-CNS injury [139].

Studies have shown that the type and amount of autoantibodies secreted from autoreactive B cells, following CNS injury may be correlated with lesion size, location, and molecular targets involved [66,136,140]. Binding of these autoantibodies to transmembrane proteins and extracellular receptors can disrupt normal cellular function. It should be noted that the activation of the complement system disturbs the functional recovery processes [134,141,142]. It has been shown that the activation of B cells post-SCI, due to the release or alteration of different self-antigens, induces a pathogenic activation of the complement cascade after the secretion of antibodies [134]. A recent study investigated the role of complement system activation in promoting the acute secondary injury which usually follows TBI. Inhibition of c3 activation prevented chronic inflammation and progressive neuronal degeneration following experimental TBI (CCI) in adult male mice. However, c3 activation reduced dendritic and synaptic density and inhibited neuroblast migration several weeks after TBI. Furthermore, sustained complement activation triggers chronic inflammatory microgliosis characterized by chronic loss of neurons, dendrites, and synapses even at 30 days post-CCI [143].

29.4 B cells as therapeutic targets for central nervous system injury

As mentioned above, recent data have accumulated evidence to suggest that overactivated B cells have an integral role in traumatic CNS injury. Overreactive B cells exacerbate the initial systemic and neurological pathology of TBI, and could impair recovery [71,134]. This crucial role of B cells in the pathogenesis of TBI, leads to the recent notion of using overreactive B cells as therapeutic targets. Since overreactive B cells contribute to TBI pathology, then targeting them will alleviate TBI outcomes attributed to B cells. Immunotherapy is one way of targeting B cells to provide a neuroprotective effect. For example, intravenous IgG administration (IVIG), which is a therapeutic preparation of polyclonal immunoglobulin G extracted from the plasma of donors [144], has neuroprotective roles and immunomodulatory effects via inhibition of inflammatory cytokine production, complement activation in the CNS, and pathogenic autoantibody production [145]. The administration of IVIG into animal models of SCI and TBI enhances the CNS functional recovery and improves the neurobehavioral and histological outcomes [146–148]. Another immunotherapy strategy targets CD20 which is a membrane-embedded surface molecule that plays a role in the development and proliferation of B cells [149]. A glycoengineered anti-CD20 antibody reduced inflammation and tissue injury by inhibiting the NFκB-dependent production of proinflammatory mediators in a mouse SCI model. Therapeutic CD20 antibodies such as rituximab or obinutuzumab may act as a novel immunotherapy strategy to improve CNS recovery [150]. However, it is still premature to predict whether anti-CD20 treatment is effective in human CNS injury models, given that anti-CD20 targets immature B that do not produce antibodies. This treatment may be effective in inhibiting de novo synthesis of more self-reactive B cells and may be beneficial if administered soon after the injury occurs [151].

Drugs that block B cell activating factor (BAFF) and a proliferation-inducing ligand (APRIL) inhibit B cell activation and differentiation and might be considered potential B cell–based therapeutic targets [152]. One study proposed the delivery of these agents, either intraspinally or intracranially, in order to evaluate their efficacy in CNS injury models [153].

29.5 Conclusion

As discussed, advanced prognostic tools, accurate disease characterization and phenotyping, and prediction of long-term complications are immensely needed for better injury management and treatment. Rigorous experimental, as well as more clinical research, is required to pin down the utility of autoantibodies for their diagnostic, prognostic, and therapy values in CNS injury paradigms. This requires a comprehensive understanding of the mechanisms involved in the production and the function of autoantibodies in CNS injury and how the CNS trauma disrupts the immune privilege of the CNS, involving the subsequent complex brain—immune system interactions that affect recovery. In addition, B cell activation represents a promising target for CNS injury treatment, which represents one main culprit involved in autoantibodies generation, which would alleviate secondary neural injury and improve TBI patient outcomes by providing a source of targeted, personalized therapy.

Acknowledgments

This work is supported by the grant support by the NIH 1 R21 NS085455-01 (PI: Kevin K. Wang). We thank all the support and contribution from all the authors for their scientific input, edits and revisions. All the figures and schematics are designed, illustrated and generated by Dr. Samar Abdelhady, MD.

References

[1] Dewan MC, Rattani A, Gupta S, et al. Estimating the global incidence of traumatic brain injury. J Neurosurg 2018;1—18.

[2] Corrigan JD, Selassie AW, Orman JA. The epidemiology of traumatic brain injury. J Head Trauma Rehab 2010;25(2):72—80.

[3] Selassie AW, Zaloshnja E, Langlois JA, Miller T, Jones P, Steiner C. Incidence of long-term disability following traumatic brain injury hospitalization, United States, 2003. J Head Trauma Rehab 2008;23(2):123—31.

[4] Wolf SJ, Bebarta VS, Bonnett CJ, Pons PT, Cantrill SV. Blast injuries. Lancet. 2009;374(9687):405—15.

[5] Malkesman O, Tucker LB, Ozl J, McCabe JT. Traumatic brain injury—modeling neuropsychiatric symptoms in rodents. Front Neurol 2013;4:157.

[6] Diamond B, Honig G, Mader S, Brimberg L, Volpe BT. Brain-reactive antibodies and disease. Annu Rev Immunol 2013;31:345—85.

[7] Bazarian JJ, Zhu T, Zhong J, et al. Persistent, long-term cerebral white matter changes after sports-related repetitive head impacts. PLoS One 2014;9(4):e94734.

[8] Angoa-Perez M, Kane MJ, Briggs DI, Herrera-Mundo N, Viano DC, Kuhn DM. Animal models of sports-related head injury: bridging the gap between preclinical research and clinical reality. J Neurochem 2014.

[9] Haring RS, Canner JK, Haider AH, Schneider EB. Ocular injury in the United States: emergency department visits from 2006—2011. Injury 2016;47(1):104—8.

[10] Albayar AA, Roche A, Swiatkowski P, et al. Biomarkers in spinal cord injury: prognostic insights and future potentials. Front Neurol 2019;10:27.

[11] Rowland JW, Hawryluk GW, Kwon B, Fehlings MG. Current status of acute spinal cord injury pathophysiology and emerging therapies: promise on the horizon. Neurosurg Focus 2008;25(5):E2.

[12] Wheaton P, Mathias JL, Vink R. Impact of pharmacological treatments on outcome in adult rodents after traumatic brain injury: a meta-analysis. J Psychopharmacol 2011;25(12):1581—99.

[13] Maas AI, Roozenbeek B, Manley GT. Clinical trials in traumatic brain injury: past experience and current developments. Neurother: J Am Soc Exp NeuroTher 2010;7(1):115—26.

[14] Loane DJ, Faden AI. Neuroprotection for traumatic brain injury: translational challenges and emerging therapeutic strategies. Trends Pharmacol Sci 2010;31(12):596—604.

[15] Beauchamp K, Mutlak H, Smith WR, Shohami E, Stahel PF. Pharmacology of traumatic brain injury: where is the "golden bullet"? Mol Med 2008;14(11—12):731—40.

[16] Polinder S, Cnossen MC, Real RGL, et al. A multidimensional approach to post-concussion symptoms in mild traumatic brain injury. Front Neurol 2018;9:1113.

[17] Ahmed S, Venigalla H, Mekala HM, Dar S, Hassan M, Ayub S. Traumatic brain injury and neuropsychiatric complications. Indian J Psychol Med 2017;39(2):114—21.

[18] Pouw MH, Hosman AJ, van Middendorp JJ, Verbeek MM, Vos PE, van de Meent H. Biomarkers in spinal cord injury. Spinal Cord 2009;47(7):519—25.

[19] Robb MA, McInnes PM, Califf RM. Biomarkers and surrogate endpoints: developing common terminology and definitions. Jama. 2016;315(11):1107—8.

[20] NIH. NIH-FDA conference: biomarkers and surrogate endpoints: advancing clinical research and applications. Abstracts. Dis Markers 1998;14(4):187—334.

[21] Wagner JA, Ball JR. Implications of the institute of medicine report: evaluation of biomarkers and surrogate endpoints in chronic disease. Clin Pharmacol Ther 2015;98(1):12—15.

[22] Papa L, Ramia MM, Kelly JM, Burks SS, Pawlowicz A, Berger RP. Systematic review of clinical research on biomarkers for pediatric traumatic brain injury. J Neurotrauma 2013;30(5):324—38.

[23] Gadani SP, Walsh JT, Lukens JR, Kipnis J. Dealing with danger in the CNS: the response of the immune system to injury. Neuron. 2015;87(1):47—62.

[24] Peruzzotti-Jametti L, Donega M, Giusto E, Mallucci G, Marchetti B, Pluchino S. The role of the immune system in central nervous system plasticity after acute injury. Neuroscience. 2014.

[25] Loane DJ, Kumar A. Microglia in the TBI brain: the good, the bad, and the dysregulated. Exp Neurol 2016;275(Pt 3):316—27.

[26] McDonald B, Kubes P. Innate immune cell trafficking and function during sterile inflammation of the liver. Gastroenterology. 2016;151(6):1087—95.

[27] Corps KN, Roth TL, McGavern DB. Inflammation and neuroprotection in traumatic brain injury. JAMA Neurol 2015;72(3):355—62.

[28] Jassam YN, Izzy S, Whalen M, McGavern DB, El Khoury J. Neuroimmunology of traumatic brain injury: time for a paradigm shift. Neuron. 2017;95(6):1246—65.

[29] Braun M, Vaibhav K, Saad NM, et al. White matter damage after traumatic brain injury: A role for damage associated molecular patterns. Biochim Biophys Acta Mol Basis Dis 2017;1863(10 Pt B):2614—26.

[30] Clausen F, Hanell A, Bjork M, et al. Neutralization of interleukin-1beta modifies the inflammatory response and improves histological and cognitive outcome following traumatic brain injury in mice. Eur J Neurosci 2009;30(3):385—96.

[31] Adamczak SE, de Rivero Vaccari JP, Dale G, et al. Pyroptotic neuronal cell death mediated by the AIM2 inflammasome. J Cereb Blood Flow Metab 2014;34(4):621—9.

[32] de Rivero Vaccari JP, Lotocki G, Alonso OF, Bramlett HM, Dietrich WD, Keane RW. Therapeutic neutralization of the NLRP1 inflammasome reduces the innate immune response and improves histopathology after traumatic brain injury. J Cereb Blood Flow Metab 2009;29(7):1251—61.

[33] Brickler T, Gresham K, Meza A, et al. Nonessential role for the NLRP1 inflammasome complex in a murine model of traumatic brain injury. Mediators Inflamm 2016;2016:6373506.

[34] Walsh JG, Muruve DA, Power C. Inflammasomes in the CNS. Nat Rev Neurosci 2014;15(2):84—97.

[35] Liu HD, Li W, Chen ZR, et al. Expression of the NLRP3 inflammasome in cerebral cortex after traumatic brain injury in a rat model. Neurochem Res 2013;38(10):2072—83.

[36] Kuwar R, Rolfe A, Di L, et al. A novel small molecular NLRP3 inflammasome inhibitor alleviates neuroinflammatory response following traumatic brain injury. J Neuroinflammation 2019;16(1):81.

[37] Fourgeaud L, Traves PG, Tufail Y, et al. TAM receptors regulate multiple features of microglial physiology. Nature. 2016;532(7598):240—4.

[38] Gomes C, Ferreira R, George J, et al. Activation of microglial cells triggers a release of brain-derived neurotrophic factor (BDNF) inducing their proliferation in an adenosine A2A receptor-dependent manner: A2A receptor blockade prevents BDNF release and proliferation of microglia. J Neuroinflammation 2013;10:16.

[39] Roth TL, Nayak D, Atanasijevic T, Koretsky AP, Latour LL, McGavern DB. Transcranial amelioration of inflammation and cell death after brain injury. Nature. 2014;505(7482):223—8.

[40] Koizumi S, Shigemoto-Mogami Y, Nasu-Tada K, et al. UDP acting at P2Y6 receptors is a mediator of microglial phagocytosis. Nature. 2007;446(7139):1091—5.

[41] Lou N, Takano T, Pei Y, Xavier AL, Goldman SA, Nedergaard M. Purinergic receptor P2RY12-dependent microglial closure of the injured blood-brain barrier. Proc Natl Acad Sci USA 2016;113(4):1074—9.

[42] Caplan HW, Cox CS, Bedi SS. Do microglia play a role in sex differences in TBI? J Neurosci Res 2017;95 (1—2):509—17.

[43] Koellhoffer EC, McCullough LD, Ritzel RM. Old maids: aging and its impact on microglia function. Int J Mol Sci 2017;18(4).

[44] Walker CL, Fry CME, Wang J, et al. Functional and histological gender comparison of age-matched rats after moderate thoracic contusive spinal cord Injury. J Neurotrauma 2019;36(12):1974−84.

[45] Donat CK, Scott G, Gentleman SM, Sastre M. Microglial activation in traumatic brain injury. Front Aging Neurosci 2017;9:208.

[46] Kong X, Gao J. Macrophage polarization: a key event in the secondary phase of acute spinal cord injury. J Cell Mol Med 2017;21(5):941−54.

[47] Tang Y, Le W. Differential roles of M1 and M2 microglia in neurodegenerative diseases. Mol Neurobiol 2016;53(2):1181−94.

[48] Zhang L, Zhang J, You Z. Switching of the microglial activation phenotype is a possible treatment for depression disorder. Front Cell Neurosci 2018;12:306.

[49] Xu H, Wang Z, Li J, et al. The polarization states of microglia in TBI: a new paradigm for pharmacological intervention. Neural Plasticity 2017;2017:5405104.

[50] McKee CA, Lukens JR. Emerging roles for the immune system in traumatic brain injury. Front Immunol 2016;7:556.

[51] Huber-Lang M, Lambris JD, Ward PA. Innate immune responses to trauma. Nat Immunol 2018;19 (4):327−41.

[52] Ling C, Sandor M, Suresh M, Fabry Z. Traumatic injury and the presence of antigen differentially contribute to T-cell recruitment in the CNS. J Neurosci 2006;26(3):731−41.

[53] Popovich PG, Stokes BT, Whitacre CC. Concept of autoimmunity following spinal cord injury: possible roles for T lymphocytes in the traumatized central nervous system. J Neurosci Res 1996;45(4):349−63.

[54] Cohen IR, Schwartz M. Autoimmune maintenance and neuroprotection of the central nervous system. J Neuroimmunol 1999;100(1−2):111−14.

[55] Weckbach S, Neher M, Losacco JT, et al. Challenging the role of adaptive immunity in neurotrauma: Rag1 (-/-) mice lacking mature B and T cells do not show neuroprotection after closed head injury. J Neurotrauma 2012;29(6):1233−42.

[56] Fee D, Crumbaugh A, Jacques T, et al. Activated/effector CD4 + T cells exacerbate acute damage in the central nervous system following traumatic injury. J Neuroimmunol 2003;136(1−2):54−66.

[57] Held KS, Steward O, Blanc C, Lane TE. Impaired immune responses following spinal cord injury lead to reduced ability to control viral infection. Exp Neurol 2010;226(1):242−53.

[58] Moalem G, Leibowitz-Amit R, Yoles E, Mor F, Cohen IR, Schwartz M. Autoimmune T cells protect neurons from secondary degeneration after central nervous system axotomy. Nat Med 1999;5(1):49−55.

[59] Dalakas MC. Invited article: inhibition of B cell functions—implications for neurology. Neurology. 2008;70 (23):2252−60.

[60] Waubant E. Spotlight on anti-CD20. Int MS J 2008;15(1):19−25.

[61] Stefanova I, Dorfman JR, Germain RN. Self-recognition promotes the foreign antigen sensitivity of naive T lymphocytes. Nature. 2002;420(6914):429−34.

[62] Jones TB, McDaniel EE, Popovich PG. Inflammatory-mediated injury and repair in the traumatically injured spinal cord. Curr Pharm Des 2005;11(10):1223−36.

[63] Trivedi A, Olivas AD, Noble-Haeusslein LJ. Inflammation and spinal cord injury: infiltrating leukocytes as determinants of injury and repair processes. Clin Neurosci Res 2006;6(5):283−92.

[64] Diamond B, Huerta PT, Mina-Osorio P, Kowal C, Volpe BT. Losing your nerves? Maybe it's the antibodies. Nat Rev Immunol 2009;9(6):449−56.

[65] de Rivero Vaccari JP, Lotocki G, Marcillo AE, Dietrich WD, Keane RW. A molecular platform in neurons regulates inflammation after spinal cord injury. J Neurosci 2008;28(13):3404−14.

[66] Archelos JJ, Hartung HP. Pathogenetic role of autoantibodies in neurological diseases. Trends Neurosci 2000;23(7):317−27.

[67] Lopez-Escribano H, Minambres E, Labrador M, Bartolome MJ, Lopez-Hoyos M. Induction of cell death by sera from patients with acute brain injury as a mechanism of production of autoantibodies. Arthritis Rheum 2002;46(12):3290−300.

[68] Wright BR, Warrington AE, Edberg DD, Rodriguez M. Cellular mechanisms of central nervous system repair by natural autoreactive monoclonal antibodies. Arch Neurol 2009;66(12):1456−9.

[69] Stein TD, Fedynyshyn JP, Kalil RE. Circulating autoantibodies recognize and bind dying neurons following injury to the brain. J Neuropathol Exp Neurol 2002;61(12):1100–8.

[70] Cox AL, Coles AJ, Nortje J, et al. An investigation of auto-reactivity after head injury. J Neuroimmunol 2006;174(1–2):180–6.

[71] Ankeny DP, Lucin KM, Sanders VM, McGaughy VM, Popovich PG. Spinal cord injury triggers systemic autoimmunity: evidence for chronic B lymphocyte activation and lupus-like autoantibody synthesis. J Neurochem 2006;99(4):1073–87.

[72] Okonkwo DO, Yue JK, Puccio AM, et al. GFAP-BDP as an acute diagnostic marker in traumatic brain injury: results from the prospective transforming research and clinical knowledge in traumatic brain injury study. J Neurotrauma 2013;30(17):1490–7.

[73] Hook GR, Yu J, Sipes N, Pierschbacher MD, Hook V, Kindy MS. The cysteine protease cathepsin B is a key drug target and cysteine protease inhibitors are potential therapeutics for traumatic brain injury. J Neurotrauma 2014;31(5):515–29.

[74] Auer L. Brain protease activity after experimental head injury. J Neurosurg Sci 1979;23(1):23–8.

[75] Takala RS, Posti JP, Runtti H, et al. Glial fibrillary acidic protein and ubiquitin C-terminal hydrolase-L1 as outcome predictors in traumatic brain injury. World Neurosurg 2016;87:8–20.

[76] Marchi N, Bazarian JJ, Puvenna V, et al. Consequences of repeated blood-brain barrier disruption in football players. PLoS One 2013;8(3):e56805.

[77] Zhang Z, Zoltewicz JS, Mondello S, et al. Human traumatic brain injury induces autoantibody response against glial fibrillary acidic protein and its breakdown products. PLoS One 2014;9(3):e92698.

[78] Goryunova AV, Bazarnaya NA, Sorokina EG, et al. Glutamate receptor autoantibody concentrations in children with chronic post-traumatic headache. Neurosci Behav Physiol 2007;37(8):761–4.

[79] Buonora JE, Mousseau M, Jacobowitz DM, et al. Autoimmune profiling reveals peroxiredoxin 6 as a candidate traumatic brain injury biomarker. J Neurotrauma 2015;32(22):1805–14.

[80] Tanriverdi F, De Bellis A, Ulutabanca H, et al. A five year prospective investigation of anterior pituitary function after traumatic brain injury: is hypopituitarism long-term after head trauma associated with autoimmunity? J Neurotrauma 2013;30(16):1426–33.

[81] Tanriverdi F, De Bellis A, Bizzarro A, et al. Antipituitary antibodies after traumatic brain injury: is head trauma-induced pituitary dysfunction associated with autoimmunity? Eur J Endocrinol 2008;159(1):7–13.

[82] De Bellis A, Bellastella G, Maiorino MI, et al. The role of autoimmunity in pituitary dysfunction due to traumatic brain injury. Pituitary. 2019;22(3):236–48.

[83] Tanriverdi F, De Bellis A, Battaglia M, et al. Investigation of antihypothalamus and antipituitary antibodies in amateur boxers: is chronic repetitive head trauma-induced pituitary dysfunction associated with autoimmunity? Eur J Endocrinol 2010;162(5):861–7.

[84] Arevalo-Martin A, Grassner L, Garcia-Ovejero D, et al. Elevated autoantibodies in subacute human spinal cord injury are naturally occurring antibodies. Front Immunol 2018;9:2365.

[85] Hergenroeder GW, Redell JB, Choi HA, et al. Increased levels of circulating glial fibrillary acidic protein and collapsin response mediator protein-2 autoantibodies in the acute stage of spinal cord injury predict the subsequent development of neuropathic pain. J Neurotrauma 2018;35(21):2530–9.

[86] Iliff JJ, Wang M, Liao Y, et al. A paravascular pathway facilitates CSF flow through the brain parenchyma and the clearance of interstitial solutes, including amyloid beta. Sci Transl Med 2012;4(147) 147ra111.

[87] Takano T, Tian GF, Peng W, et al. Astrocyte-mediated control of cerebral blood flow. Nat Neurosci 2006;9(2):260–7.

[88] Schummers J, Yu H, Sur M. Tuned responses of astrocytes and their influence on hemodynamic signals in the visual cortex. Science. 2008;320(5883):1638–43.

[89] Arighi A, Di Cristofori A, Fenoglio C, et al. Cerebrospinal fluid level of aquaporin4: a new window on glymphatic system involvement in neurodegenerative disease? J Alzheimers Dis 2019;69(3):663–9.

[90] Verheggen ICM, Van Boxtel MPJ, Verhey FRJ, Jansen JFA, Backes WH. Interaction between blood-brain barrier and glymphatic system in solute clearance. Neurosci Biobehav Rev 2018;90:26–33.

[91] Wang LH, Wang ZL, Chen WY, Chen MJ, Xu GY. The glymphatic system: concept, function and research progresses. Sheng Li Xue Bao 2018;70(1):52–60.

[92] Xie L, Kang H, Xu Q, et al. Sleep drives metabolite clearance from the adult brain. Science. 2013;342(6156):373–7.

[93] Larson EB. Sleep disturbance and cognition in people with TBI. Neuro Rehab. 2018;43(3):297−306.

[94] Barshikar S, Bell KR. Sleep disturbance after TBI. Curr Neurol Neurosci Rep 2017;17(11):87.

[95] Rao V, McCann U, Han D, Bergey A, Smith MT. Does acute TBI-related sleep disturbance predict subsequent neuropsychiatric disturbances? Brain Inj 2014;28(1):20−6.

[96] Iliff JJ, Chen MJ, Plog BA, et al. Impairment of glymphatic pathway function promotes tau pathology after traumatic brain injury. J Neurosci 2014;34(49):16180−93.

[97] Sullan MJ, Asken BM, Jaffee MS, DeKosky ST, Bauer RM. Glymphatic system disruption as a mediator of brain trauma and chronic traumatic encephalopathy. Neurosci Biobehav Rev 2018;84:316−24.

[98] Hui FK. Clearing your mind: a glymphatic system? World Neurosurg 2015;83(5):715−17.

[99] Jessen NA, Munk AS, Lundgaard I, Nedergaard M. The glymphatic system: a beginner's guide. Neurochem Res 2015;40(12):2583−99.

[100] Tarasoff-Conway JM, Carare RO, Osorio RS, et al. Clearance systems in the brain-implications for Alzheimer disease. Nat Rev Neurol 2015;11(8):457−70.

[101] Kanaan NM, Cox K, Alvarez VE, Stein TD, Poncil S, McKee AC. Characterization of early pathological Tau conformations and phosphorylation in chronic traumatic encephalopathy. J Neuropathol Exp Neurol 2016;75(1):19−34.

[102] Prochazka M, Voltnerova M, Stefan J. Studies of immunologic reactions after brain injury. II. Antibodies against brain tissue lipids after blunt head injury in man. Int Surg 1971;55(5):322−6.

[103] Shamrei RK. The value of determining autoantibodies in the diagnosis and expertise of closed brain injury. Voen Med Zh 1969;4:39−43.

[104] Bartanusz V, Jezova D, Alajajian B, Digicaylioglu M. The blood-spinal cord barrier: morphology and clinical implications. Ann Neurol 2011;70(2):194−206.

[105] Marchi N, Granata T, Janigro D. Inflammatory pathways of seizure disorders. Trends Neurosci 2014;37(2):55−65.

[106] Sorokina EG, Vol'pina OM, Semenova Zh B, et al. Autoantibodies to alpha7-subunit of neuronal acetylcholine receptor in children with traumatic brain injury. Zh Nevrol Psikhiatr Im S S Korsakova 2011;111(4):56−60.

[107] Pinelis VG, Sorokina EG. Autoimmune mechanisms of modulation of the activity of glutamate receptors in children with epilepsy and craniocerebral injury. Vestn Ross Akad Med Nauk 2008;12:44−51.

[108] Sorokina EG, Semenova Zh B, Bazarnaya NA, et al. Autoantibodies to glutamate receptors and products of nitric oxide metabolism in serum in children in the acute phase of craniocerebral trauma. Neurosci Behav Physiol 2009;39(4):329−34.

[109] Lisianyi NI, Cheren'ko TM, Terletskaia Ia T. Detection of antibodies to myelin basic proteins in patients with closed cranio-cerebral trauma. Vrach Delo 1987;10:101−4.

[110] Ngankam L, Kazantseva NV, Gerasimova MM. Immunological markers of severity and outcome of traumatic brain injury. Zh Nevrol Psikhiatr 2011;111(7):61−5.

[111] Palmers I, Ydens E, Put E, et al. Antibody profiling identifies novel antigenic targets in spinal cord injury patients. J Neuroinflammation 2016;13(1):243.

[112] Morozov SG, Asanova LM, Gnedenko BB, Panchenko LF, Lavrova TN. Autoantibodies against nerve tissue proteins long after cranio-cerebral injury. Vopr Med Khim 1996;42(2):147−52.

[113] De Bellis A, Sinisi AA, Pane E, et al. Involvement of hypothalamus autoimmunity in patients with autoimmune hypopituitarism: role of antibodies to hypothalamic cells. J Clin Endocrinol Metab 2012;97(10):3684−90.

[114] Li W, Chen SC, Wang ZG, Song XB, Wang YP, Zhang M. Relationship between anti-myelin basic protein antibody and myelinoclasis in rat brain stem after brain trauma. Nan Fang Yi Ke Da Xue Xue Bao 2008;28(6):1028−30.

[115] Needham EJ, Helmy A, Zanier ER, Jones JL, Coles AJ, Menon DK. The immunological response to traumatic brain injury. J Neuroimmunol 2019;332:112−25.

[116] Kobeissy F, Moshourab RA. Autoantibodies in CNS trauma and neuropsychiatric disorders: a new generation of biomarkers. In: Kobeissy FH, editor. Brain neurotrauma: molecular, neuropsychological, and rehabilitation aspects. Boca Raton, FL; 2015.

[117] Cruz CD, Coelho A, Antunes-Lopes T, Cruz F. Biomarkers of spinal cord injury and ensuing bladder dysfunction. Adv Drug Deliv Rev 2015;82−83:153−9.

[118] Cao F, Yang XF, Liu WG, et al. Elevation of neuron-specific enolase and S-100beta protein level in experimental acute spinal cord injury. J Clin Neurosci 2008;15(5):541−4.

[119] Loy DN, Sroufe AE, Pelt JL, et al. Serum biomarkers for experimental acute spinal cord injury: rapid elevation of neuron-specific enolase and S-100beta. Neurosurgery. 2005;56(2):391−7 discussion 391−7.

[120] Ma J, Novikov LN, Karlsson K, Kellerth JO, Wiberg M. Plexus avulsion and spinal cord injury increase the serum concentration of S-100 protein: an experimental study in rats. Scand J Plast Reconstr Surg Hand Surg 2001;35(4):355−9.

[121] Kiechle K, Bazarian JJ, Merchant-Borna K, et al. Subject-specific increases in serum S-100B distinguish sports-related concussion from sports-related exertion. PLoS One 2014;9(1):e84977.

[122] Puvenna V, Brennan C, Shaw G, et al. Significance of ubiquitin carboxy-terminal hydrolase L1 elevations in athletes after sub-concussive head hits. PLoS One 2014;9(5):e96296.

[123] Bazarian JJ, Blyth BJ, He H, et al. Classification accuracy of serum apo A-I and S100B for the diagnosis of mild traumatic brain injury and prediction of abnormal initial head computed tomography scan. J Neurotrauma 2013;30(20):1747−54.

[124] Thelin EP, Nelson DW, Bellander BM. Secondary peaks of S100B in serum relate to subsequent radiological pathology in traumatic brain injury. Neurocrit Care 2014;20(2):217−29.

[125] Egea-Guerrero JJ, Murillo-Cabezas F, Gordillo-Escobar E, et al. S100B protein may detect brain death development after severe traumatic brain injury. J Neurotrauma 2013;30(20):1762−9.

[126] Thelin EP, Johannesson L, Nelson D, Bellander BM. S100B is an important outcome predictor in traumatic brain injury. J Neurotrauma 2013;30(7):519−28.

[127] Metting Z, Wilczak N, Rodiger LA, Schaaf JM, van der Naalt J. GFAP and S100B in the acute phase of mild traumatic brain injury. Neurology. 2012;78(18):1428−33.

[128] Berg DK, Conroy WG. Nicotinic alpha 7 receptors: synaptic options and downstream signaling in neurons. J Neurobiol 2002;53(4):512−23.

[129] Drisdel RC, Green WN. Neuronal alpha-bungarotoxin receptors are alpha7 subunit homomers. J Neurosci 2000;20(1):133−9.

[130] Bien CG, Vincent A, Barnett MH, et al. Immunopathology of autoantibody-associated encephalitides: clues for pathogenesis. Brain 2012;135(Pt 5):1622−38.

[131] Petit-Pedrol M, Armangue T, Peng X, et al. Encephalitis with refractory seizures, status epilepticus, and antibodies to the GABAA receptor: a case series, characterisation of the antigen, and analysis of the effects of antibodies. Lancet Neurol 2014;13(3):276−86.

[132] Yang Z, Zhu T, Weissman AS, et al. Autoimmunity and traumatic brain injury. Curr Phys Med Rehab Rep 2017;5(1):22−9.

[133] Vadasz Z, Haj T, Kessel A, Toubi E. Age-related autoimmunity. BMC Med 2013;11:94.

[134] Ankeny DP, Guan Z, Popovich PG. B cells produce pathogenic antibodies and impair recovery after spinal cord injury in mice. J Clin Invest 2009;119(10):2990−9.

[135] Bao F, Bailey CS, Gurr KR, et al. Increased oxidative activity in human blood neutrophils and monocytes after spinal cord injury. Exp Neurol 2009;215(2):308−16.

[136] Ankeny DP, Popovich PG. B cells and autoantibodies: complex roles in CNS injury. Trends Immunol 2010;31(9):332−8.

[137] Gris D, Hamilton EF, Weaver LC. The systemic inflammatory response after spinal cord injury damages lungs and kidneys. Exp Neurol 2008;211(1):259−70.

[138] Liu J, An H, Jiang D, et al. Study of bacterial translocation from gut after paraplegia caused by spinal cord injury in rats. Spine (Phila Pa 1976) 2004;29(2):164−9.

[139] Kobayashi T, Takahashi K, Nagai Y, et al. Tonic B cell activation by Radioprotective105/MD-1 promotes disease progression in MRL/lpr mice. Int Immunol 2008;20(7):881−91.

[140] Popovich PG, Longbrake EE. Can the immune system be harnessed to repair the CNS? Nat Rev Neurosci 2008;9(6):481−93.

[141] Abdul-Majid KB, Stefferl A, Bourquin C, et al. Fc receptors are critical for autoimmune inflammatory damage to the central nervous system in experimental autoimmune encephalomyelitis. Scand J Immunol 2002;55(1):70−81.

[142] Qiao F, Atkinson C, Song H, Pannu R, Singh I, Tomlinson S. Complement plays an important role in spinal cord injury and represents a therapeutic target for improving recovery following trauma. Am J Pathol 2006;169(3):1039−47.

[143] Alawieh A, Langley EF, Weber S, Adkins D, Tomlinson S. Identifying the role of complement in triggering neuroinflammation after traumatic brain injury. J Neurosci 2018;38(10):2519−32.

[144] Thom V, Arumugam TV, Magnus T, Gelderblom M. Therapeutic potential of intravenous immunoglobulin in acute brain injury. Front Immunol 2017;8:875.

[145] Putatunda R, Bethea JR, Hu WH. Potential immunotherapies for traumatic brain and spinal cord injury. Chin J Traumatol 2018;21(3):125−36.

[146] Brennan FH, Kurniawan ND, Vukovic J, et al. IVIg attenuates complement and improves spinal cord injury outcomes in mice. Ann Clin Transl Neurol 2016;3(7):495−511.

[147] Kasai T, Kondo M, Ishii R, et al. Abeta levels in the jugular vein and high molecular weight Abeta oligomer levels in CSF can be used as biomarkers to indicate the anti-amyloid effect of IVIg for Alzheimer's disease. PLoS One 2017;12(4):e0174630.

[148] Jeong S, Lei B, Wang H, Dawson HN, James ML. Intravenous immunoglobulin G improves neurobehavioral and histological outcomes after traumatic brain injury in mice. J Neuroimmunol 2014;276(1−2):112−18.

[149] Uchida J, Lee Y, Hasegawa M, et al. Mouse CD20 expression and function. Int Immunol 2004;16(1):119−29.

[150] Casili G, Impellizzeri D, Cordaro M, Esposito E, Cuzzocrea S. B-cell depletion with CD20 antibodies as new approach in the treatment of inflammatory and immunological events associated with spinal cord injury. Neurotherapeutics 2016;13(4):880−94.

[151] Raad M, Nohra E, Chams N, et al. Autoantibodies in traumatic brain injury and central nervous system trauma. Neuroscience. 2014;281:16−23.

[152] Carson KR, Focosi D, Major EO, et al. Monoclonal antibody-associated progressive multifocal leucoencephalopathy in patients treated with rituximab, natalizumab, and efalizumab: a Review from the Research on Adverse Drug Events and Reports (RADAR) Project. Lancet Oncol 2009;10(8):816−24.

[153] Saltzman JW, Battaglino RA, Salles L, et al. B-cell maturation antigen, a proliferation-inducing ligand, and B-cell activating factor are candidate mediators of spinal cord injury-induced autoimmunity. J Neurotrauma 2013;30(6):434−40.

Index